T0394088

# Advances in Processing Technologies for Bio-based Nanosystems in Food

# Contemporary Food Engineering

**Series Editor**
**Professor Da-Wen Sun, Director**

*Food Refrigeration & Computerized Food Technology*
*National University of Ireland, Dublin*
*(University College Dublin)*
*Dublin, Ireland*
*http://www.ucd.ie/sun/*

**Emerging Technologies for Food Quality and Food Safety Evaluation,** *edited by Yong-Jin Cho, Sukwon Kang*

**Operations in Food Refrigeration,** *edited by Rodolfo H. Mascheroni*

**Advances in Food Extrusion Technology,** *edited by Medeni Maskan and Aylin Altan*

**Modified Atmosphere and Active Packaging Technologies,** *edited by Ioannis Arvanitoyannis*

**Juice Processing: Quality, Safety and Value-Added Opportunities,** *edited by Victor Falguera and Albert Ibarz*

**Physical Properties of Foods: Novel Measurement Techniques and Applications,** *edited by Ignacio Arana*

**Fermentation Processes Engineering in the Food Industry,** *edited by Carlos Ricardo Soccol, Ashok Pandey, and Christian Larroche*

**Engineering Aspects of Cereal and Cereal-Based Products,** *edited by Raquel de Pinho Ferreira Guine, and Paula Maria dos Reis Correia*

**Enhancing Extraction Processes in the Food Industry,** *edited by Nikolai Lebovka, Eugene Vorobiev, and Farid Chemat*

**Thermal Food Processing: New Technologies and Quality Issues, Second Edition,** *edited by Da-Wen Sun*

**Advances in Fruit Processing Technologies,** *edited by Sueli Rodrigues and Fabiano Andre Narciso Fernandes*

**Engineering Aspects of Membrane Separation and Application in Food Processing,** *edited by Robert W. Field, Erika Bekassy-Molnar, Frank Lipnizki, and Gyula Vatai*

**Edible Oils: Extraction, Processing, and Applications,** *edited by Smain Chemat*

**Engineering Aspects of Food Biotechnology,** *edited by José A. Teixeira and António A. Vicente*

**Engineering Aspects of Food Emulsification and Homogenization,** *edited by Marilyn Rayner and Petr Dejmek*

**Advances in Postharvest Fruit and Vegetable Technology,** *edited by Ron B.H. Wills and John Golding*

**Advances in Meat Processing Technology,** *by Alaa El-Din A. Bekhit*

**High Pressure Processing of Fruit and Vegetable Juices,** *edited by Milan Houška and Filipa Vinagre Marques da Silva*

**Trends in Fish Processing Technologies,** *edited by Daniela Borda, Anca I. Nicolau, and Peter Raspor*

**Food Biofortification Technologies,** *edited by Agnieszka Saeid*

**Trends in Fish Processing Technologies,** *edited by Daniela Borda, Anca I. Nicolau, and Peter Raspor*

**Computational Fluid Dynamics in Food Processing, Second Edition,** *edited by Da-Wen Sun*

**Advances in Processing Technologies for Bio-based Nanosystems in Food,** *edited by Óscar L. Ramos, Ricardo N. Pereira, Miguel A. Cerqueira, José A. Teixeira, and António A. Vicente*

For more information about this series, please visit: https://www.crcpress.com/Contemporary-Food-Engineering/book-series/CRCCONFOOENG

# Advances in Processing Technologies for Bio-based Nanosystems in Food


Edited by

Óscar L. Ramos

Ricardo N. Pereira

Miguel A. Cerqueira

José A. Teixeira

António A. Vicente


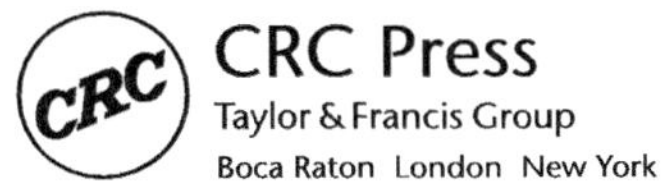



CRC Press

Taylor & Francis Group

Boca Raton London New York

CRC Press is an imprint of the

Taylor & Francis Group, an **informa** business

CRC Press
Taylor & Francis Group
6000 Broken Sound Parkway NW, Suite 300
Boca Raton, FL 33487-2742



Printed on acid-free paper

International Standard Book Number-13: 978-1-138-03730-4 (Hardback)



**Library of Congress Cataloging-in-Publication Data**

Names: Ramos, Óscar L., editor.
Title: Advances in processing technologies for bio-based nanosystems in food / editor(s): Óscar L. Ramos, Ricardo N. Pereira, Miguel A. Cerqueira, José A. Teixeira, and António A. Vicente.
Description: Boca Raton, FL : CRC Press, Taylor & Francis Group, 2020. | Includes index.
Identifiers: LCCN 2019008521 | ISBN 9781138037304 (978-1-138-03730-4)
Subjects: LCSH: Food--Biotechnology. | Food industry and trade. | Nanotechnology.
Classification: LCC TP248.65.F66 R366 2020 | DDC 664/.024--dc23
LC record available at https://lccn.loc.gov/2019008521

**Visit the Taylor & Francis Web site at**
**http://www.taylorandfrancis.com**

**and the CRC Press Web site at**
**http://www.crcpress.com**

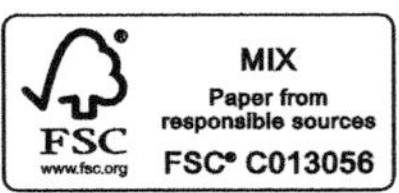


Printed and bound in Great Britain by
TJ International Ltd, Padstow, Cornwall

# Contents

## *SECTION V Future Perspectives*

# Series Preface

Food engineering is the multidisciplinary field of applied physical sciences combined with the knowledge of product properties. Food engineers provide the technological knowledge transfer essential to the cost-effective production and commercialization of food products and services. In particular, food engineers develop and design processes and equipment in order to convert raw agricultural materials and ingredients into safe, convenient, and nutritious consumer food products. However, food engineering topics are continuously undergoing changes to meet diverse consumer demands, and the subject is being rapidly developed to reflect market needs.

In the development of food engineering, one of the many challenges is to employ modern tools and knowledge, such as computational materials science and nanotechnology, to develop new products and processes. Simultaneously, improving quality, safety, and security remain critical issues in food engineering study. New packaging materials and techniques are being developed to provide more protection to foods, and novel preservation technologies are emerging to enhance food security and defense. Additionally, process control and automation regularly appear among the top priorities identified in food engineering. Advanced monitoring and control systems are developed to facilitate automation and flexible food manufacturing. Furthermore, energy saving and minimization of environmental problems continue to be important food engineering issues, and significant progress is being made in waste management, efficient utilization of energy, and reduction of effluents and emissions in food production.

Consisting of edited books, the Contemporary Food Engineering book series attempts to address some of the recent developments in food engineering. Advances in classical unit operations in engineering applied to food manufacturing are covered as well as such topics as progress in the transport and storage of liquid and solid foods; heating, chilling, and freezing of foods; mass transfer in foods; chemical and biochemical aspects of food engineering and the use of kinetic analysis; dehydration, thermal processing, nonthermal processing, extrusion, liquid food concentration, membrane processes and applications of membranes in food processing; shelf-life, electronic indicators in inventory management, and sustainable technologies in food processing; and packaging, cleaning, and sanitation. The books are aimed at professional food scientists, academics researching food engineering problems, and graduate level students.

The editors of the books are leading engineers and scientists from many parts of the world. All the editors were asked to present their books in a manner that will address the market need and pinpoint the cutting-edge technologies in food engineering. Furthermore, all contributions are written by internationally renowned experts who have both academic and professional credentials. All authors have attempted to provide critical, comprehensive, and readily accessible information on the art and science of a relevant topic in each chapter, with reference lists to be used by readers for further information. Therefore, each book can serve as an essential reference source to students and researchers in universities and research institutions.

**Da-Wen Sun**
*Series Editor*

# Series Editor

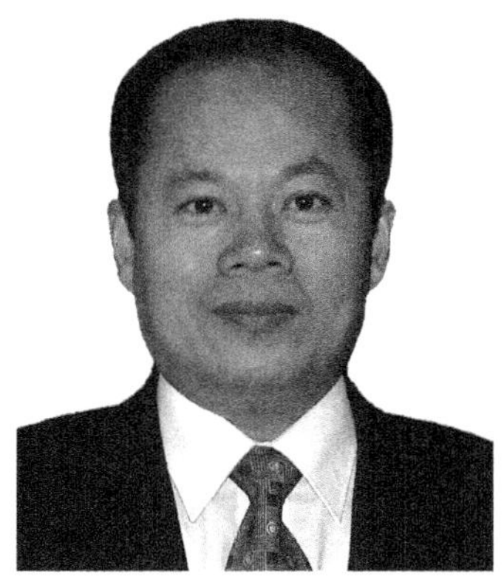

Born in Southern China, Professor Da-Wen Sun is a global authority in food engineering research and education. He is an Academician of six academies, including a Member of the Royal Irish Academy, the highest academic honour in Ireland; a Member of Academia Europaea (The Academy of Europe), one of the most prestigious academies in the world; a Foreign Member of the Polish Academy of Sciences; a Fellow of the International Academy of Food Science and Technology; a Fellow of the International Academy of Agricultural and Biosystems Engineering; and a Full Member of International Academy of Refrigeration. He is also the founder and Editor-in-Chief of *Food and Bioprocess Technology*, one of the most prestigious food science and technology journals; Series Editor of Contemporary Food Engineering book series with already over 50 volumes published; and the founder and President of the International Academy of Agricultural and Biosystems Engineering (iAABE). In addition, he served as the President of the International Commission of Agricultural and Biosystems Engineering (CIGR), the world's largest organization in the field, in 2013–2014, and is now Honorary President of CIGR. He has significantly contributed to the field of food engineering as a researcher, as an academic authority, and as an educator.

His main research activities include cooling, drying, and refrigeration processes and systems; quality and safety of food products; bioprocess simulation and optimization; and computer vision/image processing and hyperspectral imaging technologies. Especially, his many scholarly works have become standard reference materials for researchers in the areas of hyperspectral imaging, computer vision, ultrasonic freezing, vacuum cooling, computational fluid dynamics modeling, etc. Results of his work have been published in over 1000 papers including more than 500 peer-reviewed journal papers indexed by Web of Science, with an average citation of more than 40 per paper (Web of Science h-index = 95, SCOPUS h-index = 101, Google Scholar = 110). Among them, 38 papers have been selected by Thomson Reuters's Essential Science Indicators$^{SM}$ as highly cited papers, ranking him No. 2 in the world in Agricultural Sciences. He has also edited 17 authored books. In addition, Professor Sun has been named Highly Cited Researcher in the last three consecutive years (2015–2018) by Clarivate Analytics (formerly Thomson Reuters).

He received a first-class BSc Honours and MSc in Mechanical Engineering, and a PhD in Chemical Engineering in China before working in various universities in Europe. He became the first Chinese national to be permanently employed in an Irish University when he was appointed College Lecturer at National University of Ireland, Dublin (University College Dublin), in 1995, and was then continuously promoted in the shortest possible time to Associate Professor, Professor, and Full Professor. Dr. Sun is now a Full Professor of Food and Biosystems Engineering and Director of the Food Refrigeration and Computerised Food Technology Research Group at University College Dublin (UCD).

As a leading educator in food engineering, Professor Sun has significantly contributed to the field of food engineering. He has trained many PhD students, who have made their own contributions to the industry and academia. He has also given lectures on advances in food engineering on a regular basis in academic institutions internationally and delivered keynote speeches at international conferences. As a recognized authority in food engineering, he has been conferred adjunct/visiting/consulting professorships from ten top universities in China including Zhejiang University, Shanghai Jiaotong University, Harbin Institute of Technology, China Agricultural University, South China University of Technology, Jiangnan University, and so on. In recognition of his significant contribution to Food Engineering worldwide and for his outstanding leadership in the field, the CIGR awarded him the "CIGR Merit Award" in 2000, in 2006, and again in 2016. The Institution of Mechanical Engineers (IMechE) based in the UK named him "Food Engineer of the Year 2004." In 2007 he was presented with the only "AFST(I) Fellow Award" in that year by the Association of Food Scientists and Technologists (India). In 2008 he was awarded "CIGR Recognition Award" in honour of his distinguished achievements as the top 1 percent of Agricultural Engineering scientists in the world. In 2010 he received the "CIGR Fellow Award"; the title of Fellow is the highest honour in CIGR, and is conferred to individuals who have made sustained, outstanding contributions worldwide. In March 2013, he was presented with the "You Bring Charm to the World Award" by Hong Kong-based Phoenix Satellite Television, with other award recipients including the 2012 Nobel Laureate in Literature and the Chinese Astronaut Team for Shenzhou IX Spaceship. In July 2013 he received "The Frozen Food Foundation Freezing Research Award" from the International Association for Food Protection (IAFP) for his significant contributions to enhancing the field of food freezing technologies, the first time that this prestigious award was presented to a scientist outside the USA, and in June 2015 he was presented with the "IAEF Lifetime Achievement Award." This IAEF (International Association of Engineering and Food) award highlights the lifetime contribution of a prominent engineer in the field of food, and in February 2018, he was conferred with the honorary doctorate degree by Universidad Privada del Norte in Peru.

# Preface

*Advances in Processing Technologies for Bio-based Nanosystems in Food* represents an overview of the most recent advances made in the field of nanoscience and nanotechnology that significantly influenced the food industry.

The advent of nanotechnology coupled with innovative approaches and processing technologies has enabled crucial advances that led to novel applications in a variety of industrial and consumer products, including food and food packaging.

Nanotechnology can be used to address challenges faced by the food and bioprocessing industries for developing and implementing improved or novel systems that can produce safer, nutritious, healthier, sustainable, and environmental-friendly food products.

The complex mechanisms involved in the research, development, production, and legislation of food containing nanostructures systems are comprehensively reviewed under multi- and inter-disciplinary scopes. Bearing this in mind, this book was conceived. This book is divided into 15 chapters that aim to contribute to advance knowledge on topics of food nanoscience and nanotechnology. The first chapter presents an overview to the book topics; the following four chapters discuss the main nanostructured systems made from bio-based materials, techniques for their production (with particular focus in innovative), and examples of bioactive compounds that can be entrapped into, for food applications. Chapter 6 is focused in bio-nanosystems developed through electrohydrodynamic techniques, whereas Chapter 7 is devoted to comprehensively review specific techniques employed in the characterization of bio-nanosystems (including the most frequently used, and the most recent and innovative ones). The book continues with three chapters dedicated to evaluate the behavior of bio-nanosystems containing bioactive compounds, which include their functionality as delivery systems, their *uptake and digestion through in vitro* and *in vivo* experiments, and *toxicological studies.* Three chapters selecting examples of nanotechnology applications in food industry are shown, focusing on advanced aspects of food packaging, processing, and preservation. Finally, two chapters, one addressing the *advanced methods for detection and quantification of nanosystems in food*, and the other overviewing the future trends and perspectives.

In this book, international experts will be in charge of each chapter and critical reviews of each topic will be presented together with the most recent research results. It is expected that this book will provide a source of much needed and up-to-date information on the use of emergent technologies in bio-based nanosystems for foods, ideal for scientists, regulators, industrialists, and consumers that aim at doing research and development in the food processing industry.

# Acknowledgments

Óscar L. Ramos and Ricardo N. Pereira gratefully acknowledge their post-doctoral grants (SFRH/BPD/80766/2011 and SFRH/BPD/81887/2011, respectively) to Fundação para a Ciência e Tecnologia (FCT, Portugal). The authors thank FCT under the scope of the strategic funding of UID/BIO/04469 unit and COMPETE 2020 (POCI-01-0145-FEDER-006684) and BioTecNorte operation (NORTE-01-0145-FEDER-000004) funded by the European Regional Development Fund under the scope of Norte2020–Programa Operacional Regional do Norte.

# About the Editors

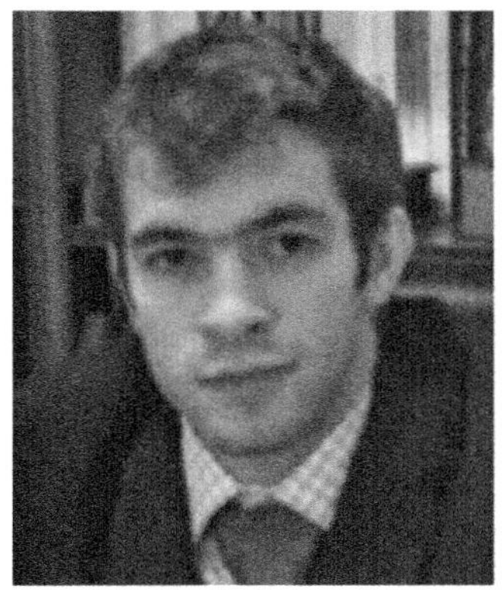

**Óscar L. Ramos** graduated in Microbiology in 2005 from the Portuguese Catholic University in Porto, Portugal and finished his PhD in Technological and Engineering Sciences, with a specialization in Biochemical Engineering, in 2011 at the New University of Lisbon in Lisboa, Portugal. He was postdoctoral researcher, between 2012 and 2018, and invited Assistant Professor, between 2015 and 2018, of classes of PhD program in Food Science and Technology and Nutrition, both at Centre Biological Engineering of University Minho in Braga, Portugal. He co-edited a book *Edible Food Packaging: Materials and Processing Technologies* and co-authored 35 scientific papers in peer reviewed journals, 14 chapters in edited books, and a National Patent (Invention N° 105852) entitled "Revestimento comestível para alimentos" in the Food Science and Technology field. Until now, he did more than 50 oral and poster presentations and had co-supervised 1 post-doctoral, 3 PhD, 6 MSc, and 10 undergraduate students. He also participated in several R&D of independent national and international projects and worked as a consultant for several private food industry companies related to food technology. Currently, he is Senior Research in Alchemy Project at Centre of Biotechnology and Fine Chemistry of Biotechnology School of Portuguese Catholic University in Porto, Portugal, and in parallel, he is the Guest Editor of a special issue in Food Science and Technology field and member of the Directive Board of National Association of Science and Technology Researchers (ANICT).

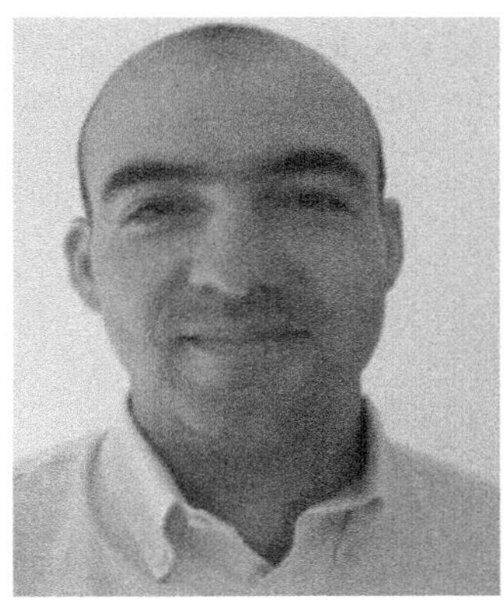

**Ricardo N. Pereira** graduated in 2003 in Food Engineering from the Portuguese Catholic University in Porto, Portugal, obtained MSc degree in Biotechnology-Bioprocess Engineering in 2007 from the University of Minho (UM) in Braga, Portugal and finished his PhD in Chemical and Biological Engineering in 2011 also at the UM. During his early career as researcher, he has participated in several research projects, both national and international, in the food industry and worked as a consultant for a number of private and public sector clients (professional and educational) related to food technology and innovative food processing. He has published more than 30 research articles in international peer-reviewed journals (Scopus *h*-index of 12), 5 book chapters in international books, and become editor of the book *Edible Food Packaging: Materials and Processing Technologies.* Since

2013, his scientific merit and leadership lead to more than 10 oral presentations and more than 20 publications in proceedings international meetings and supervision of national/international master, doctoral, and post-doctoral students. From 2016 to 2019 he was Guest Professor at the Department of Biological Engineering (UM) and lectured the classes of Laboratories of Food Technology (4th year discipline), in Integrated Master of Biological Engineering and Food Technology (from Master Programme in Food Science and Technology). He is presently a postdoctoral researcher working in the field of electro-thermal food processing, at the Centre for Biological Engineering (CEB) in UM.

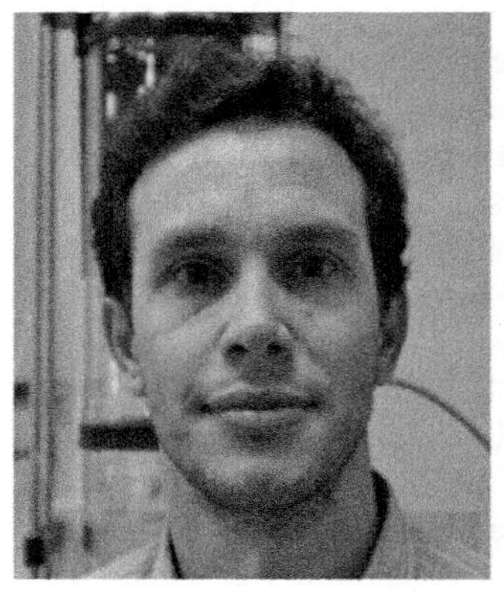

**Miguel A. Cerqueira** is graduated in Chemical and Biological Engineering (2005), at the University of Minho (UM) where he received two scholar merit awards and a scholarship merit award. He finished his PhD in December 2010 and from the developed work, he received the award for the best PhD Thesis 2011 by the School of Engineering of UM. From April 2011 to February 2016, he was postdoctoral researcher at UM focused on the development of bio-based nanostructures for food applications. In 2013, he co-founded Improveat, Lda, a spin-off company of University of Minho, and in 2014, he was selected as one of the winners of the Young Scientist Award of the 17th IUFoST World Congress of Food Science and Technology. Since March 2016, he is researcher in the Food Processing Group at the International Iberian Nanotechnology Laboratory, and till now he published more than 85 papers in peer-reviewed journals; 2 patents; 6 papers in non-peer-reviewed journals; 2 books, 20 chapters; 15 extended abstracts in international conferences; 81 abstracts in international conferences; and 22 abstracts in national conferences. In 2018, he join the list of "Highly Cited Researchers" by Clarivate Analytics (http://orcid.org/0000-0001-6614-3942). He has expertise on edible and biodegradable films and coatings for food packaging, encapsulation of functional compounds using emergent encapsulation technologies, and on the development and characterization of emulgels and oleogels for functional foods.

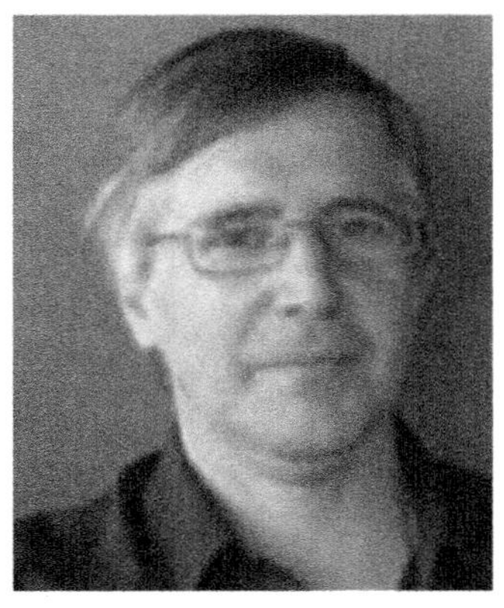

**José A. Teixeira** is a full professor at Biological Engineering Department, Minho University. He is responsible for scientific research and advanced formation in the areas of biological and chemical engineering and carries out research in industrial and food biotechnology and bioengineering.

His research activities have been focused on two main topics: fermentation and food technology. He is also interested in food nanotechnology, as well as in the extraction/production of bioactive compounds for food and medical applications. He has been the scientific coordinator of 31 research projects, including two Alfa networks. He (co)-authored 550 peer-reviewed papers and is coeditor of the books *Reactores Biológicos-Fundamentos e Aplicações* (in Portuguese), *Engineering Aspects of Milk and Dairy Products*, *Engineering Aspects of Food Biotechnology*, *Current Developments in Biotechnology and Bioengineering: Foundations of Biotechnology*, and *Bioengineering and Lignocellulosic Materials and Their Use in Bio-based Packaging.*

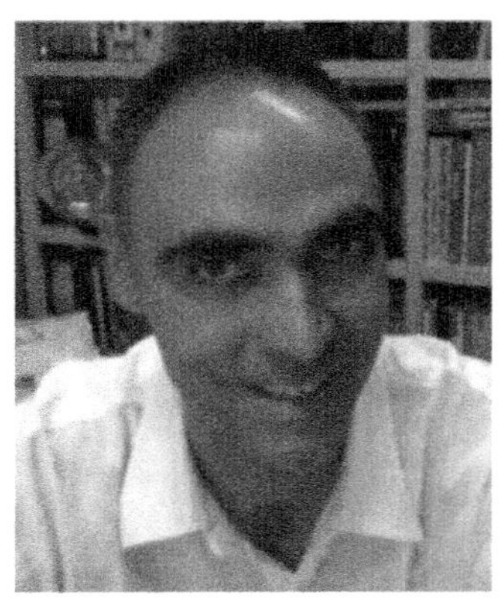

**António A. Vicente** graduated in Food Engineering in 1994 from the Portuguese Catholic University in Porto, Portugal, and finished his PhD in Chemical and Biological Engineering in 1998 at the University of Minho. He has received his habilitation in Chemical and Biological Engineering from the University of Minho in 2010. From an early stage of his career, he has kept close contact with the food industry, and he is involved in several research projects, both national and international, together with industrial partners either as a participant or as a project leader. Currently, he has collaborations established in countries such as Brazil, France, Germany, Ireland, Italy, Mexico, New Zealand, Slovakia, Spain, Sweden, United Kingdom, and the United States. His main research interests are: food processing by ohmic heating/moderate electric fields (namely, the study of the effects of electric currents on biomolecules and cells); edible films and coatings for food products (chemical, physical, and functional characterization); nanotechnology applied to food technology (nano-multilayered films and coatings, nanoparticles, and nanogels, all from food-grade materials); and fermentation technology (including design and operation of bioreactors). He has supervised 27 PhD theses; he has also supervised several MSc theses and 15 postdoctoral fellows. He has published approximately 230 research articles in international peer-reviewed journals and approximately 25 book chapters in international books and 4 patents.

# Contributors

**Edgar Acosta**
Department of Chemical Engineering and Applied Chemistry
University of Toronto
Toronto, Ontario, Canada

**José C. Andrade**
CESPU
Instituto de Investigação e Formação Avançada em Ciências e Tecnologias da
Gandra, Portugal

**Ana I. Bourbon**
CEB, Centre of Biological Engineering
University of Minho
Braga, Portugal

**Adriano Brandelli**
Laboratório de Bioquímica e Microbiologia Aplicada
Instituto de Ciência e Tecnologia de Alimentos
Universidade Federal do Rio Grande do Sul
Porto Alegre, Brazil

**María A. Busolo**
Novel Materials and Nanotechnology Group
IATA-CSIC
Paterna, Spain

**Rosa Busquets**
Faculty of Science, Engineering and Computing
Kingston University
Kingston upon Thames, United Kingdom

**Maria G. Carneiro-da-Cunha**
Laboratório de Imunopatologia Keizo Asami
Departamento de Bioquímica
Centro de Biociências
Universidade Federal de Pernambuco (UFPE)
Recife, Brazil

**Miguel A. Cerqueira**
INL, International Iberian Nanotechnology Laboratory
Braga, Portugal

**Peter X. Chen**
School of Pharmacy
University of Waterloo
Kitchener, Ontario, Canada

**Adriane Cherpinski**
Novel Materials and Nanotechnology Group
IATA-CSIC
Paterna, Spain

**M. Cornejo-Mazón**
Departamento de Graduados e Investigación en Alimentos
Escuela Nacional de Ciencias Biológicas
Instituto Politécnico Nacional
México, Mexico

**Ana C. Fortuna**
Department of Pharmacology
Faculty of Pharmacy
University of Coimbra (FFUC)
and
CIBIT, Coimbra Institute for Biomedical Imaging and Translational Research
University of Coimbra
Coimbra, Portugal

**Pablo Fuciños**
INL, International Iberian Nanotechnology Laboratory
Braga, Portugal

**S. García-Pinilla**
Departamento de Graduados e Investigación en Alimentos
Escuela Nacional de Ciencias Biológicas
Instituto Politécnico Nacional
México, Mexico

**G.F. Gutiérrez-López**
Departamento de Graduados e Investigación en Alimentos
Escuela Nacional de Ciencias Biológicas
Instituto Politécnico Nacional
México, Mexico

**Jose M. Lagaron**
Novel Materials and Nanotechnology Group
IATA-CSIC
Paterna, Spain

**Adriana Lima**
CESPU
Instituto de Investigação e Formação Avançada em Ciências e Tecnologias da
Gandra, Portugal

**Cristina Prieto López**
Novel Materials and Nanotechnology Group
IATA-CSIC
Paterna, Spain

**Nathalie A. Lopes**
Laboratório de Bioquímica e Microbiologia Aplicada
Instituto de Ciência e Tecnologia de Alimentos
Universidade Federal do Rio Grande do Sul
Porto Alegre, Brazil

**Alan R. Mackie**
School of Food Science and Nutrition
University of Leeds
Leeds, United Kingdom

**Joana T. Martins**
CEB, Centre of Biological Engineering
University of Minho
Braga, Portugal

**Beatriz Melendez-Rodriguez**
Novel Materials and Nanotechnology Group
IATA-CSIC
Paterna, Spain

**Mehdi Nouraei**
Department of Chemical Engineering and Applied Chemistry
University of Toronto
Toronto, Ontario, Canada

**Lorenzo M. Pastrana**
INL, International Iberian Nanotechnology Laboratory
Braga, Portugal

**Ricardo N. Pereira**
CEB, Centre of Biological Engineering
University of Minho
Braga, Portugal

**Dmitri Y. Petrovykh**
INL, International Iberian Nanotechnology Laboratory
Braga, Portugal

**Ana C. Pinheiro**
CEB, Centre of Biological Engineering
University of Minho
Braga, Portugal

and

Instituto de Biologia Experimental e Tecnológica
Estação Agronómica Nacional
Oeiras, Portugal

**Cristian M.B. Pinilla**
Laboratório de Bioquímica e Microbiologia Aplicada
Instituto de Ciência e Tecnologia de Alimentos
Universidade Federal do Rio Grande do Sul
Porto Alegre, Brazil

**Óscar L. Ramos**
CEB, Centre of Biological Engineering
University of Minho
Braga, Portugal

and

CBQF, Centro de Biotecnologia e Química Fina Laboratório Associado
Escola Superior de Biotecnologia
Universidade Católica Portuguesa/Porto
Porto, Portugal

**Philippe E. Ramos**
CEB, Centre of Biological Engineering
University of Minho
Braga, Portugal

**Michael A. Rogers**
Department of Food Science
University of Guelph
Guelph, Ontario, Canada

**Bruno Sarmento**
CESPU
Instituto de Investigação e Formação Avançada em Ciências e Tecnologias da
Gandra, Portugal

and

INEB, Instituto Nacional de Engenharia Biomédica
Universidade do Porto

and

i3S, Instituto de Investigação e Inovação em Saúde
Universidade do Porto
Porto, Portugal

**Amélia M. Silva**
Department of Biology and Environment
University of Trás-os Montes e Alto Douro (UTAD)

and

Centre for Research and Technology of Agro-Environmental and Biological Sciences (CITAB-UTAD)
Vila Real, Portugal

**Francisco Silva**
CESPU
Instituto de Investigação e Formação Avançada em Ciências e Tecnologias da
Gandra, Portugal

**Cláudia Sousa**
INL, International Iberian Nanotechnology Laboratory
Braga, Portugal

**Eliana B. Souto**
Department of Pharmaceutical Technology
Faculty of Pharmacy
University of Coimbra (FFUC)
Coimbra, Portugal

and

CEB, Centre of Biological Engineering
University of Minho
Braga, Portugal

**Selma B. Souto**
Department of Endocrinology
Braga Hospital
Braga, Portugal

**José A. Teixeira**
CEB, Centre of Biological Engineering
University of Minho
Braga, Portugal

**Amelia Torcello-Gómez**
School of Food Science and Nutrition
University of Leeds
Leeds, United Kingdom

**Sergio Torres-Giner**
Novel Materials and Nanotechnology Group
IATA-CSIC
Paterna, Spain

**António A. Vicente**
CEB, Centre of Biological Engineering
University of Minho
Braga, Portugal

**Raquel Vieira**
Department of Pharmaceutical Technology
Faculty of Pharmacy
University of Coimbra (FFUC)
Coimbra, Portugal

**J.C. Villalobos-Espinosa**
Instituto Tecnológico Superior de Teziutlán
Teziutlán, México

and

Departamento de Graduados e Investigación en Alimentos
Escuela Nacional de Ciencias Biológicas
Instituto Politécnico Nacional
México City, Mexico

# *Section I*

## *Overview*

# 1 Nanotechnology in Food
## *Introduction, Context, and Concepts*

*Óscar L. Ramos, José A. Teixeira, and António A. Vicente*

**CONTENTS**



## 1.1 INTRODUCTION

Nanoscience and nanotechnology link distinct, but complementary, areas of knowledge such as physics, chemistry, life sciences, medicine, engineering, information and communication technologies, thus potentiating the share of knowledge between these fields, while offering a broad number of opportunities and applications. Among them, the impact of nanoscience and nanotechnology in fields related to health and well-being is currently very strong and their applications are expected to bring large benefits to the food and nutrition sector (Rossi et al. 2014, Ranjan et al. 2014). This book highlights the most recent advances and promising technologies used in the design, fabrication, characterization, and utilization of nanosystems, manufactured from bio-based materials to add value to the food and food-related industries through the whole food chain. Nonetheless, a significant part of the information covered within this book can be also usefully applied to other fields, including health and personal care products, cosmetics, pharmaceuticals, and agrochemicals. It is well recognized by the scientific community that many challenges found in nanoscience and nanotechnology are shared in different fields of application. Equally, the potential solutions to overcome such challenges can be applied in different types of products. Thus, the scope of this book, although with a clear focus in food applications, goes far beyond this field of knowledge.

In recent years, the development of novel nanosystems and their application by the food industry has been growing fast to face the current challenges found in processing, production, nutrition, preservation and safety of food products, aiming at the sustainable supply of the population needs. This growing trend is clearly showed by the increasing number of publications and issued patents in this field, particularly during recent years, and it is corroborated also by the increasing amount of companies applying nanotechnology to the development of their products (Cerqueira et al. 2017).

In the food industry (Figure 1.1), nanotechnology can be applied to improve quality, shelf life, safety, cost, and nutritional benefits of foods (McClements and Xiao 2017).

Nanosystems, such as nanohydrogels, nanoparticles, lipid-based nanosystems, and nanolaminates (subjects addressed in Chapters 2 through 5, respectively) can also be used as delivery systems (discussed in Chapter 8) to protect and improve the stability of active ingredients (e.g., colors, flavors, nutraceuticals, antimicrobials, antioxidants, and preservatives) added to foods during processing and storage, thus enhancing their effectiveness and bioavailability, while improving the nutritional value of foods (Cerqueira et al. 2017). Active ingredients such as vitamins (e.g., vitamins E, $B_2$, and $B_{12}$), polyphenols (e.g., curcumin, resveratrol, and quercetin), fatty acids (e.g., ω-3 and ω-6), and minerals (e.g., iron) are examples of poorly water-soluble substances that have a relatively low stability during digestion and gastrointestinal (GI) absorption. So, they may be highly degraded when subjected to extreme environmental conditions (e.g., temperature, light, and oxygen), thus affecting their

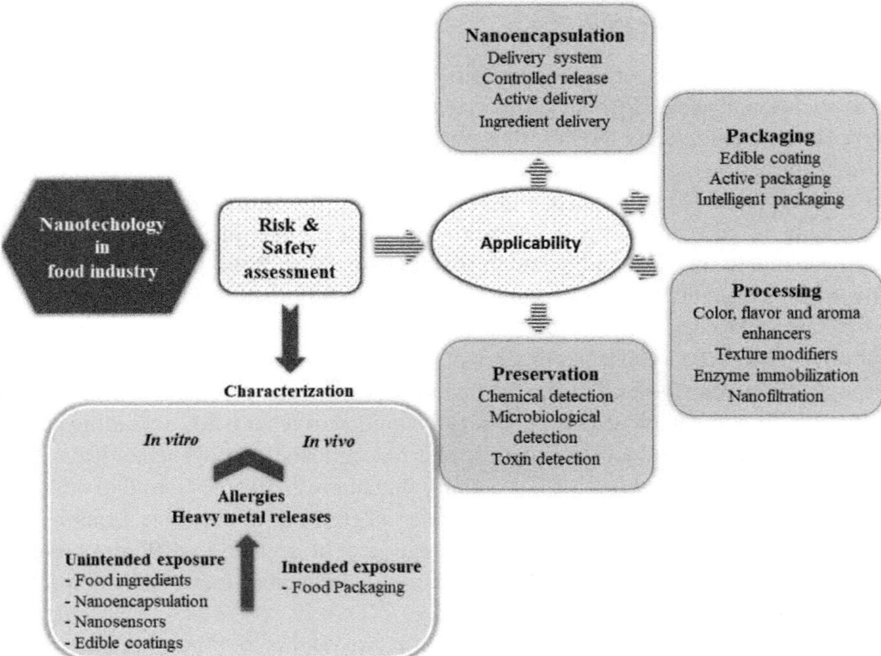


**FIGURE 1.1** Schematic representation of the major applications of nanotechnology in different food sectors.

effectiveness (de Souza Simões et al. 2017, Madalena et al. 2018). Therefore, the nanoencapsulation (Figure 1.1) of these ingredients through top-down or bottom-up strategies, or the combination of both, may allow overcoming these issues (de Souza Simões et al. 2017).

In this sense, nanoencapsulation technologies (topic discussed in Chapter 3) provide promising solutions to inherent issues characteristic of higher size systems (i.e., macro- and microsystems). This happens because reducing the size to nanoscale range allows a large surface area-to-volume ratio, but also distinct physicochemical interactions between materials, which significantly impact the final properties and functionalities of those systems. Thus, it is expected that nanotechnology will solve compatibility problems (e.g., aggregation or coalescence phenomena) occurring with the food matrix, and improve the final product attributes (e.g., flavor, texture, color, and appearance), while allowing a controlled release of active ingredients entrapped into the nanostructures, in specific sites of action, as a response to external stimuli. This means that, i.e., bioactives that are absorbed in the intestine should be released there in order to avoid possible degradation provoked by undesired conditions (e.g., pH, temperature, and presence of enzymes) (de Souza Simões et al. 2017). Together with all mentioned advantages, the use of tailor-made delivery systems may also allow designing personalized nutrition/supplementation programs to face public health global requirements or consumer demands for safer, healthier, and nutritious food products.

The use of nanosystems in food packaging (Figure 1.1), mainly through the incorporation of nanocomposites, allows the improvement of mechanical, barrier, and optical properties, while imparting antimicrobial and antioxidant capacity, thus contributing to the development of active and intelligent packaging systems (subject addressed in Chapter 11). These systems actively contribute to extend food shelf life by improving food safety, stability, and nutritional value during transportation and storage conditions (Cerqueira et al. 2017). Intelligent packaging has the ability to, e.g., control the release of food preservatives in response to external stimuli (e.g., presence of microorganisms) and/or incorporate nanosensors that will inform, control, and monitor the quality or freshness of the sealed food products. The main concern regarding the use of active and intelligent packaging systems, which is common to any food contact materials, is the possible migration to food. These concerns are covered by Commission Regulation (European Union, EU) No 10/2011 (European Union 2011b).

In food processing (Figure 1.1), nanosystems can also be used as effective tools to enhance food manufacturing, encapsulation and filtration conditions, or the final features of foods such as sensorial attributes (e.g., through color, flavor, and aroma enhancers) and rheological properties (indirectly influencing sensorial attributes, e.g., through the use of texture modifiers) (subject discussed in Chapter 12). In respect to food preservation, nanotechnologies can potentiate the development of detection tools and analytical systems (e.g., nanosensors) to control and monitor food quality or the presence of potential chemical and microbiological hazards along the food chain (topic discussed in Chapter 13). This will promote food safety, while contributing to potentiate the market value of foods (Cerqueira et al. 2017).

Nevertheless, one of the major challenges toward the successful application of nanotechnology for food purposes comprises the use of food-grade materials as an alternative to replace the non-food-grade polymers (Cerqueira et al. 2014, de Souza Simões et al. 2017). Polysaccharides (e.g., cellulose, alginate, pectin, and chitosan), proteins (e.g., whey proteins, zein, and casein), and lipids (e.g., medium chain triglycerides, oleic acid tristearin, and corn oil), or combinations of these materials can be used to address such challenges, as these materials are biodegradable, devoid of toxicity, and thus generally recognized as safe with potential to be functionalized in order to display novel or improved properties.

In respect to the use of nanosystems in food applications, it is of utmost importance to clarify the existence of four main groups of nanomaterials, as reported by several authors (Morris 2011, Chaudhry and Castle 2011, McClements and Xiao 2017), namely: (i) naturally occurring materials from proteins (e.g., casein micelles formed by protein-mineral clusters), polysaccharides (cell organelles such as ribosomes, vacuoles, and lysosomes), or lipids (e.g., oil bodies composed by phospholipid/protein-coated triglyceride droplets); (ii) new or modified materials resulting from processing, such as cooking, grinding, or homogenization (e.g., the network structures present in food gels, the crystalline structures of starch-based foods, or the crystalline structures of fats); (iii) substances and molecules (e.g., nanoparticles, nutrients, and vitamins) present in the body as result of digestion; and (iv) engineered nanomaterials deliberately added either as additives (e.g., titanium dioxide and iron oxide nanoparticles as whitening agents or carriers of iron, respectively) to food products, as anticaking agents (e.g., synthetic amorphous silicon to control powder flowability) in food processing, or as antimicrobial agents (e.g., silver and zinc oxide nanoparticles) in food packaging.

Regarding the nanosystems deliberately added, they are specifically developed to have one or more functionalities (e.g., act as delivery systems or applied to improve stability and appearance, or to alter the texture of foods). However, some of them have poor solubility or are at least partially digested through the GI tract, therefore they may be absorbed, retained, or accumulated within the body (topic discussed in Chapter 9). This subject has concerned the scientific community and the public in general, due to the lack of knowledge on how new or modified physicochemical properties arising from engineered nanosystems may enhance their bioavailability which, in turn, may have an impact in their toxicological properties.

Hence, despite all the great benefits that nanotechnology can bring to the food industry through the use of engineered nanosystems, potential risks need to be exhaustively evaluated, namely, those related with potential side effects to human health including oxidative damage, inflammation of the GI tract, cancer, as well as lesions due to toxicity (either acute or chronic) in organs such as liver and kidneys (Dasgupta et al. 2015, Neethirajan and Jayas 2011). In the case of food consumption, the most relevant for consumers is the chronic toxicity, since relatively low quantities of nanosystems can be ingested during longer time periods. The potential toxicity provoked by the prolonged consumption of foods containing nanosystems can affect human health either by directly affecting cells and organs, or indirectly by impacting the normal microbial population within the GI tract, thus dangerously impacting human health or well-being (Buzea et al. 2007).

In this sense, the safety and risk assessment of nanosystems (Figure 1.1), as well as the evaluation of their potential toxic effects is fundamental, and therefore this subject has been the focus of many recent studies (Jantunen et al. 2018, Rossi et al. 2014). Research works in this field have shown that specific types of nanosystems added to food products, and some physicochemical and physiological mechanisms involved, are more prone to provoke adverse health effects than others. Nonetheless, there is no consensus among the scientific community regarding this matter and many contradictory results exist with studies showing that a specific nanosystem causes toxicity, while other studies suggest just the opposite (McClements and Xiao 2017). These discrepancies may be explained mainly by the different legislations or regulatory definitions of nanomaterial adopted by different countries. Furthermore, the physicochemical properties (e.g., composition, shape, size, physical state, purity, and aggregation state) of the nanosystems studied, as well as the methodologies employed in toxicity evaluation (e.g., *in vitro* or *in vivo* experiments) vary considerably from laboratory to laboratory, which hinder the establishment of correlations among the results. On the other hand, the lack of studies available evaluating the nanosystems' behavior, fate, and toxicity when added to food matrices or after oral ingestion and passage through the GI tract, limits further conclusions (McClements et al. 2016). It is therefore crucial that standardized techniques and methodologies are adequately used to evaluate the nanosystems' behavior, characteristics, and toxicity under accurate, reproducible, and realistic conditions. In order to fulfill this gap, Chapter 7 overviews a multiple set of complementary techniques needed to extensively characterize nanosystems, which is fundamental in the process of standardization of the classification and definition of nanomaterials. Chapter 14 comprehensively reviews the most advanced methods for detection of micro- and nanosystems in foods and in its last chapter (Chapter 15), this book shows the most recent trends and advances toward the use of nanosystems in the food industry.

## 1.2 DEFINITIONS

The term nanotechnology has been widely used to define the deliberate synthesis and use of nano-sized objects to produce materials with new properties and functions, in order to address specific scientific and technological purposes (Rossi et al. 2014). However, the definition that is more widely used and accepted is that of The Royal Society and The Royal Academy of Engineering (2004), which defines nanotechnology as the design, manufacture, characterization, processing, and application of structures, materials, devices, and systems by controlling the shape and size of matter at the nanometer scale (McClements and Xiao 2017, Cerqueira et al. 2014, de Souza Simões et al. 2017). Regarding this topic, it is also essential to define which length scale is being considered of interest for nanoscience and nanotechnologies and within which a nanomaterial can be considered as such. A nanometer is one-billionth of a meter ($10^{-9}$), and the nanoscale is thus referred to structures with a length between 1 and 100 nm, thus including distinct structures such as atoms, molecules, nanoparticles, and carbon nanotubes (Villena de Francisco and García-Estepa 2018, Engineering 2004). Nanomaterials are engineered constructions or particles with size properties smaller than a micrometer wherein at least one dimension of the material is less than or equivalent to 100 nm (Rossi et al. 2014).

However, this definition is used only as a guide because there is no consensus in this matter among different countries (Amenta et al. 2015).

The EU is, until now, the only region that adopted a clear regulatory definition of nanomaterials through their commission recommendation (2011/696/EU), as being: "*A natural, incidental or manufactured material containing particles, in an unbound state or as an aggregate or as an agglomerate and where, for 50% or more of the particles in the number size distribution, one or more external dimensions is in the size range 1 nm–100 nm*" (European Union 2011a). In specific cases, the threshold of 50% can be reduced as follows: "*In specific cases and where warranted by concerns for the environment, health, safety or competitiveness the number size distribution threshold of 50% may be replaced by a threshold between 1 and 50%.*" and if "*By derogation from the above, fullerenes, graphene flakes and single wall carbon nanotubes with one or more external dimensions below 1 nm should be considered as nanomaterials.*"

This definition intends to clarify, while providing a binding framework for manufacturers, importers, and users in the EU region and ensure the safety of substances and products in different regulatory sectors, including the agri/feed/food sector.

*In Canada*, nanomaterials have been defined as "*any manufactured substance or product and any component material, ingredient, device, or structure [.] if it is at or within the nanoscale in at least one external dimension, or has internal or surface structure at the nanoscale, or it is smaller or larger than the nanoscale in all dimensions and exhibits one or more nanoscale properties/phenomena*" (Canada 2011). This last definition is more general and includes larger or smaller materials than the nanoscale range, as long as they display properties or functionalities typical of the nano dimension.

On the other hand, in the United States, the *Federal Food, Drug, and Cosmetic Act*, responsible for the supervision of the Food and Drug Administration (FDA) that is in turn responsible to guarantee the safety of food additives/food contact materials/feed additives that are placed on the market, did not issue any regulatory definition for nanomaterials (Amenta et al. 2015). Instead, FDA published several guidelines addressing the nanomaterials/nanotechnology issues to support the industry (US-FDA 2014) and for food players, recommending a preliminary safety assessment of "Food Ingredients and Food Contact Substances produced at nanoscale." Therefore, for FDA, the products containing nanomaterials are not considered, *a priori*, intrinsically hazardous, but should be subjected to a case-by-case evaluation in respect to their safety and expected use (Tyler 2012, Amenta et al. 2015).

Despite the significant debates and discussion, particularly in the recent years, over the need of establishing standardized regulations for nanotechnology use in food products, the regulatory agencies and governmental entities have not yet reached an agreement on worldwide-applicable rules (Coles and Frewer 2013, Amenta et al. 2015).

## 1.3 TERMINOLOGY

The following terms/concepts associated with the use of nanosystems for food applications are recurrently employed throughout this book, so it was considered useful to define them here for clarity:

*Nanotechnology*—The process of designing, manufacturing, characterizing, processing, and applying structures, materials, devices, and systems by controlling the shape and size of matter at the nanometer scale.

*Nanosystems*—Particles, structures, and materials with size properties smaller than a micrometer, wherein at least one dimension of the material is sized between 1 and 100 nm.

*Engineered nanosystems*—Engineered constructions or particles, structures, and materials with size properties smaller than a micrometer, wherein at least one dimension of the material is sized between 1 and 100 nm, specific developed, and deliberately added to have one or more functionalities.

*Nanoscale*—Refers to systems, structures, and materials with a length scale between 1 and 100 nanometers.

*Encapsulation*—The process of incorporating a specific component ("active ingredient" or "bioactive compound") within a matrix (the "encapsulant"). This matrix can be composed by single or multiple components, and it can display a homogeneous or heterogeneous structure, depending on the materials and methodologies employed in their design and production.

*Delivery*—The process of carrying an encapsulated "active ingredient" or "bioactive compound" to the specific site of action [e.g., the human stomach or small intestine (for a "nutrient" or "nutraceutical") or the colon (for "probiotic" or "prebiotic")]. Once an active component has been encapsulated, it is "maintained" or "retained" inside the delivery system for a certain period of time under specific conditions until its release occurs.

*Delivery system*—A system designed to encapsulate, protect, and release one or more "active ingredients" or "bioactive compounds."

*Controlled release*—The process of releasing an encapsulated "active ingredient" or "bioactive compound" with a specific concentration–time profile at the desired site of action.

*Bioaccessibility*—The fraction of an "active ingredient" or "bioactive compound" that is released from the matrix (either food or encapsulated) in the gastrointestinal lumen and is thereby made available for intestinal absorption.

*Bioavailability*—The fraction of an "active ingredient" or "bioactive compound" that is absorbed into a living system or is made available at the site of physiological activity.

## 1.4 CONCLUSION AND FUTURE PERSPECTIVES

The application of nanotechnology in the food industry is expected to bring numerous potential benefits to the whole food chain and consequently to the final consumer. From the current commercial applications, it is possible to realize that the major areas in this industry, as shown by their faster increase, include the supplementation of foods through nanoencapsulation of active ingredients to improve their nutritional value, and the application of nanocomposites to develop active and intelligent food packaging systems.

Despite the great potential offered by nanotechnology to the food sector, the acceptance by consumers is relatively low. This behavior is highly related with the risk perception associated to the consumption of food products containing engineered nanosystems. Studies performed to evaluate the social impacts of nanotechnology show that a well-established regulation is fundamental to obtaining confidence and ensuring acceptance of this technology by consumers. The consumer-safety implications from the use of nanosystems in food are highly related to the reduced size of materials at nanoscale range and consequently to their new physicochemical properties and to possibility of prolonged consumption of foods containing nanomaterials. The potential risks coming from continuous ingestion of nanomaterials have been recently the object of numerous debates and discussions, but there is a lack of knowledge that needs to be filled before nanotechnology can be fully applied. For instance, currently there is rather poor information about the toxicity, fate, and behavior of most food-grade nanomaterials, and it is not possible to issue a single and general recommendation about the safety of all nanosystems. In turn, the risk and safety assessment of nanosystems must be evaluated on a case-by-case basis depending on their nature, size, shape, and physicochemical properties, as well as the features of the food matrices where they are added.

The major challenge regarding the safety assessment is the accurate characterization of the nanomaterials' properties, namely in terms of size, size distribution, concentration, composition, surface shape and charge, and stability under standardized testing conditions. In the case of toxicity evaluation, the use of standards and validated methods is crucial.

Therefore, it is obvious that the use of nanotechnology in foods cannot advance independently of the progress in nanometrology, the science that measures and characterizes the materials at the nanoscale. The lack of an adequate link between nanotechnology and nanometrology could compromise the successful use of nanotechnology or at least retard significantly the time to market for many applications.

Regarding the regulatory aspects of nanotechnology, although the framework on the use of nanosystems in food products is progressing, it is expected that in the near future the regulatory agencies and governmental entities will increase initiatives to better monitor, regulate, and standardize nanosystems' proper design and use in foods.

## ACKNOWLEDGMENTS

This work was supported by the Portuguese Foundation for Science and Technology under the scope of the strategic funding of UID/Multi/50016/2019 and UID/BIO/04469/2013 units and COMPETE 2020 (POCI-01-0145-FEDER-006684) and BioTecNorte operation (NORTE-01-0145-FEDER-000004) funded by European Regional Development Fund under the scope of Norte2020, Programa Operacional Regional do Norte. Óscar L. Ramos gratefully acknowledge Portuguese Foundation for Science and Technology for his financial grant with reference SFRH/BPD/80766/2011.

## REFERENCES


Amenta, Valeria, Karin Aschberger, Maria Arena, Hans Bouwmeester, Filipa Botelho Moniz, Puck Brandhoff, Stefania Gottardo, et al. 2015. "Regulatory aspects of nanotechnology in the agri/feed/food sector in EU and non-EU countries." *Regulatory Toxicology and Pharmacology* no. 73 (1):463–476.

Buzea, C., I. I. Pacheco, and K. Robbie. 2007. "Nanomaterials and nanoparticles: Sources and toxicity." *Biointerphases* no. 2 (4):Mr17–71.

Baughan, J. S. (2015) 3 - Future trends in global food packaging regulation. Baughan, In *Woodhead Publishing Series in Food Science, Technology and Nutrition, Global Legislation for Food Contact Materials*, ed. J. Sylvain, pp. 65–74. Woodhead Publishing.

Cerqueira, Miguel A., Ana C. Pinheiro, Hélder D. Silva, Philippe E. Ramos, Maria A. Azevedo, María L. Flores-López, Melissa C. Rivera, Ana I. Bourbon, Óscar L. Ramos, and António A. Vicente. 2014. "Design of bio-nanosystems for oral delivery of functional compounds." *Food Engineering Reviews* no. 6 (1):1–19.

Cerqueira, Miguel Ângelo, Ana C. Pinheiro, Oscar L. Ramos, Hélder Silva, Ana I. Bourbon, and Antonio A. Vicente. 2017. "Chapter two–Advances in food nanotechnology." In *Emerging Nanotechnologies in Food Science*, edited by Rosa Busquets, 11–38. Boston: Elsevier.

Chaudhry, Qasim, and Laurence Castle. 2011. "Food applications of nanotechnologies: An overview of opportunities and challenges for developing countries." *Trends in Food Science & Technology* no. 22 (11):595–603.

Coles, David, and Lynn J. Frewer. 2013. "Nanotechnology applied to European food production—A review of ethical and regulatory issues." *Trends in Food Science & Technology* no. 34 (1):32–43.

Dasgupta, Nandita, Shivendu Ranjan, Deepa Mundekkad, Chidambaram Ramalingam, Rishi Shanker, and Ashutosh Kumar. 2015. "Nanotechnology in agro-food: From field to plate." *Food Research International* no. 69:381–400.

de Souza Simões, Lívia, Daniel A. Madalena, Ana C. Pinheiro, José A. Teixeira, António A. Vicente, and Óscar L. Ramos. 2017. "Micro- and nano bio-based delivery systems for food applications: In vitro behavior." *Advances in Colloid and Interface Science* no. 243:23–45.

The Royal Society and The Royal Academy of Engineering. 2004. "Nanoscience and nanotechnologies: Opportunities and uncertainties." In Royal Society, pp. 1–11. Cardiff: Clyvedon Press.

European Union. 2011a. "Commission recommendation of 18 October 2011 on the definition of nanomaterial (2011/696/EU)." *Official Journal of the European Union* no. L 275:38–40.

European Union. 2011b. "Commission Regulation (EU) No 10/2011 of 14 January 2011 on plastic materials and articles intended to come into contact with food." *Official Journal of the European Union* no. L12/1.

Jantunen, A. Paula K., Stefania Gottardo, Kirsten Rasmussen, and Hugues P. Crutzen. 2018. "An inventory of ready-to-use and publicly available tools for the safety assessment of nanomaterials." *NanoImpact* no. 12:18–28.

Madalena, Daniel A., Ricardo N. Pereira, António A. Vicente, and Óscar L. Ramos. 2018. "New insights on bio-based micro- and nanosystems in food." In *Reference Module in Food Science*. Elsevier.

McClements, David Julian, Glen DeLoid, Georgios Pyrgiotakis, Jo Anne Shatkin, Hang Xiao, and Philip Demokritou. 2016. "The role of the food matrix and gastrointestinal tract in the assessment of biological properties of ingested engineered nanomaterials (iENMs): State of the science and knowledge gaps." *NanoImpact* no. 3–4:47–57.

McClements, David Julian, and Hang Xiao. 2017. "Is nano safe in foods? Establishing the factors impacting the gastrointestinal fate and toxicity of organic and inorganic food-grade nanoparticles." *npj Science of Food* no. 1 (1):6.

Morris, V. J. 2011. "Emerging roles of engineered nanomaterials in the food industry." *Trends in Biotechnology* no. 29 (10):509–516.

Neethirajan, Suresh, and Digvir S. Jayas. 2011. "Nanotechnology for the food and bioprocessing industries." *Food and Bioprocess Technology* no. 4 (1):39–47.

Ranjan, Shivendu, Nandita Dasgupta, Arkadyuti Roy Chakraborty, S. Melvin Samuel, Chidambaram Ramalingam, Rishi Shanker, and Ashutosh Kumar. 2014. "Nanoscience and nanotechnologies in food industries: opportunities and research trends." *Journal of Nanoparticle Research* no. 16 (6):2464.

Rossi, M., F. Cubadda, L. Dini, M. L. Terranova, F. Aureli, A. Sorbo, and D. Passeri. 2014. "Scientific basis of nanotechnology, implications for the food sector and future trends." *Trends in Food Science & Technology* no. 40 (2):127–148.

Tyler, L. C.. 2012. "FDA issues draft guidance on use of nanotechnology in food and food packaging." *Nanotechnology Law & Business* no. 9:149–155.

US-FDA. 2014. "Guidance for Industry—Considering whether an FDA-regulated product involves the application of nanotechnology." *Silver Spring* no. 20993, http://www.fda.gov/regulatoryinformation/guidances/ucm257698.htm. (accessed on November 13, 2018).

Villena de Francisco, Elena, and Rosa M. García-Estepa. 2018. "Nanotechnology in the agro-food industry." *Journal of Food Engineering* no. 238:1–11.

# *Section II*

## *Production and Characterization of Bio-nanosystems Focusing Emerging Processing Technologies*

# 2 Nanohydrogels Production

*Ricardo N. Pereira and Óscar L. Ramos*

**CONTENTS**



## 2.1 INTRODUCTION

Nanohydrogels can be considered as superabsorbent materials composed of three-dimensional crosslinked polymer networks at nanoscale size. These polymeric and highly hydrophilic materials have a high swelling capacity, retaining large amounts of water (the preferential dispersion medium) within a very flexible stable structure, which can resemble a natural tissue (Ahmed 2015). Over the past few years, the interest in the development of nanohydrogel matrices has been growing, particularly in the field of biomedical sciences for drug delivery applications (Dalwadi and Patel 2015). Presently, nanohydrogels prepared from natural and biodegradable polymeric sources—i.e., proteins and polysaccharides—are establishing a strong foothold not only in medicine (e.g., cancer therapy and tissue engineering), but also in other fields of science such as agriculture and food technology, in particular for the development of functional foods, active or smart food packaging systems, and biosensing elements (Akram and Hussain 2017). Protein-based nanohydrogels are drawing huge attention due to their biological value and different possibilities of structural design, which offers an innumerous potential for the encapsulation, association, or biocomplexation with active ingredients. These features place protein nanohydrogels in the frontline of bio-systems that can deliver enhanced functionality to the food by carrying, protecting, and delivering bioactive compounds for an intended purpose in a safe way (Bourbon et al. 2015). Currently, nanohydrogel research is emerging in the food science triggering the development of nanosystems with new and varied functionalities, innovative production strategies, and development of characterization tools. But toward a successful commercialization of these nanosystems a wide gap still needs to be filled. Aspects related with production scale, public perception, and, particularly, the lack of knowledge of the long-term effects of these nanomaterials on human safety are restraining its practical application.

This chapter intends to give an overview about the use of biopolymers from food sources for the production of bio-based nanohydrogel systems, addressing aspects related with preparation, most promising applications, as well as challenges to overcome and future perspectives.

## 2.2 CLASSIFICATION AND DIFFERENT TYPES OF NANOHYDROGELS

Nanohydrogels can be classified based on their origin source (e.g., natural or synthetic), type of crosslinking (e.g., chemical, physical, or even both), stimuli responsiveness (e.g., biochemical, physical, or chemical), among others ways.

Natural nanohydrogels can be prepared through the use of promising sources such as proteins (e.g., protein fractions from whey including β-lactoglobulin and lactoferrin) and polysaccharides from animal (e.g., chitosan), vegetal (e.g., alginate), and microbial (e.g., pullulan) origins. These natural and emergent origins bring advantageous aspects which include biodegradability, lack of toxicity, good biocompatibility, and tunable mechanical properties. Hydrogels can also be distinguished from the type of network crosslinking that can be physical or chemical. Chemical crosslinked hydrogels are prepared through covalent bonding—e.g., disulfide formation, while physical hydrogels are molecular rearrangements which can involve non-covalent bonding (i.e., hydrogen bonds, hydrophobic interactions and van der Waals forces) resulting from external stimuli such as pH, temperature, and ionic balance. The interest in physically crosslinked hydrogel networks is increasing. Once they were weaker structures, and thus more susceptible to mechanical forces, and avoided the use of crosslinking agents which are often toxic compounds that impair biomedical and food applications (Jonker et al. 2012, Ullah et al. 2015). The composition of crosslinked networks of nanohydrogels can also be classified as: (i) homopolymeric—with one type of hydrophilic monomer unit; (ii) copolymeric—with two co-monomer units in which at least one should be hydrophilic thus assuring swelling behavior; and (iii) interpenetrating polymeric networks—consist in a combination of polymer networks to produce an advanced multicomponent polymeric system that can also involve the entrapment of a linear polymer into prepared polymer networks, also known by semi-interpenetrating polymeric networks (Dragan 2014, Ullah et al. 2015, Akram and Hussain 2017).

Another way to distinguish nanohydrogels is measured by its ability of swelling or deswelling as a response to physical trigger such as light, pH, temperature, pressure, and electric field. These are commonly called as smart or stimuli-responsive nanohydrogels (Xia et al. 2013) that are emerging as innovative materials in food packaging for development of active packaging (Fuciños et al. 2012) and in food processing for design of delivery systems intended for the controlled released of nutraceuticals in specific sites of action in the body (Zimet and Livney 2009, Ramos et al. 2017). One of the major challenges of food nanotechnology in relation to the development of bio-nanosystems to improve food functionality relies in the use of food source macromolecules. In this sense, protein-based materials are being used for the production of nanohydrogels offering the possibility of multivalent bioconjugation and diversified structural networks through simple thermal and salt addition methods for example (Cerqueira et al. 2014).

## 2.3 NATURAL NANOHYDROGELS

Polysaccharides and proteins occur naturally in food as nanoscale structures or building blocks and in reason of that have been inspiring the development of innovative nanostructured materials with fascinating architectural designs and functionalities (Wendell et al. 2006). Table 2.1 summarizes examples of nanohydrogels produced using biopolymers such as food proteins and polysaccharides.

### 2.3.1 Polysaccharides-Based Nanohydrogels

Bulk hydrogels of polysaccharides have been produced since a long time, but only a limited number of polysaccharides have been studied for the development of nanohydrogels systems (Alhaique et al. 2015). Further, most of the applications developed are still intended to the biomedical, pharmaceutical, and cosmetic fields of science (Wang et al. 2012). However, some of most common examples of the use of polysaccharides include the use of alginate and chitosan, which have recognized potential to produce nanosystems that can entrap in their nanogel matrix bioactive compounds, showing non-toxicity and low price together with a high biodegradability and excellent biocompatibility (Abreu et al. 2012). Chitosan is a cationic polysaccharide derived from the N-deacetylation of chitin, which is one of the most abundant natural polysaccharides on earth and extracted from exoskeletons of marine arthropods. Chitosan exhibits interesting biological properties such as adsorption, mucoadhesive, and immunogenic. Regarding composition, it is a linear copolymer with several free amino groups that allow the establishment of covalent or ionic crosslinking (Brunel et al. 2010, Wang et al. 2012, Liu et al. 2016). Alginate, an anionic polysaccharide extracted from marine seaweed, is being extensively used as thickening and stabilizing agent in food processing, but can also render nanohydrogels when an appropriate concentration of divalent counterions (e.g., $Ca^{2+}$) is added to a dilute dispersion. Pistone et al. have developed stable alginate nanoparticles ranging from 200 to 230 nm through crosslinking with divalent cation zinc (Pistone et al. 2015)—Table 2.1. Through a methodology that involves a pre-gel state step—through the interaction between alginate and calcium ions—followed by the addition of a polycationic molecule such as chitosan, it is possible to produce nanoparticles with a alginate nanohydrogel nucleus stabilized by chitosan layer (Rajaonarivony et al. 1993, Sarmento et al. 2007). Through this approach, it has been possible to fabricate different food nanosystems with intended functionalities.

**TABLE 2.1**
**Examples of Nanohydrogels and Nanostructures and Its Respective Production Method and Main Features (Size and Associated Bioactivity)**

| Method | Main Biomaterials | Bioactive Compound | Approximate Network Size (nm) | References |
|---|---|---|---|---|
| Electrostatic interaction | Alginate | — | 200–300 | Pistone et al. (2015) |
| | Alginate-chitosan | Crocin | | Rahaiee et al. (2015) |
| | Alginate-chitosan | Vitamin $B_2$ | 40–70 | Azevedo et al. (2014) |
| Enzymatic hydrolysis | α-lactalbumin $Mn^{2+}$ | Caffeine | — | Fuciños et al. ( 2017) |
| Heat-induced gelation and pH acidification | β-Lg | Epigallocatechin-3-gallate | 7–10 | Li et al. (2012) |
| Heat induced gelation | β-Lg | Epigallocatechin-3-gallate | <50 | Shpigelman et al. (2012) |
| | LF-glycomacropeptide | — | ~170 | Bourbon et al. (2015) |
| Physical self-assembly | β-Lg–Pectin | ω– -3 fatty acids | 100 | Zimet and Livney (2009) |
| Desolvation | Bovine serum albumin | — | 260–919 | Jun et al. (2011) |
| | β-Lg | Curcumin | 142 | Sneharani et al. (2010) |
| Heat and salt induced gelation | LF | $Fe^{2+}$ | 107–110 | Martins et al. (2016) |
| Ohmic heating and salt induced gelation | WPI | $Fe^{2+}$ | 90–200 | Pereira et al. (2017) |
| Ohmic heating induced gelation | WPI | | 50–150 | Pereira et al. (2016) |
| Heat and ultrasound induced gelation | WPI | Totarol | 20–30 | Ma et al. (2017) |

*Source:* Cerqueira, M. Â. et al., Chapter two—Advances in food nanotechnology, in *Emerging Nanotechnologies in Food Science*, edited by Rosa Busquets, pp. 11–38. Elsevier, Boston, MA, 2017.

Through a ionic gelation method, spherical nanoparticles, with the size range of 165–230 nm in weight ratio of chitosan:alginate (1:1.25) and pH 4.7, served as encapsulating agents of a saffron carotenoid (crocin) improving its stability (Rahaiee et al. 2015). Nanoparticles of alginate/chitosan were used as encapsulating agents of vitamin B2, presenting a hydrodynamic average size ranging approximately between 40 and 170 nm with an polydispersity index below 0.5 (Azevedo et al. 2014)—Table 2.1. These systems showed higher stability as well as encapsulation efficiency and loading capacity of 55% and 2%, respectively. More recently, chitosan was also used as coating material aiming to protect protein-based nanohydrogels from gastric digestibility (Bourbon et al. 2016). In this study, chitosan coating was applied in protein nanohydrogels by layer-by-layer technique, and a model compound (caffeine) was encapsulated within the nanosystem in an attempt to evaluate caffeine stability and release mechanisms. It was concluded that chitosan was able to improve the stability of produced nanohydrogels during gastric digestion by reducing protein hydrolysis, without affecting caffeine.

### 2.3.2 Protein-Based Nanohydrogels

Proteins are one of the most important structural elements in life, playing an important role in food either derived from animal or plants. Food proteins provide nutritional quality and life support, supplying essential amino acids, but also bringing important functional and biological properties (Li-Chan and Lacroix 2018). Major food proteins, their main properties and functions, as well as trends and opportunities regarding innovative food processing have been excellently reviewed recently (McSweeney and Fox 2013, Nadathur et al. 2017, Martins et al. 2018, Yada 2018). Milk proteins from whey and casein fractions due to their biological value and technological versatility are being consistently used for development of unique functional networks at nanoscale size. β-Lactoglobulin (β-Lg), a globular protein from whey, can be found or designed in an aggregate form in the size order of a few nanometers (Madalena et al. 2016, Ramos et al. 2017) to design functional hydrogels. Other proteins such as: (i) α-lactalbumin can be used to produce nanotubes as encapsulating agents (Fuciños et al. 2017); (ii) lactoferrin (LF) can be tailored at nanometric scale in the size range below 200 nm to produce functional nanohydrogels as delivery systems or stable emulsions (Bourbon et al. 2015, de Figueiredo Furtado et al. 2018); (iii) bovine serum albumin has great potential for the preparation of nanoparticles with size ranging from 260 to 919 nm, which can be used as nanovehicles (Jun et al. 2011)—Table 2.1; and (iv) casein micelle, which is natural colloidal system from milk that can unevenly range from 20 to 300 nm, can be used to produce acidified gel systems or to carry/delivery of nutrients (Singh 2016).

In particular, whey ingredients rich in β-Lg—i.e., whey protein concentrate and isolate (WPI)—due to their high availability, reduced cost, and generally recognized as safe character are being used for the design of nanostructures for incorporation and release of nutraceutical compounds in food (Ramos et al. 2017), production of whey protein isolate aggregates at nanoscale with different size ranges (Pereira et al. 2016), or even for the development of food nanocoatings through controlled aggregation (Ramos et al. 2014).

The spontaneous binding between β-Lg through docosahexaenoic acid at a 1:2 (β-Lg:docosahexaenoic acid) molar ratio was used to produce transparent dispersions with an average particle size of ~100 nm, showing new perspectives to nanoencapsulate long chain polyunsaturated fatty acids (Zimet and Livney 2009). Epigallocatechin-3-gallate was loaded in heat treated β-Lg allowing to produce stable and clear solution system with particle sizes less than 10 nm at pH 6.4–7.0 with the molar ratio of 1:2 (β-Lg:epigallocatechin-3-gallate) (Li et al. 2012). These systems offer potential to serve as nanovehicles to carry functional bioactive compounds such as polyunsaturated fatty acids, polyphenols, and vitamins in foods and clear drinks.

In another study, β-Lg nanoparticles (<50 nm) produced through heat-denaturation, were used to encapsulate epigallocatechin-3-gallate with a loading efficiency ranging from 60% to 70%, inhibiting its associated bitterness and astringency (Shpigelman et al. 2012). The binding ability of the central cavity (calyx) of β-Lg is being used to successfully carry small hydrophobic molecules, such as curcumin. Nanoparticles of β-Lg with particle size of 142 nm can encapsulate curcumin enhancing its solubility and stability (Sneharani et al. 2010). Other authors have used WPI to produce nanohydrogels through a two-step process, which involve thermal unfolding of the protein followed by cold gelation through addition salts. These protein systems can be used to transport iron presenting network structures at nanoscale size range (Martins et al. 2016, Pereira et al. 2017). Martins et al. produced stable and pH-responsive β-Lg nanoparticles with iron binding efficiency value of ca. 20% (Martins et al. 2016). Pereira et al. produced WPI nanohydrogels capable of incorporating ca. 33 mmol $L^{-1}$ of $Fe^{2+}$ in the produced protein network, corresponding to iron intake of 9 mg/day through a daily teaspoon dose (~5 mL) (Pereira et al. 2017). Thermal gelation has also been used to encapsulate (with high efficiency >90%) both hydrophilic and lipophilic compounds (i.e., caffeine and curcumin, respectively) through LF-glycomacropeptide nanohydrogel (Bourbon et al. 2016a).

In general, the preparation of these nanohydrogels involves low-cost materials and dispensable use of extra crosslinking materials. Protein network is usually established through thermal gelation and often requires addition of polysaccharides, as pectin and alginate, to serve as coating materials, thus protecting encapsulating materials from degradation (Somchue et al. 2009, Zimet and Livney 2009). The factors and techniques that can affect the gelation, and thus the preparation of protein-based nanohydrogels will be discussed in the next section.

## 2.4 BIOPOLYMER INTERACTIONS

Depending on physical/chemical environment and processing techniques, different types of biopolymers interactions and thus nanostructures can be developed. Preparation of nanostructures is dependent of intrinsic or molecular *per se* features and extrinsic factors (such as environment and processing). Intrinsic characteristics are mainly related with molecular mass, conformation, and molecular composition—i.e., amino acids profile, hydrophobicity, charge distribution, presence of free sulfhydryl's groups and disulfide bonds, among others. Extrinsic or environment factors such as biopolymer concentration, pH, type of solvent, ionic strength, and type of ions can be imposed, while processing involves temperature, method of acidification and mixing, application of external electrical and electromagnetic fields, and high pressure (Totosaus et al. 2002, Ramos et al. 2017, Jafari 2017). These intrinsic and extrinsic features can be strategically combined to modulate interactions and thus design functional aqueous nanosystems.

The main crosslinking methods used for the preparation of nanohydrogels comprise two main types of interactions: (i) non-covalent interactions, such as hydrogen bonding, electrostatic intermolecular hydrophobic interactions, van der Waals forces among others; and (ii) covalent interactions, such as disulfide bonding. Self-assembling of different biopolymers can occur through thermodynamic compatibility when they have electrical net charges of opposite sign. This assembling is governed by electrostatic interactions and commonly results in an associative phase separation or complex coacervation, giving rise to biopolymer coacervate-rich phase (i.e., soluble and insoluble complexes and gels) and a solvent-rich phase (Singh et al. 2007, Klemmer et al. 2012). Whey protein ingredients (e.g., WPI and purified forms of β-Lg) are usually assembled with polysaccharides, such as alginate, through complex coacervation, allowing the production of functional nanocomplexes, which in turn are able to encapsulate hydrophilic and lipophilic bioactive compounds (Singh et al. 2007, Jafari 2017). The successful establishment of electrostatic interactions between these biopolymers is strongly dependent of the pH of solution, which should be between the isoelectric point of protein and the pKa of polysaccharide. This reinforces the importance of controlling the intrinsic and extrinsic factors on the modulation of biopolymers interaction.

Covalent bonding is of crucial relevance in protein-protein interactions and thus in the development of protein-based nanohydrogels. When protein is exposed to any external stress (imposed by chemical environment and temperature for example), due to molecular unfolding, starts to expose reactive group's precursors of covalent bonds that were initially buried within its native conformation. The extensive use of β-Lg in the production of nanohydrogels can be related with this aptitude. For example, at temperature above 60°C β-Lg molecule undergoes conformational unfolding exposing its free sulfhydryl group and hydrophobic core to aqueous phase, which facilitates the establishment of sulfhydryl/disulfide interchange reactions and non-covalent hydrophobic interactions resulting in the formation of primary aggregates recognized as the building blocks of protein gelation (Gupta and Nayak 2015, Pereira et al. 2016, Ramos et al. 2017). In this sense, controlled aggregation and gelation are the most common strategies to produce protein-based nanohydrogels that can incorporate or encapsulate bioactive compounds (Totosaus et al. 2002, Cerqueira et al. 2014, 2017). To achieve a tailored development, it is important to choose the adequate physical and chemical mechanisms of protein unfolding, taking into account the following assumptions: (i) protein concentration and ionic strength can drastically change the rate of protein aggregation; (ii) depending on the pH value, the balance between electrostatic and covalent bonding can be changed, as well as different morphologies of protein aggregates can be obtained (i.e., spherical or fibrillar structures, for example). For instance, at pH $> 5.7$, thermal aggregation of β-Lg is mainly governed by disulfide bonding, while at low pH ($<3.5$) no covalent bonding have been observed within the produced aggregates (Nicolai et al. 2011).

## 2.5 PREPARATION TECHNIQUES

Protein gelation results from previous unfolding, interaction, and thus aggregation of protein molecules. Currently, several gelation techniques have been employed to produce protein structures from macro- to nanosize with intended functionalities. Physical processing mechanisms in combination with chemical environment (intrinsic factors) will define protein entanglements and thus the final properties of a given nanohydrogel such as structure (e.g., particle size distribution), water holding capacity, and viscosity. Recently, Martins et al. (2018) have reviewed the use of protein-based structures for innovative applications that addresses the fact that the protein nanohydrogels are often produced through heat alone or in combination with other techniques such as salt induced gelation and pH acidification. Thermal denaturation is still the most common way to achieve protein gelation and an efficient way of producing nanohydrogels as encapsulating agents of bioactive compounds. After unfolding and onset of thermal denaturation with disruption of native protein conformation, thermal gelation comprises three steps as follows: (1) primary aggregation (through disulfide bridges and non-covalent bonds); (2) propagation or secondary aggregation driven through hydrophobic and disulfide interactions between the protein primary-aggregates; and (3) formation of an intended protein network structure (i.e., when secondary aggregates exceed a critical concentration) with swelling capacity that can range from nanoscale (such as nanohydrogels, nanofibrils, and nanotubes) to macroscale, depending on the conditions already aforementioned.

Innovative and emergent processes of gelation have been arising with promising results regarding process control and functionality. One of these approaches is related with electrical food processing such as pulsed electric fields (PEF) and Ohmic heating. PEF is known by a non-thermal techniques consisting in the application of electric fields of high intensity (dozens of kV/cm) in a very short time interval (<1s). PEF pulses with an intensity of 16 $kVcm^{-1}$ applied at temperatures below 35°C induce changes in the whey protein surface hydrophobicity, as well as conformational alterations in tryptophan region (Xiang et al. 2011). These structural modifications under PEF should be better exploited, and may give rise to a new strategy of producing nanohydrogels with distinct functionalities, thus avoiding the use of heat. Ohmic heating, which differs from PEF given its electric fields of low intensity (<1 kV/cm), frequency modulation (from Hz to kHz), and prominent Joule effect (heat dissipation), allows to rapidly heat in a volumetric way protein solutions, thus influencing unfolding, denaturation, and size of protein aggregates. Figure 2.1 shows a schematic representation of Ohmic heating way of application and alleged effects on protein denaturation.

Ohmic heating at 90°C (for 5 min) allowed to produce WPI-based aggregates resembling a fibrillar structure with particle size ranging from approximately 50–150 nm, depending on come-up-time of heating process and electric field applied (Pereira et al. 2016). In another study, Ohmic heating (at 90°C for 5 min) under moderate electric fields was combined with salt-induced gelation to produce WPI nanohydrogels rich in iron (Pereira et al. 2017). It was shown that by varying $Fe^{2+}$ concentration (0–50 mmol/L) and intensity of moderate electric fields applied (e.g., ranging from 0 to 12 V/cm), it was possible to modulate particle size

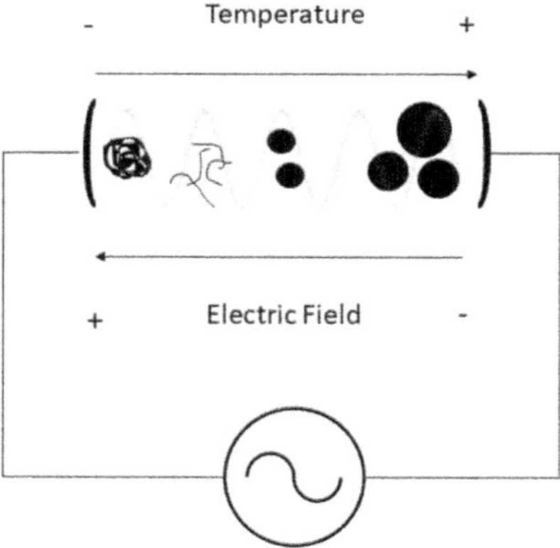


**FIGURE 2.1** Ohmic heating effects on protein aggregation showing relationship between temperature and electric field effects.

distribution (i.e., approximately ranging from 90 to 200 nm), network structure viscosity of the produced protein systems. Ultrasound treatment in combination with the use of heat allowed to narrow the size of protein nanoparticles (e.g., from 31.24 ± 5.31 to 24.20 ± 4.02 nm) which were used to encapsulate an antimicrobial compound, pointing out an increased antibacterial effectiveness with increasing ultrasonic treatment time (Ma et al. 2017).

Electrospinning is novel drying processing technique that is gaining increased visibility in food processing. Through this processing method, a biopolymeric solution is delivered through a millimeter-scale nozzle or charged syringe needle in which a high voltage is applied allowing solvent evaporation. Electrostatic forces between needle and grounded collector plate allow solvent evaporation and the production of ultra-fine solid biopolymer fibers (Frenot and Chronakis 2003, Sullivan et al. 2014). These fibers can be designed from micro- to nanoscale size, such as nanofibers with diameter below 100 nm. In this sense, electrospinning is being used as tool to modulate biopolymer nanostructures enhancing its stability, as well as a way for an efficient encapsulation of bioactive compounds within dried biopolymer network. For example, electrospinning in combination with use of glycerol as co-solvent can help to improve the flexibility entanglements of alginate chains (Nie et al. 2008). In another work, electrospinning allowed to obtain WPI-based nanofibers with diameters ranging between 312 and 690 nm, depending on the biopolymer solution properties (e.g., composition, concentration, among others). Prolonged heat treatment of these nanofibers above protein gelation temperature resulted in formation of additional protein crosslinks and increase of thermal stability and swelling properties (Sullivan et al. 2014). The latest findings about use of electrospinning technology on development of proteins (such as casein, whey protein, gelatin, soy and wheat protein, among others) and polysaccharides (such as chitosan, cellulose, alginate, among others) nanofibers have been recently reviewed (Mendes et al. 2017). Through this technology, it will be possible to change structural properties of major food proteins (e.g., conformation and protein-protein interactions) and with that, the functional and technological aspects—i.e., aggregation and gelation. Regarding polysaccharides, its chemical and structural properties, in particular the level of chain entanglement seem to be crucial for the successful development of nanofibers.

Processing methods based on electricity such as PEF, Ohmic heating, and electrospinning bring a new enthusiasm in the design of nanohydrogels based on proteins, polysaccharides, or mixtures of both. The effects of electric variables of these methods such as levels of applied voltage, electric field, current density, or even electrical frequency still need more fundamental research once they can change the way how biopolymers interact with each other resulting in the production of a given network. But for the effectiveness of these methods biopolymer solutions should present minimum value for electrical conductivity which traduces the ability of the biopolymers to act as semi-conductors and carry electricity. Electrical conductivity can easily be modulated by addition of salts and depending on its value, different electric fields strengths can be generated which can result in protein aggregates with different morphologies and sizes. It seems clear that electric processing methods can offer a platform to a wide range of food processing applications including development of tailored biopolymer food nanohydrogels with distinctive features.

## 2.6 CONCLUSIONS AND FUTURE PERSPECTIVES

As outlined in the previous sections, the research and development of bio-based nanohydrogels for innovative food applications is increasing rapidly. Most of these nanostructures are being customized as nanovehicles for the carry and delivery systems of functional or bioactive compounds. Protein and polysaccharides have rich fractions that can be extracted from low-cost food sources or wastes (e.g., whey resulting from cheese production) are the most promising candidates to be used in the formulation of natural-based nanohydrogels for food applications. In particular, the knowledge about structure and function of major food proteins regarding the development of functional systems at nanoscale has been matured and extensively researched throughout the latest years. Whey is a typical case of food waste valorization. Proteins from whey can be designed through fine-tune control of their aggregation, gelation, and bioconjugation properties to produce nanohydrogels with an intended functionality to human body, while preserving high nutritional value. However, still exits many challenges to overcome toward disseminated practical application of these systems. One of the most limiting one is related with the lack of understanding about the supposed toxicological effects of nanoparticles in biological systems (Busquets and Mbundi 2017). In this sense, the safety and toxicity of nano food requires case-by-case safety evaluation and its acceptance for human consumption should be checked in the applicable regulatory legislation. Currently there is about one hundred of entities around the world struggling to establish risk assessment and legislation for applying food nanotechnology (Jafari et al. 2017). The European Food Safety Authority in Europe, the Food and Drug Administration in the United States, and Food Standards Australia and New Zealand in Australia and New Zealand are some examples of the regulatory organizations that approve the use nanomaterials in food. The several definitions and legislations and way of communicating nanotechnology among the world are sometimes ambiguous, which turn out much more complex the commercialization and widespread of these products, as well as influences the public perception that, in general, it is already negative. All the involved parties such as scientists, governmental, regulatory entities, and food industry should work together addressing risk and safety assessment, a clear regulatory framework of applicability, and communication of the potential benefits of the products developed. Another question is also related with alleged functional claims of these nanostructures. It is crucial to understand the effectiveness of natural-based nanohydrogels as vehicle of bioactive compounds by evaluating how these systems behave under conventional food processing unit operations (such as pasteurization, sterilization among others) and during human gastrointestinal digestion. Assessment of the bioavailability of these nanosystems still a complex but necessary challenge to overcome (Pinheiro et al. 2017). The scale-up of developed systems at laboratory is another issue, in particular the costs of large-scale implementation and production, and the chemical heterogeneity of natural macromolecules (such as food proteins), which result in variability in the performance properties of the produced systems (Martins et al. 2018). An interdisciplinary expertise is then necessary to rapidly reduce the gap between research and finalized products reaching commercialization, which in turn will contribute to foster the appearance of specialized small-companies and increase of competitiveness and market acceptance (Cerqueira et al. 2017). Once this gap has been narrowed and given the high number of scientific publications and patents published over the last decade, innovative food products incorporating nanotechnology are expected to be rapidly disseminated in the market. Food leading companies such as Unilever, Nestle, Kraft, and Heinz are now strategically investing in the development of food nanotechnology aiming innovative products that can promote health and create a difference in terms of texture and flavor for example (Jafari et al. 2017).

Overall bio-based nanohydrogels present a recognized potential offering interesting solutions for development of innovative and functional food products aiming at health and well-being in a sustainable way. A long but exciting path is still necessary to demonstrate that these systems are safe and that can comprise intended function in human body.

## ACKNOWLEDGMENTS

This work was supported by the Portuguese Foundation for Science and Technology under the scope of the strategic funding of UID/BIO/04469/2013 unit and COMPETE 2020 (POCI-01-0145-FEDER-006684) and by BioTecNorte operation (NORTE-01-0145-FEDER-000004) funded by the European Regional Development Fund under the scope of Norte2020—Programa Operacional Regional do Norte. The author Ricardo N. Pereira, also thank to Portuguese Foundation for Science and Technology financial grant with reference SFRH/BPD/81887/2011.

## REFERENCES

Abreu, F. O. M. S., E. F. Oliveira, H. C. B. Paula, and R. C. M. de Paula. 2012. "Chitosan/cashew gum nanogels for essential oil encapsulation." *Carbohydrate Polymers* no. 89 (4):1277–1282.

Ahmed, E. M. 2015. "Hydrogel: Preparation, characterization, and applications: A review." *Journal of Advanced Research* no. 6 (2):105–121.

Akram, M., and R. Hussain. 2017. "Nanohydrogels: History, development, and applications in drug delivery." In *Nanocellulose and Nanohydrogel Matrices*, edited by Mohammad Jawaid. Wiley.

Alhaique, F., P. Matricardi, C. Di Meo, T. Coviello, and E. Montanari. 2015. "Polysaccharide-based self-assembling nanohydrogels: An overview on 25-years research on pullulan." *Journal of Drug Delivery Science and Technology* no. 30:300–309.

Azevedo, M. A., A. I. Bourbon, A. A. Vicente, and M. A. Cerqueira. 2014. "Alginate/chitosan nanoparticles for encapsulation and controlled release of vitamin B2." *International Journal of Biological Macromolecules* no. 71:141–146.

Bourbon, A. I., A. C. Pinheiro, M. G. Carneiro-da-Cunha, R. N. Pereira, M. A. Cerqueira, and A. A. Vicente. 2015. "Development and characterization of lactoferrin-GMP nanohydrogels: Evaluation of pH, ionic strength and temperature effect." *Food Hydrocolloids* no. 48:292–300.

Bourbon, A. I., A. C. Pinheiro, M. A. Cerqueira, and A. A. Vicente. 2016. "Influence of chitosan coating on protein-based nanohydrogels properties and in vitro gastric digestibility." *Food Hydrocolloids* no. 60:109–118.

Brunel, F., L. Véron, L. David, A. Domard, B. Verrier, and T. Delair. 2010. "Self-assemblies on chitosan nanohydrogels." *Macromolecular Bioscience* no. 10 (4):424–432.

Busquets, R., and L. Mbundi. 2017. "Chapter one—Concepts of nanotechnology." In *Emerging Nanotechnologies in Food Science*, edited by Rosa Busquets, pp. 1–9. Boston, MA: Elsevier.

Cerqueira, M. Â., A. C. Pinheiro, O. L. Ramos, H. Silva, A. I. Bourbon, and A. A. Vicente. 2017. "Chapter two—Advances in food nanotechnology." In *Emerging Nanotechnologies in Food Science*, edited by Rosa Busquets, pp. 11–38. Boston, MA: Elsevier.

Cerqueira, M. A., A. C. Pinheiro, H. D. Silva, P. E. Ramos, M. A. Azevedo, M. L. Flores-López, M. C. Rivera, A. I. Bourbon, Ó. L. Ramos, and A. A. Vicente. 2014. "Design of bio-nanosystems for oral delivery of functional compounds." *Food Engineering Reviews* no. 6 (1):1–19.

Dalwadi, C., and G. Patel. 2015. "Application of nanohydrogels in drug delivery systems: Recent patents review." *Recent Patents on Nanotechnology* no. 9 (1):17–25.

de Figueiredo Furtado, G., R. N. C. Pereira, A. A. Vicente, and R. L. Cunha. 2018. "Cold gel-like emulsions of lactoferrin subjected to ohmic heating." *Food Research International* no. 103:371–379.

Dragan, E. S. 2014. "Design and applications of interpenetrating polymer network hydrogels: A review." *Chemical Engineering Journal* no. 243:572–590.

Frenot, A., and I. S. Chronakis. 2003. "Polymer nanofibers assembled by electrospinning." *Current Opinion in Colloid & Interface Science* no. 8 (1):64–75.

Fuciños, C., N. P. Guerra, J. M. Teijón, L. M. Pastrana, M. L. Rúa, and I. Katime. 2012. "Use of poly(N-isopropylacrylamide) nanohydrogels for the controlled release of pimaricin in active packaging." *Journal of Food Science* no. 77 (7):N21–N28.

Fuciños, C., M. Míguez, P. Fuciños, L. M. Pastrana, M. L. Rúa, and A. A. Vicente. 2017. "Creating functional nanostructures: Encapsulation of caffeine into α-lactalbumin nanotubes." *Innovative Food Science & Emerging Technologies* no. 40:10–17.

Gupta, P., and K. K. Nayak. 2015. "Characteristics of protein-based biopolymer and its application." *Polymer Engineering & Science* no. 55 (3):485–498.

Jafari, S. M., I. Katouzian, and S. Akhavan. 2017. "15—Safety and regulatory issues of nanocapsules." In *Nanoencapsulation Technologies for the Food and Nutraceutical Industries*, edited by Seid Mahdi Jafari, pp. 545–590. Amsterdam, the Netherlands: Academic Press.

Jafari, S. M. 2017. "Chapter 1—An introduction to nanoencapsulation techniques for the food bioactive ingredients." In *Nanoencapsulation of Food Bioactive Ingredients*, edited by Seid Mahdi Jafari, pp. 1–62. San Diego, CA: Academic Press.

Jonker, A. M., D. W. P. M. Löwik, and J. C. M. van Hest. 2012. "Peptide- and protein-based hydrogels." *Chemistry of Materials* no. 24 (5):759–773.

Jun, J. Y., H. H. Nguyen, S.-Y.-R. Paik, H. S. Chun, B.-C. Kang, and S. Ko. 2011. "Preparation of size-controlled bovine serum albumin (BSA) nanoparticles by a modified desolvation method." *Food Chemistry* no. 127 (4):1892–1898.

Klemmer, K. J., L. Waldner, A. Stone, N. H. Low, and M. T. Nickerson. 2012. "Complex coacervation of pea protein isolate and alginate polysaccharides." *Food Chemistry* no. 130 (3):710–715.

Li, B., W. Du, J. Jin, and Q. Du. 2012. "Preservation of (–)-epigallocatechin-3-gallate antioxidant properties loaded in heat treated β-lactoglobulin nanoparticles." *Journal of Agricultural and Food Chemistry* no. 60 (13):3477–3484.

Li-Chan, E. C. Y., and I. M. E. Lacroix. 2018. "1—Properties of proteins in food systems: An introduction." In *Proteins in Food Processing* (2nd ed.), edited by Rickey Y. Yada, pp. 1–25. Oxford, UK: Woodhead Publishing.

Liu, S., J. Zhang, X. Cui, Y. Guo, X. Zhang, and W. Hongyan. 2016. "Synthesis of chitosan-based nanohydrogels for loading and release of 5-fluorouracil." *Colloids and Surfaces A: Physicochemical and Engineering Aspects* no. 490:91–97.

Ma, S., C. Shi, C. Wang, and M. Guo. 2017. "Effects of ultrasound treatment on physiochemical properties and antimicrobial activities of whey protein-totarol nanoparticles." *Journal of Food Protection* no. 80 (10):1657–1665.

Madalena, D. A., Ó. L. Ramos, R. N. Pereira, A. I. Bourbon, A. C. Pinheiro, F. X. Malcata, J. A. Teixeira, and A. A. Vicente. 2016. "*In vitro* digestion and stability assessment of β-lactoglobulin/riboflavin nanostructures." *Food Hydrocolloids* no. 58:89–97.

Martins, J. T., A. I. Bourbon, A. C. Pinheiro, L. H. Fasolin, and A. A. Vicente. 2018. "Protein-based structures for food applications: From macro to nanoscale." *Frontiers in Sustainable Food Systems* no. 2 (77).

Martins, J. T., S. F. Santos, A. I. Bourbon, A. C. Pinheiro, Á. González-Fernández, L. M. Pastrana, M. A. Cerqueira, and A. A. Vicente. 2016. "Lactoferrin-based nanoparticles as a vehicle for iron in food applications—Development and release profile." *Food Research International* no. 90:16–24.

McSweeney, P. L. H., and P. F. Fox. 2013. *Advanced Dairy Chemistry*. 4th ed. Vol. 1, Volume 1A: Proteins: Basic Aspects, New York: Springer US.

Mendes, A. C., K. Stephansen, and I. S. Chronakis. 2017. "Electrospinning of food proteins and polysaccharides." *Food Hydrocolloids* no. 68:53–68.

Nadathur, S. R., J. P. D. Wanasundara, and L. Scanlin. 2017. In *Sustainable Protein Sources*, edited by Sudarshan R. Nadathur, Janitha P. D. Wanasundara, and Laurie Scanlin. San Diego, CA: Academic Press.

Nicolai, T., M. Britten, and C. Schmitt. 2011. "β-Lactoglobulin and WPI aggregates: Formation, structure and applications." *Food Hydrocolloids* no. 25 (8):1945–1962.

Nie, H., A. He, J. Zheng, S. Xu, J. Li, and C. C. Han. 2008. "Effects of chain conformation and entanglement on the electrospinning of pure alginate." *Biomacromolecules* no. 9 (5):1362–1365.

Pereira, R. N., R. M. Rodrigues, E. Altinok, Ó. L. Ramos, F. X. Malcata, P. Maresca, G. Ferrari, J. A. Teixeira, and A. A. Vicente. 2017. "Development of iron-rich whey protein hydrogels following application of ohmic heating—Effects of moderate electric fields." *Food Research International* no. 99:435–443.

Pereira, R. N., R. M. Rodrigues, Ó. L. Ramos, F. X. Malcata, J. A. Teixeira, and A. A. Vicente. 2016. "Production of whey protein-based aggregates under ohmic heating." *Food and Bioprocess Technology* no. 9 (4):576–587.

Pinheiro, A. C., R. F. S. Gonçalves, D. A. Madalena, and A. A. Vicente. 2017. "Towards the understanding of the behavior of bio-based nanostructures during in vitro digestion." *Current Opinion in Food Science* no. 15:79–86.

Pistone, S., D. Qoragllu, G. Smistad, and M. Hiorth. 2015. "Formulation and preparation of stable cross-linked alginate-zinc nanoparticles in the presence of a monovalent salt." *Soft Matter* no. 11 (28):5765–5774.

Rahaiee, S., S. A. Shojaosadati, M. Hashemi, S. Moini, and S. H. Razavi. 2015. "Improvement of crocin stability by biodegradeble nanoparticles of chitosan-alginate." *International Journal of Biological Macromolecules* no. 79:423–432.

Rajaonarivony, M., C. Vauthier, G. Couarraze, F. Puisieux, and P. Couvreur. 1993. "Development of a new drug carrier made from alginate." *Journal of Pharmaceutical Sciences* no. 82 (9):912–917.

Ramos, O. L., R. N. Pereira, A. Martins, R. Rodrigues, C. Fucinos, J. A. Teixeira, L. Pastrana, F. X. Malcata, and A. A. Vicente. 2017. "Design of whey protein nanostructures for incorporation and release of nutraceutical compounds in food." *Critical Reviews in Food Science and Nutrition* no. 57 (7):1377–1393.

Ramos, O. L., R. N. Pereira, R. Rodrigues, J. A. Teixeira, A. A. Vicente, and F. X. Malcata. 2014. "Physical effects upon whey protein aggregation for nano-coating production." *Food Research International* no. 66:344–355.

Sarmento, B., A. J. Ribeiro, F. Veiga, D. C. Ferreira, and R. J. Neufeld. 2007. "Insulin-loaded nanoparticles are prepared by alginate ionotropic pre-gelation followed by chitosan polyelectrolyte complexation." *Journal of Nanoscience and Nanotechnology* no. 7 (8):2833–2841.

Shpigelman, A., Y. Cohen, and Y. D. Livney. 2012. "Thermally-induced β-lactoglobulin–EGCG nanovehicles: Loading, stability, sensory and digestive-release study." *Food Hydrocolloids* no. 29 (1):57–67.

Singh, H. 2016. "Nanotechnology applications in functional foods; opportunities and challenges." *Preventive Nutrition and Food Science* no. 21 (1):1–8.

Singh, S. S., A. K. Siddhanta, R. Meena, K. Prasad, S. Bandyopadhyay, and H. B. Bohidar. 2007. "Intermolecular complexation and phase separation in aqueous solutions of oppositely charged biopolymers." *International Journal of Biological Macromolecules* no. 41 (2):185–192.

Sneharani, A. H., J. V. Karakkat, S. A. Singh, and A. G. A. Rao. 2010. "Interaction of curcumin with beta-lactoglobulin-stability, spectroscopic analysis, and molecular modeling of the complex." *Journal of Agricultural and Food Chemistry* no. 58 (20):11130–11139.

Somchue, W., W. Sermsri, J. Shiowatana, and A. Siripinyanond. 2009. "Encapsulation of α-tocopherol in protein-based delivery particles." *Food Research International* no. 42 (8):909–914.

Sullivan, S. T., C. Tang, A. Kennedy, S. Talwar, and S. A. Khan. 2014. "Electrospinning and heat treatment of whey protein nanofibers." *Food Hydrocolloids* no. 35:36–50.

Totosaus, A., J. G. Montejano, J. A. Salazar, and I. Guerrero. 2002. "A review of physical and chemical protein-gel induction." *International Journal of Food Science & Technology* no. 37 (6):589–601.

Ullah, F., M. B. Othman, F. Javed, Z. Ahmad, and H. M. Akil. 2015. "Classification, processing and application of hydrogels: A review." *Materials Science and Engineering C: Materials for Biological Applications* no. 57:414–433.

Wendell, D. W., J. Patti, and C. D. Montemagno. 2006. "Using biological inspiration to engineer functional nanostructured materials." *Small* no. 2 (11):1324–1329.

Wang, Y., F. Bamdad, Y. Song, and L. Chen. 2012. "14—Hydrogel particles and other novel protein-based methods for food ingredient and nutraceutical delivery systems." In *Encapsulation Technologies and Delivery Systems for Food Ingredients and Nutraceuticals*, edited by Nissim Garti and David Julian McClements, pp. 412–450. Cambridge, UK: Woodhead Publishing.

Xia, L.-W., R. Xie, X.-J. Ju, W. Wang, Q. Chen, and L.-Y. Chu. 2013. "Nano-structured smart hydrogels with rapid response and high elasticity." *Nature Communications* no. 4:2226. https://www.nature.com/articles/ncomms3226#supplementary-information.

Xiang, B. Y., M. O. Ngadi, L. A. Ochoa-Martinez, and M. V. Simpson. 2011. "Pulsed electric field-induced structural modification of whey protein isolate." *Food and Bioprocess Technology* no. 4 (8):1341–1348.

Yada, R. Y. 2018. In *Proteins in Food Processing*, edited by Rickey Y. Yada, 2nd ed.: Oxford, UK: Woodhead Publishing.

Zimet, P., and Y. D. Livney. 2009. "Beta-lactoglobulin and its nanocomplexes with pectin as vehicles for ω-3 polyunsaturated fatty acids." *Food Hydrocolloids* no. 23 (4):1120–1126.

# 3 Nanoparticles Production Methods

*Adriana Lima, Francisco Silva, Bruno Sarmento, and José C. Andrade*

## CONTENTS



## 3.1 INTRODUCTION

Nanoencapsulation, a field of nanotechnology, is emerging in the food area opening new perspectives in the development of new food products and in the improvement of the existing ones. The term nanoencapsulation is related to the entrapping of several substances (bioactive compounds) within another material (encapsulant). This process forms nanoparticles with sizes ranging from 1 to 1000 nm (Quintanilla-Carvajal et al. 2010, Suganya and Anuradha 2017). However, this size threshold is controversial and is not unanimous, for instance, the European Food Safety Authority (EFSA 2011) refers to nanoparticles as engineered nanomaterials that have at least one dimension in the range of 1–100 nm. Nanoparticles can be defined as solid nanocarriers and divided into nanospheres (matrix systems where the bioactive substances are uniformly dispersed) and nanocapsules (vesicular systems in which the bioactive compound is confined to a cavity surrounded by a unique polymer membrane) (Suganya and Anuradha 2017). In the food industry these delivery systems, due to their small size, can carry and release functional ingredients, nutraceuticals, and supplements within cells in a more controlled manner, mainly improving solubility and bioavailability, preventing biodegradation and undesirable chemical reactions (Acosta 2009, Cerqueira et al. 2014). A wide variety of encapsulation technologies and carrier materials has been reported in the scientific literature. However, for food industry application, the material used to produce a delivery system should be generally recognized as safe, relatively inexpensive, easy to use, and readily available. Moreover, the production methods to create the delivery system should be cost-effective, reproducible, and suitable for large-scale production. The most suitable nanoscale carrier materials for food applications are biopolymers, such as carbohydrates and proteins along with lipids (e.g., fatty acids and natural esters), as they are biodegradable, biocompatible, and present functional properties (Cerqueira et al. 2014).

This chapter presents an overview of some manufacturing methods (see also Chapters 2, 4 through 6) used to produce nanoparticles with emphasis on those using biopolymers. A compilation of recently published papers is also presented in order to highlight the latest progress and to envisage outline future trends and challenges.

## 3.2 NANOENCAPSULATION METHODS

In the scope of nanoparticles development, choosing the production method is a crucial step in order to produce a nanocarrier structurally functional and effective (Livney 2017, Rao and Geckeler 2011). Therefore, several aspects must be considered before the production process: the desired characteristics for the nanoparticle (size, shape, solubility, efficiency, and releasing mechanism, which affects the choice of the polymer to be used), the physicochemical properties of the chosen polymer, the nature of the bioactive compound to be encapsulated, and the final application (Cerqueira et al. 2014, Ezhilarasi et al. 2013, Lal Pal et al. 2011, Rao and Geckeler 2011).

Nanoencapsulation production techniques are classically divided into "top-down" and "bottom-up" approaches, wherein the particle size is respectively reduced or increased during the process of nanoparticle formation, however, a combination of both approaches is also possible (McClements 2015). Regarding the final application of the nanomaterials being developed, the top-down approach (e.g., homogenization, emulsification, ultrasonification) requires the application of mechanical actions, which consequently leads to size reduction and structure shaping (McClements 2015, Komaiko and McClements 2015). When a bottom-up approach is used, construction of the materials is given by self-assembly and self-organization of molecules, which were influenced by many factors including pH, temperature, concentration, and ionic strength (Acosta 2009, Cerqueira et al. 2014, Ezhilarasi et al. 2013, Komaiko and McClements 2015, Livney 2017). Nowadays, it is better to categorize nanoparticle production techniques in more groups based on some other indices.

### 3.2.1 Emulsification

Emulsification is one of the first methods for production of nanocapsules, also known as nanoemulsions (Borthakur et al. 2016, Vauthier and Bouchemal 2009). This method is fast, readily scalable, and is usually applied to encapsulate bioactive compounds in aqueous solutions, which can either be used directly after emulsification process or further be dried to form powders (e.g., by spray, roller, or freeze drying) (Fang and Bhandari 2010, Vauthier and Bouchemal 2009, Vrignaud et al. 2011). In an emulsion at least two immiscible liquids, such as oil and water, are used with one of the liquids being dispersed as small spherical droplets in the other, with sizes ranging between 50 and 1000 nm (Ezhilarasi et al. 2013, Fang and Bhandari 2010). The classification of an emulsion system is based in the spatial organization of the oil and water phases. A system that consists of oil droplets dispersed in an aqueous phase is called an oil-in-water (O/W) emulsion and is generally used for the encapsulation of lipophilic active agents, such as carotenoids, plant sterols, and dietary fats. A system that consists of water droplets dispersed in an oil phase is called a water-in-oil (W/O) emulsion, which is commonly used to encapsulate hydrophilic food active agents like polyphenols (Ezhilarasi et al. 2013, Fang and Bhandari 2010, Joye and McClements 2014). Moreover, multiple emulsions can be developed, such as oil-in-water-in-oil (O/W/O) or water-in-oil-in-water (W/O/W) emulsions (Ito et al. 2012). Multiple emulsions are more complexed and more advantageous, when compared with conventional emulsion systems, since it can enable the encapsulation of multiple active ingredients using a single delivery system. Hydrophilic bioactive compounds (e.g., vitamins, minerals, proteins, and bioactive peptides) can be immobilized within the internal water phase, while hydrophobic ones (e.g., antioxidants and bioactive lipids) can be immobilized within the oil phase, being possible to prevent undesired reactions between ingredients of the different phases (McClements 2015).

High levels of kinetic stability are due to the emulsions of extremely reduced size and are closely correlated to the retention of surface oil content of the product (Ezhilarasi et al. 2013). Therefore, to obtain a kinetically stable solution, stabilizers, such as emulsifiers (e.g., monoglycerides, polyol esters of fatty acids, and lecithin) or texture modifiers (e.g., milk and egg proteins, and gum arabic) are commonly added in the emulsion systems (Galanakis 2018). The delivery of food compounds and nutraceuticals using this technology has already been reviewed by Augustin and Hemar (2009), McClements et al. (2009) and Silva et al. (2012). Nanoemulsions can be achieved by high-energy or low-energy methods (Gupta et al. 2016). Through high-energy methods, the dispersed phase is disrupted by a mechanical device (Figure 3.1), like high shear mixer, high-speed or high-pressure homogenizer, ultrasonicator, and micro-fluidizer, which applies intensive forces to the emulsion (Ezhilarasi et al. 2013, Jafari 2017a, McClements 2015). These methods require significant energy input to create larger surface area, to produce extremely small size droplets, and to overcome cohesive energy holding the molecules together in solid and liquid states. In this technique, the droplet size depends on the design of the mechanical device, operation and environmental conditions, emulsion composition, and physicochemical properties of mixture's components (Anu Bhushani

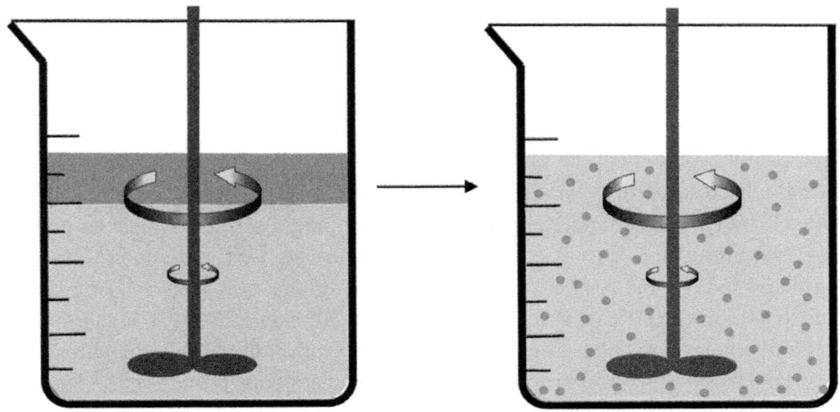

**FIGURE 3.1** Schematic representation of oil-in-water system showing oil droplets (represented in dark grey circles) dispersed in an aqueous phase (represented in light grey) after a mechanical action.

and Anandharamakrishnan 2014, Borthakur et al. 2016). Self-emulsification, phase inversion, and emulsion inversion point are low-energy methods where emulsification occurs itself by altering environmental conditions of the mixture, such as temperature (Choi and Kwak 2014, Jafari 2017a). These techniques are more economic and simple than those requiring high-energy in-put, and droplet size of the emulsion depends on the composition of phases, type, and amount of surfactant, environmental factors, and mixing conditions (Jafari 2017a).

#### 3.2.1.1 Emulsion Polymerization

Many bioactives, such as fish oils that are rich in omega-3 fatty acids, are generally unstable and interact with oxygen or with other components in the food matrix. Protection by encapsulation using synthetic or natural degradable polymers may be required from storage to processing to product consumption (Sanguansri and Augustin 2006).

This technique involves an O/W system, in which the emulsification of hydrophobic polymers occurs (Cerqueira et al. 2014). Nanocapsules are formed due to the polymerization of a monomer with low water solubility, generating a large oil-water interface (Figure 3.2) (Choi and Kwak 2014, Reis et al. 2006). The polymerization reaction only can be accomplished with the addition of a water-soluble initiator (e.g., ammonium persulfate) (Cerqueira et al. 2014, Zhang and Yu 2007). This technique can be classified as conventional emulsion polymerization (if a surfactant such as sodium dodecyl sulfate is added to the system), surfactant-free emulsion polymerization (if no surfactant is used), as well as mini- (or nano-emulsions) and microemulsions polymerization (which differ in terms of kinetic and thermodynamic behaviors) (Cerqueira et al. 2014, Choi and Kwak 2014).

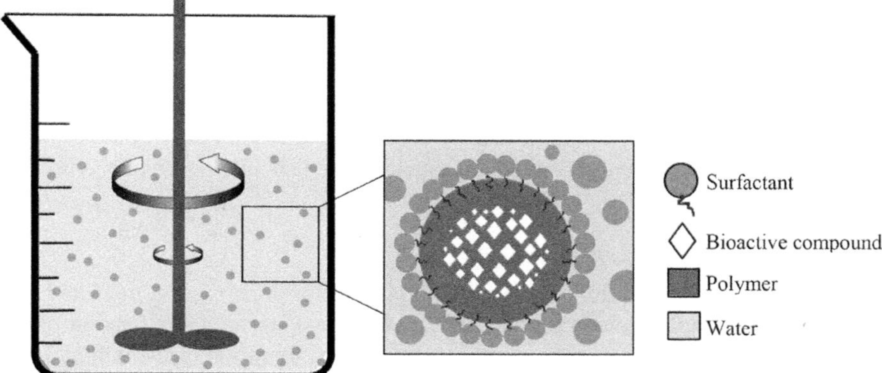


**FIGURE 3.2** Schematic illustration of encapsulation of a bioactive compound by emulsion polymerization technique.

Mini-emulsions are critically stabilized, requiring the use of a low molecular mass compound as the co-stabilizer and the use of a high-shear device, being this is the major difference from conventional emulsion polymerization (Landfester 2009, Nagavarma et al. 2012, Ziegler et al. 2009). Micro-emulsions form spontaneously, without the need of high energy processes, which is a major advantage when compared to emulsions and mini-emulsions (Vrignaud et al. 2011). Micro-emulsion polymerization is a new and effective approach to produce nanosized polymer particles. When compared with emulsion polymerization, it differs entirely from the kinetic point of view, once that both particle size and the average number of chains per particle are considerably smaller in micro-emulsion polymerization (Khanjani et al. 2017). In this technique, an initiator is added to the aqueous phase of a thermodynamically stable micro-emulsion containing swollen micelles (Kumar et al. 2013). The polymerization starts from this spontaneously formed and thermodynamically stable state and relies on high quantities of surfactant systems. At the end, because high amounts of surfactant are used, particles are completely covered with this compound (Aguilar and Román 2014). Surfactants (e.g., sorbintan esters and polysorbates) or protective soluble polymers (e.g., polyethylene glycol) can be used to prevent nanocapsules aggregation in the early stages of reaction, however, the type of surfactants can affect their size (Nagavarma et al. 2012). It should be noted that in the micro-emulsion polymerization, as already referred, a large quantity of surfactant is needed to produce smaller nanocapsules. The addition of a surfactant limits both polymer solid content in the dispersion and, most importantly, their application, its removal without affecting the stability of the emulsion is extremely difficult (Choi and Kwak 2014). After the reaction, nanocapsules can be separated by centrifugation and/or filtration and then washed using water and organic solvents (Cerqueira et al. 2014, Zhang and Yu 2007).

Jafari and coworkers (2008) used maltodextrin combined with a surface-active biopolymer (modified starch or whey protein concentrate) at a ratio of 3:1, as a wall material, to encapsulate fish oil, maximizing its encapsulation and increasing the process efficiency. High energy emulsifying (i.e., micro-fluidization and ultra-sonication) and spray-drying techniques were used and results showed that micro-fluidization is an efficient technique to encapsulate fish oil, producing emulsion droplets at the range of 210–280 nm.

### 3.2.1.2 Emulsion Solvent-Evaporation

Emulsion-solvent evaporation, also known as "in-water drying," is a modified version of solvent evaporation technique and involves two steps: emulsification of the polymer solution into an aqueous phase followed by evaporation of the polymer solvent, thus inducing polymer precipitation as nanoparticles (Ezhilarasi et al. 2013, Nagavarma et al. 2012, Reis et al. 2006). In this procedure, water acts as a non-solvent to the polymer. The polymer and the bioactive compound are dissolved in an organic solvent (e.g., ethyl acetate, methylene chloride, or chloroform), and then the entire mixture is emulsified in an aqueous solution containing an appropriate surfactant (Deshmukh et al. 2016, Jafari 2017b, Wang et al. 2016). The solvent is subsequently evaporated by increasing the temperature under pressure or by continuous stirring, which leads to polymer precipitation and formation of nanoparticles (Figure 3.3) (Soppimath et al. 2001, Wang et al. 2016). The size can be controlled by adjusting the stir rate, type and amount of dispersing agent, viscosity

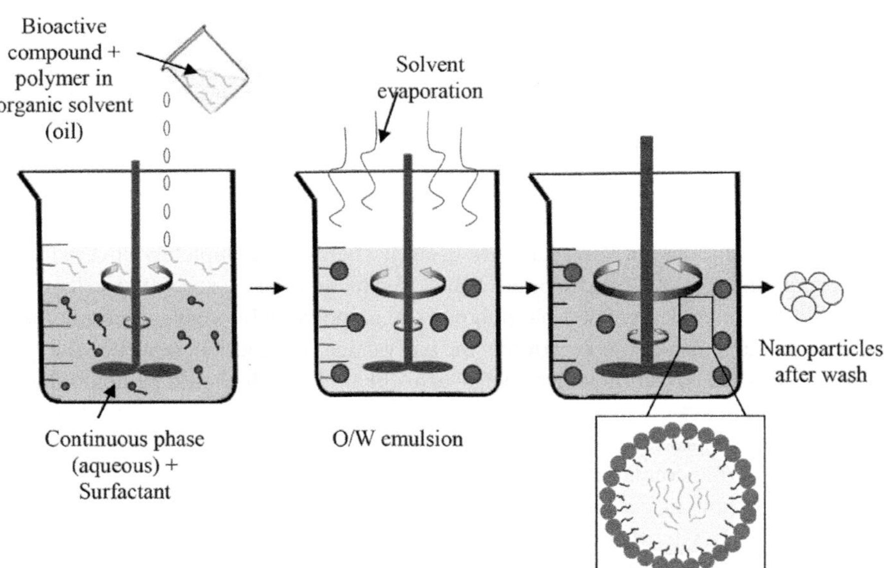


**FIGURE 3.3** Schematic illustration of the encapsulation of a bioactive compound by emulsion solvent evaporation technique.

of organic and aqueous phases, and temperature (Reis et al. 2006, Tice and Gilley 1985). Developed to encapsulate lipophilic bioactive compounds, this method is very economical and eliminates recycling of an external phase, thus facilitating the washing step and minimizing agglomeration (Aftabrouchad and Doelker 1992). Some limitations are imposed by the scale-up of the high-energy requirements in homogenization (Lal Pal et al. 2011, Reis et al. 2006).

Through this technique, Dandekar and collaborators (2010) produced curcumin nanoparticles using a combination of (hydroxylpropyl)methyl cellulose and polyvinyl pyrrolidone as the wall material. In this research work, they studied the size and hydrophilic nature of the nanocarriers to enhance absorption and prolong the rapid clearance of curcumin due to possible evasion of the reticulo-endothelial system. The produced nanoparticles presented sizes around 100 nm and an encapsulation efficiency of 72%. Troncoso et al. (2011) also applied emulsion solvent-evaporation technique to produce nanoparticles. Nanoemulsions were formed by homogenizing the organic phase, composed by corn oil and hexane, and the emulsifier solution containing Tween 20 or β-lactoglobulin (β-Lg) protein. Before hexane evaporation, diameters of the nanoparticles prepared with Tween 20 ranged from 171 to 95 nm, while those using β-Lg ranged from 170 to 125 nm. In the end, after hexane evaporation, the smallest particle diameters obtained using Tween 20 and β-Lg were 60 and 97 nm, respectively.

#### 3.2.1.3 Emulsion Solvent-Diffusion

Preparation of nanocapsules by the emulsion solvent-diffusion technique allows the nanoencapsulation of both lipophilic and hydrophilic active substances and requires three phases: organic, aqueous, and dilution (Mora-Huertas et al. 2010, Reis et al. 2006). Regarding the nanoencapsulation of lipophilic bioactive compounds through this widely used method, the organic phase (which contains the polymer, the active substance, oil, and a partially water-miscible organic solvent) is saturated with water, ensuring the initial thermodynamic equilibrium of both liquids (Battaglia et al. 2007). Then, the organic phase is emulsified in an aqueous solution containing a stabilizing agent, leading to solvent diffusion to the external phase (Figure 3.4) and consequent formation of nanoparticles (Lal Pal et al. 2011, Mora-Huertas et al. 2010, Reis et al. 2006). Diffusion of the solvent is accomplished by dilution of the system (dilution phase) with an excess of water and leads to the precipitation of the polymer (Reis et al. 2006). High encapsulation efficiencies (usually above 70%), no need of homogenization, high batch-to-batch reproducibility, ease of scale-up, simplicity, and narrow size distribution are some of the many advantages of this technique (Liu et al. 2010). However, some disadvantages may exist and therefore reduce the encapsulation efficiency, such as high volumes of water to be eliminated from the suspension and the leakage of water-soluble bioactive substance into the saturated-aqueous external phase during emulsification (Bhatia 2016, Reis et al. 2006).

By using this technique, Poletto et al. (2008) produced oily nanocapsules both of caprylic/capric triglyceride or mineral oil with poly(hydroxybutyrate-co-hydroxyvalerate) as the wall material. Controlled particle sizes were obtained employing different mixtures of chloroform and ethanol in the organic phase: the smaller nanoparticles, with sizes between 253 and 493 nm, were obtained using 70%

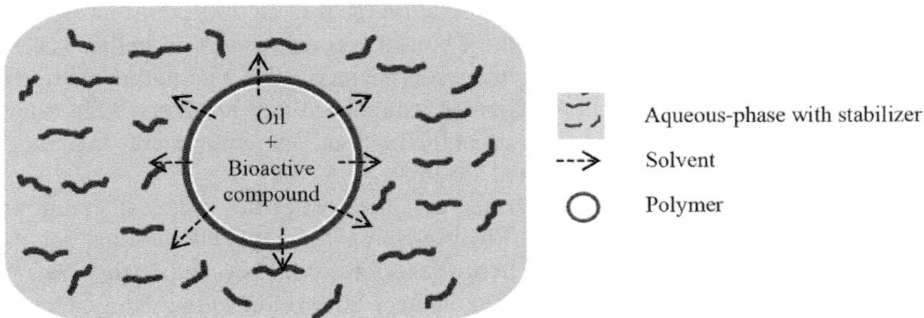


**FIGURE 3.4** Diffusion of the solvent to the external phase, in emulsion solvent-diffusion technique, after dilution of the system.

of ethanol and 30% of chloroform (v/v), and the largest nanocapsules, with a size range of 896–1568 nm, were obtained using chloroform exclusively.

#### 3.2.1.4 Salting-Out

This technique is considered a modification of the emulsion solvent diffusion method and is based on the separation of a water-miscible solvent from aqueous solution via a salting-out effect (Fang and Bhandari 2010, Reis et al. 2006). In the first step, the polymer and the lipophilic bioactive compound are dissolved in an organic solvent such as acetone (Cerqueira et al. 2014). The organic phase is then emulsified into the aqueous-phase, which contains the salting-out agent and colloidal stabilizer (e.g., polyvinylpyrrolidone or hydroxyethylcellulose) (Jafari 2017b). Electrolytes (namely, magnesium chloride, calcium chloride, and magnesium acetate) and non-electrolytes (e.g., sucrose) can be used as salting-out agents (Jafari 2017b, Soppimath et al. 2001). In a final stage, diffusion of acetone into the aqueous phase is enhanced by diluting the O/W emulsion system with water or an aqueous solution, leading to the formation of nanoparticles (Choi and Kwak 2014). At the end of the process, both solvent and salting-out agent are then eliminated by cross-flow filtration. This technique is useful to encapsulate heat sensitive bioactive compounds once it does not require an increase of temperature (Lal Pal et al. 2011, Reis et al. 2006). In addition, the high efficiency of the process and the ease to scale-up are other advantages of this technology. Despite the mentioned benefits there are some disadvantages such as exclusive application to lipophilic substances and large number of washing steps (Lal Pal et al. 2011).

### 3.2.2 Drying Techniques

Conversion of nanoparticle suspensions into a dried form has been reported and widely used in order to maintain their stability (Nakagawa et al. 2011). Chemical and enzymatic hydrolysis of polymeric substances, causing leakage of the encapsulated bioactive compound, is one of the major problems of polymeric nanoparticles, once that leads to chemical instability and irreversible aggregation (Chacon et al. 1999,

Ezhilarasi et al. 2013, Joye and McClements 2014). Therefore, drying techniques have been used to produce or stabilize particles. Drying also decreases nanoparticles volume and mass, thus reducing storage and transport costs (Joye and McClements 2014). However, it is necessary to investigate the relationship between the drying process parameters and the nanoparticles stability, due to the additional stress induced by these techniques (Ezhilarasi et al. 2013, Nakagawa et al. 2011).

#### 3.2.2.1 Spray-Drying

Spray-drying is an economical, simple, fast, and easy to scale-up encapsulation operation, which is widely used in the food industry to encapsulate flavors, vitamins, minerals, colors, fats, and oil, since the late 1950s (Pillai et al. 2012, Wang et al. 2016). This technique uses water-based dispersions, avoiding the use of organic solvents, and produces particles of good quality with low moisture content and extended shelf life stability during storage (Joye and McClements 2014, Pillai et al. 2012). Fine droplets are obtained by atomizing solutions and suspensions of bioactive compounds and polymeric substances, and then feeding them into a flow of hot air. Evaporation of the solvent, which is most often water, quickly occurs and the encapsulation of the interest compound occurs almost instantaneously (Gharsallaoui et al. 2007, Joye and McClements 2014). The resulting dried particles, with spherical shape and diameters between 1 and 10 μm, are then collected after they fall to the bottom of the dryer (Fang and Bhandari 2010, Joye and McClements 2014, Wang et al. 2016). This technique can be considered as a micro-encapsulation method and, by itself, cannot be used for nanoencapsulation purposes, once it is just capable of converting a suspension of colloidal nanoparticles into a nanostructured powder form (Ezhilarasi et al. 2013). Consequently, it is necessary the application of another nanoencapsulation technique, like emulsion, prior to spray-drying. Regarding the drying of nanoemulsions and suspensions, spray-drying method needs suitable modifications to retain particles of nanometer size (Anandharamakrishnan et al. 2008; Ezhilarasi et al. 2013). Despite this, in 2009, the introduction of the Büchi nanospray drier came to revolutionize the spray-drying technology. Due to its vibration, mesh spray technology is possible to create tiny droplets before the evaporation step, generating ultrafine powders in the submicron size range with very narrow distributions and high formulation yields (Jafari 2017b, Li et al. 2010).

Lee and coworkers (2011) showed that nanospray-drying approach is effective to prepare bovine serum albumin nanoparticles. By using a 4 μm spray mesh at bovine serum albumin concentration of 0.1% (w/v), a surfactant concentration of 0.05% (w/v), a drying gas flow rate of 150 L/min, and an inlet temperature of 120°C, they produced spherical nanoparticles with median size of 460 $\pm$ 10 nm with a yield of 72 $\pm$ 4%.

#### 3.2.2.2 Freeze-Drying

Freeze-drying technique, also known as lyophilization, is used for the dehydration of heat-sensitive materials and aromas. Procedure comprises three different steps: freezing, sublimation or primary drying, and desorption or secondary drying (Ezhilarasi et al. 2013, Reis et al. 2006). In the freezing step, the nanoparticles are cooled below their triple point, the temperature and pressure at which the three fundamental states (gas, liquid, and solid) coexist in thermodynamic equilibrium, ensuring that sublimation, rather than melting, will occur in the following steps. During the primary drying phase, the pressure is lowered, and enough heat is supplied to the material for the ice to sublime. In the secondary drying phase, the removal of unfrozen water molecules occurs leading to the separation of the nanoparticles previously produced by other nanoencapsulation methods (Al-Muhteseb and Emeish 2015, Ezhilarasi et al. 2013, Fang and Bhandari 2010). Freeze-drying is not considered a nanoencapsulation method once that pores are formed, due to the ice sublimation process, and the bioactive substances are exposed to the atmosphere. Moreover, particle's high porosity can significantly affect the stability of the enclosed component (Ezhilarasi et al. 2013, Joye and McClements 2014). This technique, currently used to remove water from nanocapsules without alter their shape and structure, results in high-quality products with longer shelf life. However, when compared to spray-drying, it is more expensive and the drying process is much slower (Ciurzyńska and Lenart 2011, Joye and McClements 2014). A possible alternative to freeze-drying technique is spray-freeze-drying, regarding the reduction of the pore size and drying time (Joye and McClements 2014).

Choi et al. (2010) showed the encapsulation of fish oil by self-aggregation and emulsion solvent-diffusion methods, using β-cyclodextrin and polycaprolactone, respectively, followed by freeze drying process. The results showed that polycaprolactone/fish oil particles, with less than 200 nm, had higher fish oil loading, higher encapsulation efficiency, and lower fish oil leakage than β-cyclodextrin/fish oil nanoparticles, which presented sizes between 250 and 700 nm. Nakagawa and coworkers (2011) also used polycaprolactone, stabilized with gelatin, as the encapsulating material to create capsicum oleoresin nanocapsules. In this work, freeze-drying was used after emulsion-diffusion technique and nanocapsules dispersibility was studied. Results suggested that gelatin's arrangement in the nanocapsules could be advantageous, largely increasing dispersion patterns after the drying process. The average diameter of the produced nanocapsules was lower than 200 nm.

### 3.2.3 Nanoprecipitation

The nanoprecipitation method, also known as antisolvent precipitation or solvent displacement, is suitable to form both nanocapsules and nanospheres (Barreras-Urbina et al. 2016, Ezhilarasi et al. 2013). This technique has several advantages compared with other methods, among which stand out the fact that it does not require expensive or specialized equipment or the use of complex operating conditions, low cost, and the ease of scaling-up (Joye and McClements 2014, Thorat and Dalvi 2012). In this method, the bioactive compound and the polymer are first dissolved in organic solvent and then mixed into an aqueous water solution while stirring or sonicating (Recharla et al. 2017). Thus, the nanoparticles formed are dispersed in the water solution. The procedure is based on the spontaneous emulsification of the organic internal phase containing the dissolved bioactive compound, polymer, and organic solvent into the aqueous external phase (Figure 3.5). It involves the precipitation of polymer from an organic solution and the diffusion of the organic solvent in the

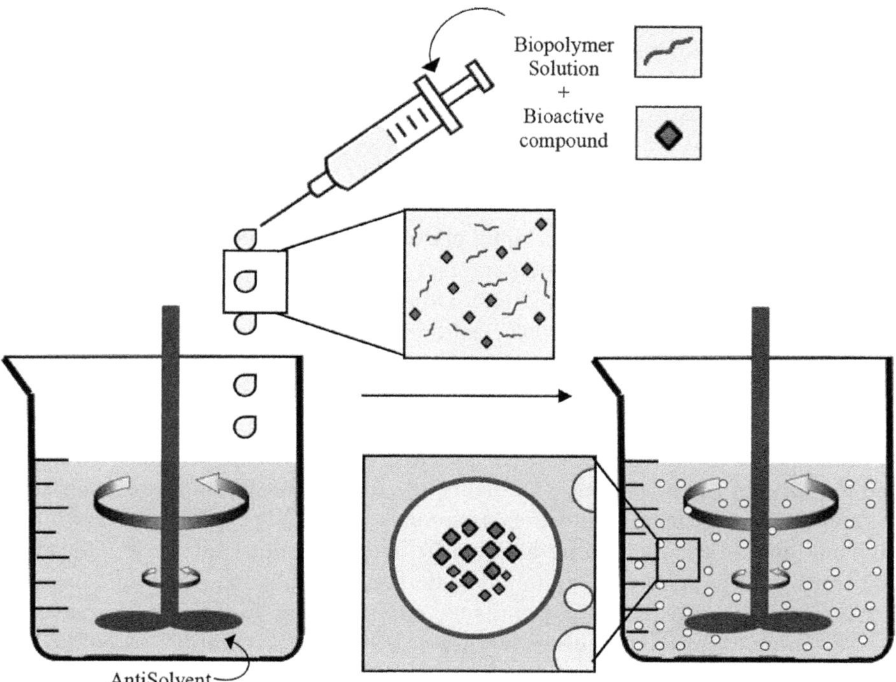


**FIGURE 3.5** Schematic illustration of bioactive compound encapsulation by the nanoprecipitation method.

aqueous medium (Galindo-Rodriguez et al. 2004). Several liquids are usually used as both solvents and antisolvents, such as water, organic solvents (acetone, ethanol, or hexane) or supercritical $CO_2$ (Joye and McClements 2014).

Nanoprecipitation technique was used mainly for the encapsulation of lipophilic compounds. Biodegradable polymers such as polycaprolactone, poly(lactide), poly(lactide-co-glicolide), Eudragit, and poly(alkylcyanoacrylate) are often used, but food-grade polymers such as polysaccharides and proteins are preferred for food applications (Ezhilarasi et al. 2013, Joye and McClements 2014). Noronha et al. (2014) used nanoprecipitation method to prepare α-tocopherol nanocapsules for incorporation of this antioxidant with methylcellulose films that enhance the solubility and protect them from oxidation. Nanoprecipitation has been pointed out as a suitable method for the preparation of α-tocopherol-loaded polycaprolactone nanocapsules, to produce nanoparticles and to improve the encapsulation efficacy (Noronha et al. 2013). Davidov-Pardo et al. (2015) investigated the possibility of encapsulating resveratrol in biopolymer particles produced using liquid antisolvent precipitation. The particles were produced with gliadin or zein in the absence or presence of pectin or sodium caseinate (hydrophilic biopolymers), which were used as coating. Encapsulation efficiencies were higher for coated than bare particles with 53% and 86% in coated gliadin and zein particles, respectively. These particles seem promising encapsulation systems to stabilize resveratrol upon supplementation to functional foods (Joye et al. 2015). da Rosa et al. (2015) also used zein to encapsulate thymol and carvacrol phenolics by a nanoprecipitation method. Zein nanoparticles were shown to be able to maintain antioxidant and antimicrobial activities during storage at 4°C and 20°C, for 90 days.

### 3.2.4 Complex Coacervation

Complex coacervation is a liquid-liquid phase separation process that occurs when two oppositely charged biopolymers interact with each other by electrostatic interactions (Eghbal and Choudhary 2018). Other forces such as hydrogen bonding, hydrophobic interactions, and polarization-induced attractive interactions may also be involved. Coacervates for encapsulation are usually formed from polysaccharides and proteins, but may be also formed from the interaction of a charged bioactive component and an oppositely charged biopolymer (simple coacervation). Several factors including biopolymer type and concentration, pH, ionic strength, and the ratio of the biopolymers influence the formation of complex coacervates. In order to improve its integrity, the coacervates are usually covalently crosslinked by using glutaraldehyde, tannic acid, gallic acid, or transglutaminase. However, due to its high toxicity risk, glutaraldehyde is not suitable for food applications. Coacervation is considered a promising encapsulation technology because of the very high encapsulation efficiency (up to 99%), the possibilities of controlled and sustained release, and the thermal and mechanical resistance (Gouin 2004). Nevertheless, some disadvantages of this method have been identified such as the difficulty to strictly control particle size and to prevent particle agglomeration, as well as the limited stability of some particles in various aqueous matrices (Joye and McClements 2014).

Complex coacervation has been used for nanoencapsulation of various active agents as shown in Table 3.1.

### 3.2.5 Inclusion Complexation

Inclusion complexation usually designates the molecular encapsulation of a guest molecule (bioactive compound) into a cavity bearing host molecule through hydrogen bonding, van der Waals force, or hydrophobic interaction. For food applications, cyclodextrins, β-Lg, and starch are the only host molecules that are considered appropriated (Joye and McClements 2014). Inclusion complexation-based delivery systems for food derived ingredients are given in Table 3.2.

Cyclodextrins (CDs) are cyclic oligomers of α-d-glucopyranose consisting of 6, 7, or 8 units (α-, β-, and γ-CDs, respectively), which enclose cavities of approximately 0.6, 0.8, and 1.0 nm in diameter (Marques 2010). CDs have a truncated cone shape, with a hydrophobic zone inside and a hydrophilic external surface. Therefore, they are able to form inclusion complexes with hydrophobic molecules improving molecules' solubility. Moreover, complexation with cyclodextrin can also improve chemical stability, protect bioactive compounds from external environment, and promote taste modification and controlled release of bioactive compounds (Marques 2010, Pinho et al, 2014). For these reasons, CDs have been widely used in the food

**TABLE 3.1**
**Coacervation-Based Delivery Systems of Selected Bioactive Compounds**

| Bioactive Compound | Encapsulating Materials | Particle Size (nm) | Effect/Objective | References |
|---|---|---|---|---|
| Docosahexaenoic acid | β-Lactoglobulin and low methoxyl pectin | 100 | Increased stability | Zimet and Livney (2009) |
| Capsaicin | Gelatin and acacia gum | 100 | Masking of pungent odor Increased stability | Jincheng et al. (2010) |
| Vitamin D3 | Whey protein isolate | 80–260 | Increased stability | Abbasi et al. (2014) |
| Folic acid (vitamin B9) | Casein | 150 | Increased oral bioavailability | Penalva et al. (2015) |
| Astaxanthin containing lipid extract | Gelatin and cashew gum | 32,7 | Increased stability | Gomez-Estaca et al. (2016) |
| Oenothein B (polyphenol) | Caseinophosphopeptides and chitosan | 200–300 | Enhanced protection through gastrointestinal tract | Lan et al. (2017) |

**TABLE 3.2**
**Inclusion Complexation-Based Delivery Systems of Selected Food-Derived Compounds**

| Bioactive Compound | Encapsulating Materials | Particle Size | Effect/Objective | References |
|---|---|---|---|---|
| Linoleic acid | α- and β-cyclodextrin | n.a. | Improved thermal stability | Hădărugă et al. (2006) |
| Resveratrol | β-Cyclodextrin | n.a. | Improved stability | Lucas-Abellán et al. (2007) |
| Lycopene | β-Cyclodextrin | 40 nm | Improved water-solubility | Nerome et al. (2013) |
| Red bell pepper carotenoids | β-Cyclodextrin | 562 nm | Improved stability<br>Improved water-solubility | Gomes et al. (2014) |
| Curcumin | β-Cyclodextrin | n.a. | Improved stability<br>Improved water-solubility | Mangolim et al. (2014) |
| Essential oils | β-Cyclodextrin | n.a. | Improved antioxidant activity | Kfoury et al. (2015) |
| α-Tocopherol | β-Lactoglobulin | n.a. | Improved stability<br>Improved water-solubility | Liang et al. (2011) |
| Vitamin D3 | β-Lactoglobulin | | Improved stability<br>Improved water-solubility | Diarrassouba et al. (2013) |
| Naringenin | β-Lactoglobulin | 10 nm | Improved water-solubility | Shpigelman et al. (2014) |
| Genistein | High amylose corn starch | n.a | Improved bioavailability | Cohen et al. (2011) |
| Flax seed oil | High amylose corn starch | 20 nm | Improved thermal stability<br>Reduction of off-flavors | Gökmen et al. (2011) |
| Ascorbyl palmitate | High amylose maize starch | n.a | Improved stability | Kong et al. (2014a) |
| Coenzyme Q10 | High amylose maize starch | <150 nm | Improved water-solubility | Yoon et al. (2014) |
| Zinc | Amylose from potato starch | n.a. | Zinc nutrition fortifier | Luo et al. (2016) |
| Garlic bioactive components | Amylose from potato starch | n.a. | Improved stability | Zhang et al. (2018) |
| β-Carotene | High-amylose corn starch | n.a. | Improved stability | Kong et al. (2018) |

*Note:* n.a.—not available.

industry as food additives, for stabilization of flavors, elimination of undesired tastes, or other unwanted compounds (e.g., cholesterol, mycotoxins, and allergens) and to avoid micro-biological contaminations and browning reactions (Astray et al. 2009, Fenyvesi et al. 2016). There are several methods for obtaining CDs inclusion complexes, namely: (i) physical blending; (ii) kneading method; (iii) co-precipitation method; (iv) milling technique; (v) spray-drying method; (vi) freeze-drying/lyophilization technique; and (vii) supercritical antisolvent technique (Marques 2010, Recharla et al. 2017). The choice of the method will depend on the properties of the guest molecule and on the nature of the CD chosen. Pinho et al. (2014) have recently reviewed the application of CDs as encapsulation agents for plant bioactive compounds.

β-Lg is the major whey protein with high nutritional value and excellent functional properties (Rodrigues and Andrade 2015). It has been extensively studied for its capacity to bind hydrophobic and amphiphilic compounds such as flavors, vitamins, fatty acids, and polyphenols (Tavares et al. 2014). Complexation typically occurs via hydrophobic interactions and hydrogen bonding. β-Lg has a conical β-barrel structure with a large central hydrophobic cavity (calyx), which has been proposed as the main binding site (Shpigelman et al. 2014). Nevertheless, other binding sites in the cavity near to the α-helix and in the external surface of the β-barrel have also been reported (Kontopidis et al. 2004, Shpigelman et al. 2014). Shpigelman et al. (2014) explored the use of β-Lg-based nanovehicles to facilitate a citrus flavonoid, naringenin, solubilization, and delivery. Naringenin was shown to form complexes with preheated and non-preheated β-Lg probably by binding at the two main hydrophobic binding sites of the protein, the calyx and the cleft near the α-helix. The formation of such complexes between naringenin and β-Lg enabled solubilization and prevented crystallization of the flavonoid up to three times its solubility limit.

Starch comprises two polysaccharides, amylose [a α-(1-4) linear glucan] and amylopectin [a α-(1-4), α-(1-6) branched glucan]. Amylose molecules are known to form single-helical inclusion complexes with different ligands such as iodine, linear, or fatty acids (Putseys et al. 2010). In the presence of such molecules, amylose can form a left-handed single helix, which has a hydrophilic outer surface and a hydrophobic helical channel that accommodates the guest molecules (Lesmes et al. 2009). The amylose helices then form a crystalline structure known as V-amylose. Two methods are normally used, co-precipitation and acidification of an alkaline solution (Zhu 2017). In the co-precipitation method, starch (normally purified amylose or high amylose maize starch) is dissolved in water at a high temperature (e.g., 145°C) and maintained at 90°C (Zhu 2017). The guest molecule is added dissolved in an organic solvent and the whole system maintained at 90°C before slowly cooling down to room temperature to form the inclusion complexes. In the acidification of an alkaline solution method, starch is dissolved in an alkaline solution at 90°C. The bioactive molecules dissolved in solvent are added and mixed with the starch solution. Then, the whole system is slightly acidified (pH 5 to 6) to facilitate the formation of inclusion complexes. An electrospinning-based complexation method was also recently reported (Kong and Ziegler 2014b). Amylose-guest inclusion complexes may be useful as a delivery composition for bioactive guest molecules such as fatty acids, vitamins, or soy isoflavones (Table 3.2). The inclusion complexes are expected to protect the bioactive compounds against the acidic conditions of the stomach and improve their bioavailability by releasing them in the lower gastrointestinal tract after amylose hydrolysis by endogenous enzymes or saccharolytic bacteria (Kong and Ziegler 2018).

### 3.2.6 Supercritical Fluids

A supercritical fluid (SCF) can either be a liquid or gas used above its thermodynamic critical point of temperature and pressure (Jung and Perrut 2001). SCFs have properties intermediate between those of liquids and gases like low viscosity and density and high solvating power, diffusivities, and mass transfer rates (above the critical point). Moreover, physical properties such as density, dielectric constant, and polarity may be modified by changing operating conditions (e.g., pressure and/or temperature) around the critical point. Due to their high pressure and high temperatures, the SCFs exhibit greater solvating capabilities than the normal liquids (Reverchon et al. 2003). Supercritical carbon dioxide is the most commonly used SCF due to its low critical temperature (i.e., $Tc = 31.10°C$) and pressure ($Pc = 7.3$ MPa) (Recharla et al. 2017). Moreover, it is considered an alternative to hazardous solvents as it is nontoxic, non-flammable, and is available in large quantities with low cost and high purity. The most common methods to prepare particles under SCF technology are: (i) rapid expansion of supercritical solutions; (ii) precipitation with supercritical antisolvent; and (iii) solution enhanced dispersion by SCF (Recharla et al. 2017).

For application in the food industry, nanoparticles production by SCFs technology presents some disadvantages related to some steps and materials (non-food grade) used (Cerqueira et al. 2014). Using supercritical antisolvent precipitation, Heyang et al. (2009) encapsulated lutein in hydroxylpropyl methylcellulose phthalate to maintain its bioactivity and to avoid thermal/light degradation. The mean diameter of a lutein-loaded hydroxylpropyl methylcellulose phthalate nanocapsule ranged from 163 to 219 nm and an encapsulation efficiency of 88% was achieved. Using rapid expansion from SCF technique, Türk and Lietzow (2004) synthesized phytosterol nanoparticles (below 500 nm) with long-term stability.

## 3.3 CONCLUSION AND FUTURE PERSPECTIVES

There is an increasing interest in the development of nanoparticle-based delivery systems appropriate for utilization in the food industry. The nanoparticles may be used to encapsulate, protect, and release bioactive ingredients including lipids, vitamins, minerals, and nutraceuticals such as polyphenols and antioxidants. Accordingly, nanoencapsulation may contribute to produce new (functional) food products and/or to improve the existing ones by addressing issues such as nutrient loss, low bioavailability, flavor loss, and texture deterioration during processing and storage. However, for this to materialize is still necessary to search and develop new materials and production methods suitable and compatible to uses in foods and beverages. Moreover, these ingredients and processing methods must also to be economically feasible and appropriate for large-scale production.

Another important aspect to consider before widespread application is health and safety factors. The use of nano-sized particles may alter the biological fate of the ingested encapsulating materials and bioactive compounds, which may have potentially adverse effects on human health. Therefore, toxicological studies must be undertaken in order to ensure nanodelivery systems safe for application in food products.

## ACKNOWLEDGMENTS

This work was supported by CESPU/IINFACTS under the project MicelCampt-CESPU-2017 and MicroFluiPro-CESPU-2017. This work was financed by FEDER–Fundo Europeu de Desenvolvimento Regional funds through the COMPETE 2020—Operacional Programme for Competitiveness and Internationalisation (POCI), Portugal 2020 (NORTE-01-0145-FEDER-000012), and by Portuguese funds through Fundação para a Ciência e a Tecnologia/Ministério da Ciência, Tecnologia e Inovação in the framework of the project "Institute for Research and Innovation in Health Sciences" (POCI-01-0145-FEDER-007274).

## REFERENCES

Abbasi, A., Z. Emam-Djomeh, M. A. E. Mousavi, and D. Davoodi, 2014. "Stability of vitamin D3 encapsulated in nanoparticles of whey protein isolate." *Food Chemistry* 143:379–383.

Acosta, E. 2009. "Bioavailability of nanoparticles in nutrient and nutraceutical delivery." *Current Opinion in Colloid & Interface Science* 14:3–15.

Aftabrouchad, C., and E. Doelker. 1992. "Preparation methods for biodegradable microparticles loaded with water-soluble drugs." *STP Pharma Sciences* 2:365–365.

Aguilar, M. R., and J. S. Román. 2014. *Smart Polymers and Their Applications*. Cambridge, UK: Woodhead Publishing.

Al-Muhteseb, S. I., and S. Emeish. 2015. "Producing natural mixed carotenoids from *Dunaliella salina*." *Journal of Natural Sciences Research* 5:53–59.

Anandharamakrishnan, C., C. D. Rielly, and A. G. F. Stapley. 2008. "Loss of solubility of α-lactalbumin and β-lactoglobulin during the spray drying of whey proteins." *LWT-Food Science and Technology* 41:270–277.

Anu Bhushani, J., and C. Anandharamakrishnan. 2014. "Electrospinning and electrospraying techniques: Potential food based applications." *Trends in Food Science & Technology* 38:21–33.

Astray, G., C. Gonzalez-Barreiro, J. C Mejuto, R. Rial-Otero, and J. Simal-Gándara. 2009. "A review on the use of cyclodextrins in foods." *Food Hydrocolloids* 23:1631–1640.

Augustin, M. A., and Y. Hemar. 2009. "Nano-and micro-structured assemblies for encapsulation of food ingredients." *Chemical Society Reviews* 38:902–912.

Barreras-Urbina, C. G., B. Ramírez-Wong, G. A. López-Ahumada, et al. 2016. "Nano-and micro-particles by nanoprecipitation: Possible application in the food and agricultural industries." *International Journal of Food Properties* 19:1912–1923.

Battaglia, L., M. Trotta, M. Gallarate, M. E. Carlotti, G. P. Zara, and A. Bargoni. 2007. "Solid lipid nanoparticles formed by solvent-in-water emulsion–diffusion technique: Development and influence on insulin stability." *Journal of Microencapsulation* 24:672–684.

Bhatia, S. 2016. "Nanoparticles types, classification, characterization, fabrication methods and drug delivery applications." In *Natural Polymer Drug Delivery Systems*, pp. 33–93. Cham, Switzerland: Springer.

Borthakur, P., P. K. Boruah, B. Sharma, and M. R. Das. 2016. "Nanoemulsion: Preparation and its application in food industry." In *Emulsions*, ed. A. M. Grumezescu, pp. 153–191. London, UK: Academic Press.

Cerqueira, M. A., A. C. Pinheiro, H. D. Silva, et al. 2014. "Design of bio-nanosystems for oral delivery of functional compounds." *Food Engineering Reviews* 6:1–19.

Chacon, M., J. Molpeceres, L. Berges, M. Guzman, and M. R. Aberturas. 1999. "Stability and freeze-drying of cyclosporine loaded poly (D, L lactide–glycolide) carriers." *European Journal of Pharmaceutical Sciences* 8:99–107.

Choi, M. J., and H. S. Kwak. 2014. "Advanced approaches of nano- and microencapsulation for food ingredients." In *Nano- and Microencapsulation for Foods*, ed. H.-S. Kwak, pp. 95–116. Chichester, UK: John Wiley & Sons.

Choi, M. J., U. Ruktanonchai, S. G. Min, J. Y. Chun, and A. Soottitantawat. 2010. "Physical characteristics of fish oil encapsulated by β-cyclodextrin using an aggregation method or polycaprolactone using an emulsion–diffusion method." *Food Chemistry* 119:1694–1703.

Ciurzyńska, A., and A. Lenart. 2011. "Freeze-drying-application in food processing and biotechnology-A review." *Polish Journal of Food and Nutrition Sciences* 61:165–171.

Cohen, R., B. Schwartz, I. Peri, and E. Shimoni. 2011. "Improving bioavailability and stability of genistein by complexation with high-amylose corn starch." *Journal of Agricultural and Food Chemistry* 59: 7932–7938.

da Rosa, C. G., M. V. D. O. B. Maciel, S. M. de Carvalho. et al. 2015. "Characterization and evaluation of physicochemical and antimicrobial properties of zein nanoparticles loaded with phenolics monoterpenes." *Colloids and Surfaces A: Physicochemical and Engineering Aspects* 481:337–344.

Dandekar, P. P., R. Jain, S. Patil, et al. 2010. "Curcumin-loaded hydrogel nanoparticles: Application in anti-malarial therapy and toxicological evaluation." *Journal of Pharmaceutical Sciences* 99:4992–5010.

Davidov-Pardo, G., I. J. Joye, and D. J. McClements. 2015. "Encapsulation of resveratrol in biopolymer particles produced using liquid antisolvent precipitation. Part 1: Preparation and characterization." *Food Hydrocolloids* 45:309–316.

Deshmukh, R., P. Wagh, and J. Naik. 2016. "Solvent evaporation and spray drying technique for micro- and nanospheres/particles preparation: A review." *Drying Technology* 34:1758–1772.

Diarrassouba, F., G. Remondetto, L. Liang, G. Garrait, E. Beyssac, and M. Subirade. 2013. "Effects of gastrointestinal pH conditions on the stability of the β-lactoglobulin/vitamin D3 complex and on the solubility of vitamin D3." *Food Research International* 52:515–521.

EFSA Scientific Committee. 2011. "Scientific opinion on guidance on the risk assessment of the application of nanoscience and nanotechnologies in the food and feed chain." *EFSA Journal* 9:2140 doi:10.2903/j.efsa.2011.214

Eghbal, N., and R. Choudhary. 2018. "Complex coacervation: Encapsulation and controlled release of active agents in food systems." *LWT-Food Science and Technology*. 90:254–264.

Ezhilarasi, P. N., P. Karthik, N. Chhanwal, and C. Anandharamakrishnan. 2013. "Nanoencapsulation techniques for food bioactive components: A review." *Food and Bioprocess Technology* 6:628–647.

Fang, Z., and B. Bhandari. 2010. "Encapsulation of polyphenols: A review." *Trends in Food Science & Technology* 21:510–523.

Fenyvesi, E., M. A. Vikmon, and L. Szente. 2016. "Cyclodextrins in food technology and human nutrition: Benefits and limitations." *Critical Reviews in Food Science and Nutrition* 56:1981–2004.

Galanakis, C. M. 2018. *Polyphenols: Properties, Recovery, and Applications*. Cambridge, UK: Woodhead Publishing.

Galindo-Rodriguez, S., E. Allémann, H. Fessi, and E. Doelker. 2004. "Physicochemical parameters associated with nanoparticle formation in the salting-out, emulsification-diffusion, and nanoprecipitation methods." *Pharmaceutical Research* 21:1428–1439.

Gharsallaoui, A., G. Roudaut, O. Chambin, A. Voilley, and R. Saurel. 2007. "Applications of spray-drying in microencapsulation of food ingredients: An overview." *Food Research International* 40:1107–1121.

Gökmen, V., B. A. Mogol, R. B. Lumaga, V. Fogliano, Z. Kaplun, and E. Shimoni. 2011. "Development of functional bread containing nanoencapsulated omega-3 fatty acids". *Journal of Food Engineering* 105:585–591.

Gomes, L. M. M., N. Petito, V. G. Costa, D. Q. Falcão, and K. G. de Lima Araújo. 2014. "Inclusion complexes of red bell pepper pigments with β-cyclodextrin: Preparation, characterization and application as natural colorant in yogurt." *Food Chemistry* 148:428–436.

Gomez-Estaca, J., T. A. Comunian, P. Montero, R. Ferro-Furtado, and C. S. Favaro-Trindade. 2016. "Encapsulation of an astaxanthin-containing lipid extract from shrimp waste by complex coacervation using a novel gelatin–cashew gum complex." *Food Hydrocolloids* 61:155–162.

Gouin, S. 2004. "Microencapsulation: Industrial appraisal of existing technologies and trends." *Trends in Food Science & Technology*, 15:330–347.

Gupta, A., H. B. Eral, T. A. Hatton, and P. S. Doyle. 2016. "Nanoemulsions: Formation, properties and applications." *Soft Matter* 12:2826–2841.

Hădărugă, N. G., D. I. Hădărugă, V. Păunescu, et al. 2006. "Thermal stability of the linoleic acid/α-and β-cyclodextrin complexes." *Food Chemistry* 99: 500–508.

Heyang, J. I. N., X. I. A. Fei, C. Jiang, Z. H. A. O. Yaping, and H. E. Lin. 2009. "Nanoencapsulation of lutein with hydroxypropylmethyl cellulose phthalate by supercritical antisolvent." *Chinese Journal of Chemical Engineering* 17: 672–677.

Ito, T., Y. Tsuji, K. Aramaki, and N. Tonooka. 2012. "Two-step emulsification process for water-in-oil-in-water multiple emulsions stabilized by lamellar liquid crystals." *Journal of Oleo Science* 61 (8):413–420.

Jafari, S. M. 2017a. *Nanoencapsulation of Food Bioactive Ingredients: Principles and Applications*. London, UK: Academic Press.

Jafari, S. M. 2017b. *Nanoencapsulation Technologies for the Food and Nutraceutical Industries*. London, UK: Academic Press.

Jafari, S. M., E. Assadpoor, B. Bhandari, and Y. He. 2008. "Nano-particle encapsulation of fish oil by spray drying." *Food Research International* 41:172–183. Ed. Jincheng, W., Z. Xiaoyu, and C. Sihao. 2010. "Preparation and properties of nanocapsulated capsaicin by complex coacervation method." *Chemical Engineering Communications* 197:919–933.

Joye, I. J., and D. J. McClements. 2014. "Biopolymer-based nanoparticles and microparticles: Fabrication, characterization, and application." *Current Opinion in Colloid & Interface Science* 19:417–427.

Joye, I. J., G. Davidov-Pardo, and D. J. McClements. 2015. "Encapsulation of resveratrol in biopolymer particles produced using liquid antisolvent precipitation. Part 2: Stability and functionality." *Food Hydrocolloids* 49:127–134.

Jung, J., and M. Perrut. 2001. "Particle design using supercritical fluids: Literature and patent survey." *The Journal of Supercritical Fluids* 20:179–219.

Kfoury, M., L. Auezova, H. Greige-Gerges, and S. Fourmentin. 2015. "Promising applications of cyclodextrins in food: Improvement of essential oils retention, controlled release and antiradical activity." *Carbohydrate Polymers* 131:264–272.

Khanjani, J., M. Zohuriaan-Mehr, and S. Pazokifard. 2017. "Microemulsion and macroemulsion polymerization of octamethylcyclotetrasiloxane: A comparative study." *Phosphorus, Sulfur, and Silicon and the Related Elements* 192:967–976.

Komaiko, J., and D. J. McClements. 2015. "Low-energy formation of edible nanoemulsions by spontaneous emulsification: Factors influencing particle size." *Journal of Food Engineering* 146:122–128.

Kong, L., and G. R. Ziegler. 2014a. "Molecular encapsulation of ascorbyl palmitate in preformed V-type starch and amylose." *Carbohydrate Polymers* 111:256–263.

Kong, L., and G. R. Ziegler. 2014b. "Formation of starch-guest inclusion complexes in electrospun starch fibers." *Food Hydrocolloids* 38:211–219.

Kong, L., R. Bhosale, and G. R. Ziegler. 2018. "Encapsulation and stabilization of β-carotene by amylose inclusion complexes." *Food Research International* 105:446–452.

Kontopidis, G., C. Holt, and L. Sawyer. 2004. "Invited review: β-lactoglobulin: Binding properties, structure, and function." *Journal of Dairy Science* 87:785–796.

Kumar, A., H. M. Mansour, A. Friedman, and E. R. Blough. (Eds.). 2013. *Nanomedicine in Drug Delivery*. Boca Raton, FL: CRC Press/Taylor & Francis Group.

Lan, Y., L. Wang, S. Cao, et al. 2017. "Rational design of food-grade polyelectrolyte complex coacervate for encapsulation and enhanced oral delivery of oenothein B." *Food & Function* 8:4070–4080.

Landfester, K. 2009. "Miniemulsion polymerization and the structure of polymer and hybrid nanoparticles." *Angewandte Chemie International Edition* 48:4488–4507.

Lee, S. H., D. Heng, W. K. Ng, H. K. Chan, and R. B. Tan. 2011."Nano spray drying: A novel method for preparing protein nanoparticles for protein therapy." *International Journal of Pharmaceutics* 403:192–200.

Lesmes, U., S. H. Cohen, Y. Shener, and E. Shimoni. 2009. "Effects of long chain fatty acid unsaturation on the structure and controlled release properties of amylose complexes." *Food Hydrocolloids* 23:667–675.

Li, X., N. Anton, C. Arpagaus, F. Belleteix, and T. F. Vandamme. 2010. "Nanoparticles by spray drying using innovative new technology: The Büchi Nano Spray Dryer B-90." *Journal of Controlled Release* 147:304–310.

Liang, L., V. Tremblay-Hébert, and M. Subirade. 2011. "Characterization of the β-lactoglobulin/α-tocopherol complex and its impact on α-tocopherol stability." *Food Chemistry* 126:821–826.

Liu, J., Z. Qiu, S. Wang, L. Zhou, and S. Zhang. 2010. "A modified double-emulsion method for the preparation of daunorubicin-loaded polymeric nanoparticle with enhanced in vitro anti-tumor activity." *Biomedical Materials* 5:065002.

Livney, Y. D. 2017. Nanoencapsulation technologies. In *Engineering Foods for Bioactives Stability and Delivery*, ed. Y. H. Roos and Y. D. Livney, pp. 143–169. New York: Springer.

Lucas-Abellán, C., I. Fortea, J. M. López-Nicolás, and E. Núñez-Delicado. 2007. "Cyclodextrins as resveratrol carrier system." *Food Chemistry* 104:39–44.

Luo, Z., J. Zou, H. Chen, W. Cheng, X. Fu, and Z. Xiao. 2016. "Synthesis and characterization of amylose–zinc inclusion complexes." *Carbohydrate Polymers* 137:314–320.

Mangolim, C. S., C. Moriwaki, A. C. Nogueira. et al. 2014. "Curcumin–β-cyclodextrin inclusion complex: Stability, solubility, characterization by FT-IR, FT-Raman, X-ray diffraction and photoacoustic spectroscopy, and food application." *Food Chemistry* 153:361–370.

Marques, H. M. C. 2010. "A review on cyclodextrin encapsulation of essential oils and volatiles." *Flavour and Fragrance Journal* 25:313–326.

McClements, D. J., E. A. Decker, Y. Park, and J. Weiss. 2009. "Structural design principles for delivery of bioactive components in nutraceuticals and functional foods." *Critical Reviews in Food Science and Nutrition* 49:577–606.

McClements, D.J. 2015. *Nanoparticle- and Microparticle-Based Delivery Systems: Encapsulation, Protection and Release of Active Compounds*. Boca Raton, FL: CRC Press/Taylor & Francis Group.

Mora-Huertas, C. E., H. Fessi, and A. Elaissari. 2010. "Polymer-based nanocapsules for drug delivery." *International Journal of Pharmaceutics* 385:113–142.

Nagavarma, B. V. N., H. K. S. Yadav, A. Ayaz, L. S. Vasudha, and H. G. Shivakumar. 2012. "Different techniques for preparation of polymeric nanoparticles-a review." *Asian Journal of Pharmaceutical and Clinical Research* 5:16–23.

Nakagawa, K., S. Surassmo, S. G. Min, and M. J. Choi. 2011. "Dispersibility of freeze-dried poly(epsilon-caprolactone) nanocapsules stabilized by gelatin and the effect of freezing." *Journal of Food Engineering* 102:177–188.

Nerome, H., S. Machmudah, R. Fukuzato, et al. 2013. "Nanoparticle formation of lycopene/β-cyclodextrin inclusion complex using supercritical antisolvent precipitation." *The Journal of Supercritical Fluids* 83:97–103.

Noronha, C. M., A. F. Granada, S. M. de Carvalho, R. C. Lino, M. V. de O. B. Maciel, and P. L. M. Barreto. 2013. "Optimization of α-tocopherol loaded nanocapsules by the nanoprecipitation method." *Industrial Crops and Products* 50:896–903.

Noronha, C. M., S. M. de Carvalho, R. C. Lino, and P. L. M. Barreto. 2014. "Characterization of antioxidant methylcellulose film incorporated with α-tocopherol nanocapsules." *Food Chemistry* 159:529–535.

Pal, S. L., U. Jana, P. K. Manna, G. P. Mohanta, and R. Manavalan. 2011. "Nanoparticle: An overview of preparation, characterization and application." *Journal of Applied Pharmaceutical Science* 01:228–234.

Penalva, R., I. Esparza, M. Agüeros, C. J. Gonzalez-Navarro, C. Gonzalez-Ferrero, and J. M. Irache. 2015. "Casein nanoparticles as carriers for the oral delivery of folic acid." *Food Hydrocolloids* 44:399–406.

Pillai, D. S., P. Prabhasankar, B. S. Jena, and C. Anandharamakrishnan. 2012. "Microencapsulation of Garcinia cowa fruit extract and effect of its use on pasta process and quality." *International Journal of Food Properties* 15:590–604.

Pinho, E., M. Grootveld, G. Soares, and M. Henriques. 2014. "Cyclodextrins as encapsulation agents for plant bioactive compounds." *Carbohydrate Polymers* 101:121–135.

Poletto, F. S., L. A. Fiel, B. Donida, M. I. Ré, S. S. Guterres, and A. R. Pohlmann. 2008. "Controlling the size of poly (hydroxybutyrate-co-hydroxyvalerate) nanoparticles prepared by emulsification–diffusion technique using ethanol as surface agent." *Colloids and Surfaces A: Physicochemical and Engineering Aspects* 324:105–112.

Putseys, J. A., L. Lamberts, and J. A. Delcour, 2010. "Amylose-inclusion complexes: Formation, identity and physico-chemical properties." *Journal of Cereal Science* 51:238–247.

Quintanilla-Carvajal, M. X., B. H. Camacho-Díaz, L. S. Meraz-Torres. et al. 2010. "Nanoencapsulation: A new trend in food engineering processing." *Food Engineering Reviews* 2:39–50.

Rao, J. P., and K. E. Geckeler. 2011. "Polymer nanoparticles: Preparation techniques and size-control parameters." *Progress in Polymer Science* 36:887–913.

Recharla, N., M. Riaz, S. Ko, and S. Park. 2017. "Novel technologies to enhance solubility of food-derived bioactive compounds: A review." *Journal of Functional Foods* 39:63–73.

Reis, C. P., R. J. Neufeld, A. J. Ribeiro, and F. Veiga. 2006. "Nanoencapsulation I. Methods for preparation of drug-loaded polymeric nanoparticles." *Nanomedicine* 2:8–21.

Reverchon, E., and G. Della Porta. 2003. "Particle design using supercritical fluids." *Chemical Engineering & Technology* 26:840–845.

Rodrigues, C. F., and J. C. Andrade. 2015. Milk proteins. In *Encyclopedia of Biomedical Polymers and Polymeric Biomaterials*, ed. M. Mishra, pp. 4756–4766. New York: Taylor & Francis Group.

Sanguansri, P., and M. A. Augustin. 2006. "Nanoscale materials development–A food industry perspective." *Trends in Food Science & Technology* 17:547–556.

Shpigelman, A., Y. Shoham, G Israeli-Lev, and Y. D. Livney. 2014. "β-Lactoglobulin–naringenin complexes: Nano-vehicles for the delivery of a hydrophobic nutraceutical." *Food Hydrocolloids* 40:214–224.

Silva, H. D., M. A. Cerqueira, and A. A. Vicente. 2012. "Nanoemulsions for food applications: Development and characterization." *Food and Bioprocess Technology* 5:854–867.

Soppimath, K. S., T. M. Aminabhavi, A. R. Kulkarni, and W. W. E. Rudzinski. 2001. "Biodegradable polymeric nanoparticles as drug delivery devices." *Journal of Controlled Release* 70:1–20.

Suganya, V., and V. Anuradha. 2017. "Microencapsulation and nanoencapsulation: A Review." *International Journal of Pharmaceutical and Clinical Research* 9:233–239

Tavares, G. M., T. Croguennec, A. F. Carvalho, and S. Bouhallab. 2014. "Milk proteins as encapsulation devices and delivery vehicles: Applications and trends." *Trends in Food Science & Technology* 37:5–20.

Thorat, A. A., and S. V. Dalvi. 2012. "Liquid antisolvent precipitation and stabilization of nanoparticles of poorly water soluble drugs in aqueous suspensions: Recent developments and future perspective." *Chemical Engineering Journal* 181:1–34.

Tice, T. R., and R. M. Gilley. 1985. "Preparation of injectable controlled-release microcapsules by a solvent-evaporation process." *Journal of Controlled Release* 2:343–352.

Troncoso, E., J. M. Aguilera, and D. J. McClements. 2011. "Development of nanoemulsions by an emulsification-evaporation technique." In *Proceedings of the 11th International Congress on Engineering and Food* (ICEF11), ed. P. S. Taoukis, N. G. Stoforos, V. T. Karathanos and G. D. Saravacos, pp. 929–930. Athens, Greece: Cosmosware.

Türk, M., and R. Lietzow. 2004. "Stabilized nanoparticles of phytosterol by rapid expansion from supercritical solution into aqueous solution." *Aaps PharmSciTech* 5:36–45.

Vauthier, C., and K. Bouchemal. 2009. "Methods for the preparation and manufacture of polymeric nanoparticles." *Pharmaceutical Research* 26:1025–1058.

Vrignaud, S., J. P. Benoit, and P. Saulnier. 2011. "Strategies for the nanoencapsulation of hydrophilic molecules in polymer-based nanoparticles." *Biomaterials* 32:8593–8604.

Wang, Y., P. Li, T. Truong-Dinh Tran, J. Zhang, and L. Kong. 2016. "Manufacturing techniques and surface engineering of polymer based nanoparticles for targeted drug delivery to cancer." *Nanomaterials* 6:26.

Yoon, H. K., T. R. Seo, and S. T. Lim. 2014. "Stabilization of aqueous dispersion of CoQ10 nanoparticles using maize starches." *Food Hydrocolloids*, 35:144–149.

Zhang, F. A., and C. L. Yu. 2007. "Acrylic emulsifier-free emulsion polymerization containing hydrophilic hydroxyl monomer in the presence or absence of nano-$SiO_2$." *European Polymer Journal* 43:1105–1111.

Zhang, L., P. Guan, Z. Zhang, Y. Dai, and L. Hao. 2018. "Physicochemical characteristics of complexes between amylose and garlic bioactive components generated by milling activating method." *Food Research International* 105:499–506.

Zhu, F. 2017. "Encapsulation and delivery of food ingredients using starch based systems." *Food Chemistry* 229:542–552.

Ziegler, A., K. Landfester, and A. Musyanovych. 2009. "Synthesis of phosphonate-functionalized polystyrene and poly(methyl methacrylate) particles and their kinetic behavior in miniemulsion polymerization." *Colloid and Polymer Science* 287:1261–1271.

Zimet, P., and Y. D. Livney. 2009. "Beta-lactoglobulin and its nanocomplexes with pectin as vehicles for ω-3 polyunsaturated fatty acids." *Food Hydrocolloids* 23:1120–1126.

# 4 Lipid-Based Nanosystems Production

*Peter X. Chen and Michael A. Rogers*

## CONTENTS



## 4.1 INTRODUCTION

Lipids serve a long list of biological functions from energy storage to cell signaling. In the context of foods, lipids contribute to flavor and texture, which often get their attributes from the nanoscale properties of the lipids (Forss 1969). Lipids not only impart their own unique flavor attributes, they can also absorb and preserve flavors derived from other sources and act as a flavor carrier. The long carbon chains found in lipids provide the structural framework that helps bread rise, makes whipped cream, shortens flaky pastries, and provide stability to foams (Gunstone and Norris 2013). Fats are able to form structures around air bubbles allowing for complex foams. Lipids are also of central importance for the formation of emulsions which are typically uniform dispersions of fat or oil into water and vice versa. In the culinary world, emulsions help produce flavor and texture and are often present in salad dressing, mayonnaise, gravies, sauces, among other preparations (McClements 2015). Similarly, lipid emulsions can also be employed as carrier for natural bioactive compounds with improved oral bioavailability and biological efficacies (Borel and Sabliov 2014).

Driven by increasing consumer demand for healthy food products and functional foods, advances in nanotechnology can be applied in designing novel food products containing health-promoting bioactive phytochemicals that improve well-being of consumers (Alasalvar and Bolling 2015; Pan et al. 2008). With respect to their pharmacological efficacy, absorption and bioavailability are often unpredictable and highly variable due to varying conditions throughout the gastrointestinal tract (Aditya and Ko 2015). Varied acidic medium in the stomach, first pass metabolism, presence of degrading enzymes, and the binding of the compounds to the food matrix are all factors that can affect absorption and oral bioavailability (Jiang et al. 2016; Thummel and Wilkinson 1998). The poor water solubility of some bioactives lead to low and variable oral bioavailability, which limits effectiveness.

Limitations affecting the overall effectiveness of active pharmaceutical ingredients were addressed by the pharmaceutical industry by loading the drug onto a colloidal carrier system. One of the first particulate carriers investigated was the oil-in-water (O/W) emulsion originally developed in the 1950s (Sarangi and Padhi 2016). Emulsions suffered from physical instability and poor range of drug soluble carrier oils. Phospholipids and liposomes showed some promise in the late 1980s and early 1990s, however, cost impediments and the lack of cost-effective pharmaceutical liposomes limited the total number of products on the market (Müller et al. 2000). Polymeric microparticles as a delivery system also suffered from limited product development largely due to the cytotoxicity of polymers and the absence of large scale production methods (Smith and Hunneyball 1986). In the early 1990s, research shifted to solid lipid nanoparticles (SLNs) since lipids are well tolerated by the body and large scale production was possible and cost-effective (Ekambaram and Sathali 2012; Müller et al. 2000). Lipid-based nanosystems improve stability, solubility, control delivery, enhance bioavailability, improve effectiveness, and reduce side-effects of food bioactives (Mendes et al. 2016). Nanoparticles (smaller than 100 nm in at least one dimension) show great potential to act as delivery systems due to their size-dependent properties. In particular, lipid nanoparticles exhibit advantages in terms of biocompatibility, versatility, and physicochemical and biological properties, such as, increased surface area to mass ratios compared to colloidal particles. This creates a larger reactive surface area and enhances their ability to adsorb and carry active compounds (Wilczewska et al. 2012).

Lipid delivery nanosystems vary depending on their formulation type, structure, and particle size. This chapter will examine the preparation of lipid-based nanosystems including nanoemulsions (NEs), SLNs, nanostructure lipid carriers (NLCs), and lipid nanocrystals. Nanoscale morphology greatly impacts delivery of encapsulated molecules. Therefore, the characterization of nanoparticles is significant and tools such as X-ray diffraction (XRD) and differential scanning calorimetry (DSC), to only name a few, can offer precious information on organization, shape, and dimensions of nanostructures.

## 4.2 LIPID-BASED NANOSYSTEMS

Lipid nanoscale objects are attracting significant attention due to the properties that arise at the nanoscale, which are necessary for therapeutic applications. There is a demand for safe and non-toxic delivery systems to encapsulate, protect, and release lipophilic bioactive and functional compounds that are both important for the food and pharmaceutical industries. Lipid-based delivery systems are a proven commercially viable strategy to formulate products for oral, topical, pulmonary, and parenteral delivery (Lim et al. 2012). The process involves administering the product followed by the release of the active ingredient and its subsequent transport across the biological membranes to the target site (Jain 2008). Many contentious factors are involved in developing a suitable delivery system (Table 4.1). Lipid-based nanosystems offer many advantages including (Ekambaram and Sathali 2012; Wilczewska et al. 2012): (i) controlled and targeted release of active ingredients; (ii) biocompatibility of lipid-base materials; (iii) improved stability of target compound during digestion; (iv) high loading ability; and (v) economically feasible and potential for scale-up.

### 4.2.1 Nanoemulsions

NEs are liquid-liquid dispersions developed for controlled and targeted delivery of food bioactives, improved entrapment efficiency, and protection of bioactives from degradation (Carrillo-Navas and Cruz-Olivares 2012). NEs consist of two immiscible liquids (typically water and oil) mixed to form a single thermodynamically stable phase with the aid of appropriate surfactant or stabilizing agents. Droplet size for NE is usually less than ~200 nm; to create these small droplets, high external shear energy is required to overcome the Laplace pressure that arises due to the surface free energy associated with the newly created interface (Shah et al. 2010). The characteristic size of NE enables their translucent appearance, as the diameter of the droplet is less than that of visible light and their small size provides long-term stability against sedimentation and flocculation. NEs are commonly applied to delivery of hydrophobic food bioactives and biopharmaceutical classification system class II and class IV drugs because of the high loading capacity of hydrophobic molecules in the internal organic phase of the O/W emulsion (Fong et al. 2015; Kawabata et al. 2011; Williams et al. 2013). This nano-encapsulation also provides some protection against hydrolysis and enzymatic degradation during digestion (Anthony et al. 2012). Furthermore, the controlled, sustained release of bioactives or drugs reduce the frequency of drug administration (Lovelyn and Attama 2011).

Both high and low energy methods may be employed to created NE. High-energy approaches (i.e., high-pressure valve homogenizer and sonication) or top-down approaches use mechanical devices that generate disruptive forces to break down coarse emulsions (Qian and McClements 2011). Low energy approaches or bottom-up approaches (i.e., solvent evaporation and precipitation) exploit environmental conditions to spontaneously form small oil droplets (Sun and Yeo 2012). The size of the final emulsion droplets depends on numerous factors such as the

**TABLE 4.1**
**Summary of Lipid-Based Nanosystems and Their Features**

| Lipid Nanosystems | Preparation Method | Physical State | Advantage | Disadvantage | Function | References |
|---|---|---|---|---|---|---|
| Nanoemulsions | • Homogenization<br>• Microfluidization<br>• Ultrasonication<br>• Solvent diffusion<br>• Phase inversion technique | Lipid | • Large-scale production<br>• Delivery of poorly water-soluble compounds | • Rapid release<br>• Low stability | Nutraceutical system incorporating chia essential oil and ascorbic acid | Carrillo-Navas and Cruz-Olivares (2012) |
| Solid Lipid Nanoparticle | • Hot homogenization<br>• Cold homogenization<br>• Ultrasonication<br>• Microemulsion<br>• Solvent evaporation | Solid | • Large scale production<br>• High encapsulation efficiency<br>• Controlled release profile | • Recrystallization<br>• Drug expulsion<br>• Low encapsulation load | Improving bioavailability and bioactivity of diet-derived phytochemicals | Wang et al. (2014) |
| Nanostructure Lipid Carrier | • Hot homogenization<br>• Cold homogenization<br>• Ultrasonication<br>• Solvent evaporation | Solid | • High encapsulation load<br>• High stability | • Fast release compared to SLN | Lipid carrier of β-Carotene- | Oliveira and Michelon (2016) |

*(Continued)*

**TABLE 4.1** *(Continued)*
**Summary of Lipid-Based Nanosystems and Their Features**

| Lipid Nanosystems | Preparation Method | Physical State | Advantage | Disadvantage | Function | References |
|---|---|---|---|---|---|---|
| Lipid Nanopellet and Lipospheres | • Homogenization<br>• Hot dispersion<br>• Solvent evaporation | Solid | • Physical stability<br>• Low cost of ingredients<br>• Ease of preparation and scale-up<br>• High dispersibility in an aqueous medium<br>• High entrapment of hydrophobic drugs,<br>• Controlled particle size,<br>• Extended release of entrapped drug | • Low encapsulation efficiency for hydrophilic compounds | Liposheres as a carrier of lipid-based bioactive compounds | Swain et al. (2016) |
| Nanocrystal | • Homogenization<br>• Milling<br>• Precipitation | Solid Amorphous | • 100% encapsulation<br>• No organic solvents<br>• Increased dissolution velocity<br>• Increased saturation solubility | | Carrier of bioactive compounds for food applications | Borel and Sabliov (2014) |

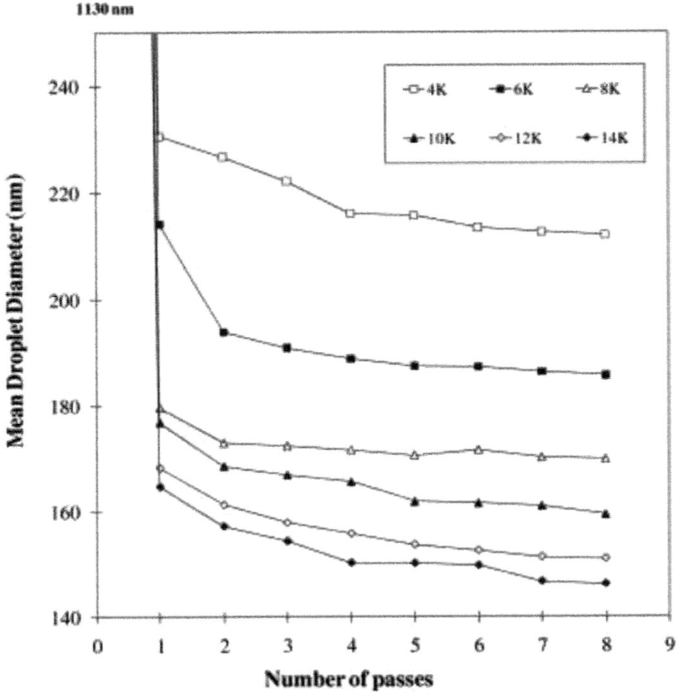


**FIGURE 4.1** Effect of microfluidization pressure (in kbar) and number of passes on the mean droplet diameter produced in 5 wt% corn oil-in-water emulsions containing 2 wt% of β-lactoglobulin. (Reproduced from Qian, C. and McClements, D.J., *Food Hydrocoll.*, 25, 1000–1008, 2011.)

type of homogenizer and its operating conditions (i.e., operating pressure, time, and temperature), as well as the sample conditions (i.e., type of surfactant added and concentration, oil type and concentration, and viscosity) (Figure 4.1).

### 4.2.2 Solid Lipid Nanoparticles

SLNs are typically made using high-melting point triglycerides or waxes which replace the liquid lipid component used in emulsions. The size of SLNs range between 80 and 1000 nm (Üner 2006). Key attributes to SLNs include good physical stability, protection of loaded compounds against degradation and hydrolysis, controlled and customizable release of bioactive compounds, and biocompatibility (Aditya and Ko 2015). SLNs are commonly 10- to 100-fold less cytotoxic than polymeric nanoparticles since the lipids used in their preparation have GRAS status (Aditya and Ko 2015). SLNs also offer a wide range of potential applications including intravenous, oral, dermal, or topical delivery. Due to the inherent crystalline structure of SLNs, they suffer from lower loading capacity and payload expulsion after crystallization (Tamjidi et al. 2013). SLNs prepared with highly purified lipids are more susceptible to crystallization in a somewhat perfect crystalline lattice structure. This limits the encapsulation potential for certain compounds. Encapsulated compounds tend to be incorporated between fatty acid chains, between lipid bilayers, or in the amorphous regions within crystal imperfections. Therefore, densely packed perfect lipid crystalline structures will limit loading and lead to expulsion during storage as the crystalline structure adopts a lower energy state, which is typically the more organized β polymorphic form (Westesen et al. 1997) (Figure 4.2).

The structure and shape of the lipid particles alters the bioactive loading efficiency and release profile. Spherically shaped isometric SLN, with minimal crystalline order, will have high loading capacities and greater controlled release of encapsulated compounds compared to thin highly ordered platelets with dense structures (Westesen et al. 2001). SLNs with α-polymorphic crystal typically undergo polymorphic transitions during storage leading to rearrangement of triacylglyceride molecules resulting in the expulsion of encapsulated compounds. Polymorphic transitions from α- to β-crystals leads to destabilization and a change from spherical to platelet shape (Helgason et al. 2008). Trujillo and Wright (2010) found that surfactant concentration and pressure plays a significant role in particle diameter, whereas the number of homogenization cycles did not. Using 10% fully hydrogenated canola stearin and 5% of Poloxamer 188 as the non-ionic surfactant, they found particles exclusively in the β form and no changes to particle size was observed over a span of 240 days at 4°C and 20°C (Trujillo and Wright 2010).

Food applications for SLNs include improving shelf life of certain fruits, stabilizing bioactives such as curcumin, resveratrol, quercetin, and epigallocatechin gallate (Ting et al. 2014; Wang et al. 2014; Zambrano-Zaragoza and

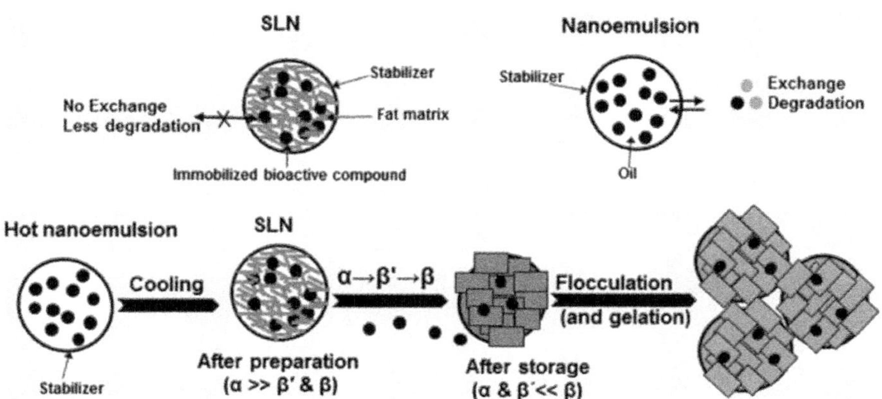


**FIGURE 4.2** Schematic presentation of defects of nanoemulsion (in comparison to SLN; Upper: Modified from Weiss, J. et al., *Food Biophys.*, 3, 146–154, 2008.) and SLN (Lower). After preparation of SLN by cooling a hot nanoemulsion, the droplets crystallize, at least partially, in higher energy modifications α and β′. During storage, these modifications transform to the low energy, more ordered β modification. A burst release is observed for nanoemulsion and for SLN during polymorphism. (Reproduced from Tamjidi, F. et al., *Innov. Food Sci. Emerg. Technol.*, 19, 29–43, 2013.)

Mercado-Silva 2013). Yu and Huang (2012) developed an organogel consisting of a non-polar semisolid gel made up of a gelator and a non-polar lipid solvent. This formulation allowed for better physical stability and loading capacity of compounds. In their study, curcumin incorporated into the organogel-derived formulation showed a 9.8-fold improvement in oral bioavailability when compared to curcumin water suspension (Yu and Huang 2012).

### 4.2.3 Nanostructure Lipid Carriers

A colloidal carrier system known as NLCs was developed to overcome some of the limitations associated with SLNs. NLCs are characterized by a solid lipid core comprised of a mixture of solid fat and liquid oil with mean particle size within the nanometer range. This nanostructure allows for increased drug loading and retention during storage compared to the SLN system by adopting a less organized solid lipid matrix (Tamjidi et al. 2013). NLCs also have low water content and are less inclined to unpredictable gelation tendencies (Tamjidi et al. 2013). Three types of NLCs have been introduced: imperfect type NLC (blended solid and fluid lipids leads to a highly disordered nanostructure allowing free spaces and amorphous clusters for the accommodation of drug/bioactive molecules); multiple type NLC (drugs are dissolved in oils and protected from degradation by the surrounding solid lipid); and amorphous type NLC (lipid matrix is solid, but in an amorphous state thereby preventing drug expulsion by crystallization) (Selvamuthukumar 2012) (Figure 4.3).

NLC have been used in encapsulating β-carotene by way of the high-pressure melt-homogenization method. The produced nanocarriers had a particle size of approximately 300 nm and displayed emulsion stability with no polymorph transitions over a period of 7 months (Hentschel et al. 2008). Tristearin/high oleic sunflower oil was used to produce β-carotene encapsulated NLC. In this study, SLNs and NLCs were produced using the solvent displacement method. The results showed NLC

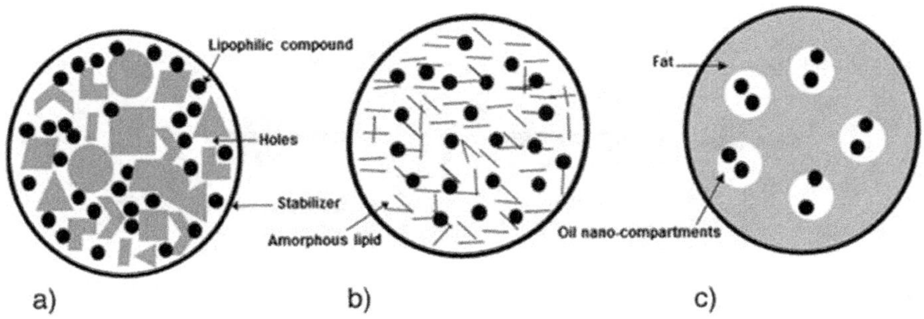


**FIGURE 4.3** Schematic presentation of three types of nanostructure lipid carriers. NLC retard polymorphic transition to more thermodynamically stable forms and reduce the overall crystallinity of lipid nanoparticles: (a) Imperfect type NLC, (b) amorphous type NLC, and (c) multiple type NLC. (Reproduced from Tamjidi, F. et al., *Innov. Food Sci. Emerg. Technol.*, 19, 29–43, 2013.)

displayed marked advantages over SLN including improvement in loading capacity and prevention of drug expulsion (Oliveira and Michelon 2016).

### 4.2.4 Lipid Nanopellets and Lipospheres

Lipid nanopellets are produced by dispersing a melted lipid in a hot surfactant solution by stirring or sonication (Speiser 1986). Solid particles are formed when the emulsion is cooled to room temperature and the lipid recrystallizes to produce lipid nanopellets. Particle diameter of the nanopellets range from 50 to 1000 nm. Intensity of stirring and surfactant concentration can influence particle size. Similarly, lipospheres are produced by dispersing a melted hydrophobic core in a hot surfactant solution and using sonication as the dispersing technique (Severino et al. 2012). Cooling to room temperature leads to the formation of solid lipospheres, which are characterized by a phospholipid layer surrounding the hydrophobic core material (Domb 2005). The suspension is solely stabilized by the phospholipid layer and as a result, lipospheres tend to have a semi-solid ointment-like consistency (Swain et al. 2016; Westesen et al. 1997). The influence of preparation parameters were studied by Cortesi et al. (2002) and included type and amount of lipids, presence and concentration of stabilizers, stirring speed, and type of stirrer. Lipospheres produced by melt dispersion with high percent recovery (82%) with a mean diameter of 80 μm and a narrow size distribution required the use of a lipid composition of cetyl alcohol/cholesterol (2:1, w/w), a 5% of 50 bloom gelatin as stabilizer, and 1000 rpm stirring speed (Cortesi et al. 2002).

Protein hydrolysates have been successfully encapsulated in lipospheres in order to reduce the perception of bitterness. The melt dispersion process was used by adding the casein hydrolysate to stearic acid melted at 70°C. Soybean phosphatidylcoline was added to the matrix and homogenized for 3 min at 9500 rpm prior to quench cooling to 20°C (Barbosa et al. 2004). Microscopy analysis revealed an average particle size of 5 μm. Encapsulation efficiency ranged between 50% and 83% depending on hydrolysis conditions. Chemical stability was achieved for a period of 60 days of refrigerated storage (Barbosa et al. 2004).

### 4.2.5 Nanocrystals

Nanocrystals offer the distinct advantage in that they can be prepared without the use of any organic solvents. Nanocrystals consist of a bioactive molecule surrounded by a surfactant. This results in 100% bioactive loading and improves the solubility of poorly water soluble bioactives (Borel and Sabliov 2014). Nanocrystals are particles within nanometer size range and have a crystalline character (Junghanns and Müller 2008). Dispersed nanocrystals in a liquid media generally require a stabilizing agent such as a surfactant or polymeric stabilizers to keep them suspended in solution. Depending on preparation techniques employed, nanocrystals can be in the crystalline or amorphous form. The latter is often referred to as nanocrystals in the amorphous state and possesses advantages such as higher saturation solubility compared to crystalline state. Nanocrystals can be used for loading of bioactives such as lutein and have been shown to enhance dissolution rate *in vivo* (Sun and Yeo 2012). Other applications in food include starch and protein nanocrystals, which were recently developed (Neto et al. 2013; Silvério et al. 2013).

## 4.3 PREPARATION TECHNIQUES

General excipients are required to prepare lipid-based nanosystems and includes: lipids, surfactants, co-emulsifiers, and water. SLN, for example, uses a solid lipid core while other colloidal carrier systems use liquid oil. Surfactants drive the desired O/W or water-in-oil type emulsion and stabilize the dispersion (Angelova et al. 2017). During homogenization, reduction in particle size leads to increased surface area and exposes new lipid surfaces. Surfactants are required at high concentrations in order to prevent agglomeration of newly uncovered lipid surfaces. Low molecular weight surfactants (e.g., polyhydroxy) have been shown to take less time for redistribution between new particle surfaces and micelles (Kovacevic et al. 2011).

Nanoparticle production can be classified as the top-down and bottom-up categories. The top-down approach involves size-reduction of large particles to nanometer range using energy intensive methods (Angelova et al. 2017). Most often, the top-down approach requires high-pressure homogenization or sonication and a general application of force either by compression, impact, or shear. In high-pressure homogenization, the formation of very fine emulsion droplets due to high shear stress occurs (Qian and McClements 2011; Yuan et al. 2008). Similarly, microfluidization utilizes shear stress, but is optimized in its design to produce higher shear and impact forces for tighter particle size distribution compared to that of traditional high-pressure homogenization (Jo and Kwon 2014). Microfluidization has already been successfully used in the production of salad dressing, syrups, chocolate and malted drinks, flavor oil emulsions, creams, yogurts, fillings, and icings (Swientek 1990).

In contrast, bottom-up approach generates nanoparticles by self-assembly properties of molecules. This requires control over thermodynamic properties and control of repulsion and attraction forces between molecules used as building blocks to form functional supramolecular structures (Chan and Kwok 2011). Temperature, concentration, pH and ionic strength, mechanical force, or electric and magnetic field strengths are common controls. Controlled precipitation or crystallization and evaporation are a few methods commonly employed. The bottom-up approach requires minimal energy input, but the resulting nanoparticles can be crystalline or amorphous and control over crystal growth rate must be in place (Angelova et al. 2017).

### 4.3.1 High-Pressure Homogenization

High-pressure homogenization is the method of choice for producing SLN, NLC, and NE (Shah et al. 2010). Homogenization occurs at elevated temperature (hot homogenization technique) or at room temperature or below (cold homogenization technique). In both cases, the bioactive is first dissolved in molten lipid at 5°C–10°C above its melting point. In the hot homogenization technique, the bioactive-lipid melt is dispersed using a high-speed stirrer in a hot aqueous surfactant solution.

This produces a coarse pre-emulsion with a desirable droplet size in the micrometer range. The pre-emulsion is then homogenized using a high-pressure homogenizer at pressures ranging from 10000 to 150000 kPa (Mehnert and Mäder 2001). It is important to note that although high temperatures generally result in lower particle sizes, this can also accelerate degradation of the drug and the carrier. The elevated pressure during the homogenization process also increases the temperature by approximately 10°C/50000 kPa. Homogenization can be repeated for consecutive cycles however, 3–5 cycles at 50000–150000 kPa is sufficient to reach the nanoscale (Muchow et al. 2008; Sarangi and Padhi 2016). Due to the small particle size and the presence of emulsifiers, the crystallization process may take several months with the sample remaining in a super cooled melt state.

Hydrophilic bioactives have a tendency to partition into the aqueous phase during hot homogenization and can result in low entrapment. Alternatively, cold homogenization technique is much more suitable for hydrophilic drugs (Aditya and Ko 2015). The bioactive-lipid melt is solidified on dry ice or liquid nitrogen to render it brittle for the milling process. This rapid cooling also allows for a more homogenous distribution of the drug in the solid matrix. A mortar mill is used to generate microparticles ranging in size between 50 and 100 μm and is dispersed in a cold aqueous surfactant solution (Üner 2006). The lipid suspension is then homogenized at room temperature or below. In general, cold homogenization produces larger particles with a wider size distribution as compared to the hot homogenization technique. The solid nature of the matrix during cold homogenization, does, however, minimize partitioning of the drug into the water phase. Heat-sensitive drugs can also take advantage of the cold homogenization technique. The cold homogenization technique also overcomes complexity of the crystallization step (Shah et al. 2015).

Homogenization conditions and emulsifier type and concentration have been shown to greatly impact particle size (Qian and McClements 2011). Increasing homogenization pressure and number of cycles can decrease mean particle diameter in a linear relationship. The study also showed that after six cycles at 1400000 kPa, the minimum achievable droplet diameter strongly depended on the type and concentration of emulsifier used. Small-molecule surfactants, e.g., Tween 20 and sodium dodecyl sulfate at high concentration (10 wt%) were found to produce smaller droplet sizes than biopolymers (e.g., β-lactoglobulin or caseinate) (Qian and McClements 2011). Similarly, O/W NE of β-carotene produced by high-pressure homogenization using Tween 20 had the smallest particle size and narrowest size distribution (Yuan et al. 2008). The particle sizes also decreased with increasing homogenization pressure and cycle. Meanwhile, the physical stability of the NE decreased at high temperature and increased at elevated pressures and increased homogenization cycles (Yuan et al. 2008).

### 4.3.2 Microemulsion

The microemulsion technique was developed by Gasco to produce SLN based on the precipitation of fine lipid droplets (Gasco 1993). A warm O/W microemulsion is produced using melted lipid at 65°C–70°C. Typically, low melting fatty acids are used such as stearic acid. Surfactants and co-surfactants include polysorbate 20, soy phosphatidylcholine sodium monocrylphosphate, and also alcohols such as butanol. Surfactants and co-surfactants are heated to the same temperature and added to the mixture under stirring. This produces a clear, optically transparent microemulsion mixture, which is then dispersed in cold water (2°C–3°C) under mechanical stirring. Ratio of warm microemulsion to cold water typically lies within the 1:25–1:50 range (Flanagan and Singh 2006). Small particle size is maintained due to precipitation as opposed to being mechanically induced by the stirring process. No energy is required to reduce particle size since the submicron droplet structure is contained within the microemulsion. Nanoparticle size has been shown to increase with increase in the alcohol chain length of the co-solvents (Chin et al. 2014). This is likely due to the lipophilicity of the co-surfactant that increases with the carbon chain length, rendering it less effective because it is more soluble in the oil phase (Chin et al. 2014). Special consideration to the regulatory process should be considered as the use of excipients such as butanol is less favorable. Disadvantages to this method include high water content and the use of surfactants and co-surfactants at high concentrations.

Preparation of anthocyanin-loaded SLN using the microemulsion dilution method was optimized in a recent study (Ravanfar et al. 2016). Based on their preliminary results, the most appropriate components for SLN preparation include palmitic acid as the lipid phase, Span 85 and lecithin as surfactants, ethanol as co-surfactant, and Pluronic $F_{127}$ as aqueous phase stabilizer (Ravanfar et al. 2016). Entrapment efficiency and particle size was evaluated using the Placket-Burman model and was reduced to highlight the significant factors (Ravanfar et al. 2016). The type of co-surfactant was a significant factor with ethanol proving to have an important effect on particle size, polydispersity, and stability of the resulting NE (Ravanfar et al. 2016). It has been reported that ethanol influences the curvature of the interface by altering the polarity of the polar and non-polar phases and increases interface flexibility of the surfactant film and, consequently, favors the formation of a microemulsion (Feng et al. 2009). According to Quintanar-Guerrero et al. solvents with higher water miscibility form smaller lipid nanoparticles likely due to different diffusion rates in contrast to low water miscible solvents which slow the transport of lipid molecules into the aqueous phase leading to aggregation resulting in large lipid nanoparticles (Quintanar-Guerrero et al. 2005).

Another factor shown to influence the entrapment efficiency was lipid concentration. This factor had a significant negative effect on entrapment with no effect on particle size. This is explained in terms of the aggregation tendency of lipids at higher concentration preventing solvent diffusion and, consequently, fewer lipid molecules are carried into the aqueous phase and inhibit the formation of small lipid aggregates (Ravanfar et al. 2016). Increased amounts of stabilizers such as the polymer Pluronic $F_{127}$ resulted in decreased particle size and increased entrapment efficiency (Ravanfar et al. 2016). Stabilizer can influence the crystallinity and lipid polymorphic transition kinetics after nanoparticle crystallization (Rizzo et al. 2015). Lastly, increasing the duration of stirring from 2 to 15 min resulted in the formation of larger particles and lower encapsulation efficiency (Blasi et al. 2011; Ravanfar et al. 2016). This is likely due to droplet size reduction generating a large interface, which is not well stabilized by the surfactant (Blasi et al. 2011).

### 4.3.3 Solvent Evaporation—Emulsification

SLN can also be produced by a precipitation method that requires the evaporation of an organic solvent. An O/W emulsion is first produced by dissolving a lipid in an organic solvent and stirring in an aqueous phase containing surfactant. Stirring is continuous and under ambient or reduced pressure conditions in order to evaporate the organic solvent. Precipitation of the lipid particle dispersion into the aqueous medium occurs upon evaporation of the solvent. Depending on the lipid and surfactant used, particles ranging from 30 to 100 nm can be produced (Siekmann and Westesen 1996). A clear disadvantage to this technique is the need for an organic solvent often times chloroform. However, the avoidance of heat is an important advantage most notably to heat labile compounds.

Similarly, solvent emulsification is based on emulsion diffusion in an aqueous system (Das et al. 2011). A lipid is dissolved in an organic solvent in a water bath. Coacervation and the formation of lipid nanoparticles occur upon addition of water to the organic phase with mechanical agitation. The obtained lipid nanoparticles are separated by centrifugation, evaporation under reduced pressure, or by filtration. In both solvent evaporation and emulsification techniques, the concentration of the obtained suspension is limited due to low solubility of lipids in the organic solvents (Üner 2006). While particle concentration can be up to 80% using the high-pressure homogenization technique, solvent evaporation and emulsification is limited to up to 15% (Üner 2006). Residual solvent toxicity is another issue plaguing these solvent techniques (Trotta et al. 2003).

Lipospheres obtained by solvent evaporation had a smaller size, but poor mechanical properties with respect to particles produced by the melt dispersion technique (Cortesi et al. 2002). In terms of liposphere recovery efficiency, size distribution, and surface morphology, the best combination of parameters consisted of a lipid composition of tristearin/monostearate (66:34, w/w) with a methacrylic polymer, a 1%(w/w) polyvinyl alcohol solution, a 750 rpm stirring speed, and a 55 mm three-blade turbine rotor (Cortesi et al. 2002).

### 4.3.4 Microfluidization

Microfluidization is used to produce uniform NE. The process uses a high-pressure pump (3447.38–137895.146 kPa) that displaces the aqueous and oily phase through the interaction chamber consisting of small channels called "microchannels." An impingement area along the microchannels produces very fine particles in the submicron range. The combination of the two phases results in a coarse emulsion that is passed through the microfluidizer repeatedly until a stable NE is attained. Filtering under nitrogen removes larger droplets. High-pressure homogenization and microfluidization are appropriate methods for production of NE at industrial scale (Shah et al. 2010).

In the preparation of β-carotene NE as an active ingredient in functional beverages, microfluidization parameters were evaluated in order to determine the optimum conditions. Pressure, number of cycles, type of emulsifier and concentration, and their effects on particles size and stability were assessed. Increase in microfluidization pressure (120 MPa), number of cycles (3), and concentration of emulsifier decreased the droplet size from 416 to 97.2 nm (Jo and Kwon 2014). Physical stability was achieved for a period of 5 weeks at room temperature with considerably slower degradation in whey protein isolate-stabilized NE compared to Tween 20-stabilized (Jo and Kwon 2014). NE of essential oils, which may serve as a preservative coating on freshly cut fruits, were prepared by microfluidization technique of a coarse emulsion. The coarse emulsion was stabilized by sodium alginate and Tween 80 and was prepared by high shear homogenization. NEs were then formed from the coarse emulsions using a microfluidization system set to a constant pressure of 150 MPa and three cycles (Salvia-Trujillo et al. 2015).

### 4.3.5 Phase Inversion Temperature

The phase inversion temperature technique is a low-energy method that makes use of the phase transitions taking place during the emulsification process. It was first introduced by Shinoda and Saito and is based on the changes in solubility of polyoxyethylene-type non-ionic surfactants with temperature (Shinoda and Saito 1968). At higher temperature, these types of surfactants become more lipophilic. At intermediate temperature, a hydrophilic-lipophilic balance temperature is achieved and a bicontinuous microemulsion phase exists. This is also referred to as the phase inversion temperature. At this temperature, the low interfacial tension promotes emulsification, however, coalescence can occur rapidly, and, consequently, the emulsion is very unstable (Friberg et al. 2011). Stable emulsions with very small droplet size and narrow size distribution can be obtained by rapidly heating or cooling (by 25°C–30°C) the emulsion from hydrophilic-lipophilic balance temperature (Lovelyn and Attama 2011). Cooling produces O/W emulsions while heating produces water-in-oil emulsions. Here, the changes in solubility of non-ionic type surfactants such as polyoxyethylene are exploited. At low temperature, the surfactant monolayer has a large positive spontaneous curvature exposing the polar head group rendering it more hydrophilic and forming oil-swollen micellar solution phases (O/W microemulsions). At high temperature, the spontaneous curvature becomes largely negative and the acyl chains are exposed and the surfactant becomes more lipophilic and as a result forms water-swollen reverse micelles (water-in-oil microemulsions) (Mouritsen 2011).

NE made using this method tends to be highly unstable and prone to droplet coalescence. A potential solution was developed using a water/surfactant/oil system (Rao and McClements 2010). A non-ionic surfactant was used (Brij 30, $C_{12}E_4$) and the oil phase consisted of a tetradecane. NEs were formed by holding water/surfactant/oil at their phase inversion temperature followed by rapid cooling. Optimum storage temperature was at 13°C while higher temperatures led to increased droplet growth due to coalescence and lower temperatures led to gelation. Stability at ambient temperature or during heating was improved by adding either a non-ionic surfactant (Tween 80) or an anionic surfactant sodium dodecyl sulfate (Rao and McClements 2010).

## 4.4 CHARACTERIZING LIPID NANOPARTICLES

Parameters that are commonly considered important in characterizing nanomaterials include zeta potential and particle size, crystallinity and lipid modification, and the co-existence of additional colloidal structures (Shah et al. 2015). Particle size and the size distribution are critical parameters used to characterize the product in terms of stability and quality. Particle charge and zeta potential are used to predict storage stability of colloidal dispersions. High zeta potential will prevent particle aggregation due to electrical repulsion (Bunjes and Unruh 2007; Mehnert and Mäder 2001). Another key determinant to quality is the lipid crystallinity of the final product. The emulsified dispersion must be cooled below the critical crystallization temperature of the lipid during production. This ensures the final product is not in the liquid state consisting of an emulsion of supercooled liquid particles. Crystallinity and lipid modification play a key role in drug incorporation and drug release rates. In brief, a less ordered lattice arrangement favors increased drug loading (Hou et al. 2003).

### 4.4.1 Particle Size and Zeta Potential

Common techniques for routine particle size measurements include photon correlation spectroscopy (PCS) and laser diffraction (LD). PCS is also known as dynamic light scattering and is used to measure the fluctuation of the scattered light intensity caused by particle movement. Particles ranging from nanometers to micrometers can be measured using this method. For larger particles the LD method, which detects size based on diffraction angle of the particle radius, is used (Keck 2010). At high angles, smaller particles will cause more intense scattering than larger particles. LD has a distinct advantage in that it can measure a broad range of particle sizes from nanometer to lower millimeter range. Sensitivity can be enhanced using polarization intensity differential scattering technology, however, it is still highly recommended to simply use both PCS and LD simultaneously (Keck 2010). PCS and LD were used to characterize SLNs and NLCs made from polyhydroxy surfactants. These techniques provided information such as particle size and polydispersity indices using PCS and unimodal size distribution using LD (Kovacevic et al. 2011).

Particle size measurements rely heavily on indirect measurement of light scattering effects which are used to calculate particle sizes. Limitations may occur when non-spherical particle shapes are present. Platelet structure, for example, is a common occurrence during lipid crystallization and in SLN (Marangoni et al. 2012). Another potential limitation is the lack of particle size uniformity. Light microscopy is useful in providing information on the presence and character of microparticles, however, it is not sensitive in the nanometer size range (Yadav et al. 2013). Particle shape can be assessed using electron microscopy, but special attention should be paid to the presence of artifacts caused by the preparation technique (Lacatusu et al. 2013). Zeta potential is an important parameter that assesses the stability of the colloidal dispersion. Zeta potential is a measure of charge derived from the particles and the electrolytes present in the dispersion medium surrounding the particles during storage. High zeta potential indicates high electric repulsion which means that particle aggregation is less likely to occur. The addition of steric stabilizers will decrease zeta potential therefore the previously mentioned statement should not be strictly applied in all cases (Schubert and Müller-Goymann 2005).

### 4.4.2 Crystallinity and Lipid Modification

Differential scanning calorimetry (DSC) is used to analyze the state and thermodynamic properties of the lipid by measuring heat exchanges that occur when the lipid is melting or crystallizing (Bunjes and Unruh 2007). Different lipid properties will imply different melting points, and thus melting enthalpies. Lipid crystallinity and lipid modification are important parameters in that they are strongly correlated with bioactive loading capacity (Müller et al. 2000). In less ordered crystal states or amorphous states, less energy is required to overcome the lattice forces (Üner 2006). Therefore, lower melting enthalpy is observed compared to higher ordered lattice arrangement. It should be noted that DSC alone cannot identify the cause of a thermal despite being able to detect even minute changes in thermal properties. For this, complementary analysis must be performed such as microscopy, XRD, or spectrometry in order to determine if the thermal events were the cause of water loss, polymorphic transitions, melting, or decomposition of the substance (Bunjes and Unruh 2007).

NLCs consisting of ω-3 fatty acid-enriched fish oils used as a delivery system for lutein were characterized by DSC in order to determine the effects of loading on melt behavior and crystallinity (Lacatusu et al. 2013). Modifications to the lipid network can be detected after lutein encapsulation underlining a less ordered crystalline structure when compared to free NLC. DSC analysis also revealed depression of the main melting points and endothermic peaks following increase in fish oil concentration. This would suggest lattice defects inside the lipid core exemplified by many imperfections present within the matrix which would consequently favor lutein entrapment amounts and efficiencies (Lacatusu et al. 2013).

XRD allows differentiation of the various polymorphs. XRD does so by characterizing the spacings of polymorphic forms distinguishing between long and short spacings of the lipid lattice. XRD is therefore only able to differentiate between amorphous and crystalline states while DSC can differentiate between amorphous solids and liquids. XRD is typically used in conjunction with DSC as a measurement used to confirm polymorphism behaviors previously established by DSC alone (Bunjes and Unruh 2007).

## 4.5 CONCLUSIONS

There is considerable interest in lipid-based nanosystems particularly as a delivery agent for bioactive compounds in foods. It has been proven to increase bioavailability, enhance solubility, and protection of food ingredients. In this chapter, we attempted to provide an overview of the most common lipid-based encapsulation systems, namely, NEs, SLNs, NLCs, lipid nanopellets and lipospheres, and nanocrystals. Recent studies have revealed that SLNs and NLCs offer considerable advantages in terms of stability, longer and sustained release profiles compared to the other aforementioned systems. Future research topics should include studies pertaining to the physicochemical properties and interaction within food systems where nanoencapsulated ingredients have been incorporated. As well, release kinetics should be ameliorated using available equations and novel modeling techniques.

## REFERENCES

Aditya, N. P., and S. Ko. 2015. "Solid lipid nanoparticles (SLNs): Delivery vehicles for food bioactives." *Rsc Advances* no. 5:30902–30911.

Alasalvar, C., and B. W. Bolling. 2015. "Review of nut phytochemicals, fat-soluble bioactives, antioxidant components and health effects." *British Journal of Nutrition* no. 113:S68–S78.

Angelova, A., V. M. Garamus, B. Angelov, and Z. Tian. 2017. "Advances in structural design of lipid-based nanoparticle carriers for delivery of macromolecular drugs, phytochemicals and anti-tumor agents." *Advances in Colloid and Interface Science* no. 249:331–345.

Anthony, A., A. Mumuni, and F. Philip. 2012. *Recent Advances in Novel Drug Carrier Systems*. Rijeka, Croatia: INTECH Open Access Publisher.

Barbosa, C., H. A. Morais, and F. M. Delvivo. 2004. "Papain hydrolysates of casein: Molecular weight profile and encapsulation in lipospheres." *Journal of the Science of Food and Agriculture* no. 84:1891–1900.

Blasi, P., S. Giovagnoli, A. Schoubben, and C. Puglia. 2011. "Lipid nanoparticles for brain targeting I. Formulation optimization." *International Journal of Pharmaceuticals* no. 419:287–295.

Borel, T., and C. M. Sabliov. 2014. "Nanodelivery of bioactive components for food applications: Types of delivery systems, properties, and their effect on ADME profiles and toxicity of nanoparticles." *Annual Review of Food Science and Technology* no. 5:197–213.

Bunjes, H., and T. Unruh. 2007. "Characterization of lipid nanoparticles by differential scanning calorimetry, X-ray and neutron scattering." *Advanced Drug Delivery Reviews* no. 59:379–402.

Carrillo-Navas, H., and J. Cruz-Olivares. 2012. "Rheological properties of a double emulsion nutraceutical system incorporating chia essential oil and ascorbic acid stabilized by carbohydrate polymer—protein blends." *Carbohydrate Polymers* no. 87:1231–1235.

Chan, H.-K., and P. Kwok. 2011. "Production methods for nanodrug particles using the bottom-up approach." *Advanced Drug Delivery Reviews* no. 63(6):406–416.

Chin, S. F., A. Azman, and S. C. Pang. 2014. "Size controlled synthesis of starch nanoparticles by a microemulsion method." *Journal of Nanomaterials* no. 9:1–7.

Cortesi, R., E. Esposito, G. Luca, and C. Nastruzzi. 2002. "Production of lipospheres as carriers for bioactive compounds." *Biomaterials* no. 23:2283–2294.

Das, S., and A. Chaudhury. 2011. "Recent advances in lipid nanoparticle formulations with solid matrix for oral drug delivery." *AAPS PharmSciTech* no. 12(1):62–76.

Domb, A. J. 2005. Lipospheres for controlled delivery of substances. In *Microencapsulation Methods and Industrial Applications, Second Edition*, Simon Benita (ed.), pp. 297–316. Informa Healthcare.

Ekambaram, P., and A. A. H. Sathali. 2012. "Solid lipid nanoparticles: A review." *Scientific Reviews and Chemical Communications* no. 2(1):80–102.

Feng, J. L., Z. W. Wang, J. Zhang, Z. N. Wang, and F. Liu. 2009. "Study on food-grade vitamin E microemulsions based on nonionic emulsifiers." *Colloids and Surfaces A: Physicochemical and Engineering Aspects* no. 339:1–6.

Flanagan, J., and H. Singh. 2006. "Microemulsions: A potential delivery system for bioactives in food." *Critical Reviews in Food Science and Nutrition* no. 46:221–237.

Fong, S. Y., A. Ibisogly, and A. Bauer-Brandl. 2015. "Solubility enhancement of BCS Class II drug by solid phospholipid dispersions: Spray drying versus freeze-drying." *International Journal of Pharmaceutics* no. 496(2):382–391.

Forss, D. A. 1969. "Role of lipids in flavors." *Journal of Agricultural and Food Chemistry* no. 4:681–685.

Friberg, S. E., R. W. Corkery, and I. A. Blute. 2011. "Phase inversion temperature (PIT) emulsification process." *Journal of Chemical & Engineering Data* no. 56(12):4282–4290.

Gasco, M. R. 1993. Method for producing solid lipid microspheres having a narrow size distribution. U.S. Patent. 5,250,236.

Gunstone, F. D., and F. A. Norris. 2013. *Lipids in Foods: Chemistry, Biochemistry and Technology*. Kent, UK: Elsevier Science.

Helgason, T., T. S. Awad, K. Kristbergsson, D. J. McClements, and J. Weiss. 2008. "Influence of polymorphic transformations on gelation of tripalmitin solid lipid nanoparticle suspensions." *Journal of the American Oil Chemists' Society* no. 85(6):501–511.

Hentschel, A., S. Gramdorf, and R. H. Müller. 2008. "β-Carotene-loaded nanostructured lipid carriers." *Journal of Food Science* no. 73(2):N1–N6.

Hou, D. Z., C. S. Xie, K. J. Huang, and C. H. Zhu. 2003. "The production and characteristics of solid lipid nanoparticles (SLNs)." *Biomaterials* no. 24(10):1781–1785.

Jain, K. K. 2008. *Drug Delivery Systems*. Vol. 2, Berlin, Germany: Springer.

Jiang, Q., X. Yang, P. Du, H. Zhang, and T. Zhang. 2016. "Dual strategies to improve oral bioavailability of oleanolic acid: Enhancing water-solubility, permeability and inhibiting cytochrome P450 isozymes." *European Journal of Pharmaceutics and Biopharmaceutics* no. 99:65–72.

Jo, Y.-J., and Y.-J. Kwon. 2014. "Characterization of -carotene nanoemulsions prepared by microfluidization technique." *Food Science and Biotechnology* no. 23(1):107–113.

Junghanns, J. U., and R. H. Müller. 2008. "Nanocrystal technology, drug delivery and clinical applications." *International Journal of Nanomedicine* no. 3(3):295–309.

Kawabata, Y., K. Wada, M. Nakatani, S. Yamada, and S. Onoue. 2011. "Formulation design for poorly water-soluble drugs based on biopharmaceutics classification system: Basic approaches and practical applications." *International Journal of Pharmaceutics* no. 420(1):1–10.

Keck, C. M. 2010. "Particle size analysis of nanocrystals: Improved analysis method." *International Journal of Pharmaceutics* no. 390:3–12.

Kovacevic, A., S. Savic, G. Vuleta, and R. H. Müller. 2011. "Polyhydroxy surfactants for the formulation of lipid nanoparticles (SLN and NLC): Effects on size, physical stability and particle matrix structure." *International Journal of Pharmaceutics* no. 406:163–172.

Lacatusu, I., E. Mitrea, N. Badea, R. Stan, O. Oprea, and A. Meghea. 2013. "Lipid nanoparticles based on omega-3 fatty acids as effective carriers for lutein delivery. Preparation and in vitro characterization studies." *Journal of Functional Foods* no. 5(3):1260–1269.

Lim, S. B., A. Banerjee, and H. Önyüksel. 2012. "Improvement of drug safety by the use of lipid-based nanocarriers." *Journal of Controlled Release* no 163(1):34–35.

Lovelyn, C., and A. A. Attama. 2011. "Current state of nanoemulsions in drug delivery." *Journal of Biomaterials and Nanobiotechnology* no. 2:626–639.

Marangoni, A. G., N. Acevedo, F. Maleky, and F. Peyronel. 2012. "Structure and functionality of edible fats." *Soft Matter* no. 8:1275–1300.

McClements, D. J. 2015. *Food Emulsions: Principles, Practices, and Techniques*, 3rd ed. Boca Raton, FL: CRC Press.

Mehnert, W., and K. Mäder. 2001. "Solid lipid nanoparticles: Production, characterization and applications." *Advanced Drug Delivery Reviews* no. 47:165–196.

Mendes, M., H. T. Soares, L. G. Arnaut, J. J. Sousa, A. A. Pais, and C. Vitorino. 2016. "Can lipid nanoparticles improve intestinal absorption?" *International Journal of Pharmaceutics* no. 515(1–2):69–83.

Mouritsen, O. G. 2011. "Lipids, curvature, and nano-medicine." *European Journal of Lipid Science and Technology* no. 113(10):1174–1187.

Muchow, M., P. Maincent, and R. H. Müller. 2008. "Lipid nanoparticles with a solid matrix (SLN, NLC, LDC) for oral drug delivery." *Drug Development and Industrial Pharmacy* no. 34(12):1394–1405.

Müller, R. H., K. Mäder, and S. Gohla. 2000. "Solid lipid nanoparticles (SLN) for controlled drug delivery: A review of the state of the art." *European Journal of Pharmaceutics and Biopharmaceutics* no. 50(1):161–177.

Neto, W. P. F., H. A. Silvério, and N. O. Dantas. 2013. "Extraction and characterization of cellulose nanocrystals from agro-industrial residue–soy hulls." *Industrial Crops and Products* no. 42:480–488.

Oliveira, D. R. B., and M. Michelon. 2016. "β-Carotene-loaded nanostructured lipid carriers produced by solvent displacement method." *Food Research International* no. 90:139–146.

Pan, M. H., G. Ghai, and C. T. Ho. 2008. "Food bioactives, apoptosis, and cancer." *Molecular Nutrition & Food Research* no. 52(1):43–52.

Qian, C., and D. J. McClements. 2011. "Formation of nanoemulsions stabilized by model food-grade emulsifiers using high-pressure homogenization: Factors affecting particle size." *Food Hydrocolloids* no. 25:1000–1008.

Quintanar-Guerrero, D., D. Tamayo-Esquivel, A. Ganem-Quintanar, E. Allemann, and E. Doelker. 2005. "Adaptation and optimization of the emulsification-diffusion technique to prepare lipidic nanospheres." *European Journal of Pharmaceutical Sciences* no. 26(2):211–218.

Rao, J., and D. J. McClements. 2010. "Stabilization of phase inversion temperature nanoemulsions by surfactant displacement." *Journal of Agricultural and Food Chemistry* no. 58:7059–7066.

Ravanfar, R., A. M. Tamaddon, M. Niakousari, and M. R. Moein. 2016. "Preservation of anthocyanins in solid lipid nanoparticles: Optimization of a microemulsion dilution method using the Placket–Burman and Box–Behnken designs." *Food Chemistry* no. 199:573–580.

Rizzo, G., J. E. Norton, and I. T. Norton. 2015. "Emulsifier effects on fat crystallisation." *Food Structure* no. 4:27–33.

Salvia-Trujillo, L., A. Rojas-Graü, and R. Soliva-Fortuny. 2015. "Physicochemical characterization and antimicrobial activity of food-grade emulsions and nanoemulsions incorporating essential oils." *Food Hydrocolloids* no. 43:547–556.

Sarangi, M. K., and S. Padhi. 2016. "Solid lipid nanoparticles—A Review." *Journal of Critical Reviews* no. 3(3):5–12.

Schubert, M. A., and C. C. Müller-Goymann. 2005. "Characterisation of surface-modified solid lipid nanoparticles (SLN): Influence of lecithin and nonionic emulsifier." *European Journal of Pharmaceutics and Biopharmaceutics* no. 61:77–86.

Selvamuthukumar, S. 2012. "Nanostructured lipid carriers: A potential drug carrier for cancer chemotherapy." *Lipids in Health and Disease* no. 11(1):159–167.

Severino, P., T. Andreani, A. S. Macedo, J. F. Fangueiro, M. H. A. Santana, A. M. Silva, and E. B. Souto. 2012. "Current state-of-art and new trends on lipid nanoparticles (SLN and NLC) for oral drug delivery." *Journal of Drug Delivery* no. 2012:1–10.

Shah, P., D. Bhalodia, and P. Shelat. 2010. "Nanoemulsion: A pharmaceutical review." *Systematic Reviews in Pharmacy* no. 1(1):24–32.

Shah, R., D. Eldridge, E. Palombo, and I. Harding. 2015. *Lipid Nanoparticles: Production, Characterization and Stability*, Springer Briefs in Pharmaceutical Science & Drug Development. Cham, Switzerland: Springer.

Shinoda, K., and H. Saito. 1968. "The effect of temperature on the phase equilibria and the types of dispersions of the ternary system composed of water, cyclohexane, and nonionic surfactant." *Journal of Colloid and Interface Science* no. 26:70–74.

Siekmann, B., and K. Westesen. 1996. "Investigations on solid lipid nanoparticles prepared by precipitation in O/W emulsions." *European Journal of Pharmaceutics and Biopharmaceutics* no. 42(2):104–109.

Silvério, H. A., W. P. F. Neto, and N. O. Dantas. 2013. "Extraction and characterization of cellulose nanocrystals from corncob for application as reinforcing agent in nanocomposites." *Industrial Crops and Products* no. 44:427–436.

Smith, A., and I. M. Hunneyball. 1986. "Evaluation of poly(lactic acid) as a biodegradable drug delivery system for parenteral administration." *International Journal of Pharmaceutics* no. 30(2):215–220.

Speiser, P. P. D. 1986. Lipid nano pellets as drug carriers for oral administration. EP0167825A3.

Sun, B., and Y. Yeo. 2012. "Nanocrystals for the parenteral delivery of poorly water-soluble drugs." *Current Opinion in Solid State and Materials Science* no. 16(6):295–301.

Swain, S., S. Beg, and S. M. Babu. 2016. "Liposheres as a novel carrier for lipid based drug delivery: Current and future directions." *Recent Patents on Drug Delivery & Formulation* no. 10(1):59–71.

Swientek, R. J. 1990. "Microfluidizing technology enhances emulsion stability." *Food Processing* no. 6:152–153.

Tamjidi, F., M. Shahedi, and J. Varshosaz. 2013. "Nanostructured lipid carriers (NLC): A potential delivery system for bioactive food molecules." *Innovative Food Science and Emerging Technologies* no. 19:29–43.

Thummel, K. E., and G. R. Wilkinson. 1998. "*In vitro* and *in vivo* drug interactions involving human CYP3A." *Annual Review of Pharmacology and Toxicology* no. 38:389–430.

Ting, Y., Y. Jiang, C. T. Ho, and Q. Huang. 2014. "Common delivery systems for enhancing in vivo bioavailability and biological efficacy of nutraceuticals." *Journal of Functional Foods* no. 7:112–128.

Trotta, M., F. Debernardi, and O. Caputo. 2003. "Preparation of solid lipid nanoparticles by a solvent emulsification–diffusion technique." *International Journal of Pharmaceutics* no. 257:153–160.

Trujillo, C. C., and A. J. Wright. 2010. "Properties and stability of solid lipid particle dispersions based on canola stearin and Poloxamer 188." *Journal of the American Oil Chemists' Society* no. 87(7):715–730.

Üner, M. 2006. "Preparation, characterization and physico-chemical properties of solid lipid nanoparticles (SLN) and nanostructured lipid carriers (NLC): Their benefits as colloidal drug carrier systems." *Die Pharmazie-An International Journal of Pharmaceutical Sciences* no. 61(5):375–386.

Wang, S., R. Su, S. Nie, M. Sun, J. Zhang, and D. Wu. 2014. "Application of nanotechnology in improving bioavailability and bioactivity of diet-derived phytochemicals." *Journal of Nutritional Biochemistry* no. 25:363–376.

Weiss, J., E. A. Decker, D. J. McClements, K. Kristbergsson, T. Helgason. 2008. "Solid lipid nanoparticles as delivery systems for bioactive food components" *Food Biophysics* no. 3(2):146–154.

Westesen, K., H. Bunjes, and M. H. J. Koch. 1997. "Physicochemical characterization of lipid nanoparticles and evaluation of their drug loading capacity and sustained release potential." *Journal of Controlled Release* no. 48:223–236.

Westesen, K., M. Drechsler, and H. Bunjes. 2001. *Colloidal Dispersions Based on Solid Lipids*. Vol. 103: Royal Society of Chemistry, Cambridge, UK.

Wilczewska, A. Z., K. Niemirowicz, and K. H. Markiewicz. 2012. "Nanoparticles as drug delivery systems." *Pharmacological Reports* no. 64:1020–1037.

Williams, H. D., N. L. Trevaskis, S. A. Charman, R. M. Shanker, W. N. Charman, C. W. Pouton, and C. J. H. Porter. 2013. "Strategies to address low drug solubility in discovery and development." *Pharmacological Reviews* no. 65(1):315–499.

Yadav, N., S. Khatak, and U. V. S. Sara. 2013. "Solid lipid nanoparticles-a review." *International Journal of Applied Pharmaceutics* no. 5(2):8–18.

Yu, H., and Q. Huang. 2012. "Improving the oral bioavailability of curcumin using novel organogel-based nanoemulsions." *Journal of Agricultural and Food Chemistry* no. 60(21):5373–5379.

Yuan, Y., Y. Gao, J. Zhao, and L. Mao. 2008. "Characterization and stability evaluation of β-carotene nanoemulsions prepared by high pressure homogenization under various emulsifying conditions." *Food Research International* no. 41:61–68.

Zambrano-Zaragoza, M. L., and E. Mercado-Silva. 2013. "Use of solid lipid nanoparticles (SLNs) in edible coatings to increase guava (*Psidium guajava* L.) shelf-life." *Food Research International* no. 51:946–953.

# 5 Nanolaminated Systems Production by Layer-by-Layer Technique

*Ana C. Pinheiro, Ana I. Bourbon, Joana T. Martins, Philippe E. Ramos, António A. Vicente, and Maria G. Carneiro-da-Cunha*

**CONTENTS**

## 5.1 INTRODUCTION

The increase in consumers' demand for health-promoting foods is stimulating food industry to pursue innovative and effective functional foods. As a consequence, there is a current trend toward the incorporation of bioactive compounds in food products, often recurring to their encapsulation. In addition, there is a growing interest in using natural alternatives to enhance food preservation while having a low impact on the organoleptic and nutritional attributes of the food product. However, the incorporation of encapsulated bioactive compounds in food products and the expected enhancement of foods' shelf life are still challenging tasks for the food industry. In recent years, the utilization of nanolaminated systems (NSs) has been investigated as a potential strategy to reach these goals. In fact, the use of NSs in food products represents a promising alternative to improve their quality, safety, and functionality.

A nanolaminate refers to two or more layers of material with nano-sized dimensions that are physically or chemically bonded to each other (Rubner 2003). NSs can be assembled on different solid supports (e.g., food products, nano-based delivery systems) and can be used in various applications such as edible films and coatings and encapsulation of bioactive compounds. Multilayer films/coatings can be applied directly onto food surfaces or to conventional packaging to functionalize their surface, as may also act as reservoirs of bioactive compounds (Acevedo-Fani et al. 2017a). As encapsulation systems, NSs present significant advantages, such as the possibility to tailor multiple functionalities—i.e., size, composition, porosity, surface functionality, and stability—in the same structure while providing protection of sensitive bioactive compounds and releasing them in response to specific triggers (e.g., pH, ionic strength, enzymes, light, and temperature). In fact, NS have been shown to have improved stability in respect to ionic strength, pH, and temperature. Also, the production of NSs may be carried out at room temperature using simple techniques [e.g., layer-by-layer (LbL) technique] and aqueous solutions of a variety of food-grade biopolymers, including several proteins and polysaccharides (Weiss et al. 2006). Nevertheless, in order to obtain these desirable characteristics, it is important to choose the right combination of polyelectrolytes and preparation conditions.

This chapter presents the recent developments concerning the formation of NSs for food applications by LbL technique, such materials and templates used, influence of environmental conditions. Examples of these systems as well as their use for encapsulation of bioactive compounds will be also addressed.

## 5.2 METHODS TO PRODUCE NANOLAMINATED SYSTEMS BY LAYER-BY-LAYER TECHNIQUE

The method selected for the development of NSs by LbL technique is a crucial step, since it allows different properties and performances. Properties such as shape, solubility, encapsulation efficiency, and release mechanism will influence the final application (Decher 2002, Pinheiro et al. 2015, Tieke et al. 2003).

LbL assembly technique consists of the alternate adsorption of polyelectrolytes using different chemical interactions—i.e., electrostatic, hydrogen bonding, hydrophobic, charge-transfer, and covalent (Acevedo-Fani et al. 2017). Electrostatic interactions between polyelectrolytes with opposite charged species are one of the most common approaches used in the LbL technique to develop stable NSs (Figure 5.1). LbL method has been widely explored for several applications in different science fields (e.g., material science, pharmacology, or biomedicine) due to its simplicity, high adaptability, and low-cost (Cerqueira et al. 2014). LbL technique is also used in food science to create interfacial coatings around different shaped templates (Bourbon

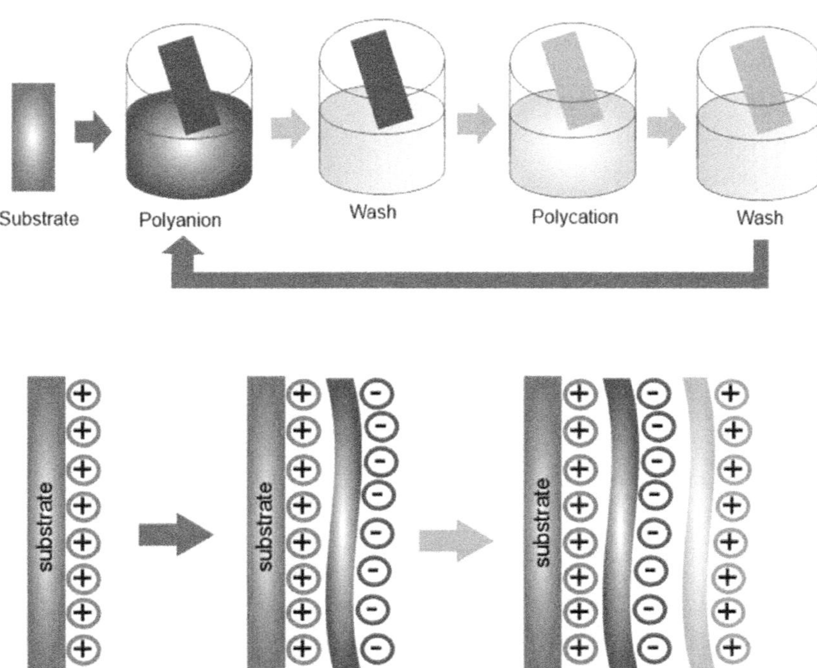


**FIGURE 5.1** Layer-by-layer deposition technique.

et al. 2016, Cerqueira et al. 2014, Pinheiro et al. 2015, Pinheiro et al. 2012, Rivera et al. 2015). Recently, some works report new strategies to improve the application of LbL technique, in order to improve the homogeneity of layers and turn this process more easily to be applied with different materials.

### 5.2.1 Dip Coating Process

One of the most commonly used methods for applying LbL is the dip coating process. During this process, the LbL technique is generally performed by manually immersing substrates into solutions where a charged polyelectrolyte is added, adsorbing to the template surface, and leading to the formation of the "first layer" by electrostatic deposition. The adsorption of the following layer is achieved by the simple addition of an oppositely charged polyelectrolyte, promoting the "second layer" adsorption on top of the first layer of polyelectrolyte. This procedure can be repeated to form three or more layers of polyelectrolytes. The number of layers will be defined by the final application of these (Cerqueira et al. 2014, Martins et al. 2015, Mora-Huertas et al. 2010). However, one of the major concerns of this procedure is the collection of unbound substrate between washing and deposition steps, which in the most cases requires centrifugation (Richardson et al. 2016). Other limitations are related with the fact that LbL technique by dip coating process typically implies long time to reach equilibrium adsorption for each coating step, and the formation of stable NS requires a high control of system composition and preparation in order to avoid aggregation (Costa et al. 2015, Pinheiro et al. 2016). One of the strategies to improve this technique is the use of automated machines such as electrically driven slide-staining robots, dipping robot, or crude robots driven by compressed air (Richardson et al. 2016).

### 5.2.2 Spin Coating

Spin coating is a useful process appointed for industrial applications. In this method, a liquid is spread onto a surface material, depositing thinner and homogeneous layers through rapid spinning (Keeney et al. 2015). The spinning process with centrifugal and viscous forces and air shear allows obtaining layers with high ordered internal structure than in dip-coated materials (Peng et al. 2017, Richardson et al. 2016). The thickness of films is controlled by the solutions viscosity, spin time, and angular speed. The disadvantage of spin coating is that the faster drying times can also lead to lower performance for some particular nano-technologies which require time to self-assemble and/or crystallize (Lee et al. 2001).

### 5.2.3 Spray Coating

Spray coating is another alternative to LbL technique. During this process, a solution is supplied by enforced spraying. One of the major advantages of this process is its ability of form homogeneous coating of 3D substrates. The deposition is faster (time needed for preparation using spraying is reduced by a factor of

64 comparing to dipping) and smoother, which turns the process high efficient. Another advantage reported to spray coating is its ability to be performed without the need of a rinsing step (Keeney et al. 2015, Richardson et al. 2016). However Kolasinska et al. (2009) observed that sprayed samples are less stable to variable external conditions when compared to dipping method. Automatic spray machines are being developed in order to optimize LbL technique, reducing the application time and improving the application on surface substrate (more homogeneous). This machine uniformly sprays aqueous mixtures containing complementary (e.g., oppositely charged, capable of hydrogen bonding, or capable of covalent bonding) species onto a large-area substrate. Between each deposition of opposite species, samples are spray-rinsed with deionized water and blow-dried with air. The spraying, rinsing, drying areas, and times are adjustable by a computer program (Seo et al. 2016).

## 5.3 MATERIALS FOR NANOLAMINATED SYSTEMS PRODUCTION

The application of layers on different systems' surfaces to improve their performance or create a new function have been explored in several works. Various adsorbing substances could be used to create the different layers, including natural polyelectrolytes (i.e., polymers with ionizable groups, that under appropriate conditions, dissociate, leaving ions on polymer chains and counterions in the solution), charged lipids (e.g., phospholipids, surfactants), and colloidal particles (e.g., micelles, vesicles, droplets). Since the key issue of LbL assembly is the need for surface recharging at each adsorption step, the materials used in each assembly should have a sufficient number of charged groups to provide stable adsorption on an oppositely charged surface and non-compensated charges exposed to the exterior (Mora-Huertas et al. 2010). Out of all the materials available for layers' formation, this section will mainly focus on the most used polyelectrolytes (either polysaccharides or proteins) to produce NSs, being some of their main characteristics are identified in Table 5.1.

### 5.3.1 Polysaccharides

Polysaccharides are carbohydrate molecules composed of several monosaccharide units connected by glyosidic bonds. These forms are constituted by several functional groups, different chemical composition, and molecular weights, being these characteristics responsible to create different properties. Polysaccharides derive from plants, animals, algae, or microbial sources (Belitz et al. 2004).

#### 5.3.1.1 Alginate

Alginate is a polysaccharide derived from algae or bacterial sources, and it is constituted by 1-4 linked $\alpha$-(L)-glucuronic and $\beta$-(D)-mannuronic acids (Rinaudo 2008). It is widely used in food because it is a powerful thickening, stabilizing, and gel-forming agent. Also, the main reason for its high utilization in NS' production is the combination of several important features, namely, its generally regarded as safe

**TABLE 5.1**
**Most Widely Used Polyelectrolytes, Polysaccharides and Proteins, in the Production of NS and Their Main Characteristics**

| | Material | Major Structure Type | *pKa/pI* | Main Functional Properties | References |
|---|---|---|---|---|---|
| Polysaccharides | Chitosan | Linear | 6.5 | Antimicrobial activity<br>Cationic polysaccharide | Pinheiro et al. (2015) |
| | Xanthan gum | Linear/helical | 4.6 | Thickening properties<br>Anionic polysaccharide | Bueno and Petri (2014) |
| | Alginate | Linear | 3.3–3.5 | Gelling and thickening properties<br>Anionic polysaccharide | Cook et al. (2012) |
| | Fucoidan | Branched random coil | 2.0 | Antioxidant, anticoagulant, anti-inflammatory, and antiviral activities<br>Anionic polysaccharide | Pinheiro et al. (2015) |
| | Pectin | Branched coil | 3.5 | Gelling and thickening properties<br>Anionic polysaccharide | Opanasopit et al. (2008) |
| | Carrageenan | Linear/helical | 2.0 | Gelling and thickening properties<br>Anionic polysaccharide | Pinheiro et al. (2012) |
| Proteins | Whey protein | Globular | 5.2 | Emulsifying, foaming, and gelling properties | Lim and Roos (2015) |
| | Gelatin | Linear | 7–9 (type A)<br>4.7–5.4 (type B) | Emulsifying, gelling properties | Shutava et al. (2009) |
| | Lactoferrin | Globular | 8.7 | Gelling, antimicrobial, anti-inflammatory, and antitumor properties | Majka et al. (2013) |
| | Lysozyme | Globular | 10.5 | Antimicrobial properties | Antonov et al. (2018) |

status, relative low cost, and lack of toxicity (Thu et al. 1996). Due to the presence of carboxylic groups on both monomers, alginate has more negative charged groups above its pKa (3.3—3.5) (Cook et al. 2012).

#### 5.3.1.2 Carrageenan

Carrageenan is a sulphated anionic polysaccharide with an approximated radius of 30 nm that is derived from seaweed, more specifically, red algae (Croguennoc et al. 2000). The pKa value of the anionic sulphate groups on carrageenan is around pH 2 (Gu et al. 2004). They are widely used in food industry for their gelling, thickening, and stabilizing properties. Also, carrageenan and modified carrageenan-based materials have proved to have several biological activities, such as antitumor, antiviral, anticoagulant, and antibacterial activity (Zhu et al. 2017).

#### 5.3.1.3 Fucoidan

Fucoidan is a sulphated polysaccharide enriched with fucose obtained from extracellular matrix of a variety of brown seaweeds (Wu et al. 2016). It presents a wide range of functional properties, such as antioxidant, anticoagulant, anti-inflammatory, and antiviral activities, exhibiting also a great potential in inhibiting cancer cell growth (Zhao et al. 2018). Its biological activity depends on its chemical composition, molecular weight, monosaccharide composition, sulphate content, and position of sulphate ester group (Ale et al. 2011). Due to the presence of sulphate groups, fucoidan exhibit negative charge at neutral pH values (pKa value of sulphate groups around 2) (Indest et al. 2009).

#### 5.3.1.4 Pectin

Pectin is a natural anionic polysaccharide extracted from plant cell walls consisting of a linear backbone of (1-4)-D-galacturonic acid residues. It has been widely used in food industry as gelling, thickening, and stabilizing (Shamsara et al. 2017). Moreover, it present excellent biocompatibility, effective bacterial inhibition ability, and biodegradability (Zhang et al. 2015). Pectin is negatively charged at neutral pH and approaches zero charge at low pH, being its pKa value about 3.5 (Opanasopit et al. 2008). The magnitude of the negative charge of pectin molecules depends on their degree of esterification: the charge density decreases with the increase of number of esterified (methoxylated) carboxyl groups. Therefore, low methoxyl pectin has a higher anionic charge density comparing to high methoxyl pectin (McClements 2014).

#### 5.3.1.5 Xanthan Gum

Xanthan gum is a high molecular weight extracellular polysaccharide produced by the bacteria *Xanthomonas campestris* (Kocherbitov et al. 2010). It is widely used in food as stabilizer and thickener agent due to its exceptional rheological properties, biodegradability, biocompatibility, and non-toxicity (Elella et al. 2017). Also, its thermal and pH stability is higher comparing with other water-soluble polysaccharides (Espert et al. 2018). Xanthan gum acts as a polyanion at $pH > 4.5$ due to the deprotonation of O-acetyl and pyruvyl residues (Petri 2015).

#### 5.3.1.6 Chitosan

Chitosan origin is chitin, a natural and linear cationic polysaccharide with glucosamine and N-acetyl glucosamine residues that are present in the cuticle of insects, shells of molluscs and crustaceans, and cell walls of fungi (Ravi Kumar 2000). Chitosan is constituted by a heterogeneous distribution of acetyl groups that depend of its origin and are present along the chain (Rinaudo 2006). Chitosan is a cationic polyelectrolyte (Peniche et al. 2003), due to the presence of amine residues, presenting a pKa around 6.5 (Sogias et al. 2010) and is insoluble at pH higher than 5.4, which is influenced by the acetylation degree (Huguet et al. 1996). Considering its origin, it might not be approved for food applications, which is the case of chitosan of animal origin that is not approved in the European Union as food additive, but presents the generally regarded as safe status in the United States. However, if its origin is fungic (*Aspergillus niger*), this polysaccharide is approved as a wine processing aid in the European Union (EU 2012) and has generally regarded as safe status under United States FDA regulation (FDA 2011) and Japan approval as a food additive (JFCRF 2011). The capacity of chitosan to resist to acidic media is an important characteristic that makes this polysaccharide one of the most used materials to form edible coatings.

### 5.3.2 Proteins

Proteins are constituted by amino acids covalently linked by peptide bonds, creating a chain, and are derived from animals or plants. There are up to 20 types of L-α-amino acids that originate several types of proteins with different and important functional and technological properties such as gelation, foaming, water binding capacity, and emulsification (Belitz et al. 2004).

#### 5.3.2.1 Whey Proteins

Milk is constituted by several proteins such as whey proteins and casein that can be used to produce high-density gel networks. These proteins are capable to create a higher local pH-value because of proteins' buffering capacity (Vidhyalakshmi et al. 2009). Whey proteins have an amphoteric character that allows their mixture with polysaccharides. At the same time, below their isoelectric point, a structural change happen in their net charges, inverting the charges to positive, which causes an interaction with negatively charged polysaccharides (Guérin et al. 2003). The isoelectric point (pI) occurs at pH 5.2 where aggregation might also occur (Ju and Kilara 1998).

#### 5.3.2.2 Gelatin

Gelatin is a natural hydrocolloid derived from the connective tissues, skin, and bones of animals such as pig, bovine, and fish. Gelatin is a fibrous protein obtained by partial denaturation of collagen, and because of this has a similar chemical structure being constituted by three α-chains in the triple helix (Etxabide et al. 2017). In food, gelatin has been used as an emulsifier, gelling and foaming agent, colloids stabilizer, fining agent, biodegradable packaging material, and micro-encapsulating agent.

The most important properties that characterize gelatin are its gel strength, viscosity, and gelling and melting points. (Gómez-Guillén et al. 2011). Acid pretreatment produces gelatin with a pI in range from 7 to 9 (type A gelatin), whereas alkaline treatment gives samples with pH ranging from 4.7 to 5.4 (type B gelatin) (Shutava et al. 2009).

#### 5.3.2.3 Lysozyme

Lysozyme is a naturally occurring enzyme with strong bactericidal and bacteriostatic activity against Gram-positive organisms, and therefore it is often used as an additive in the food industry to prevent the growth of the bacteria on food materials (Shahmohammadi 2018). This globular protein is characterized by a molecular weight of approximately 14.4 kDa and consists of a single polypeptide chain with 129 amino acids (Abeyrathne et al. 2013). It is considered a strong basic protein, having a pI of approximately 10.5 (Antonov et al. 2018). A rich and easily available source of lysozyme is the chicken egg white.

#### 5.3.2.4 Lactoferrin

Lactoferrin is an iron-binding glycoprotein, belonging to the transferrin family (Franco et al. 2018). It is produced by mucosal epithelial cells in various mammalian species and can be found in most body fluids (e.g., breast milk, tears, and saliva). This basic protein presents a pI of 8.7, a molecular weight of about 80 kDa, and shows high affinity to iron (sequestration of $Fe^{2+}$ and $Fe^{3+}$ free ions) (Majka et al. 2013). Also, it exhibits several biological functions, such as antimicrobial activity against a great variety of microorganisms, and protective activity (i.e., antitumoral, anti-inflammatory, and immunomodulatory properties) (Moreno-Expósito et al. 2018).

## 5.4 INFLUENCE OF DIFFERENT FACTORS ON NANOLAMINATED SYSTEMS' PROPERTIES

Environmental conditions have a relevant influence on the development of NSs. Factors such as pH and ionic strength can affect the amount of polyelectrolytes adsorbed in each layer, due to conformational modifications (Zhong et al. 2007).

### 5.4.1 pH

The solution pH is one of most important factors that influence the formation of multilayer systems and their final properties. During the development of a multilayer system, in the case of LbL technique, the pH of the solution should be properly selected in order to have sufficiently high opposite charges between the template surface and the adsorbing polyelectrolyte. Therefore, the charge signal of polyelectrolytes depends on the type and concentration of molecules attached to the surface, influenced by the solution conditions. The pH at which adsorption occurs depends on the magnitude and sign of the charges on the template surface and polyelectrolyte. The adsorption of a polyelectrolyte on a template with the same charge can occur at specific conditions such as, the presence of oppositely charged patches in the template surface (Gu et al. 2005, Guzey and McClements 2006). The effect of solution pH is also a relevant factor after multilayer system formation. Variations in the pH may adjust the properties of the polyelectrolyte multilayer interface that surrounds the templates. These variations can affect the electrostatic interactions between: (i) the template surface and the adsorbed polyelectrolyte, (ii) adsorbed polyelectrolytes in different layers, or (iii) adsorbed and non-adsorbed polyelectrolytes. These changes in pH can modify thickness, packing, and integrity of the new interface (Guzey and McClements 2006).

### 5.4.2 Ionic Strength

Also, ionic strength is able to rearrange the conformation of the polyelectrolytes by shielding the electrostatic repulsion within the polyelectrolytes chains. During the construction of a multilayer system, the magnitude of ionic strength may interfere with the composition, structure, and thickness of the polyelectrolyte layer, since it will determine the strength of intra- and inter-molecular electrostatic interactions (Decher et al. 1992, Guzey and McClements 2006). Generally, an increase in the ionic strength of a solution decreases the electrostatic interactions between polyelectrolytes and templates, thus occurring an electrostatic screening (Kurth et al. 2003, Pinheiro et al. 2013, Tedeschi et al. 2000). The presence of salt can also be used to control the final layers' properties. Due to weaker intra-molecular repulsion, polyelectrolyte layers are usually thicker and have a more compact conformation. Increasing the ionic strength weakens the attractive interactions between polyelectrolyte molecules in different layers, thereby causing an increase in interfacial porosity. In the absence of salt, thin layers are formed with flat chains against the colloidal template surface, once the polyelectrolyte molecules present a highly extended conformation (Guzey and McClements 2006). Ionic strength is also an important parameter on final properties of NSs. For example, the integrity of a nanolaminated coating may be greatly altered by the variations of ionic strength of a solution. These variations may cause a detaching of layers by weakening the electrostatic interactions and a loss of systems' permeability (McClements and Decker 2009).

### 5.4.3 Polyelectrolyte Properties

Polyelectrolytes properties, such as chain length, solubility, rigidity, and electrical charge, have a high relevance on the final NS. Their properties will determine the ability to be adsorbed on the template surface and will affect the system properties (e.g., thicknesses, structures, porosities, and environmental triggers sensitivity) (Guzey and McClements 2006). As reported above, environmental conditions such as pH, ionic strength, or/and temperature lead to changes in the electrical charge, conformation, and polyelectrolyte's hydrophobicity. The variation of these factors influences the amount of polyelectrolyte adsorbed to the template surface, creating new interfaces with different environmental responses that may lead to different electrical characteristics of the trapped polyelectrolyte. Finally, the amount of polyelectrolyte should be high enough to saturate the surface of the colloidal templates, reversing the charge of the templates (or previous layers), in order to create a strong electrostatic repulsion between the nanolayers. This amount will be influenced by the molecular characteristics of the polyelectrolyte, such as chain length, conformation, flexibility, and electrical charge (Guzey and McClements 2006).

## 5.5 TEMPLATES FOR LAYERS' DEPOSITION

Multilayers can be assembled on supports with different dimensions and shapes such as planar and colloidal templates (e.g., nanocapsules, nanoemulsions, nanoliposomes, and nanohydrogels) (Figure 5.2). However, the nature of the surfaces, and its surface charge density, play a major role in the layers' assembly. In fact, the homogeneity and stability of the multilayers are related to the hydrophilicity/hydrophobicity of the template, nature and density of the charged groups, as well as its roughness and presence of impurities.

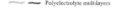

### 5.5.1 Planar Templates

Multilayer films or coatings of nanometric thickness can be produced by successive adsorption of oppositely charged polyelectrolytes on a solid planar support (Slavutsky and Bertuzzi 2016). Final films/coatings functionality, such as their permeability and mechanical properties, swelling/wetting characteristics, and their environmental sensitivity to pH and temperature, will be determined by the following aspects: (i) type of materials used to create each layer; (ii) the total number of layers; (iii) the sequence of the different layers; and (iv) by the conditions (e.g., pH and ionic strength) used in each layer deposition (Weiss et al. 2006).

Multilayer nanocoating composed of κ-carrageenan and chitosan have been assembled by LbL deposition technique on a polyethylene terephthalate support (Pinheiro et al. 2012). In this work, the authors show that the interaction between κ-carrageenan and chitosan is an exothermic process, being the formation of multilayers mainly due to electrostatic interactions existing between the two polyelectrolytes (though other types of interactions may also be involved). Also, it has been concluded that κ-carrageenan/chitosan multilayer coating presents good gas barrier properties (Pinheiro et al. 2012). Multilayer films/coatings have been successfully used to coat food products such as fruits (Medeiros et al. 2012a, Medeiros et al. 2012b) and cheese (Medeiros et al. 2014).

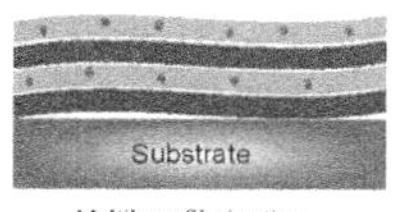

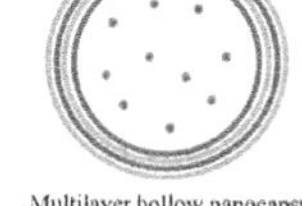

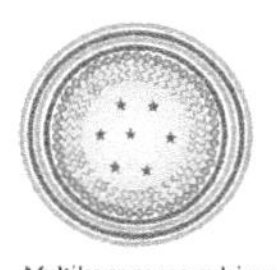

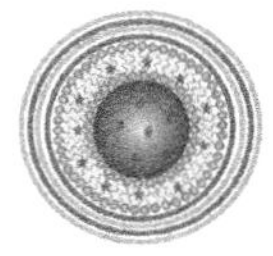

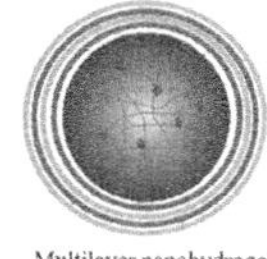


**FIGURE 5.2** Possible templates for multilayer deposition.

### 5.5.2 Colloidal Templates

The proper choice of both colloidal template and polyelectrolytes is crucial for the development of multilayer nanocapsules with specific properties, suitable for a particular application. The colloidal template choice will mainly determine the multilayer nanocapsules' size and shape, while polyelectrolytes will be the main responsible for determining the multilayer nanocapsules' properties (Cui et al. 2014).

#### 5.5.2.1 Multilayer Hollow Nanocapsules

Multilayer hollow nanocapsules are typically produced by LbL adsorption of oppositely charged polyelectrolytes on the surface of nanoscale sacrificial templates, usually carbonate (Kittitheeranun et al. 2015), silica (Shu et al. 2010), or polystyrene nanoparticles (Pinheiro et al. 2015). After polyelectrolyte multilayer deposition (multilayered shell), the sacrificial template (core) is removed by dissolution in suitable solvents (e.g., acids, bases, and chelating agents), depending on the chemical nature of the template (Pastorino et al. 2016). Subsequently, multiple centrifugation-washing cycles can be carried out to assure complete removal of the core.

In the last years, multilayer hollow nanocapsules with different polyelectrolyte pairs and core template particles and with a wide range of compositions, structures, and functionalities, have been developed. For example, polysaccharide multilayer hollow nanocapsules with a size of 150 nm, comprising chitosan and κ-carrageenan, were successfully prepared via LbL technique. These nanocapsules were found to have a dual behavior, responding to pH and ionic strength (Liu et al. 2012). Other authors successfully prepared pH-dependent multilayer nanocapsules through LbL assembly of chitosan and fucoidan (Pinheiro et al. 2015).

#### 5.5.2.2 Multilayer Nanoemulsions

Multilayer nanoemulsions can be defined as oil-in-water systems containing droplets with at least two interfacial membranes composed by emulsifiers and biopolymers, which are generally created by the LbL assembly (Acevedo-Fani et al. 2017). First, the "primary" emulsion is produced by homogenizing the oil and water phases in the presence of a charged emulsifier. Subsequently, the "secondary" emulsion is formed by mixing the primary emulsion with an oppositely charged polyelectrolyte under appropriate conditions (e.g., concentration, pH, and ionic strength). This process can be repeated numerous times by sequentially adding oppositely charged polyelectrolytes to the emulsions to form multilayer systems with tailored properties (e.g., thickness, charge, composition, and functional activity) (Chang and McClements 2015).

Different studies have shown that the addition of polyelectrolyte layers increases nanoemulsions' stability to pH changes, high ionic strength, temperature (either heating or freezing), and dehydration. Pinheiro at al. (2016) evaluated the behavior of nanoemulsions stabilized by biopolymer emulsifiers—lactoferrin and lactoferrin/alginate multilayer structure—under gastrointestinal (GI) conditions. These authors observed that the interfacial characteristics of nanoemulsions had a significant impact on their physicochemical stability within the simulated GI tract. In fact, it has been suggested that an alginate coating may allow controlling the rate of lipid digestion and free fatty acids adsorption within the GI tract (Pinheiro et al. 2016). Other authors evaluated the influence of fucoidan addition on the electrical charge, creaming stability, size, and microstructure of the particles in caseinate-stabilized nanoemulsions. They observed that the deposition of the fucoidan thin layer (with a few nanometers) improved nanoemulsions' pH stability near their isoelectric point, and that the phase behavior of droplet-polysaccharide mixtures (i.e., bridging flocculation, stabilization, and depletion flocculation) depended on lipid droplet and fucoidan concentration (Chang and McClements 2015).

### 5.5.2.3 Multilayer Nanoliposomes

Nanoliposomes are spherical vesicles that present an aqueous core enclosed by one or more phospholipid bilayers, having the ability to encapsulate both hydrophilic and hydrophobic compounds due to the presence of both lipid and aqueous phases in their structure (Lopes et al. 2017). Nanoliposomes are attractive templates for multilayer nanocapsules production via LbL, once they are typically unstable under *in vivo* conditions and present a lack of control over degradability, characteristics that can be minimized by multilayer deposition. In fact, multilayer deposition on surface of charged nanoliposomes is thought to improve their resistance to environmental stresses, as well as to enhance *in vivo* biological performance by improving characteristics such as stability and bioactive compounds' release profiles (Ramasamy et al. 2014). Hybrid nanoparticles have been produced by the electrostatic deposition of positive bovine serum albumin (BSA) and negative lactoferrin onto the surface of nanoliposomes. It was found that the resulting multilayer liposomes (with size of about 150 nm) had better stability than the bare liposomes, after heat treatment, pH variation, and long-term storage (Liu et al. 2017). Other authors formed multilayers onto soybean lecithin nanoliposomes using chitosan and dextran sulphate. They concluded that the resulting multilayer nanocapsules (with a size of about 380 nm) exhibited better stability against temperature and pH (Madrigal-Carballo et al. 2010). Also, other authors have shown that manufacturing negatively charged multilayer nanoliposomes with charged biopolymer (chitosan and λ-carrageenan) can improve their physicochemical stability (Chun et al. 2016).

### 5.5.2.4 Multilayer Nanohydrogels

Nanohydrogels are nanosized, three-dimensional networks able to absorb high amounts of water, showing swelling and de-swelling properties (Montanari et al. 2017). Protein or polysaccharide nanohydrogels are attractive delivery systems, due to their low toxicity, high biodegradability, biocompatibility, and ability to deliver bioactive compounds into and/or across the GI mucosa. However, their degradation in GI tract can be an obstacle to the delivery of the encapsulated compound at specific target (e.g., mouth, stomach, small intestine, or colon). Therefore, one of the strategies to improve nanohydrogels stability in GI conditions is the application of a coating. Recently, a chitosan coating has been applied in lactoferrin-glycomacropeptide nanohydrogels, and it was observed that the presence of chitosan improved the stability of both proteins (i.e., proteins were hydrolyzed at a slower rate and they were present in solution over a long period of time) during gastric digestion (Bourbon et al. 2016).

## 5.6 ENCAPSULATION OF BIOACTIVE COMPOUNDS IN NANOLAMINATED SYSTEMS

As previously mentioned, NSs can act as carrier systems of bioactive compounds, which open an opportunity to manufacture different systems with a significant variety of food-grade bioactive ingredients. In this section, a selected group of bioactive compounds that have been most commonly encapsulated in bio-based NSs (e.g., nanocapsules, nanoemulsions, and nanohydrogels) for food applications is reviewed.

### 5.6.1 Encapsulated Bioactive Compounds

Food grade NSs present a great potential to be applied in the design of functional foods once they could encapsulate many bioactive compounds such as vitamins, antimicrobials, antioxidants, carotenoids, prebiotics, proteins, peptides, omega-3 fatty acids, lipids, and carbohydrates. The encapsulation of such compounds could bring different achievements for food and health sectors, such as improvement of their bioavailability, absorption, stability, protection from adverse environmental conditions (e.g., temperature and pH), control release, and better solubility in aqueous solutions (Acevedo-Fani et al. 2017). Due to these properties, the functionality and stability of foods, where NSs are added, can be enhanced.

The encapsulation of a bioactive compound in a NS can be achieved using different processes such as incorporation and adsorption/absorption methods. The incorporation method consists on compound inclusion during NS formation or compound preloading in a template. On the other hand, adsorption/absorption method consists on compound entrapment through addition of a concentrated compound solution to a preformed NS (Rivera et al. 2015, Tarhini et al. 2017). Recently, many researchers have investigated encapsulation/entrapment of bioactive compounds using different types of bio-based nanolaminate systems as shown in Table 5.2. The selection of the more adequate category of NS for each compound should be made taking into consideration the compound character (e.g., lipophilic or hydrophilic), the NS purpose (e.g., increase permeability and release rate in the intestinal environment), and its particular characteristics (e.g., charge and layers composition) (Gleeson et al. 2016). For example, biopolymer-based NSs including polyelectrolyte complexes and protein- or polysaccharide-based structures are appropriate for loading hydrophilic bioactives (e.g., bioactive peptides). On the other hand, lipid-based NSs such as nanoemulsions, solid lipid nanoparticles, and nanoliposomes are appropriate for loading lipophilic bioactives (e.g., curcumin).

#### 5.6.1.1 Lipophilic Compounds

Bioactive compounds that poorly dissolve in water create a setback to oral route administration, transport, and reaching the target, resulting in a poor oral bioavailability and reduced efficacy (Matalanis et al. 2011). Phytochemicals, such as polyphenols and carotenoids, are usually poorly soluble in water. The delivery of phytochemicals is influenced by their physicochemical properties, such as water solubility, lipophilicity, and crystallinity (Dima et al. 2015). With the aim to

**TABLE 5.2**
**Selected Examples of Bioactive Compounds Encapsulated in NS for Food Applications**

| Nanolaminated System Category | Main Composition of Nanolaminate System | Bioactive Compound | Size (nm) | EE (%) | LC (%) | References |
|---|---|---|---|---|---|---|
| Nanocapsules | Pectin, zein, sodium caseinate | Curcumin | ≈117.0 | ≈92.0 | — | Chang et al. (2017) |
| | Chitosan and fucoidan | Poly-L-lysine | ≈50.0 | 45.1 ± 1.5 | ≈16.0 | Pinheiro et al. (2015) |
| | Zein, sodium caseinate, and chitosan hydrochloride | Thymol | <530.0 | ≈80.0 | — | Zhang et al. (2014) |
| | Chitosan and alginate | GMP | ≈147.0 | 49.4 ± 9.2 | — | Rivera et al. (2015) |
| | Chitosan and gum arabic | Curcumin | 250.0–290.0 | ≈90.0 | ≈3.8 | Tan et al. (2016) |
| Nanoemulsions | Chitosan and CMC | Curcumin | 159.85 ± 0.92 | — | — | Abbas et al. (2015) |
| | Lf and caseinate | ω-3 fatty acids | 9.7 | — | — | Lesmes et al. (2010) |
| | Pectin, WPC, and maltodextrin | Saffron extract (crocin, picrocrocin, and saffranal) | 536.3 ± 0.18 | 96.66 ± 0.38 (crocin); 96.82 ± 0.23 (picrocrocin); 95.94 ± 0.2 (saffranal) | — | Esfanjani et al. (2015) |
| | Chitosan and alginate | Capsaicin | >20.0 | 68.00 ± 0.34 | — | Choi et al. (2011) |
| | Lf, EGCG, and beet pectin | β-carotene | 467.0–728.0 | — | — | Liu et al. (2016) |
| Nanoliposomes | Alginate and chitosan | Vitamin C | 297.0 ± 10.0 | — | — | Liu et al. (2017) |
| | Alginate and chitosan | MCFAs | ≈330.0 | — | — | Liu et al. (2013) |
| | Chitosan and pectin | Grape seed extract | 227.0 ± 2.8 | — | — | Gibis et al. (2014) |
| | Soybean lecithin, dextran sulphate, and chitosan | Ellagic acid | 386.5 ± 25.9 | 43.6 ± 2.4 | 64.6 ± 3.5 | Madrigal-Carballo et al. (2010) |

*(Continued)*

**TABLE 5.2 (*Continued*)**
**Selected Examples of Bioactive Compounds Encapsulated in NS for Food Applications**

| Nanolaminated System Category | Main Composition of Nanolaminate System | Bioactive Compound | Size (nm) | EE (%) | LC (%) | References |
|---|---|---|---|---|---|---|
| Nanohydrogels | Chitosan, Lf, and GMP | Caffeine | 230.0 ± 12.0 | 90.02 ± 2.10 | — | Bourbon et al. (2016) |
| | WPC and alginate | Caffeine | ≈60 | — | — | Gunasekaran et al. (2007) |
| | β-LG-Pectin | DHA | ≈100 | 64 ± 10 | — | Zimet and Livney (2009) |
| Films/coatings | Alginate and zein nanocapsules | Carvacrol | 115.0 ± 10.0 | 90.0 ± 1.5 | — | Fabra et al. (2015) |
| | Alginate and chitosan | Chitosan | — | — | — | Souza et al. (2014) |
| | Alginate and lysozyme | Lysozyme | 198.2 | — | — | Medeiros et al. (2014) |
| | Pectin and chitosan | Chitosan | 266.0 (5 layers) | — | — | Medeiros et al. (2012) |
| | Alginate and chitosan | Folic acid | 2900 (20 layers) | — | ≈70 μg/cm$^2$ | Acevedo-Fani et al. (2018) |

*Note:* EE: encapsulations efficiency; LC: Loading capacity; WPC: Whey protein concentrate; EGCG: (-)-epigallocatechin-3-gallate; MCFAs: Medium-chain fatty acids; CMC: carboxymethylcellulose; Lf: Lactoferrin; β-LG: β-lactoglobulin; DHA: docosahexaenoic acid.

enhance bioavailability, to overcome instability, and poor water solubility of lipophilic compounds, one option is to entrap the compound of interest into lipid-based nanosystems (McClements 2010). Lipid-based nanoformulations have emerged as a promising approach to enhance bioavailability, solubility, and stability of foods, thus preventing unwanted interactions with other food components. However, development of these formulations involves careful design and depends on the physicochemical properties of the lipid excipients (e.g., particle size, composition, concentration, and interfacial characteristics), their compatibility with the encapsulated compounds, as well as their physiological processing in the GI tract (McClements et al. 2015, Salvia-Trujillo et al. 2017). Nanosystems such as nanoemulsions, nanoliposomes, self-emulsifying systems, and solid lipid nanoparticles have been developed as carriers for bioactive compounds (Rodríguez et al. 2016). The oral bioavailability of lipophilic compounds entrapped in the NS, such as curcumin, β-carotene, and oil-soluble vitamins, has been enhanced in various degrees through the improvement of aqueous solubility, protection against instability, and improvement of intestinal absorption and lymphatic transport (Shin et al. 2015). For instance, a recent study evaluated the efficacy of β-lactoglobulin (as a primary layer) and sodium alginate (as a secondary layer) NS, developed from electrostatic interactions, in a variety of aspects: encapsulation, protection, delivery, heat stability, and controlled release of hydrophobic curcumin (Mirpoor et al. 2017). The encapsulation efficiency of curcumin was around 98% and the NSs were efficiently able to retain the curcumin inside over time. The physical stability of curcumin toward precipitation in aqueous solution was significantly improved after introduction into NSs. Moreover, NSs conferred considerable protection to curcumin against heat-induced degradation. A sustained release behavior during 12 hours was observed in simulated intestinal fluid (78.5%), but no release occurred in simulated fasting and non-fasting gastric conditions. Table 5.2 shows other examples of poorly water-soluble compounds that have demonstrated enhanced oral bioavailability when delivered in such systems.

#### 5.6.1.2 Hydrophilic Compounds

As lipophilic compounds, the main challenges for food fortification with hydrophilic compounds are their physical and chemical vulnerability within the food matrix. For example, anthocyanins, catechins, vitamin C, and bioactive peptides are some examples of hydrophilic compounds that present high potential to be incorporated in NSs (Katouzian and Jafari 2016). Hydrophilic compounds are very sensitive to temperature, oxygen, and light conditions. They usually are quickly hydrolyzed or oxidized which lead to their degradation or non-active by-product formation during food processing (e.g., high-pressure, thermal sterilization, and blending) (Aditya et al. 2015). Another essential issue is the interaction of hydrophilic compounds with other substances in the food matrix (e.g., hydrogen ions, reducing and oxidizing substances) that could induce their chemical degradation. Moreover, bioavailability of hydrophilic compounds within the GI tract can also decrease due to their binding to proteins or to compounds enzymatic and to acidic or alkaline pH degradation before reaching the adsorption site (Aditya et al. 2017).

A number of studies have shown the capacity to encapsulate hydrophilic compounds into NSs. Water-in-oil nanoemulsions containing folic acid dispersed in canola oil by a low energy (spontaneous) emulsification technique were optimized, so that the final product could be encapsulated within maltodextrin-WPI two layer emulsions (Assadpour et al. 2016). The results showed that the optimum nanoemulsion formulation was: 12% dispersed phase volume fraction, water to surfactant ratio of 0.9, and folic acid content of 3 mg/mL of dispersed phase within maltodextrin-whey protein (in a ratio of 1:1) double emulsions. In another work, (Zhang et al. 2017) anionic carboxymethyl starch (CMS) and cationic quaternary ammonium starch were used to construct nanocapsules through LbL deposition onto colloidal BSA particles. Degree of substitution and molar mass of CMS were adjusted to obtain a BSA colon-specific delivery system. It was observed that higher degree of substitution and lower molar mass of CMS improved BSA encapsulation efficiency (45.52%). On the other hand, CMS with lower degree of substitution and molar mass showed better colon-specific delivery where 33.04% and 64.97% BSA was released in the simulated upper GI tract and in simulated colonic fluid, respectively. Other examples of nanoencapsulated hydrophilic compounds are presented in Table 5.2.

### 5.6.2 Encapsulation Efficiency and Loading Capacity of Nanolaminated Systems

When a NS is developed, it is especially important to encapsulate the highest quantity of bioactive compound. Therefore, some essential characteristics related to the encapsulation system, namely, encapsulation efficiency (EE) and loading capacity (LC), need to be considered to prove if the NS is appropriate as a carrier of a specific compound (McClements 2010).

The EE evaluates the capacity of the delivery system to hold the encapsulated bioactive compound. The EE is determined as the percentage of the entrapped compound related to its initial quantity (Eq. 5.1) (Pinheiro et al. 2015):

$$\text{EE}(\%) = \frac{\text{total mass bioactive compound-free mass bioactive compound}}{\text{total mass bioactive compound}} \times 100 \quad (5.1)$$

The LC measures the mass of encapsulated bioactive compound per unit of mass of the encapsulation system (Eq. 5.2) (Shu et al. 2010):

$$\text{LC}(\%) = \frac{\text{total mass bioactive compound-free mass bioactive compound}}{\text{total mass nanolaminated system}} \times 100 \quad (5.2)$$

To assess the total mass of bioactive compound encapsulated within the NS, the total mass of bioactive compound initial used must be determined, for example, after centrifugation of NS suspension, where non-encapsulated compounds should be present in the supernatant. The free mass of bioactive compound can be determined using different techniques such as high performance liquid chromatography or fluorescence spectrophotometry (Tarhini et al. 2017). Many features of NSs that could have an influence in EE and LC are presented below:

i. Initial bioactive compound/Nanosystem material concentration ratio. It was shown that EE increased when peppermint oil: (zein/gum arabic) mass ratio decreased (Chen and Zhong 2015).
ii. Initial ratio concentration of the materials used to produce NS. Alginate/cashew gum nanosystems encapsulating *Lippia sidoides* essential oil have been developed (de Oliveira et al. 2014). The authors showed that EE and LC values were maximum for 1:1 (alginate:cashew gum) sample and minimum for sample with a higher alginate proportion (3:1).
iii. Encapsulation method used. Higher LC and EE values have been obtained when poly-L-lysine was encapsulated during chitosan/fucoidan nanosystem formation (by adsorption of poly-L-lysine in the polystyrene nanocapsules) instead of being encapsulated after their formation (by diffusion of poly-L-lysine into the nanocapsules' interior) (Pinheiro et al. 2015).
iv. Type of template used. Hollow nanocapsules have been prepared by LbL assembly of water-soluble chitosan and dextran sulfate on BSA-entrapping silica particles (amino-functionalized or bare silica particles), which were subsequently removed (Shu et al. 2010). They reported that strong electrostatic interactions established between BSA and amino-functionalized silica particles enhanced EE, while the bare silica particles presented lower EE values, due to adsorption occurring mainly by hydrogen bonds.

Table 5.2 presents some studies of compounds encapsulated in diverse NSs and their respective EE and LC.

## 5.7 CONCLUSION AND FUTURE PERSPECTIVES

NSs can be prepared only with food-grade ingredients using the simple and cost-effective LbL method. There are a number of factors (e.g., pH, ionic strength, and polyelectrolyte properties) that can influence NS' formation and therefore should be controlled in order to obtain stable systems. These systems can act as carriers of different bioactive compounds and are able to provide enhanced physicochemical stability and functional properties to food products. In fact, their multilayer structure allows the introduction of different functionalities in the same system, and once they are generally very sensitive to environmental conditions, changes in pH or ionic strength can change their permeability, and, consequently, the release of bioactive compounds can be triggered. Therefore, NSs can be specifically designed to control the digestion, release, and absorption of bioactive compounds within the GI tract.

Different research results suggest that NSs have the potential to improve food preservation and food fortification, but there are still unknown aspects that need a deeper understanding, such as the relationship between their structure and functional properties and their safety for human consumption, mostly due to health concerns regarding the use of nanoscale systems. Therefore, further work is still needed to evaluate NSs in terms of: (i) stability and functional performance; (ii) behavior in food matrices during storage; (iii) behavior during digestion and absorption processes; and (iv) potential toxicological effects.

## ACKNOWLEDGMENTS

Ana C. Pinheiro and Joana T. Martins acknowledge the Foundation for Science and Technology for their fellowships (SFRH/BPD/101181/2014 and SFRH/BPD/89992/2012). The authors would also like to thank the Brazilian Government for support given by the Conselho Nacional de Desenvolvimento Científico e Tecnológico (CNPq). Carneiro-da-Cunha, M.G. express your gratitude to the CNPq for research grant. This work was supported by Portuguese Foundation for Science and Technology under the scope of the Project PTDC/AGR-TEC/5215/2014, of the strategic funding of UID/BIO/04469/2013 unit and COMPETE 2020 (POCI-01-0145-FEDER-006684), and BioTecNorte operation (NORTE-01-0145-FEDER-000004) funded by the European Regional Development Fund under the scope of Norte2020 - Programa Operacional Regional do Norte.

## REFERENCES

Abbas, Shabbar, Eric Karangwa, Mohanad Bashari, Khizar Hayat, Xiao Hong, Hafiz Rizwan Sharif, and Xiaoming Zhang. 2015. "Fabrication of polymeric nanocapsules from curcumin-loaded nanoemulsion templates by self-assembly." *Ultrasonics Sonochemistry* 23:81–92.

Abeyrathne, E. D. Nalaka Sandun, H. Y. Lee, and Dong Uk. Ahn. 2013. "Egg white proteins and their potential use in food processing or as nutraceutical and pharmaceutical agents—A review." *Poultry Science* 92(12):3292–3299.

Acevedo-Fani, Alejandra, Laura Salvia-Trujillo, Robert Soliva-Fortuny, and Olga Martín-Belloso. 2017a. "Layer-by-layer assembly of food-grade alginate/chitosan nanolaminates: Formation and physicochemical characterization." *Food Biophysics* 12(3):299–308.

Acevedo-Fani, Alejandra, Robert Soliva-Fortuny, and Olga Martín-Belloso. 2017b. "Nanostructured emulsions and nanolaminates for delivery of active ingredients: Improving food safety and functionality." *Trends in Food Science & Technology* 60:12–22.

Acevedo-Fani, Alejandra, Robert Soliva-Fortuny, and Olga Martín-Belloso. 2018. "Photo-protection and controlled release of folic acid using edible alginate/chitosan nanolaminates." *Journal of Food Engineering* 229:72–82.

Aditya, N. P., Sheetal Aditya, Hanjoo Yang, Hye Won Kim, Sung Ook Park, and Sanghoon Ko. 2015. "Co-delivery of hydrophobic curcumin and hydrophilic catechin by a water-in-oil-in-water double emulsion." *Food Chemistry* 173:7–13.

Aditya, N. P., Yadira Gonzalez Espinosa, and Ian T. Norton. 2017. "Encapsulation systems for the delivery of hydrophilic nutraceuticals: Food application." *Biotechnology Advances* 35 (4):450–457.

Ale, Marcel Tutor, Jørn D. Mikkelsen, and Anne S. Meyer. 2011. "Important determinants for fucoidan bioactivity: A critical review of structure-function relations and extraction methods for fucose-containing sulfated polysaccharides from brown seaweeds." *Marine Drugs* 9 (10):2106–2130.

Antonov, Yurij A., Irina L. Zhuravleva, Ruth Cardinaels, and Paula Moldenaers. 2018. "Macromolecular complexes of lysozyme with kappa carrageenan." *Food Hydrocolloids* 74:227–238.

Assadpour, Elham, Yahya Maghsoudlou, Seid-Mahdi Jafari, Mohammad Ghorbani, and Mehran Aalami. 2016. "Optimization of folic acid nano-emulsification and encapsulation by maltodextrin-whey protein double emulsions." *International Journal of Biological Macromolecules* 86:197–207.

Belitz, Hans-Dieter, Werner Grosch, and Peter Schieberle. 2004. "Coffee, tea, cocoa." In *Food Chemistry*, pp. 939–969. Berlin, Heidelberg, Germany: Springer.

Bourbon, Ana I., Ana C. Pinheiro, Miguel A. Cerqueira, and António A. Vicente. 2016. "Influence of chitosan coating on protein-based nanohydrogels properties and in vitro gastric digestibility." *Food Hydrocolloids* 60:109–118.

Bourbon, Ana I., Miguel A. Cerqueira, and António A. Vicente. 2016. "Encapsulation and controlled release of bioactive compounds in lactoferrin-glycomacropeptide nanohydrogels: Curcumin and caffeine as model compounds." *Journal of Food Engineering* 180:110–119.

Bueno, Vânia Blasques, and Denise Freitas Siqueira Petri. 2014. "Xanthan hydrogel films: Molecular conformation, charge density and protein carriers." *Carbohydrate Polymers* 101:897–904.

Cerqueira, Miguel A., Ana C. Pinheiro, Hélder D. Silva, Philippe E. Ramos, Maria A. Azevedo, María L. Flores-López, Melissa C. Rivera, Ana I. Bourbon, Óscar L. Ramos, and António A. Vicente. 2014. "Design of bio-nanosystems for oral delivery of functional compounds." *Food Engineering Reviews* 6(1–2):1–19.

Chang, Chao, Taoran Wang, Qiaobin Hu, Mingyong Zhou, Jingyi Xue, and Yangchao Luo. 2017. "Pectin coating improves physicochemical properties of caseinate/zein nanoparticles as oral delivery vehicles for curcumin." *Food Hydrocolloids* 70 (Supplement C):143–151.

Chang, Yaoguang, and David Julian McClements. 2015. "Interfacial deposition of an anionic polysaccharide (fucoidan) on protein-coated lipid droplets: Impact on the stability of fish oil-in-water emulsions." *Food Hydrocolloids* 51:252–260.

Chen, Huaiqiong, and Qixin Zhong. 2015. "A novel method of preparing stable zein nanoparticle dispersions for encapsulation of peppermint oil." *Food Hydrocolloids* 43:593–602.

Choi, Ae-Jin, Chul-Jin Kim, Yong-Jin Cho, Jae-Kwan Hwang, and Chong-Tai Kim. 2011. "Characterization of capsaicin-loaded nanoemulsions stabilized with alginate and chitosan by self-assembly." *Food and Bioprocess Technology* 4(6):1119–1126.

Chun, Ji-Yeon, Jochen Weiss, Monika Gibis, Mi-Jung Choi, and Geun-Pyo Hong. 2016. "Change of multiple-layered phospholipid vesicles produced by electrostatic deposition of polymers during storage." *International Journal of Food Engineering* 12(8):763–771.

Cook, Michael T., George Tzortzis, Dimitris Charalampopoulos, and Vitaliy V. Khutoryanskiy. 2012. "Microencapsulation of probiotics for gastrointestinal delivery." *Journal of Controlled Release* 162 (1):56–67.

Costa, Rui R., Manuel Alatorre-Meda, and João F. Mano. 2015. "Drug nano-reservoirs synthesized using layer-by-layer technologies." *Biotechnology Advances* 33(6):1310–1326.

Croguennoc, Philippe, Vincent Meunier, Dominique Durand, and Taco Nicolai. 2000. "Characterization of semidilute κ-Carrageenan solutions." *Macromolecules* 33(20):7471–7474.

Cui, Jiwei, Martin P. van Koeverden, Markus Müllner, Kristian Kempe, and Frank Caruso. 2014. "Emerging methods for the fabrication of polymer capsules." *Advances in Colloid and Interface Science* 207:14–31.

de Oliveira, Erick F., Haroldo C. B. Paula, and Regina C. M. de Paula. 2014. "Alginate/cashew gum nanoparticles for essential oil encapsulation." *Colloids and Surfaces B: Biointerfaces* 113:146–151.

Decher, Gero. 2002. "Polyelectrolyte multilayers: An overview." *Abstracts of Papers of the American Chemical Society* 223:016-COLL.

Decher, Gero, Jongdal D. Hong, and Johannes Schmitt. 1992. "Buildup of ultrathin multilayer films by a self-assembly process: III. Consecutively alternating adsorption of anionic and cationic polyelectrolytes on charged surfaces." *Thin Solid Films* 210–211, Part 2:831–835.

Dima, Ştefan, Cristian Dima, and Gabriela Iordăchescu. 2015. "Encapsulation of functional lipophilic food and drug biocomponents." *Food Engineering Reviews* 7(4):417–438.

Elella, Mahmoud H. Abu, Riham R. Mohamed, Eman Abd ElHafeez, and Magdy W. Sabaa. 2017. "Synthesis of novel biodegradable antibacterial grafted xanthan gum." *Carbohydrate Polymers* 173:305–311.

Esfanjani, Afshin Faridi, Seid Mahdi Jafari, Elham Assadpoor, and Adeleh Mohammadi. 2015. "Nano-encapsulation of saffron extract through double-layered multiple emulsions of pectin and whey protein concentrate." *Journal of Food Engineering* 165:149–155.

Espert, María, L. Constantinescu, Teresa Sanz, and Ana Salvador. 2018. "Effect of xanthan gum on palm oil in vitro digestion. Application in starch-based filling creams." *Food Hydrocolloids* 86:87–94.

Etxabide, Alaitz, Marta Urdanpilleta, Iñaki Gómez-Arriaran, Koro de la Caba, and Pedro Guerrero. 2017. "Effect of pH and lactose on cross-linking extension and structure of fish gelatin films." *Reactive and Functional Polymers* 117 (Supplement C):140–146.

EU, & Commission, T. H. E. E. 2012. "Commission Implementing Regulation (EU) No 315/2012 of 12 April 2012."

Fabra, María José, Maria L. Flores-López, Miguel A. Cerqueira, Diana Jasso de Rodriguez, Jose M. Lagaron, and António A. Vicente. 2015. "Layer-by-layer technique to developing functional nanolaminate films with antifungal activity." *Food and Bioprocess Technology* 9 (3):471–480.

FDA. 2011. "Generally Recognized as Safe (GRAS) substance under the US FDA regulation." http://www.accessdata.fda.gov/scripts/fdcc/?set=GRASNotices&id=397. (Accessed on September 2017).

Franco, Indira, María Dolores Pérez, Celia Conesa, Miguel Calvo, and Lourdes Sánchez. 2018. "Effect of technological treatments on bovine lactoferrin: An overview." *Food Research International* 106:173–182.

Gibis, Monika, Karina Thellmann, Chutima Thongkaew, and Jochen Weiss. 2014. "Interaction of polyphenols and multilayered liposomal-encapsulated grape seed extract with native and heat-treated proteins." *Food Hydrocolloids* 41:119–131.

Gleeson, John P., Sinéad M. Ryan, and David J. Brayden. 2016. "Oral delivery strategies for nutraceuticals: Delivery vehicles and absorption enhancers." *Trends in Food Science & Technology* 53:90–101.

Gómez-Guillén, M. C., Begoña Giménez, M. E. López-Caballero, and M. P. Montero. 2011. "Functional and bioactive properties of collagen and gelatin from alternative sources: A review." *Food Hydrocolloids* 25(8):1813–1827.

Gu, Yeun Suk, Eric A. Decker, and D. Julian McClements. 2004. "Influence of pH and ι-Carrageenan concentration on physicochemical properties and stability of β-lactoglobulin-stabilized oil-in-water emulsions." *Journal of Agricultural and Food Chemistry* 52(11):3626–3632.

Gu, Yeun Suk, Eric A. Decker, and D. Julian McClements. 2005. "Influence of pH and carrageenan type on properties of β-lactoglobulin stabilized oil-in-water emulsions." *Food Hydrocolloids* 19(1):83–91.

Guérin, Daniel, Jean-Christophe Vuillemard, Muriel Subirade. 2003. "Protection of bifidobacteria encapsulated in polysaccharide-protein gel beads against gastric juice and bile." *Journal of Food Protection* 66(11):2076–2084.

Gunasekaran, Sundaram, Sanghoon Ko, and Lan Xiao. 2007. "Use of whey proteins for encapsulation and controlled delivery applications." *Journal of Food Engineering* 83(1):31–40.

Guzey, Demet, and D. Julian McClements. 2006. "Formation, stability and properties of multilayer emulsions for application in the food industry." *Advances in Colloid and Interface Science* 128:227–248.

Huguet, M. L., R. J. Neufeld, and E. Dellacherie. 1996. "Calcium-alginate beads coated with polycationic polymers: Comparison of chitosan and DEAE-dextran." *Process Biochemistry* 31(4):347–353.

Indest, T., J. Laine, L. S. Johansson, K. Stana-Kleinschek, S. Strnad, R. Dworczak, and V. Ribitsch. 2009. "Adsorption of fucoidan and chitosan sulfate on chitosan modified PET films monitored by QCM-D." *Biomacromolecules* 10(3):630–637.

JFCRF. 2011. "List of existing food additives. http://www.ffcr.or.jp/zaidan/ffcrhome.nsf/pages/list-exst.add.

Ju, Zhi Yong, and Arun Kilara. 1998. "Gelation of pH-aggregated whey protein isolate solution induced by heat, protease, calcium salt, and acidulant." *Journal of Agricultural and Food Chemistry* 46(5):1830–1835.

Katouzian, Iman, and Seid Mahdi Jafari. 2016. "Nano-encapsulation as a promising approach for targeted delivery and controlled release of vitamins." *Trends in Food Science & Technology* 53:34–48.

Keeney, Matthew, Xiong-ying Jiang, M. Yamane, M. Lee, S. Goodman, and F. Yang. 2015. "Nanocoating for biomolecule delivery using layer-by-layer self-assembly." *Journal of Materials Chemistry B* 3(45):8757–8770.

Kittitheeranun, Paveenuch, Warayuth Sajomsang, Sarunya Phanpee, Alongkot Treetong, Tuksadon Wutikhun, Kunat Suktham, Satit Puttipipatkhachorn, and Uracha Rungsardthong Ruktanonchai. 2015. "Layer-by-layer engineered nanocapsules of curcumin with improved cell activity." *International Journal of Pharmaceutics* 492(1):92–102.

Kocherbitov, Vitaly, Stefan Ulvenlund, Lars-Erik Briggner, Maria Kober, and Thomas Arnebrant. 2010. "Hydration of a natural polyelectrolyte xanthan gum: Comparison with non-ionic carbohydrates." *Carbohydrate Polymers* 82(2):284–290.

Kolasinska, Marta, Rumen Krastev, Thomas Gutberlet, and Piotr Warszynski. 2009. "Layer-by-layer deposition of polyelectrolytes. Dipping versus spraying." *Langmuir* 25(2):1224–1232.

Kurth, D. G., D. Volkmer, and von R. Klitzing. 2003. *Multilayers on Solid Planar Substrates: From Structure to Function, Multilayer Thin Films*: Wiley-VCH Verlag GmbH & Co. KGaA.

Lee, Seung-Sub, Jong-Dal Hong, Chang Hwan Kim, Kwan Kim, Ja Pil Koo, and Ki-Bong Lee. 2001. "Layer-by-layer deposited multilayer assemblies of ionene-type polyelectrolytes based on the spin-coating method." *Macromolecules* 34(16):5358–5360.

Lesmes, Uri, Sandra Sandra, Eric Andrew Decker, and David Julian McClements. 2010. "Impact of surface deposition of lactoferrin on physical and chemical stability of omega-3 rich lipid droplets stabilised by caseinate." *Food Chemistry* 123 (1):99–106.

Lim, Aaron S. L., and Yrjö H. Roos. 2015. "Stability of flocculated particles in concentrated and high hydrophilic solid layer-by-layer (LBL) emulsions formed using whey proteins and gum Arabic." *Food Research International* 74:160–167.

Liu, Fuguo, Di Wang, Cuixia Sun, and Yanxiang Gao. 2016. "Influence of polysaccharides on the physicochemical properties of lactoferrin–polyphenol conjugates coated β-carotene emulsions." *Food Hydrocolloids* 52:661–669.

Liu, Weilin, Jianhua Liu, Wei Liu, Ti Li, and Chengmei Liu. 2013. "Improved physical and in vitro digestion stability of a polyelectrolyte delivery system based on layer-by-layer self-assembly alginate–chitosan-coated nanoliposomes." *Journal of Agricultural and Food Chemistry* 61 (17):4133–4144.

Liu, Weilin, Mengmeng Tian, Youyu Kong, Junmeng Lu, Na Li, and Jianzhong Han. 2017. "Multilayered vitamin C nanoliposomes by self-assembly of alginate and chitosan: Long-term stability and feasibility application in mandarin juice." *LWT—Food Science and Technology* 75:608–615.

Liu, Yuxi, Jing Yang, Ziqi Zhao, Junjie Li, Rui Zhang, and Fanglian Yao. 2012. "Formation and characterization of natural polysaccharide hollow nanocapsules via template layer-by-layer self-assembly." *Journal of Colloid and Interface Science* 379(1):130–140.

Lopes, Nathalie Almeida, Cristian Mauricio Barreto Pinilla, and Adriano Brandelli. 2017. "Pectin and polygalacturonic acid-coated liposomes as novel delivery system for nisin: Preparation, characterization and release behavior." *Food Hydrocolloids* 70:1–7.

Madrigal-Carballo, Sergio, Seokwon Lim, Gerardo Rodriguez, Amparo O. Vila, Christian G. Krueger, Sundaram Gunasekaran, and Jess D. Reed. 2010. "Biopolymer coating of soybean lecithin liposomes via layer-by-layer self-assembly as novel delivery system for ellagic acid." *Journal of Functional Foods* 2(2):99–106.

Majka, Grzegorz, Klaudyna Śpiewak, Katarzyna Kurpiewska, Piotr Heczko, Grażyna Stochel, Magdalena Strus, and Małgorzata Brindell. 2013. "A high-throughput method for the quantification of iron saturation in lactoferrin preparations." *Analytical and Bioanalytical Chemistry* 405(15):5191–5200.

Martins, Joana T., Óscar L. Ramos, Ana C. Pinheiro, Ana I. Bourbon, Hélder D. Silva, Melissa C. Rivera, Miguel A. Cerqueira, Lorenzo Pastrana, F. Xavier Malcata, África González-Fernández, and António A. Vicente. 2015. "Edible bio-based nanostructures: Delivery, absorption and potential toxicity." *Food Engineering Reviews*:1–23.

Matalanis, Alison, Owen Griffith Jones, and David Julian McClements. 2011. "Structured biopolymer-based delivery systems for encapsulation, protection, and release of lipophilic compounds." *Food Hydrocolloids* 25(8):1865–1880.

McClements, David Julian, and Eric Decker. 2009. "20—Controlling lipid bioavailability using emulsion-based delivery systems." In *Designing Functional Foods*, 502–546. Woodhead Publishing.

McClements, David Julian. 2010. "Design of nano-laminated coatings to control bioavailability of lipophilic food components." *Journal of Food Science* 75(1):R30–R42.

McClements, David Julian, Liqiang Zou, Ruojie Zhang, Laura Salvia-Trujillo, Taha Kumosani, and Hang Xiao. 2015. "Enhancing nutraceutical performance using excipient foods: Designing food structures and compositions to increase bioavailability." *Comprehensive Reviews in Food Science and Food Safety* 14(6):824–847.

McClements, David Julian. 2014. "Biopolymer-based delivery systems" In *Nanoparticle- and Microparticle-based Delivery Systems: Encapsulation, Protection and Release of Active Compounds*, 265–327. Boca Raton, FL: CRC Press.

Medeiros, Bartolomeu G. de S., Ana C. Pinheiro, J. A. Teixeira, António A. Vicente, and Maria G. Carneiro-da-Cunha. 2012a. "Polysaccharide/Protein nanomultilayer coatings: Construction, characterization and evaluation of their effect on 'Rocha' pear (Pyrus communis L.) shelf-life." *Food and Bioprocess Technology* 5(6):2435–2445.

Medeiros, Bartolomeu G. S., Ana C. Pinheiro, Maria G. Carneiro-da-Cunha, and António A. Vicente. 2012b. "Development and characterization of a nanomultilayer coating of pectin and chitosan—Evaluation of its gas barrier properties and application on 'Tommy Atkins' mangoes." *Journal of Food Engineering* 110(3):457–464.

Medeiros, Bartolomeu G. de S., Marthyna P. Souza, Ana C. Pinheiro, Ana I. Bourbon, Miguel A. Cerqueira, António A. Vicente and Maria G. Carneiro-da-Cunha. 2014. "Physical characterisation of an alginate/lysozyme nano-laminate coating and its evaluation on 'Coalho' cheese shelf life." *Food and Bioprocess Technology* 7(4):1088–1098.

Mirpoor, Seyedeh Fatemeh, Seyed Mohammad Hashem Hosseini, and Gholam Hossein Yousefi. 2017. "Mixed biopolymer nanocomplexes conferred physicochemical stability and sustained release behavior to introduced curcumin." *Food Hydrocolloids* 71:216–224.

Montanari, Elita, Chiara Di Meo, Simona Sennato, Antonio Francioso, Anna Laura Marinelli, Francesca Ranzo, Serena Schippa, Tommasina Coviello, Federico Bordi, and Pietro Matricardi. 2017. "Hyaluronan-cholesterol nanohydrogels: Characterisation and effectiveness in carrying alginate lyase." *New Biotechnology* 37:80–89.

Mora-Huertas, C. E., H. Fessi, and A. Elaissari. 2010. "Polymer-based nanocapsules for drug delivery." *International Journal of Pharmaceutics* 385(1–2):113–142.

Moreno-Expósito, Luis, Rebeca Illescas-Montes, Lucía Melguizo-Rodríguez, Concepción Ruiz, Javier Ramos-Torrecillas, and Elvira de Luna-Bertos. 2018. "Multifunctional capacity and therapeutic potential of lactoferrin." *Life Sciences* 195:61–64.

Opanasopit, Praneet, Auayporn Apirakaramwong, Tanasait Ngawhirunpat, Theerasak Rojanarata, and Uracha Ruktanonchai. 2008. "Development and characterization of pectinate micro/nanoparticles for gene delivery." *AAPS PharmSciTech* 9(1):67–74.

Pastorino, Laura, Elena Dellacasa, Mohammad Hossei Dabiri, Bruno Fabiano, and Svetlana Erokhina. 2016. "Towards the fabrication of polyelectrolyte-based nanocapsules for bio-medical applications." *BioNanoScience* 6(4):496–501.

Peng, Junbiao, Jinglin Wei, Zhennan Zhu, Honglong Ning, Wei Cai, Kuankuan Lu, Rihui Yao, Hong Tao, Yanqiong Zheng, and Xubing Lu. 2017. "Properties-adjustable alumina-zirconia nanolaminate dielectric fabricated by spin-coating." *Nanomaterials* 7(12):419.

Peniche, Carlos, Waldo Argüelles-Monal, Hazel Peniche, and Niuris Acosta. 2003. "Chitosan: An attractive biocompatible polymer for microencapsulation." *Macromolecular Bioscience* 3(10):511–520.

Petri, Denise F. S. 2015. "Xanthan gum: A versatile biopolymer for biomedical and technological applications." *Journal of Applied Polymer Science* 132(23).

Pinheiro, Ana C., Ana I. Bourbon, Bartolomeu G. de S. Medeiros, Luís H. M. da Silva, Maria C. H. da Silva, Maria G. Carneiro-da-Cunha, Manuel A. Coimbra, and António A. Vicente. 2012. "Interactions between κ-carrageenan and chitosan in nanolayered coatings—Structural and transport properties." *Carbohydrate Polymers* 87(2):1081–1090.

Pinheiro, Ana C., Ana I. Bourbon, Mafalda A. C. Quintas, Manuel A. Coimbra, and António A. Vicente. 2012. "K-carrageenan/chitosan nanolayered coating for controlled release of a model bioactive compound." *Innovative Food Science & Emerging Technologies* 16(0):227–232.

Pinheiro, Ana C., Ana I. Bourbon, Miguel A. Cerqueira, Élia Maricato, Cláudia Nunes, Manuel A. Coimbra, and António A. Vicente. 2015. "Chitosan/fucoidan multilayer nanocapsules as a vehicle for controlled release of bioactive compounds." *Carbohydrate Polymers* 115:1–9.

Pinheiro, Ana C., Manuel A. Coimbra, and António A. Vicente. 2016. "In vitro behaviour of curcumin nanoemulsions stabilized by biopolymer emulsifiers—Effect of interfacial composition." *Food Hydrocolloids* 52:460–467.

Pinheiro, Ana C., Mita Lad, Helder D. Silva, Manuel A. Coimbra, Michael Boland, and Antonio A. Vicente. 2013. "Unravelling the behaviour of curcumin nanoemulsions during in vitro digestion: Effect of the surface charge." *Soft Matter* 9(11):3147–3154.

Ramasamy, Thiruganesh, Ziyad S. Haidar, Tuan Hiep Tran, Ju Yeon Choi, Jee-Heon Jeong, Beom Soo Shin, Han-Gon Choi, Chul Soon Yong, and Jong Oh Kim. 2014. "Layer-by-layer assembly of liposomal nanoparticles with PEGylated polyelectrolytes enhances systemic delivery of multiple anticancer drugs." *Acta Biomaterialia* 10(12):5116–5127.

Ravi Kumar, Majeti N. V. 2000. "A review of chitin and chitosan applications." *Reactive and Functional Polymers* 46(1):1–27.

Richardson, Joseph J., Jiwei Cui, Mattias Björnmalm, Julia A. Braunger, Hirotaka Ejima, and Frank Caruso. 2016. "Innovation in layer-by-layer assembly." *Chemical Reviews* 116(23):14828–14867.

Rinaudo, M. 2008. "Main properties and current applications of some polysaccharides as biomaterials." *Polymer International* 57(3):397–430.

Rinaudo, Marguerite. 2006. "Chitin and chitosan: Properties and applications." *Progress in Polymer Science* 31(7):603–632.

Rivera, Melissa C., Ana C. Pinheiro, Ana I. Bourbon, Miguel A. Cerqueira, and António A. Vicente. 2015. "Hollow chitosan/alginate nanocapsules for bioactive compound delivery." *International Journal of Biological Macromolecules* 79(0):95–102.

Rodríguez, Julia, María J. Martín, María A. Ruiz, and Beatriz Clares. 2016. "Current encapsulation strategies for bioactive oils: From alimentary to pharmaceutical perspectives." *Food Research International* 83:41–59.

Rubner, M. F. 2003. "pH-controlled fabrication of polyelectrolyte multilayers: Assembly and applications." In *Multilayer Thin Films*, 133–154. Wiley-VCH Verlag GmbH & Co. KGaA.

Salvia-Trujillo, Laura, Robert Soliva-Fortuny, M. Alejandra Rojas-Graü, D. Julian McClements, and Olga Martín-Belloso. 2017. "Edible nanoemulsions as carriers of active ingredients: A review." *Annual Review of Food Science and Technology* 8(1):439–466.

Seo, Seongmin, Sangmin Lee, and Yong Tae Park. 2016. "Note: Automatic layer-by-layer spraying system for functional thin film coatings." *Review of Scientific Instruments* 87(3):036110.

Shahmohammadi, Azin. 2018. "Lysozyme separation from chicken egg white: A review." *European Food Research and Technology* 244(4):577–593.

Shamsara, Omid, Seid Mahdi Jafari, and Zayniddin Kamarovich Muhidinov. 2017. "Development of double layered emulsion droplets with pectin/β-lactoglobulin complex for bioactive delivery purposes." *Journal of Molecular Liquids* 243:144–150.

Shin, Gye Hwa, Jun Tae Kim, and Hyun Jin Park. 2015. "Recent developments in nanoformulations of lipophilic functional foods." *Trends in Food Science & Technology* 46(1):144–157.

Shu, Shujun, Chunyang Sun, Xinge Zhang, Zhongming Wu, Zhen Wang, and Chaoxing Li. 2010. "Hollow and degradable polyelectrolyte nanocapsules for protein drug delivery." *Acta Biomaterialia* 6 (1):210–217.

Shutava, Tatsiana G., Shantanu S. Balkundi, and Yuri M. Lvov. 2009. "(–)-Epigallocatechin gallate/gelatin layer-by-layer assembled films and microcapsules." *Journal of Colloid and Interface Science* 330(2):276–283.

Slavutsky, Aníbal M., and María A. Bertuzzi. 2016. "Improvement of water barrier properties of starch films by lipid nanolamination." *Food Packaging and Shelf Life* 7:41–46.

Sogias, Ioannis A., Vitaliy V. Khutoryanskiy, and Adrian C. Williams. 2010. "Exploring the factors affecting the solubility of chitosan in water." *Macromolecular Chemistry and Physics* 211(4):426–433.

Souza, Marthyna P., Antônio F. M. Vaz, Miguel A. Cerqueira, José A. Texeira, António A. Vicente, and Maria G. Carneiro-da-Cunha. 2014. "Effect of an edible nanomultilayer coating by electrostatic self-assembly on the shelf life of fresh-cut mangoes." *Food and Bioprocess Technology* 8(3):647–654.

Tan, Chen, Jiehong Xie, Xiaoming Zhang, Jibao Cai, and Shuqin Xia. 2016. "Polysaccharide-based nanoparticles by chitosan and gum arabic polyelectrolyte complexation as carriers for curcumin." *Food Hydrocolloids* 57:236–245.

Tarhini, Mohamad, Hélène Greige-Gerges, and Abdelhamid Elaissari. 2017. "Protein-based nanoparticles: From preparation to encapsulation of active molecules." *International Journal of Pharmaceutics* 522(1):172–197.

Tedeschi, Concetta, Frank Caruso, Helmuth Möhwald, and Stefan Kirstein. 2000. "Adsorption and desorption behavior of an anionic pyrene chromophore in sequentially deposited polyelectrolyte-dye thin films." *Journal of the American Chemical Society* 122(24):5841–5848.

Thu, Beate, Per Bruheim, Terje Espevik, Olav Smidsrød, Patrick Soon-Shiong, and Gudmund Skjåk-Bræk. 1996. "Alginate polycation microcapsules: II. Some functional properties." *Biomaterials* 17(11):1069–1079.

Tieke, B., Mario Pyrasch, and A. Toutianoush. 2003. Functional layer-by-layer assemblies with photo- and electrochemical response and selective transport of small molecules and ions, In *Multilayer Thin Films*, Wiley-VCH Verlag GmbH & Co. KGaA.

Vidhyalakshmi, R., R. Bhakyaraj, R. S. Subhasree. 2009. "Encapsulation "The future of probiotics"-A review." *Advances in Biological Research* 3(3–4):96–103.

Weiss, Jochen, Paul Takhistov, and D. Julian McClements. 2006. "Functional materials in food nanotechnology." *Journal of Food Science* 71(9):R107–R116.

Wu, Lei, Jing Sun, Xitong Su, Qiuli Yu, Qiuyang Yu, and Peng Zhang. 2016. "A review about the development of fucoidan in antitumor activity: Progress and challenges." *Carbohydrate Polymers* 154:96–111.

Zhang, Tingting, Panghu Zhou, Yingfei Zhan, Xiaowen Shi, Jinyou Lin, Yumin Du, Xiuhong Li, and Hongbing Deng. 2015. "Pectin/lysozyme bilayers layer-by-layer deposited cellulose nanofibrous mats for antibacterial application." *Carbohydrate Polymers* 117:687–693.

Zhang, Yaqiong, Yuge Niu, Yangchao Luo, Mei Ge, Tian Yang, Liangli Yu, and Qin Wang. 2014. "Fabrication, characterization and antimicrobial activities of thymol-loaded zein nanoparticles stabilized by sodium caseinate–chitosan hydrochloride double layers." *Food Chemistry* 142:269–275.

Zhang, Yiping, Chengdeng Chi, Xiaoyi Huang, Qin Zou, Xiaoxi Li, and Ling Chen. 2017. "Starch-based nanocapsules fabricated through layer-by-layer assembly for oral delivery of protein to lower gastrointestinal tract." *Carbohydrate Polymers* 171:242–251.

Zhao, Dong, Jian Xu, and Xia Xu. 2018. "Bioactivity of fucoidan extracted from Laminaria japonica using a novel procedure with high yield." *Food Chemistry* 245:911–918.

Zhong, Yang, Catherine F. Whittington, Ling Zhang, and Donald T. Haynie. 2007. "Controlled loading and release of a model drug from polypeptide multilayer nanofilms." *Nanomedicine: Nanotechnology, Biology and Medicine* 3(2):154–160.

Zhu, Mingjin, Liming Ge, Yongbo Lyu, Yaxin Zi, Xinying Li, Defu Li, and Changdao Mu. 2017. "Preparation, characterization and antibacterial activity of oxidized κ-carrageenan." *Carbohydrate Polymers* 174:1051–1058.

Zimet, Patricia, and Yoav D. Livney. 2009. "Beta-lactoglobulin and its nanocomplexes with pectin as vehicles for ω-3 polyunsaturated fatty acids." *Food Hydrocolloids* 23(4):1120–1126.

# 6 Bio-nanosystems Resorting to Electrohydrodynamic Processing

*Sergio Torres-Giner, Beatriz Melendez-Rodriguez, Adriane Cherpinski, and Jose M. Lagaron*

**CONTENTS**



## 6.1 INTRODUCTION TO ELECTROHYDRODYNAMIC PROCESSING

Over the past decade, electrohydrodynamic processing (EHDP) has gained a great interest in both scientific community and industry for fabrication of ultrathin polymer structures in the field of food technology (Echegoyen et al. 2017). EHDP is a straightforward, versatile, and low-cost technique that employs a high-voltage electrostatic field into a polymer solution or melt *via* a metallic capillary orifice to fabricate ultrathin polymer structures with diameters ranging from below 100 nm to above some microns (Reneker and Chun 1996). Polymer micro-, submicro-, and nanostructures obtained by EHDP offer notable physicochemical characteristics, including a significantly large surface-to-mass ratio, great porosity, and remarkable mechanical performance (Ramakrishna et al. 2006).

EHDP basic setup consists of four main components:

- A plastic or glass syringe containing the polymer solution
- A high-voltage power supply, typically up to 30 kV
- A spinneret, which is usually made of a metallic needle
- A grounded or an oppositely charged collector surface that is based on a single piece of conductive substrate either in the form of a static flat plate or of a rotating mandrel.

Briefly, the power supply is connected to the needle while the polymer solution is pumped at a steady flow-rate. The application of high voltage results in several instabilities (e.g., whipping or bending motions) within the polymer solution due to the presence of two electrostatic forces playing an antagonist role—the electrostatic repulsion between the surface charges tends to break the biopolymer solution drop while the surface tension acts as an attracting force maintaining their shape. If the strength of the electrical field continues to increase, the repulsive forces overcome the surface tension of the polymer solution. This produces the deformation of the spherical droplet to a conical shape, leading to the eruption of an electrically charged jet from the conical polymer droplet, i.e., the so-called "Taylor cone" (Li and Xia 2004). As the jet accelerates toward regions of lower potential, the solvent rapidly evaporates, whereas the entanglements of the polymer chains prevent the jet from breaking up. Finally, the polymer nanostructures are deposited on the metallic collector, which can be either a static flat plate or a rotating mandrel, placed at a suitable distance from the needle.

The morphology of electrospun nanostructures is affected by different processing conditions (Doshi and Reneker 1995). Indeed, for a given polymer, different morphologies can co-exist. The most relevant factors can be divided into two main categories: (i) those dependent on the intrinsic properties of the polymer solution, and (ii) those related to the operational conditions during EHDP. As a result, by changing these parameters multiple morphologies can be attained. Mainly, two "sister" technologies or variants of EHDP can be defined, namely, electrospinning and electrospraying. Both processes are illustrated in Figure 6.1. In the electrospinning process a mat of continuous ultrathin fibers is obtained, which can be seen in the scanning electron microscopy inset included in Figure 6.1a. This can comprise different fiber-like morphologies, such as tubular and flat nanofibers, as well as microfibers of above 1 μm with ribbon-like profiles and rough surfaces. In the case of electrospraying, round-like submicron or nanocapsules are obtained, as shown in Figure 6.1b. For electrospraying, the expression electrohydrodynamic atomization is also used due to the formation of non-continuous structures.

Firstly, solution properties, namely, viscosity, surface tension, and conductivity, certainly have a strong influence on the resultant polymer morphology (Torres-Giner et al. 2008a, 2008b). In particular, solution viscosity, which is in turn related to both polymer molecular weight and concentration, plays the main role in defining

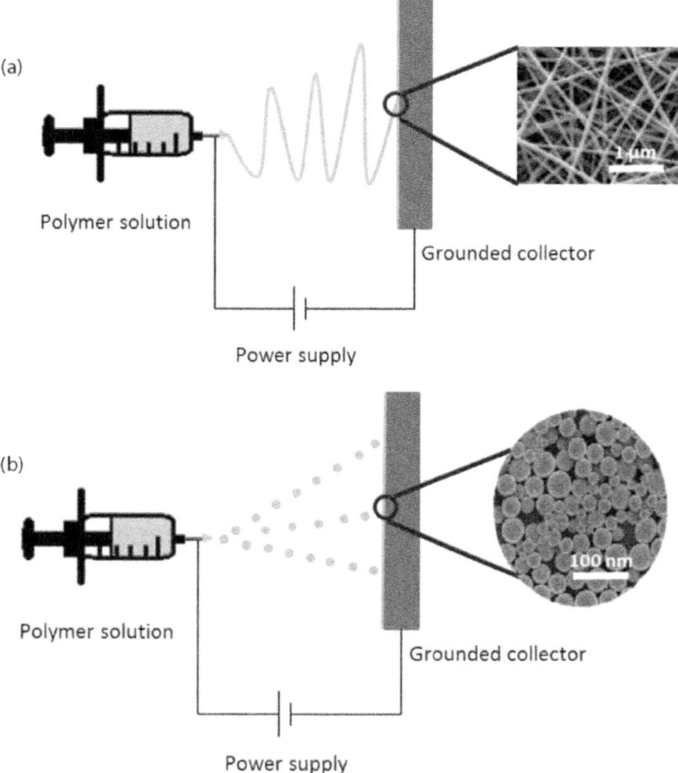


**FIGURE 6.1** Schematic illustration displaying the process of electrospinning (a) and electrospraying (b). The scanning electron microscopy images display the resultant morphology obtained for each process. Scale markers are 1 µm and 100 nm, respectively.

both optimum electrospinnability conditions for the polymer solution as well as the final particle morphology attained (Frenot and Chronakis 2003). As solution viscosity increases, more force is required to overcome both the surface tension and the viscoelastic force, i.e., to attenuate the jet and favor electrospinning. In particular, it has been found that low polymer concentrations generally tend to yield capsules, i.e., electrospraying, whereas higher values of viscosity lead to the formation of continuous polymer fibers, i.e., electrospinning. Indeed, electrospinning is often improved by reducing surface tension of a given polymer solution (Doshi and Reneker 1993). Similarly, polymer solutions with higher conductivities, i.e., with a higher charge density, tend to produce electrospun fibers with smaller diameter (Tan et al. 2005). For most natural polymers, which are generally "polyelectrolytic" in nature, the ions increase the charge-carrying ability of the polymer jet, subjecting the polymer solution to a higher tension under the electric field. This habitually results in a poor degree of fiber formation when compared to synthetic polymer counterparts (Zong et al. 2002). To improve solution conductivity, both the addition of a salt and/or the use of organic acids as solvents can enhance electrospinnability as these can function as carriers of the electric charges (Chaobo et al. 2006).

Secondly, the above-described process parameters, i.e., applied voltage, solution flow-rate, and tip-to-collector distance, obviously have also a great impact on the fabricated polymer nanostructures. Among them, applied voltage is often considered to have the strongest influence on nanofibers diameter, though this is varying from polymer to polymer and is also highly dependent on the solution properties. For instance, an increase in the applied voltage typically produces nanofibers with smaller diameters, which is related to the stretching of the polymer solution in correlation with the charge repulsion within the polymer jet (Sill and von Recum 2008). However, an extremely high voltage can potentially result in formation of beads or beaded nanofibers that are attributed to an increase in the jet length (Deitzel et al. 2001). Concerning flow-rate, its proper adjustment allows obtaining nanofibers with uniform bead-free shapes (Pillay et al. 2013). In general, a positive relation between flow-rate and fibers diameter is usually established, which is attributed to a higher volume of solution available (Megelski et al. 2002). However, excessively high values of flow-rate can also lead to the formation of beaded fibers, being associated with wet jets due to the presence of the remaining solvent (Torres-Giner et al. 2009). Changing the tip-to-collector distance can additionally affect the morphology of the resulting polymer nanostructures. Different studies have shown that, for a given polymer solution concentration, fibers or capsules with diameters in the nanoscale range can be obtained by increasing the tip-to-collector distance (Wang and Kumar 2006; Torres-Giner et al. 2008a, 2008b).

Finally, in addition to the solution properties and process parameters, environmental factors, such as temperature and relative humidity, can also exert a significant effect on the process and the resultant polymer nanostructures (De Vrieze et al. 2008). On the one hand, high temperature can increase the evaporation rate of the solvent and, hence, reduce solution viscosity (Su et al. 2011). On the other hand, different values of relative humidity can influence the control of the solidification process of the charged jet, affecting the morphology of the electrospun or electrosprayed materials (Park and Lee 2010). Thus, precise controls of solution parameters, operating conditions, and also environmental factors are required to obtain smooth and defect-free polymer nanostructures.

The morphology of the electrospun structures plays an important role in the material physical properties and in the encapsulation efficiency (Pérez-Masiá et al. 2014b). Interestingly, electrospun nanofibers are comparatively much thinner in diameter and, accordingly, with greater surface-to-volume ratios than fibers produced using classical melt spinning processes. This fact is due to the elongation process, which is accomplished *via* a contactless scheme. Indeed, individual fiber diameters can be around 10–1000 times smaller than synthetic fibers produced by melt extrusion and also than naturally occurring fibers such as cotton, wool, and silk. The formed fibers within the electrospun mat are all fully interconnected to form a tridimensional network, in which a high density of pores is formed as a result of fiber entanglements. Regarding the electrosprayed capsules, these are also considerably smaller than capsules obtained through other conventional encapsulation technologies (e.g., spray drying and fluidized bed coating). Such smaller dimensions lead to higher specific surface areas and, particularly, provide extraordinary functionalities, which otherwise could not be found in equivalent materials of larger sizes.

## 6.2 FUNCTIONALIZATION TECHNIQUES BY ELECTROHYDRODYNAMIC PROCESSING

Regarding the incorporation of functional agents, three main different strategies during EHDP can be considered, namely, blending, coaxial, and emulsion (Rieger et al. 2013). Figure 6.2 illustrates the configuration process setup and cross-section of an individual polymer particle, either a fiber or capsule, fabricated *via* these three methods. It can be seen that, whereas the blend-electrospun materials contain the functional agents dispersed throughout the whole polymer matrix, the structures obtained by the other two EHDP methods, i.e., coaxial and emulsion, lead to the formation of a core-shell morphology. In the next subsections, the different strategies are summarized.

### 6.2.1 Blending

In this configuration, usually also called single-step electrospinning, the active agent molecules (e.g., drugs or nutraceuticals) are dissolved or dispersed (in terms of lacking solubility) in the polymer solution used for EHDP. The distribution of the functional agent inside the electrospun material is highly dependent on the physico-chemical properties of the polymer solution and the agent interaction with the solution (Zamani et al. 2013). Although this technique is relatively simple in comparison with the coaxial and emulsion configurations, its application has its own limitations.

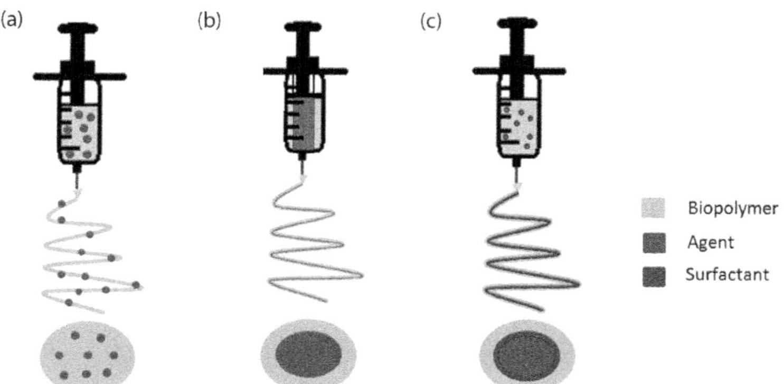


**FIGURE 6.2** Schematic illustration of the different strategies for functionalization of electrospun/electrosprayed biopolymers and the expected distribution of the agent molecules in the resultant structures: (a) blending; (b) coaxial; and (c) emulsion.

For instance, in the context of food ingredients, sensitive bioactive agents (e.g., antioxidants or proteins) may degrade or denature in the presence of the harsh solvents and lose their bioactivity (Szentivanyi et al. 2011). Moreover, regarding substance distribution, most bioactive molecules are typically charged molecules that, hence, migrate toward the jet surface due to charge repulsion during EHDP. As a result, instead of a uniform distribution of the functional molecules within the polymer structure, a surface enrichment is generally observed. This can potentially result in the formation of beaded fibers and/or severe burst releases of the agent molecules when the electrospun mats are exposed to the release media. In general, blending easily yields a dispersed functional agent, but, in order to achieve higher protections or sustained release capacities, it certainly requires the use of other EHDP configurations.

### 6.2.2 Coaxial

The coaxial configuration implies the use of two concentrically arranged needles that are connected to two reservoirs containing different polymer solutions. Typically, one solution includes the polymer matrix (shell), and the other solution is based on a different polymer containing the functional additive (core). The two polymer solutions, generally made of different polymers, though this is not a necessary condition, are pumped *via* the two nozzles above-mentioned in a concentric arrangement and connected to the same high voltage source. This results in a ultrathin polymer structure with a core-shell morphology. To avoid the contact between polymer solutions, the two solutions are kept separated in different reservoirs until drop formation occurs, i.e., prior to the eruption of an electrically charged jet. In coaxial electrospinning, also referred as co-electrospinning, the functional agent, which is usually fed through the inner core polymer solution, is protected both from the electric field and solvents by the outer polymer shell (Torres-Giner et al. 2012). The core and shell phases interaction certainly has an important effect on the electrospinnability during coaxial electrospinning, and the best results are generally achieved by adding a common solvent into the two immiscible solvents of the core and sheath solutions. In this regard, to avoid the jet break-up and uneven fiber deposition, i.e., fibers without uniform core or sheath layers, the flow-rate ratios of the shell and core solutions are typically adjusted between 3:1 and 6:1, respectively (Chakraborty et al. 2009).

The coaxial configuration certainly opens up new routes for encapsulation of biologically active compounds by EHDP. However, application of this method also suffers from certain disadvantages, including design complexity and requirement of precise control of processing variables such as interfacial tension and viscoelasticity of the two polymers. In any case, coaxial electrospinning can be a very powerful tool when properly controlled, particularly to control the release of active agents.

### 6.2.3 Emulsion

In a sense, emulsion electrospinning can be considered an extension of the blending strategy because it requires the same basic setup. However, it involves processing two immiscible solutions simultaneously. In this method, one solution, which contains the core material in the appropriate solvent, is dispersed into the other solution until a stable emulsion is formed. For this, a surfactant, also referred to as emulsifier, is used to disperse the two distinct phases. According to the spatial organization of the oil- and water-based phases, emulsion systems can be conveniently categorized into oil-in-water and water-in-oil emulsions. In an oil-in-water emulsion, oil droplets are dispersed in a continuous water phase, whereas water-in-oil emulsions are dispersions of aqueous droplets in a continuous oil phase. For instance, in the formulation of a water-in-oil emulsion, the water phase is prepared by dissolving both a hydrophilic (or low hydrophobic) polymer and a hydrophilic additive or food ingredient in a water-based solvent, whereas the oil phase is composed of a hydrophobic polymer dissolved in an organic solvent. Once both polymer solutions are fully dissolved, these are mixed in the presence of the surfactant. Therefore, during the emulsion method, common solvents are eliminated, and the solubility and compatibility of the functional agents in the polymer-solvent system is not a decisive factor. During fiber stretching in emulsion electrospinning, water rapidly evaporates and the aqueous phase droplets containing the active ingredients migrate to the center of the jet due to a viscosity gradient. Depending on the molecular weight of the bioactive molecules, they can be placed on the fiber surfaces, remain indifferently distributed within the polymer matrix, or form a core-shell structure (Sy et al. 2009). For instance, active molecules with high molecular weight tend to be encapsulated inside the formed fibers, by which burst release can be avoided (Xu et al. 2005).

In the field of food technology, a large amount of research has been lately performed, being focused on the incorporation of functional materials (e.g., bioactive compounds, enzymes, proteins, drugs, etc.) into biodegradable polymer nanostructures by means of the emulsion configuration (Nikmarama et al. 2017). Compared to the single-step EHDP technique, the use of emulsion systems is a promising alternative since it allows the encapsulation of lipophilic compounds using low-cost hydrophilic polymers and avoids the use of organic solvents that are highly restricted in food systems (Arecchi et al. 2010). Nevertheless, in comparison to the coaxial arrangement, this technique may still damage the active components due to the interface tension between the aqueous and the organic phases of the emulsion. Still, both its basic setup and the simplicity of the process itself make emulsion electrospinning a relatively versatile technique to successfully produce relative bead-free fibers with sustained release capacity. Moreover, this enables optimal loadings of functional agents.

## 6.3 ELECTROHYDRODYNAMIC PROCESSING OF FOOD-GRADE POLYMERS

One of the main advantages of EHDP is the wide range of types of wall polymer materials that can be used. The most common materials used for EHDP are synthetic polymers, which can easily produce fibers. However, these are usually not permitted for direct use in food and are very restricted for pharma or cosmetic applications. Therefore, aiming at the development of electrospun structures for food applications (e.g., encapsulation of food bioactives), biopolymers, including food-grade polymers such as carbohydrate polymers and proteins as well as biodegradable polymers are usually the most preferred choice because they may be non-toxic, and even in some cases, edible and digestible.

Interestingly, electrospun or electrosprayed carbohydrate polymers and proteins can interact with a wide range of active and bioactive compounds *via* their functional groups. This makes these bio-nanosystems versatile carriers to bind and entrap a variety of hydrophilic and hydrophobic active food ingredients. In the case of carbohydrates, they also show higher temperature stability compared to lipids or proteins. Moreover, many biopolymers can be easily dissolved in water-based solvents, or create hydrocolloids, for a stable process. This is of special interest in food-related applications, where the use of organic solvents for the development of edible food additives can pose reasonable concerns regarding the toxic effects due to the presence of remaining solvents (Pérez-Masiá et al. 2015). The high surface tension of water as well as the ionization of water molecules at high voltages in an air environment usually complicate EHDP. Nevertheless, this issue can be solved by addition of surfactants (e.g., polyoxyethylenesorbitan monooleate) in relatively low concentrations (1%–2% wt.) (Pérez-Masiá et al. 2015; Torres-Giner et al. 2017). Moreover, as outlined above, by adjusting the process parameters, the morphology (i.e., size and shape) of the encapsulation structures can be easily controlled.

As a result, the EHDP technology has expanded the use of polysaccharide-based wall materials, like chitosan, alginates, celluloses, starches, or malto- and cyclodextrins (Stijnman et al. 2011). Likewise, proteins, such as whey protein isolate, whey protein concentrate (WPC), soy protein isolate, egg albumen, collagen, gelatine, zein, or casein are a very interesting group of food-grade polymers to be processed by EHDP (Nieuwland et al. 2013). Among food hydrocolloids, WPC deserves a greater interest and attention because of its valuable dietary supplement and functional food enhancement properties. In particular, the secondary structure of the proteins in WPC leads to the formation of a globular quaternary structure, which can create closed and impenetrable capsule walls after electrospraying (López-Rubio and Lagaron 2012). In addition, electrosprayed WPC capsules offer UV-blocking capacity and oxygen barrier properties that show a great deal of potential in the protection of functional foods and nutraceuticals (Torres-Giner et al. 2017). Similarly, zein prolamine, a hydrophobic protein extracted from corn by solvation in ethanol, is also a promising protein in the food technology and related areas. In particular, electrospun zein nanofibers combine high biological value with good physical properties, such as high thermal resistance (Torres-Giner et al. 2008a) and water entrapping enhancement (Yao et al. 2007). In relation to carbohydrates, chitosan is a linear polysaccharide composed of D-glucosamine and N-acetyl-D-glucosamine units that are obtained by partial or full deacetylation of naturally occurring chitin. In this sense, electrospun chitosan nanofibers (Torres-Giner et al. 2008b) and electrosprayed submicron chitosan capsules (Sreekumar et al. 2017) can be targeted to encapsulate food ingredients and to develop novel functional packaging structures. For instance, due to the inherent antimicrobial properties of this polysaccharide, films coated by these chitosan layers are envisaged to potentially prevent food spoilage produced by microorganisms during transportation and storage, expanding the shelf life of packaged foodstuffs and consumer food safety (Torres-Giner 2011b).

## 6.4 BIO-NANOSYSTEMS IN THE FOOD INDUSTRY

Food industry is undoubtedly one of the major fields that may benefit from EHDP using biopolymers, especially for the development of functional foods containing active ingredients. The physiological benefits of the latter, which are particularly expected to impart a health benefit to consumers in addition to the nutrition that the food itself offers, are highly dependent on preserving their bioavailability. This represents a formidable challenge for scientists in the food science and technology field, as most of these functional substances are known to lose effectiveness during processing, storage, and/or in the gastrointestinal tract. The development of nanostructures by EHDP provide a carrier to stabilize labile food ingredients and protect them from diverse factors such as pH and temperature changes, and also to act as delivery vehicles for controlled release is, therefore, of high interest. This can lead to the protection and controlled release of bioactive compounds at the right time and place. In addition, is it also a potential approach to transform liquids into stable and free-flowing powders, which become easier to handle and could be directly incorporated into dry food systems. These novel bio-nanosystems can be particularly formulated to survive travel through the gastrointestinal system to deliver their payload at a particular point, thus maximizing its effectiveness in reducing risk of diseases. Moreover, in the case of non-solid and semi-solid foods, the matrix size reduction of the electrosprayed capsules would allow their incorporation with minimal input in food quality aspects (López-Rubio and Lagaron 2012). More importantly, by decreasing the matrix size to the nano-sized range, improved vehicles with highly controllable delivery-rate can be developed. In particular, particle size reduction is considered to introduce several bio-adhesive improvement factors, including increased adhesive force and thence prolonged gastrointestinal transit time, leading to a higher bioavailability of the encapsulated compound (Chen et al. 2006).

EHDP presents advantages to preserve food ingredients over other well-established encapsulation technologies, for instance, emulsification, coacervation, complexation nanoprecipitation, inclusion, emulsification-solvent evaporation, supercritical fluids, and drying techniques (e.g., freeze drying and spray drying) (Ezhilarasi et al. 2013). Obviously, each technique has its own advantages and disadvantages. Some of these techniques are not suitable for sensitive bioactive ingredients as they apply simultaneous dehydration, thermal, and oxygen stresses that can cause viability/activity loss. In other cases, these processes are expensive, have a low throughput, and, more importantly, require a long processing time. In comparison, if properly designed, EHDP typically offers higher encapsulation efficiency, sustained release capacity, greater thermal, light, and storage stabilities, and enhanced protection from chemical degradation for the encapsulated active ingredients (Pérez-Mariá et al. 2013). Additionally, since no high temperatures are needed in EHDP, temperature-sensitive ingredients can be encapsulated with no thermal exposure (Pérez-Masiá et al. 2014a).

Because of their extremely high surface area and trapping efficiency, different electrospun and electrosprayed nanostructures have been proposed for a huge range of active and bioactive applications (Torres-Giner et al. 2016). When food-grade polymers are applied, resultant bio-nanosystems span from the stabilization of antioxidants to the release of antimicrobials and to the protection of probiotics. Some of these bio-nanosystems can also show enhanced stability and functionality if stored at different conditions of temperature and relative humidity. There is no limitation in terms of the substance to encapsulate, independently of the chemical nature of the encapsulating matrix, as emulsion or coaxial electrospinning/electrospraying might be employed. The following subsections describe different applications in which novel bio-nanosystems obtained by EHDP can result beneficial to the food industry.

### 6.4.1 Antioxidants

Antioxidants are naturally present in foods or can be intentionally added to minimize changes in flavor, aroma, color, or nutritional value. These can protect the body against damages caused by free radicals and degenerative diseases, and thus, are increasingly studied for their inclusion in functional foods. However, due to their intrinsic sensitivity to several environmental factors, such as light, oxygen, or temperature, natural antioxidants should be protected from the surrounding medium or the processing conditions during food production. In addition, the poor solubility of some antioxidants may impede their dissolution and absorption and thus result in poor bioavailability. In recent years, EHDP has been evaluated for the encapsulation of antioxidants aiming at preserving their bioactivity.

An interesting natural antioxidant is β-carotene, a terpene with pro-vitamin A activity. The oxidative and light stability of β-carotene has been enhanced when encapsulated *via* EHDP in zein (Fernandez et al. 2009), WPC (López-Rubio and Lagaron 2012) and, more recently, polyvinyl alcohol (PVOH), and polyethylene oxide (PEO) biopolymers (de Freitas Zômpero et al. 2015), giving rise to both fiber and capsule morphologies. These recent works have demonstrated an increased stability of the antioxidant within the encapsulation in these electrospun or electrosprayed matrices in comparison with the non-encapsulated compound. In particular, a very high encapsulation efficiency was obtained when using glycerol as a vehicle for β-carotene incorporation into WPC. The resultant nanocapsules are shown in Figure 6.3, where it can be seen that the antioxidant is properly encapsulated in single capsules. In contrast, Figure 6.4 shows the encapsulation of β-carotene in ultrathin zein fiber. In this case, it can be observed that the antioxidant is nanodispersed along the fibers.

Zein nanofibers have been also developed to encapsulate and protect some polyphenolic compounds. As an example, Li et al. (2009) encapsulated epigallocatechin gallate (EGCG), a catechin extracted from green tea with diverse health benefits (e.g., oxidative stress protection, reduced risk of cardiovascular diseases, and certain types of cancer) in ultrathin zein fibers by electrospinning. It was observed that both relative humidity and aging time after electrospinning were important in determining the stability of EGCG upon subsequent contact with water. Freshly electrospun ultrathin fibers were less effective at immobilizing the EGCG upon immersion in water (82% recovery) as compared to fibers that were aged at 0% relative humidity for at least 1 day (>98% recovery) before water immersion. In another work, gallic acid, which is a naturally occurring phenolic acid that exhibits anti-inflammatory and antimicrobial properties, has been also successfully incorporated into submicron zein fibers by Neo et al. (2013). The antioxidant was loaded at different amounts (5%–20% wt.), as shown in Figure 6.5. The obtained results indicate that

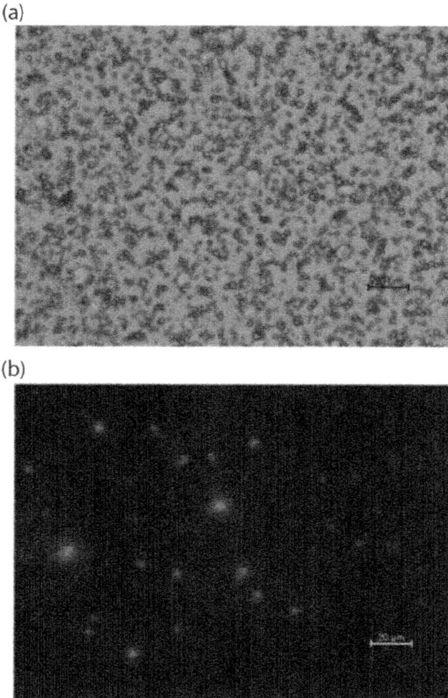


**FIGURE 6.3** Optical images of electrosprayed capsules of WPC containing β-carotene using normal illumination (a) and fluorescence source (b). (Reproduced with permission from López-Rubio, A. and Lagaron, J.M., *Innov. Food Sci. Emerg. Technol.*, 13, 200–206, 2012. Scale bars are 20 μm.)

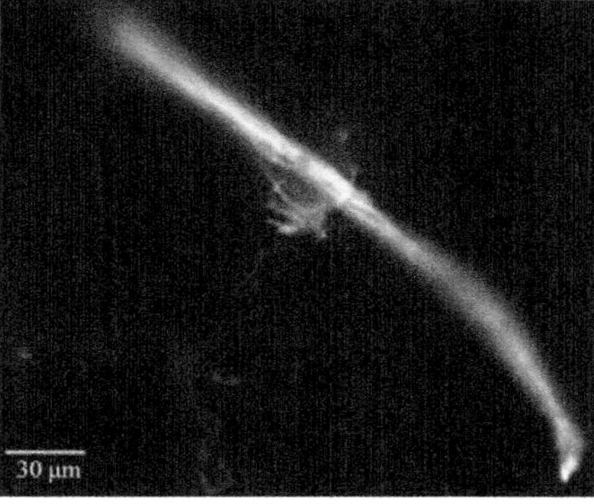


**FIGURE 6.4** Optical image of electrospun zein/β-carotene ultrathin fibers. This was obtained by means of fluorescence filters to enhance the phase contrast between the encapsulated bioactive ingredient and the biopolymer. Excitation at 450–490 nm and emission up 525 nm. (Reproduced with permission from Fernandez, A. et al., *Food Hydrocoll.*, 23, 1427–1432, 2009. Scale bar is 30 μm.)

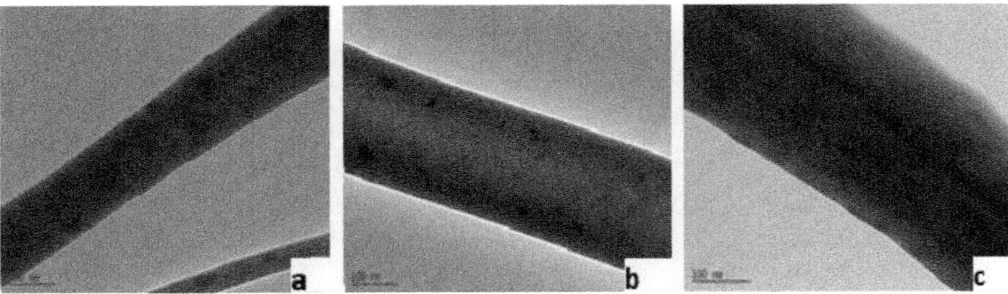


**FIGURE 6.5** Transmission electron microscopy (TEM) images of electrospun zein nanofibers with varying gallic acid weight content: (a) 5% wt.; (b) 10% wt.; and (c) 20% wt. (Adapted from Neo, Y. P. et al., *Food Chem.*, 136, 1013–1021, 2013. Scale bars are 100 nm.)

the loaded gallic acid preserved its phenolic character and antioxidant activity after electrospinning. The optimal properties of zein prolamine in enhancing the stability and bioavailability of other antioxidants, such as curcumin (Dhandayuthapani et al. 2012), α-tocopherol (Wongsasulak et al. 2014), ferulic acid (Yang et al. 2013), or tannin (de Oliveira Mori et al. 2014), have also been demonstrated. These electrospun nanofiber mats show a great deal of potential to constitute coatings and interlayers for active packaging functions, such as antioxidant, antimicrobial, etc.

The importance of developing the above antioxidant-loaded bio-based materials could not be only relevant for food applications, but also regarding the potential to create a completely new market for other materials arising from wastes and agro-based products. In this context, amaranth protein isolate is obtained from *Amaranthus hypochondriacus*, a traditional Mexican plant that remains as an underutilized crop. Amaranth protein isolate is of particular interest as it provides both grains and tasty leaves of high nutritional value due to its amino acid composition. Amaranth protein isolate has been recently electrospun into ultrathin fibers and used to encapsulate quercetin and ferulic acid (Aceituno-Medina et al. 2015b) as well as folic acid (Aceituno-Medina et al. 2015a). A sustained release of the bioactives was revealed during *in-vitro* digestion, which contributes to its improved antioxidant capacity in comparison with the free compounds.

### 6.4.2 Nutraceuticals

Nutraceuticals are nutritional products that provide health benefits, including the prevention and treatment of disease. In contrast to pharmaceuticals, these are not synthetic chemicals formulated for specific indications. Among them, polyunsaturated fatty acids, and more specifically, omega-3 fatty acids, have become popular as food supplements due to the beneficial health effects supported by a variety of epidemiological and interventional studies of fish consumption. This includes a reduction in blood pressure, modulation of the response to endogenous and exogenous thrombolytic agents, antiarrhythmic actions, inhibition of platelet activation, modulation of inflammation, triglycerides reduction, and decrease of cardiovascular diseases (Horrocks and Yeo 1999). Polyunsaturated fatty acids, such as eicosapentaenoic acid, C20:5n-3, and docosahexaenoic acid (DHA), C22:6n-3, which are known to occur naturally in foods such as oily fish and some plant and seed oils, are one of the last substances to be added to a variety of food products including margarine, milk, fruit juice, and eggs to develop functional foods for cardiovascular risk reduction effect. In the EHDP field, DHA has been encapsulated in ultrathin zein capsules produced by electrospraying (Torres-Giner et al. 2010). This process was analyzed by infrared spectroscopy, and it was observed that the DHA encapsulated in the zein capsules was more efficient against degradation under both ambient conditions and in a confined space, i.e., the so-called headspace experiment. In the latter case, which more closely simulates a sealed food packaging situation, the bioactive DHA was considerably more stable, showing up to 2.5-fold reduction in the degradation rate as compared to the free omega-3 fatty acids. Moreover, DHA was more protected from oxidation when the zein capsules were exposed to high humidity values than under dry conditions, releasing much less off-flavors. In a more recent work, cod liver oil was encapsulated by emulsion electrospinning using PVOH as polymer and whey protein isolate or fish protein hydrolysate as emulsifiers (García-Moreno et al. 2016). Resultant bio-nanosystems presented high encapsulation efficiency (>92%), and the encapsulated oil was randomly distributed as small droplets inside the fibers. However, also a higher content of hydroperoxides and secondary oxidation products (e.g., 1-penten-3-ol, hexanal, octanal, and nonanal) was observed when compared to emulsified and unprotected fish oil. This was related to the presence of traces of metals (e.g., iron) in PVOH, which could catalyze lipid oxidation. This result was in agreement with the previous findings of Moomand and Lim (2014), who observed a higher oxidative stability of fish oil when encapsulated in electrospun nanofibers made of zein *versus* PVOH over a period of 14 days.

Vitamin and mineral mixtures are also in the list of the most popular forms of food supplements. Some of these have been encapsulated by EHDP and added to enrich foods aiming at raising dietary levels in a target population. For instance, vitamins A and E were incorporated by Taepaiboon et al. (2007) into electrospun cellulose acetate nanofibers, showing a smooth and round cross-sectional morphology. The immobilization of these food supplements onto the nanofibers provided a more controlled release over the test period compared to the burst release that was observed in control cast films of cellulose acetate. Folic acid (vitamin B) without any coating is susceptible to degradation when exposed to light and acidic condition. However, when it was encapsulated in electrospun sodium alginate-pectin-PEO nanofibers, almost 100% of the folic acid was retained after 41 days of storage in the dark at pH 3 (Alborzi et al. 2013).

### 6.4.3 Flavors

Encapsulation by EHDP not only improves stability, bioavailability, and release properties of bioactive molecules, but also masks unwanted odor and taste. Flavors are very valuable ingredients in any food formula. Even small amounts of flavors or aroma substances can be expensive and, due to they are usually delicate and volatile, preserving them is often a top concern of food manufacturers. Some flavors have been also encapsulated using EHDP. For instance, Alborzi et al. (2013)

immobilized perillaldehyde aroma compound directly onto an edible blend of pullulan/β-cyclodextrin (β-CD) by a single-step electrospinning process. Resultant bio-nanosystems allowed a humidity-triggered release of the aroma compounds, which can be of interest in the design of new food applications. In another study, solid lipid nanoparticles based on stearic acid and ethyl cellulose were prepared by Eltayeb et al. (2013) to encapsulate maltol flavor without chemical interaction among the ingredients. Specifically, the encapsulated nanoparticles, in range of 10–100 nm, showed enhanced stability and resisted flavor loss or degradation during processing and storage.

Cyclodextrin inclusion complexes (CD-IC), such as α-CD, β-CD, and γ-CD of vanilla, menthol, and eugenol flavor compounds can be used in the food industry to improve flavor stability. In the research works carried out by Kayaci and Uyar (2012a, 2012b) the encapsulation of these cyclodextrin inclusion complexes in electrospun nanofibers of both PVOH and zein proved to enhance the durability and provided high temperature stability of flavors, specifically of vanillin. Among them, γ-CD was observed to be most effective in their stabilization and controlled release. Similarly, the successful application of emulsion electrospinning for the encapsulation of highly volatile fragrances, namely, limonene, in electrospun PVOH nanofibers has been presented (Camerlo et al. 2013). The release profile of the fragrance from the electrospun mats was sustained for a period of over 15 days. These bio-nanosystems may find practical application in the food industry, especially in designing active food packaging materials, such as food containers with enhanced or modified organoleptic characteristics and antimicrobial performance.

### 6.4.4 Antimicrobials

Bio-nanosystems developed through EHDP can improve food safety by means of the encapsulation of antimicrobial compounds (Torres-Giner 2011b). Moreover, these can be used to develop active packaging materials, for instance, biocide coatings, which involve the usage of antimicrobial agents capable of diffusing into the food product and inhibiting the proliferation of microorganisms during storage (Torres-Giner 2011a). However, the use of some of these food bioactive compounds in active packaging is yet to be investigated on the basis of the activation mechanism for controlled release. Sun et al. (2011) incorporated EGCG–$Cu^{II}$ complex into 210-nm electrospun PVOH fibers, which exhibited potent and broad antibacterial activity. Similarly, electrospun PVOH fibers containing nanosized of Pu-erh tea powder, a variety of fermented dark tea, were prepared by Su et al. (2012). The resulting nanofibers mat showed a minimum inhibitory concentration of 13.5 mg/mL against *Escherichia coli*, rendering encouraging results for novel antibacterial materials. Previously, Kriegel et al. (2009) incorporated eugenol, a lipophilic antimicrobial phytophenol that is the predominant constituent of clove (*Syzygium aromaticum*) essential oil, into a blend of PVOH and cationic chitosan by emulsion electrospinning. Antimicrobial activity of fabricated nanofibers was higher against *Salmonella typhimurium* (Gram-negative bacterium) than *Listeria monocytogenes* (Gram-positive bacterium). In addition, the eugenol-loaded nanofibers, with diameters ranging from 57 to 126 nm, were found to have stronger antimicrobial effect when compared to an equivalent pure eugenol microemulsion. This was particularly attributed to faster exhaustion and loss of antimicrobial activity of the free system.

In the active packaging area, allyl isothiocyanate (AITC), a naturally occurring compound with known bactericidal activity, has been electrospun using fiber forming solutions of soy protein isolate and polylactide, by making use of β-CD inclusion complex (Vega-Lugo and Lim 2009). A controlled release of the antimicrobial from the fibers, presenting diameters ranging from 200 nm to 2 μm, was achieved, and it was induced by moisture sorption. Similarly, zein/chitosan electrospun insoluble nanofiber mats were produced, which can be mainly aimed to packaging applications (Torres-Giner et al. 2009). The obtained biocide properties were ascribed to both the intrinsic antimicrobial activity of chitosan and to the strong acid solvent used during electrospinning, that remained trapped inside the structure. In a more recent work, zein nanocomposite mats containing thymol also showed antimicrobial capacity against foodborne bacteria, i.e., *Listeria monocytogenes*, when these were particularly employed as coatings on polylactide films prepared by solvent casting (Torres-Giner et al. 2014). The interactive behavior of these antimicrobial nanofibers may be promising in bioactive applications for single and multilayer food packaging.

### 6.4.5 Enzymes

Enzymes, which are biocatalysts with high specificity and efficiency, can be also efficiently immobilized by EHDP, being the coaxial configuration probably the best choice (Wang et al. 2009). It is widely recognized that enzymes immobilization confines enzymes either in a physical support or encapsulated within solid matrices for retention of their catalytic activities and also serves as a medium for controlled release, which increases its usage for commercial purposes. The use of EHDP for hosting enzymes has gained increasing attention for several reasons (Dror et al. 2008): (i) the ultrathin size of the electrospun materials confers a large surface area that makes possible the creation of systems with higher enzyme concentrations and efficiency; (ii) the porosity of the nanofiber mats can be tailored and, thus, the movement of molecules into and out of the electrospun mats can be controlled according to specific requirements; (iii) the use of non-soluble electrospun nanofibers in aqueous medium provides the ability to recover the mat for reuse; and (iv) multiple enzymes from diverse sources can be simultaneously encapsulated. In addition to encapsulation, enzymes can be physically adsorbed or covalently attached to the nanofibers, commonly referred as "surface attachment" (Kim et al. 2008). In this case, the electrospun nanofibers act as a merely structural support for enzyme immobilization, but with the benefit to offer an increase function due to the increased surface area and porosity of the nanofibers.

Enzymes have multiple applications in the food area, not only for food processing, but also for use as antioxidant or antimicrobial additives and food quality control. Immobilization of enzymes by EHDP such as β-galactosidase and chymotrypsin, which are used chiefly in the dairy and meat industries, could potentially aid in their effective utilization by increasing enzyme stability against denaturation and facilitating continuous enzymatic reactions (Anu Bhushani and Anandharamakrishnan 2014). Another example is cellulase, which was immobilized by Wu et al. (2005) onto PVOH nanofibers, showing 65% of the free enzyme activity. The resulting bio-nanosystem can be employed, for instance, in food biotechnology and fruit and vegetable juice processing. Various works have been also carried out to immobilize laccase, an unspecific copper-containing oxidase. For instance, Dai et al. (2010) successfully encapsulated this enzyme in electrospun ultrathin fibers made of poly(D, L-lactide) and a triblock copolymer based on PEO by emulsion electrospinning. It was found that up to 67% of enzyme activity remained after the electrospinning process, maintaining 50% of its initial activity after ten successive runs. Moreover, the work demonstrated that the obtained core–shell structure and porosity of the electrospun fibers were beneficial for preserving the activity and stability of this enzyme in a wide range of pH values. In another work, Liu et al. (2011) also developed laccase-containing electrospun structures as biosensors for phenolic compounds using PVOH as the encapsulation matrix. The results showed that the enzyme retained its high activity and good sensing performance for several polyphenolic compounds. Furthermore, porous silica electrospun PVOH fibers containing horseradish peroxidase were also developed for use as biosensors, also demonstrating a good catalytic activity (Patel et al. 2006).

Glucose oxidase (GOD), which can be used in glucose biosensors of importance in, for instance, food and fermentation industries, has been successfully immobilized onto electrospun PVOH-based matrices (Ren et al. 2006; Wu and Yin 2013). In another study, Ge et al. (2012) electrospun GOD along with PVOH, chitosan, and green tea extract solution. As illustrated on Figure 6.6, the enzyme was embedded in nanofibers in the form of beads. The activity of immobilized GOD in the electrospun membranes was over 68% of that of the free enzyme. In addition, the obtained

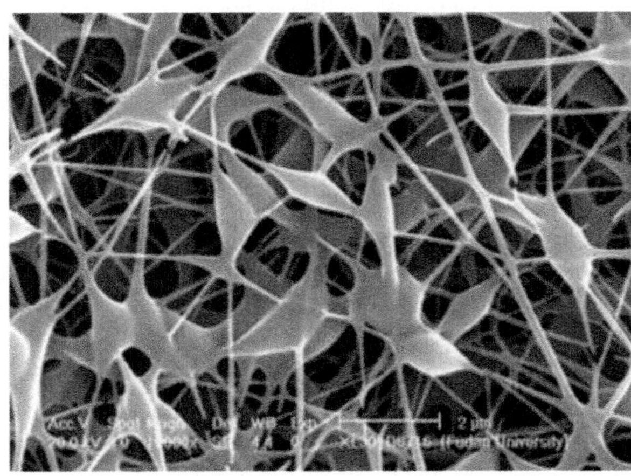


**FIGURE 6.6** Scanning electron microscopy image of electrospun polyvinyl alcohol (PVOH)/chitosan/tea extract nanofibers employed for the immobilization of glucose oxidase (GOD). (Reproduced with permission from Ge, L. et al., *Food Control*, 26, 188–193, 2012. Scale bar is 2 μm.)

electrospun membrane was observed to exert 73% deoxidization to the food samples tested, i.e., haw jelly and cream cake, as the growth and reproduction of microorganisms were significantly inhibited when the oxygen concentration was ≤1%. Though its effect on sugar-rich foods or semi-solid foods was observed to be still low, its potential might be explored in food preservation. Other relevant enzymes that have been encapsulated by EHDP for bioconversion reactions in the food industry are lipases, which have high interest in fats and oils, dairy, and bakery processes. In this sense, Xie and Hsieh (2003) encapsulated lipase in PVOH or in mixture of PEO and casein. In particular, the highest catalytic activity of immobilized lipase in hydrolyzing olive oil was observed for the PVOH/lipase membrane. Though the bioactivity of the immobilized enzyme was lower than that of the free enzyme, this was found to be 6-fold greater than that in an equivalent cast membrane. Similarly, literature reveals the formation of bio-nanosystems using stabilized chitosan from a mixed chitosan/PVA solution and post-treatment with alkaline solution (Huang et al. 2007). The immobilized lipase onto electrospun fibers with diameters of 80–150 nm also showed enhanced storage stability when compared to free lipase.

### 6.4.6 Probiotics

Probiotics are defined as living microorganisms which, when properly administered in adequate amounts, confer health benefits to the host, including the prevention and treatment of some pathologies. These include reduction of gastrointestinal infections, improvement of lactose metabolism, reduction of serum cholesterol, and improvement of immune system defenses (Kechagia et al. 2013). EHDP can be an ideal tool to ensure microorganisms survival during product storage and marketing since it does not involve severe conditions, both in terms of temperature and solvents used. For instance, the suitability of electrospinning for generating probiotic-containing nanostructures was proven by Fung et al. (2011) using PVOH and soluble dietary fiber from agricultural wastes, namely, okara (soybean solid waste), oil palm trunk, and oil palm frond obtained *via* alkali treatment, with *Lactobacillus acidophilus*. In particular, viability studies showed bacterial survival in the range of 78%–90% under EHDP conditions, retaining viability at refrigeration temperature during the 21-day storage study.

Among probiotics, the genus *Bifidobacterium* has been the subject of intense research due to its predominance in breastfed infants and the beneficial effects attributed to some strains, leading to their incorporation into diverse food products and pharmaceutical formulations for commercialization. In a first attempt, the feasibility and potential of electrospinning for nanoencapsulation of *Bifidobacterium animalis* subsp. *lactis* Bb12 was initially proven using 150-nm PVOH fibers by means of the coaxial configuration (López-Rubio et al. 2009). The process did not affect the viability of the probiotics, and the viability of encapsulated bacteria was significantly higher than that of non-encapsulated bacteria after 40 days of storage at room temperature (~20°C) and 130 days at refrigerated temperature (4°C). Later on, WPC- and pullulan-based electrosprayed capsules were developed for the encapsulation of a bifidobacterial strain (López-Rubio et al. 2012). Comparison of optical images taken using a digital microscopy system under polarized light and an epifluorescence illuminator, as shown in Figure 6.7, revealed that bacteria were

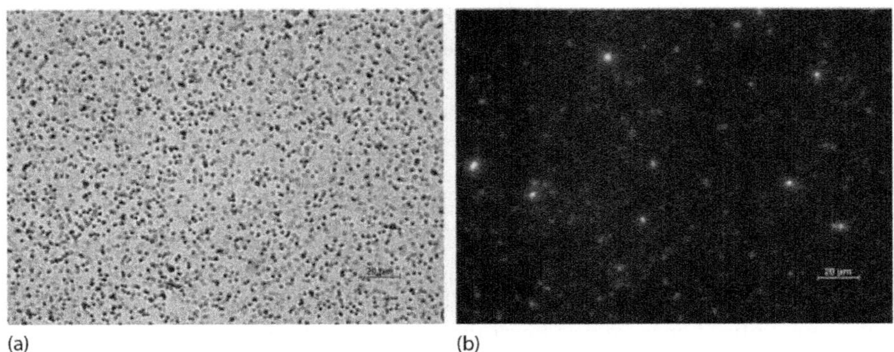

(a) (b)

**FIGURE 6.7** Optical images of pullulan capsules containing encapsulated *B. animalis* Bb12 under polarized light (a) and using a fluorescence source (b). (Reproduced with permission from López-Rubio, A. et al., *Food Hydrocoll.*, 28, 159–167, 2012. Scale bars are 20 μm.)

effectively encapsulated in the pullulan capsules. In some cases, bacteria were forced to bend in order to accommodate inside the electrosprayed capsules. The resultant electrosprayed hydrocolloids demonstrated the ability to prolong probiotics survival during storage at 4°C and 20°C. Interestingly, WPC presented greater protection as encapsulation matrix than pullulan as it effectively prolonged the survival of bacteria even at high relative humidity. In summary, the above studies gave rise to probiotics metabolically active and abundant in the materials obtained by EHDP.

## 6.5 CONCLUSIONS AND FUTURE TRENDS

Encapsulation of bioactive compounds and probiotics for protection and delivery purposes is an area of great interest for both academia and food industry. To this regard, EHDP, which is based on the application of electrostatic forces to polymer solutions, is beneficial for entrapping the active ingredients in or into solid nanostructures, either in the form fibers or capsules. In the food industry, the use of biopolymers that are water soluble or that create hydrocolloids opens up new possibilities since these are perfect non-toxic shells for the encapsulation of sensitive actives substances. Resulting bio-nanosystems can be particularly useful to control the release of food ingredients in the gut and can thus be used as novel delivery systems in the body while stabilizing the components during food processing and storage.

As outlined above, the main advantages offered by electrospun food-grade polymers for the stabilization and protection of food active ingredients are the use of water-based solvents, room temperature processes, reduced denaturation, efficient encapsulation, enhanced stability of actives, and sustained and controlled release capacity. Due to these advantages, in addition to the ease of the process, the number of research papers dealing with the EHDP technique in the food area has exponentially increased in the last decade and new applications are being continuously envisioned. Production of these novel bio-nanosystems can be of high interest in the food sector, for instance, to develop new formulas, bioactive packaging, biosensors, or delivery systems.

Nevertheless, the industrial-scale application of the EHDP technology in the food and food packaging sectors is still limited and some issues need to be addressed. The main reason by which the potentialities of these bio-nanosystems have not been widely adopted in the food industry is the prevalence of research studies on synthetic polymers rather than on biopolymers, which has reduced their appeal. Secondly, the low throughput of common EHDP devices restricts its commercial exploitation at a large scale for most conventional purposes, and, therefore, new high-value applications should be initially explored. Finally, many food-grade polymer systems, particularly carbohydrate polymers, can be difficult to prepare optimally by EHDP. This is related to their limited solubility, poor viscoelastic behavior, or lack of sufficient molecular entanglement, and, more commonly, because only a few processing parameters can be controlled directly since some of them are either highly interdependent or derive from the properties of the biopolymer solution used (Ghorani and Tucker 2015).

Therefore, one of the most important challenges related with the large production of these bio-nanosystems is the implementation of new methods, allowing increase of the process and product reproducibility and also extending the types of materials that can be used. In order to deal with the low productivity of solution electrospinning, the number of jets can be efficiently increased by different approaches, including multi-jets from single or multiple needles and needleless systems (Yarin and Zussman 2004). Moreover, significant advances in both the EHDP technique and design of equipment, in combination with new strategies that allow generating different encapsulation morphologies and even simultaneously encapsulate diverse active substances, will certainly expand the use of this novel technology for encapsulation purposes in the food area. Furthermore, the extrapolation from the electrospun and electrosprayed structures developed in the laboratory at the early research stage for a commercial scale can be carried out rather easily. Therefore, fabrication of bioactive materials by EHDP at industrial scale is really feasible.

Currently, there are already some industrial EHDP devices and contract manufacturing plants (see www.bioinicia.com) available in the market. A few companies are also globally supplying either laboratory or large-scale EHDP equipment and also, in some cases, electrospun products for well-defined market segments (e.g., filtration and medical industry). To stimulate future developments, a tighter interaction between academic and industrial communities as well as a critical assessment of the weaknesses and strengths of the EHDP technologies, including coaxial and emulsion electrospinning, for industrial processes can be certainly useful. In particular, the format in which the electrospun materials are industrially provided, in terms of both their physical form and their subsequent methods of incorporation into the functional foods, will take a considerable research effort in the near future.

## REFERENCES

Aceituno-Medina, M., S. Mendoza, B. A. Rodríguez, J. M. Lagaron, and A. López-Rubio. 2015b. 'Improved antioxidant capacity of quercetin and ferulic acid during in-vitro digestion through encapsulation within food-grade electrospun fibers', *Journal of Functional Foods*, 12: 332–341.

Aceituno-Medina, M., S. Mendoza, J. M. Lagaron, and A. López-Rubio. 2015a. 'Photoprotection of folic acid upon encapsulation in food-grade amaranth (Amaranthus hypochondriacus L.) protein isolate—Pullulan electrospun fibers', *LWT—Food Science and Technology*, 62: 970–975.

Alborzi, S., L.-T. Lim, and Y. Kakuda. 2013. 'Encapsulation of folic acid and its stability in sodium alginate-pectin-poly(ethylene oxide) electrospun fibres', *Journal of Microencapsulation*, 30: 64–71.

Anu Bhushani, J., and C. Anandharamakrishnan. 2014. 'Electrospinning and electrospraying techniques: Potential food based applications', *Trends in Food Science & Technology*, 38: 21–33.

Arecchi, A., S. Mannino, and J. Weiss. 2010. 'Electrospinning of Poly(vinyl alcohol) nanofibers loaded with hexadecane nanodroplets', *Journal of Food Science*, 75: N80–N88.

Camerlo, A., C. Vebert-Nardin, R. M. Rossi, and A. M. Popa. 2013. 'Fragrance encapsulation in polymeric matrices by emulsion electrospinning', *European Polymer Journal*, 49: 3806–3813.

Chakraborty, S., I. C. Liao, A. Adler, and K. W. Leong. 2009. 'Electrohydrodynamics: A facile technique to fabricate drug delivery systems', *Advanced Drug Delivery Reviews*, 61: 1043–1054.

Chaobo, H., C. Shuiliang, L. Chuilin, H. R. Darrell, Q. Haiyan, Y. Ying, and H. Haoqing. 2006. 'Electrospun polymer nanofibres with small diameters', *Nanotechnology*, 17: 1558.

Chen, L., G. E. Remondetto, and M. Subirade. 2006. 'Food protein-based materials as nutraceutical delivery systems', *Trends in Food Science & Technology*, 17: 272–283.

Dai, Y., J. Niu, J. Liu, L. Yin, and J. Xu. 2010. 'In situ encapsulation of laccase in microfibers by emulsion electrospinning: Preparation, characterization, and application', *Bioresource Technology*, 101: 8942–8947.

de Freitas Zômpero, R. H., A. López-Rubio, S. C. de Pinho, J. M. Lagaron, and L. G. de la Torre. 2015. 'Hybrid encapsulation structures based on β-carotene-loaded nanoliposomes within electrospun fibers', *Colloids and Surfaces B: Biointerfaces*, 134: 475–482.

de Oliveira Mori, C. L. S., N. A. dos Passos, J. E. Oliveira, L. H. C. Mattoso, F. A. Mori, A. G. Carvalho, A. de Souza Fonseca, and G. H. D. Tonoli. 2014. 'Electrospinning of zein/tannin bio-nanofibers', *Industrial Crops and Products*, 52: 298–304.

De Vrieze, S., T. Van Camp, A. Nelvig, B. Hagström, P. Westbroek, and K. De Clerck. 2008. 'The effect of temperature and humidity on electrospinning', *Journal of Materials Science*, 44: 1357.

Deitzel, J. M., J. Kleinmeyer, D. Harris, and N. C. Beck Tan. 2001. 'The effect of processing variables on the morphology of electrospun nanofibers and textiles', *Polymer*, 42: 261–272.

Dhandayuthapani, B., M. Anila, A. R. Girija, N. Yutaka, K. Venugopal, Y. Yasuhiko, M. Toru, and D. Sakthikumar. 2012. 'Hybrid fluorescent curcumin loaded zein electrospun nanofibrous scaffold for biomedical applications', *Biomedical Materials*, 7: 045001.

Doshi, J., and D. H. Reneker. 1993. "Electrospinning process and applications of electrospun fibers." In *Conference Record of the 1993 IEEE Industry Applications Conference Twenty-Eighth IAS Annual Meeting*, pp. 1698–1703 vol.3.

Doshi, J., and D. H. Reneker. 1995. 'Electrospinning process and applications of electrospun fibers', *Journal of Electrostatics*, 35: 151–160.

Dror, Y., J. Kuhn, R. Avrahami, and E. Zussman. 2008. 'Encapsulation of enzymes in biodegradable tubular structures', *Macromolecules*, 41: 4187–4192.

Echegoyen, Y., M. J. Fabra, J. L. Castro-Mayorga, A. Cherpinski, and J. M. Lagaron. 2017. 'High throughput electro-hydrodynamic processing in food encapsulation and food packaging applications: Viewpoint', *Trends in Food Science & Technology*, 60: 71–79.

Eltayeb, M., P. K. Bakhshi, E. Stride, and M. Edirisinghe. 2013. 'Preparation of solid lipid nanoparticles containing active compound by electrohydrodynamic spraying', *Food Research International*, 53: 88–95.

Ezhilarasi, P. N., P. Karthik, N. Chhanwal, and C. Anandharamakrishnan. 2013. 'Nanoencapsulation techniques for food bioactive components: A review', *Food and Bioprocess Technology*, 6: 628–647.

Fernandez, A., S. Torres-Giner, and J. M. Lagaron. 2009. 'Novel route to stabilization of bioactive antioxidants by encapsulation in electrospun fibers of zein prolamine', *Food Hydrocolloids*, 23: 1427–1432.

Frenot, A., and I. S. Chronakis. 2003. 'Polymer nanofibers assembled by electrospinning', *Current Opinion in Colloid & Interface Science*, 8: 64–75.

Fung, W.-Y., K.-H. Yuen, and M.-T. Liong. 2011. 'Agrowaste-based nanofibers as a probiotic encapsulant: Fabrication and characterization', *Journal of Agricultural and Food Chemistry*, 59: 8140–8147.

García-Moreno, P. J., K. Stephansen, J. van der Kruijs, A. Guadix, E. M. Guadix, I. S. Chronakis, and C. Jacobsen. 2016. 'Encapsulation of fish oil in nanofibers by emulsion electrospinning: Physical characterization and oxidative stability', *Journal of Food Engineering*, 183: 39–49.

Ge, L., Y.-sheng Zhao, Ting Mo, Jian-rong Li, and Ping Li. 2012. 'Immobilization of glucose oxidase in electrospun nanofibrous membranes for food preservation', *Food Control*, 26: 188–193.

Ghorani, B., and N. Tucker. 2015. 'Fundamentals of electrospinning as a novel delivery vehicle for bioactive compounds in food nanotechnology', *Food Hydrocolloids*, 51: 227–240.

Horrocks, L. A., and Y. K. Yeo. 1999. 'Health benefits of docosahezaenoic acid (DHA)', *Pharmacological Research*, 40: 211–225.

Huang, X.-J., D. Ge, and Z.-K. Xu. 2007. 'Preparation and characterization of stable chitosan nanofibrous membrane for lipase immobilization', *European Polymer Journal*, 43: 3710–3718.

Kayaci, F., and T. Uyar. 2012a. 'Encapsulation of vanillin/cyclodextrin inclusion complex in electrospun polyvinyl alcohol (PVA) nanowebs: Prolonged shelf-life and high temperature stability of vanillin', *Food Chemistry*, 133: 641–649.

Kayaci, F., and T. Uyar. 2012b. 'Electrospun zein nanofibers incorporating cyclodextrins', *Carbohydrate Polymers*, 90: 558–568.

Kechagia, M., D. Basoulis, S. Konstantopoulou, D. Dimitriadi, K. Gyftopoulou, N. Skarmoutsou, and E. M. Fakiri. 2013. 'Health benefits of probiotics: A review', *ISRN Nutrition*, 2013: 481651.

Kim, J., J. W. Grate, and P. Wang. 2008. 'Nanobiocatalysis and its potential applications', *Trends in Biotechnology*, 26: 639–646.

Kriegel, C., K. M. Kit, D. J. McClements, and J. Weiss. 2009. 'Nanofibers as carrier systems for antimicrobial microemulsions. Part I: Fabrication and characterization', *Langmuir*, 25: 1154–1161.

Li, D., and Y. Xia. 2004. 'Electrospinning of nanofibers: Reinventing the wheel?', *Advanced Materials*, 16: 1151–1170.

Li, Y., L. T. Lim, and Y. Kakuda. 2009. 'Electrospun zein fibers as carriers to stabilize (–)-epigallocatechin gallate', *Journal of Food Science*, 74: C233–C240.

Liu, J., J. Niu, L. Yin, and F. Jiang. 2011. 'In situ encapsulation of laccase in nanofibers by electrospinning for development of enzyme biosensors for chlorophenol monitoring', *Analyst*, 136: 4802–4808.

López-Rubio, A., E. Sanchez, Y. Sanz, and J. M. Lagaron. 2009. 'Encapsulation of living bifidobacteria in ultrathin PVOH electrospun fibers', *Biomacromolecules*, 10: 2823–2829.

López-Rubio, A., and J. M. Lagaron. 2012. 'Whey protein capsules obtained through electrospraying for the encapsulation of bioactives', *Innovative Food Science & Emerging Technologies*, 13: 200–206.

López-Rubio, A., E. Sanchez, S. Wilkanowicz, Y. Sanz, and J. M. Lagaron. 2012. 'Electrospinning as a useful technique for the encapsulation of living bifidobacteria in food hydrocolloids', *Food Hydrocolloids*, 28: 159–167.

Megelski, S., J. S. Stephens, D. B. Chase, and J. F. Rabolt. 2002. 'Micro- and nanostructured surface morphology on electrospun polymer fibers', *Macromolecules*, 35: 8456–8466.

Moomand, K., and L.-T. Lim. 2014. 'Oxidative stability of encapsulated fish oil in electrospun zein fibres', *Food Research International*, 62: 523–532.

Neo, Y. P., S. Ray, J. Jin, M. Gizdavic-Nikolaidis, M. K. Nieuwoudt, D. Liu, and S. Y. Quek. 2013. 'Encapsulation of food grade antioxidant in natural biopolymer by electrospinning technique: A physicochemical study based on zein–gallic acid system', *Food Chemistry*, 136: 1013–1021.

Nieuwland, M., P. Geerdink, P. Brier, P. van den Eijnden, J. T. M. M. Henket, M. L. P. Langelaan, N. Stroeks, H. C. van Deventer, and A. H. Martin. 2013. 'Food-grade electrospinning of proteins', *Innovative Food Science & Emerging Technologies*, 20: 269–275.

Nikmarama, N., S. Roohinejad, S. Hashemi, M. Koubaa, F. J. Barba, A. Abbaspourrad, and R. Greiner. 2017. 'Emulsion-based systems for fabrication of electrospun nanofibers: Food, pharmaceutical and biomedical applications', *RSC Advances*, 7: 28951–28964.

Park, J. Y., and I. H. Lee. 2010. 'Relative humidity effect on the preparation of porous electrospun polystyrene fibers', *Journal of Nanoscience and Nanotechnology*, 10: 3473–3477.

Patel, A. C., S. Li, J. M. Yuan, and Y. Wei. 2006. 'In situ encapsulation of horseradish peroxidase in electrospun porous silica fibers for potential biosensor applications', *Nano Letters*, 6: 1042–1046.

Pérez-Mariá, R., M. J. Fabra, J. M. Lagarón, and A. López-Rubio. 2013. 'Use of electrospinning for encapsulation' in, *Encapsulation Nanotechnologies* edited by Vikas Mittal (John Wiley & Sons: Hoboken, NJ).

Pérez-Masiá, R., J. M. Lagaron, and A. López-Rubio. 2014a. 'Development and optimization of novel encapsulation structures of interest in functional foods through electrospraying', *Food and Bioprocess Technology*, 7: 3236–3245.

Pérez-Masiá, R., J. M. Lagaron, and A. López-Rubio. 2014b. 'Surfactant-aided electrospraying of low molecular weight carbohydrate polymers from aqueous solutions', *Carbohydrate Polymers*, 101: 249–255.

Pérez-Masiá, R., R. López-Nicolás, M. J. Periago, G. Ros, J. M. Lagaron, and A. López-Rubio. 2015. 'Encapsulation of folic acid in food hydrocolloids through nanospray drying and electrospraying for nutraceutical applications', *Food Chemistry*, 168: 124–133.

Pillay, V., C. Dott, Y. E. Choonara, C. Tyagi, L. Tomar, P. Kumar, L. C. du Toit, and Valence M. K. Ndesendo. 2013. 'A review of the effect of processing variables on the fabrication of electrospun nanofibers for drug delivery applications', *Journal of Nanomaterials*, 2013: 22.

Ramakrishna, S., K. Fujihara, W.-E. Teo, T. Yong, Z. Ma, and R. Ramaseshan. 2006. 'Electrospun nanofibers: Solving global issues', *Materials Today*, 9: 40–50.

Ren, G., X. Xu, Q. Liu, J. Cheng, X. Yuan, L. Wu, and Y. Wan. 2006. 'Electrospun poly(vinyl alcohol)/glucose oxidase biocomposite membranes for biosensor applications', *Reactive and Functional Polymers*, 66: 1559–1564.

Reneker, D. H., and I. Chun. 1996. 'Nanometre diameter fibres of polymer, produced by electrospinning', *Nanotechnology*, 7: 216–223.

Rieger, K. A., N. P. Birch, and J. D. Schiffman. 2013. 'Designing electrospun nanofiber mats to promote wound healing—A review', *Journal of Materials Chemistry B*, 1: 4531–4541.

Sill, T. J., and H. A. von Recum. 2008. 'Electrospinning: Applications in drug delivery and tissue engineering', *Biomaterials*, 29: 1989–2006.

Sreekumar, S., P. Lemke, B. Moerschbacher, S. Torres-Giner, and J. M. Lagaron. 2017. 'Preparation and optimization of submicron chitosan capsules by water-based electrospraying for food and bioactive packaging applications.', *Food Additives & Contaminants: Part A*. 34: 1795–1806.

Stijnman, A. C., I. Bodnar, and R. H. Tromp. 2011. 'Electrospinning of food-grade polysaccharides', *Food Hydrocolloids*, 25: 1393–1398.

Su, Y., B. Lu, Y. Xie, Z. Ma, L. Liu, H. Zhao, J. Zhang, H. Duan, H. Zhang, J. Li, Y. Xiong, and E. Xie. 2011. 'Temperature effect on electrospinning of nanobelts: The case of hafnium oxide', *Nanotechnology*, 22: 285609.

Su, Y., C. Zhang, Y. Wang, and P. Li. 2012. 'Antibacterial property and mechanism of a novel Pu-erh tea nanofibrous membrane', *Applied Microbiology and Biotechnology*, 93: 1663–1671.

Sun, L.-M., C.-L. Zhang, and P. Li. 2011. 'Characterization, antimicrobial activity, and mechanism of a high-performance (–)-epigallocatechin-3-gallate (EGCG)–CuII/polyvinyl alcohol (PVA) nanofibrous membrane', *Journal of Agricultural and Food Chemistry*, 59: 5087–5092.

Sy, J. C., A. S. Klemm, and V. P. Shastri. 2009. 'Emulsion as a means of controlling electrospinning of polymers', *Advanced Materials*, 21: 1814–1819.

Szentivanyi, A., T. Chakradeo, H. Zernetsch, and B. Glasmacher. 2011. 'Electrospun cellular microenvironments: Understanding controlled release and scaffold structure', *Advanced Drug Delivery Reviews*, 63: 209–220.

Taepaiboon, P., U. Rungsardthong, and P. Supaphol. 2007. 'Vitamin-loaded electrospun cellulose acetate nanofiber mats as transdermal and dermal therapeutic agents of vitamin A acid and vitamin E', *European Journal of Pharmaceutics and Biopharmaceutics*, 67: 387–397.

Tan, S. H., R. Inai, M. Kotaki, and S. Ramakrishna. 2005. 'Systematic parameter study for ultra-fine fiber fabrication via electrospinning process', *Polymer*, 46: 6128–6134.

Torres-Giner, S. 2011a. 'Electrospun nanofibers for food packaging applications' in, *Multifunctional and Nanoreinforced Polymers for Food Packaging* edited by Jose-Maria Lagaron (Woodhead Publishing Limited: Cambridge, UK).

Torres-Giner, S. 2011b. 'Novel antimicrobials obtained by electrospinning methods' in, *Antimicrobial Polymers* edited by Jose Maria Lagaron, Maria Jose Ocio, and Amparo López-Rubio (John Wiley & Sons: Hoboken, NJ).

Torres-Giner, S., A. Martinez-Abad, and J. M. Lagaron. 2014. 'Zein-based ultrathin fibers containing ceramic nanofillers obtained by electrospinning. II. Mechanical properties, gas barrier, and sustained release capacity of biocide thymol in multilayer polylactide films', *Journal of Applied Polymer Science*, 131: 9270–9276.

Torres-Giner, S., A. Martinez-Abad, J. V. Gimeno-Alcañiz, M. J. Ocio, and J. M. Lagaron. 2012. 'Controlled delivery of gentamicin antibiotic from bioactive electrospun polylactide-based ultrathin fibers', *Advanced Engineering Materials*, 14: B112–B122.

Torres-Giner, S., A. Martinez-Abad, M. J. Ocio, and J. M. Lagaron. 2010. 'Stabilization of a nutraceutical omega-3 fatty acid by encapsulation in ultrathin electrosprayed zein prolamine', *Journal of Food Science*, 75: N69–N79.

Torres-Giner, S., E. Gimenez, and J. M. Lagaron. 2008a. 'Characterization of the morphology and thermal properties of zein prolamine nanostructures obtained by electrospinning', *Food Hydrocolloids*, 22: 601–614.

Torres-Giner, S., M. J. Ocio, and J. M. Lagaron. 2008b. 'Development of active antimicrobial fiber based chitosan polysaccharide nanostructures using electrospinning', *Engineering in Life Sciences*, 8: 303–314.

Torres-Giner, S., M. J. Ocio, and J. M. Lagaron. 2009. 'Novel antimicrobial ultrathin structures of zein/chitosan blends obtained by electrospinning', *Carbohydrate Polymers*, 77: 261–266.

Torres-Giner, S., R. Pérez-Masiá, and J. M. Lagaron. 2016. 'A review on electrospun polymer nanostructures as advanced bioactive platforms', *Polymer Engineering and Science*, 56: 500–527.

Torres-Giner, S., S. Wilkanowicz, B. Meléndez-Rodríguez, and J. M. Lagaron. 2017. 'Nanoencapsulation of *Aloe vera* in synthetic and naturally occurring polymers by electrohydrodynamic processing of interest in food technology and bioactive packaging', *Journal of Agricultural and Food Chemistry*, 65: 4439–4448.

Vega-Lugo, A. C., and L. T. Lim. 2009. 'Controlled release of allyl isothiocyanate using soy protein and poly(lactic acid) electrospun fibers', *Food Research International*, 42: 933–940.

Wang, T., and S. Kumar. 2006. 'Electrospinning of polyacrylonitrile nanofibers', *Journal of Applied Polymer Science*, 102: 1023–1029.

Wang, Z.-G., L.-S. Wan, Z.-M. Liu, X.-J. Huang, and Z.-K. Xu. 2009. 'Enzyme immobilization on electrospun polymer nanofibers: An overview', *Journal of Molecular Catalysis B: Enzymatic*, 56: 189–195.

Wongsasulak, S., S. Pathumban, and T. Yoovidhya. 2014. 'Effect of entrapped α-tocopherol on mucoadhesivity and evaluation of the release, degradation, and swelling characteristics of zein–chitosan composite electrospun fibers', *Journal of Food Engineering*, 120: 110–117.

Wu, J., and F. Yin. 2013. 'Sensitive enzymatic glucose biosensor fabricated by electrospinning composite nanofibers and electrodepositing Prussian blue film', *Journal of Electroanalytical Chemistry*, 694: 1–5.

Wu, L., X. Yuan, and J. Sheng. 2005. 'Immobilization of cellulase in nanofibrous PVA membranes by electrospinning', *Journal of Membrane Science*, 250: 167–173.

Xie, J., and Y.-L. Hsieh. 2003. 'Ultra-high surface fibrous membranes from electrospinning of natural proteins: Casein and lipase enzyme', *Journal of Materials Science*, 38: 2125–2133.

Xu, X., L. Yang, X. Xu, X. Wang, X. Chen, Q. Liang, J. Zeng, and X. Jing. 2005. 'Ultrafine medicated fibers electrospun from W/O emulsions', *Journal of Controlled Release*, 108: 33–42.

Yang, J.-M., L.-S. Zha, D.-G. Yu, and J. Liu. 2013. 'Coaxial electrospinning with acetic acid for preparing ferulic acid/zein composite fibers with improved drug release profiles', *Colloids and Surfaces B: Biointerfaces*, 102: 737–743.

Yao, C., X. Li, and T. Song. 2007. 'Electrospinning and crosslinking of zein nanofiber mats', *Journal of Applied Polymer Science*, 103: 380–385.

Yarin, A. L., and E. Zussman. 2004. 'Upward needleless electrospinning of multiple nanofibers', *Polymer*, 45: 2977–2980.

Zamani, M., M. P. Prabhakaran, and S. Ramakrishna. 2013. 'Advances in drug delivery via electrospun and electrosprayed nanomaterials', *International Journal of Nanomedicine*, 8: 2997–3017.

Zong, X., K. Kim, D. Fang, S. Ran, B. S. Hsiao, and B. Chu. 2002. 'Structure and process relationship of electrospun bioabsorbable nanofiber membranes', *Polymer*, 43: 4403–4412.

# 7 Characterization of Bio-nanosystems

*Cláudia Sousa and Dmitri Y. Petrovykh*

**CONTENTS**



## 7.1 INTRODUCTION

In the context of food research and applications, the objectives of characterizing nanoparticles are primarily derived from the guidance (EFSA et al. 2018) issued by the European Food Safety Authority (EFSA). And while the ultimate properties of interest for food materials and substances are related to their interactions with human senses and bodies, the characterization of these materials—and any nanomaterial components thereof—must begin with their physicochemical properties (Gioria et al. 2018; Rasmussen et al. 2018). The resulting need to adapt and extend various analytical methods from their traditional use on relatively well-defined nanomaterials encountered in physics and chemistry to characterization of the more complex and heterogeneous nanomaterials in food creates well-recognized, if not yet fully understood, challenges (Rasmussen et al. 2018). A provocative editorial recently highlighted this perspective of challenges that arise when working with "messy systems" and trying to obtain reliable and reproducible results (Harris 2017).

These daunting challenges notwithstanding, the regulatory needs (EFSA 2018) and requirements in both food (EFSA et al. 2018) and biomedical (Gioria et al. 2018; Pita et al. 2016) applications of nanomaterials have motivated the development and validation of analytical techniques and methodologies that enable characterization of increasingly more complex nanomaterials (Table 7.1). The most significant progress has been made in characterization of solid nanoparticles that are subject to the more extensive regulations across various application areas. The resulting methodologies are being successfully adapted to related nanomaterials that are composed of a solid-core and a shell of "softer" organic or biological material. Important advances are being made in characterization of soft nanoparticles as well, however, both regulators and practitioners agree that the inherent flexibility and responsiveness of soft nanomaterials make them particularly challenging targets for robust and unambiguous measurements.

The two types of nanomaterials outlined above—solid-core and soft nanoparticles—are discussed in the two sections of the following brief overview, with each section organized by the individual physicochemical properties and parameters that need to be characterized within the context of the EFSA guidance (EFSA et al. 2018). More extensive overviews of the physicochemical properties and characterization methods have been recently provided for edible nanoparticles (McClements and McClements 2016) and for general nanocharacterization, based on the Organisation for Economic Co-operation and Development Testing Program (Rasmussen et al. 2018).

**TABLE 7.1**
**International Projects Addressing Regulatory and Metrology Aspects of Nanocharacterization**

| Name | URL | Description |
|---|---|---|
| NANoREG | www.nanoreg.eu | A common European approach to the regulatory testing of manufactured nanomaterials.[a] |
| DaNa$^{2.0}$ | www.nanopartikel.info/en/ | Information about nanomaterials and their safety assessment. |
| NanoDefine | www.nanodefine.eu | Methods for the implementation of the European definition of a nanomaterial.[b] |
| InNanoPart | empir.npl.co.uk/innanopart | Measuring the concentration and surface chemistry of nanoparticles. |

[a] The Dutch National Institute for Public Health and the Environment (RIVM) maintains the *NANoREG Results Repository*: http://www.rivm.nl/en/About_RIVM/International/International_Projects/Completed/NANoREG

[b] Results from the NanoDefine project are summarized in Babick et al. 2016 and Wohlleben et al. 2017.

## 7.2 SOLID-CORE NANOPARTICLES

Among various complex nanomaterials, solid-core nanoparticles benefit from availability and applicability of some of the most advanced nanocharacterization techniques, many of which have been adapted from the decades of extensive research on characterization of solid nanoparticles (Bowen 2002). Solid nanoparticles are typically sufficiently stable in terms of size, morphology, and composition that the appropriate variants of electron microscopy, mass spectrometry, spectroscopy, adsorption, diffraction, light scattering, gravimetry, thermal, and sedimentation measurements can be used to obtain complementary information about their properties (Rasmussen et al. 2018). And while only some of the methods, typically those that are optimized for speed and simplicity rather than high information content, can be readily employed by practitioners in research and industry, the more advanced and information-rich techniques are available as an analytical "backstop," when lower uncertainty is required or ambiguity/inconsistency in results needs to be resolved. Serendipitously, the insight into the properties of a nanomaterial derived from long-term multi-technique characterization (Nurmi et al. 2005) often can be used to identify the two or three techniques that provide sufficient information for routine analysis of the material (Baer et al. 2013).

In characterization of solid-core nanoparticles, the explicit inclusion of surface modification and coatings into consideration requires the use of surface-analysis techniques (Baer and Engelhard 2010; Baer et al. 2010; Rasmussen et al. 2018) and the consideration of how the changes in the environment and preparation of nanoparticles affect their surfaces (Baer 2018; Rasmussen et al. 2018). The need to understand the surfaces of nanoparticles is not qualitatively a new requirement for characterization of solid-core nanoparticles, but rather an enhancement of the well-established caveats to the assumptions of stability and uniformity for nominally solid nanoparticles, which in practice are never completely stable or uniform all the way from the core to the surface (Baer et al. 2008, 2016). The effects on the surfaces of nanoparticles of the exposure to a complex environment or matrix become particularly significant for characterization of nanomaterials in the environmental (Domingos et al. 2009; Hassellöv et al. 2008), food (Linsinger et al. 2013; McClements and McClements 2016; Peters et al. 2014), and biomedical (Lynch et al. 2007; Wohlleben 2012; Wu et al. 2011; Zhang et al. 2011) contexts.

### 7.2.1 Definition of a Nanomaterial

EFSA guidance (EFSA et al. 2018) follows the classification and definitions from the International Organization for Standardization to establish the vocabulary for nanomaterials, whereby *nanoscale* is defined as ranging from approximately 1 to 100 nm and *nanoparticles* are defined as objects with all three external dimensions on the nanoscale (ISO 2015); objects with only one or two external dimensions on the nanoscale are referred to as *nanoplates* and *nanofibers*, respectively. The definitive role of the size in the classification of nanomaterials is further emphasized in the definition recommended by the European Commission (EC), whereby *nanomaterial* means a natural, incidental, or manufactured material containing particles 50% or more of which in the number-size distribution have one or more external dimensions in the size range of 1–100 nm (EC 2011).

EFSA guidance, however, considers the specific cutoff at 100 nm in the above definitions to be not fully justified from a risk assessment perspective, noting that biological effects, such as toxicokinetic behavior and particle–cell interactions, "are not rigidly related to specific size thresholds" and may occur for particles that are either smaller or larger than 100 nm in size (EFSA et al. 2018). The guidance also explicitly includes materials that are not engineered as nanomaterial, but contain a nanomaterial fraction as a result of manufacturing processes for powdered or particulate food. This broad interpretation of the nanomaterial definition in the food safety context effectively increases the range of sizes across which the particle size distribution needs to be determined, as measuring the fraction of particles with sizes <100 nm may not be sufficient for interpreting the results of subsequent risk assessment measurements.

### 7.2.2 Size

Following the above definitions, the particle size (distribution) is the first parameter that needs to be measured in order to determine whether a given material is classified as a nanomaterial. The primary conceptual challenge in implementing the size measurements in this context is the need to measure specifically the *number-size* distribution, which can be directly measured for nanomaterials only by inherently particle-counting, mainly imaging, techniques, such as electron (Hodoroaba et al. 2014; Rice et al. 2013) or scanning probe (Baalousha et al. 2014) microscopy. As the authoritative review produced by the NanoDefine project (Table 7.1) noted, such definition "was a paradigm change without metrological guidance" (Babick et al. 2016). Furthermore, the advanced as well as time- and resource-intensive nature of electron microscopy measurements often make them impractical for routine characterization of particles. Accordingly, the metrology community has attempted to investigate and validate the use of specific surface area (Hackley and Stefaniak 2013; Lecloux et al. 2017; Wohlleben et al. 2017) and solution-based (Anderson et al. 2013) measurements as proxies for obtaining particle size distributions around and below 100 nm threshold of the EC definition. Such proxy measurements evaluate the particle sizes and particle size distributions indirectly and often with size-dependent sensitivity (Anderson et al. 2013), so a calibration against the appropriate reference materials or electron microscopy measurements is typically required to validate their ability to produce a *number-size* distribution for a given material system and to establish any necessary correction factors (Babick et al. 2016).

The two-tiered approach to particle size measurements (Babick et al. 2016) recommended by the NanoDefine project (Table 7.1) should be generally applicable for implementing the EFSA guidelines (EFSA et al. 2018). The simpler *Tier 1* techniques provide estimates of particle size distributions that either clearly identify a material as a nanomaterial or reveal the need for follow-up by the *Tier 2* imaging techniques to resolve borderline or ambiguous cases.

#### 7.2.2.1 Tier 1 Techniques for Particle Sizing: Powders

The volume-specific surface area (VSSA) measurements are the primary recommended *Tier 1* technique for materials in powder form (Babick et al. 2016). As detailed in validation studies of VSSA (Lecloux et al. 2017; Wohlleben et al. 2017), the most common implementation of VSSA relies on measuring gas adsorption, via the Brunauer-Emmett-Teller method (Hackley and Stefaniak 2013), to determine the specific surface area (SSA), which is then multiplied by the density of the material from a He-pycnometry measurement. The VSSA measurements fundamentally cannot provide information about the distribution of the particle sizes, but assuming some independent knowledge of the form-factor of particles in a material (nanoparticles, nanofibers, nanoplates), can provide an estimate of the smallest dimension ($d_{VSSA}$) of a representative particle. This $d_{VSSA}$ size estimate is strongly correlated (an agreement within a factor of 2 for many materials) with the median size of the number-size distribution obtained from electron microscopy (Babick et al. 2016; Lecloux et al. 2017; Wohlleben et al. 2017). This good agreement was observed for samples with 20%–60% polydispersity of organic, inorganic, metal-organic, and metallic substances, porosity being one of the main caveats that required a more complex analysis procedure (Lecloux et al. 2017; Wohlleben et al. 2017). Given the definition of a nanoparticle (Section 7.2.1), $d_{VSSA}$ effectively provides the estimate of the median particle size for a material in nanoparticle form.

For classification under the EFSA guidelines (EFSA et al. 2018), the following basic recommendations can be adapted from the VSSA validation study (Wohlleben et al. 2017). Materials with a VSSA > 60 $m^2/cm^3$ (and thus a $d_{VSSA}$ < 100 nm) can be classified as nanomaterials. Materials with a $d_{VSSA}$ > 1000 nm (assuming spherical form-factor) can be classified as non-nanomaterials, subject to the EFSA-specific classification caveats summarized in Section 7.2.1. Materials with a $d_{VSSA}$ between 100 and 1000 nm need to be further investigated by at least one of the *Tier 2* imaging techniques.

#### 7.2.2.2 Tier 1 Techniques for Particle Sizing: Suspensions

Dynamic light scattering (DLS) is one of the most popular techniques for sizing particles in suspensions (Rasmussen et al. 2018), including in the context of food materials (Linsinger et al. 2013; McClements and McClements 2016). The size of colloidal particles in DLS measurements is not measured directly, but estimated as the hydrodynamic equivalent diameter from their diffusion coefficient under Brownian motion. Accordingly, the size distributions obtained from DLS are intrinsically intensity-weighted, which for polydisperse materials requires specialized algorithms to extract reliable particle size distributions and can result in a few large particles dominating the signal (Anderson et al. 2013; Kato et al. 2014; Lamberty et al. 2011; Meli et al. 2012). For monodisperse samples of solid spherical reference nanoparticles, therefore, the mean diameters measured by DLS and electron microscopy typically agree very well (e.g., within 5%–10% for ca. 33 nm silica particles in Lamberty et al. 2011), but in polydisperse samples—even simple mixed/multimodal ones—some of the sub-populations are not identified by DLS (Anderson et al. 2013).

For realistic polydisperse samples of various size ranges in the NanoDefine survey, number-weighted medians obtained from DLS ($d_{DLS}$) are typically >50% larger than those from electron microscopy ($d_{EM}$) (Babick et al. 2016). This overestimation is typically by less than a factor of 2.5, resulting in the adjusted thresholds recommended for material classification based on DLS data: $d_{DLS} < 40$ nm strongly indicates a nanomaterial, while $d_{DLS} > 250$ nm implies that it may not be a nanomaterial and additional characterization is needed (Babick et al. 2016). Subject to these caveats, DLS is recommended by the NanoDefine project as a *Tier 1* technique for screening particles in suspensions (Babick et al. 2016).

Analytical centrifugation is the second class of *Tier 1* sizing techniques for suspensions recommended by the NanoDefine project (Babick et al. 2016). Centrifugation produces differential sedimentation of suspended particles based on their density and hydrodynamic mobility, which can be particularly beneficial for characterization of complex polydisperse samples (Wohlleben 2012), such as those encountered in food or biomedical applications. The two popular implementations of analytical centrifuges use disc or cuvette configurations and intrinsically measure, respectively, a scaled density function or the cumulative function of the size distribution; the use of turbidity or refractive index measurements (currently available in the cuvette configuration) to monitor the sedimentation also adds a weighting to the recorded size distribution (Anderson et al. 2013; Babick et al. 2016; Wohlleben 2012).

In multimodal suspensions of reference materials, analytical centrifugation demonstrates excellent performance in terms of separating and identifying the sub-populations in the particle size distribution, which for well-defined nanoparticles can be readily converted into number-size distributions (Anderson et al. 2013; Wohlleben 2012). The recently reported capability of analytical centrifugation to detect the presence of dimers and multimers can be beneficial for identifying the origin of such multimodal sub-populations in samples of nominally monomodal particles (Mehn et al. 2017a). For most of the more realistic polydisperse materials in the NanoDefine survey, number-weighted medians obtained from analytical centrifugation ($d_{AC}$) differ by <50% from $d_{EM}$ (Babick et al. 2016; Ullmann et al. 2017). While $d_{AC}$ values exhibit a better agreement with $d_{EM}$ than do $d_{DLS}$ ones, the discrepancies (including occasional major ones) between $d_{AC}$ and $d_{EM}$ are difficult to rationalize, so the same adjusted thresholds are recommended for material classification based on analytical centrifugation or DLS data (Babick et al. 2016).

### 7.2.2.3 Tier 1 Techniques for Particle Sizing: Limitations

Three potential *Tier 1* techniques were not recommended by the NanoDefine project for classification or screening measurements of particle size distributions in suspensions—particle tracking analysis (PTA), small angle X-ray scattering (SAXS), and angular light scattering—due to limitations summarized below (Babick et al. 2016).

PTA relies on tracking the Brownian motion of individual particles based on their visualization by the light they scatter when illuminated against a dark background (Saveyn et al. 2010). Accordingly, PTA measurements at nanoscale are currently reliable only within a small range just below 100 nm (extended to smaller sizes only for strongly scattering materials) (Babick et al. 2016). Furthermore, even for larger particles in the 200–400 nm range, PTA failed to resolve populations in a multimodal sample (Anderson et al. 2013). Future improvements in the instrumentation may be able to address both the sensitivity and resolution limitations of PTA.

SAXS takes advantage of the small wavelengths of X-rays to characterize nanoscale objects and structures (Meli et al. 2012), including unique modalities for distinguishing between aggregates and constituent particles as well as roughly resolving the shape of the constituent particles (Babick et al. 2016). Another unique modality of SAXS allows the measurement of the SSA of the (constituent) particles in suspension (Babick et al. 2016; Rasmussen et al. 2018). The effective upper limit of size measurements by SAXS, however, is about 100 nm, diminishing its usefulness for classification of nanomaterials as a stand-alone technique (Babick et al. 2016; Rasmussen et al. 2018).

Angular light scattering was originally developed for measurements of microparticles, and its performance for particles in the sub-micron size range is reported to be inconsistent (Babick et al. 2016; Kuchenbecker et al. 2012). These limitations of angular light scattering appear to be fundamental, related to relatively weak and unstructured light scattering by nanoparticles *versus* microparticles, so any future improvements may require the development of dedicated instruments for the sub-micron size range.

#### 7.2.2.4 Tier 2 Techniques for Particle Sizing: Electron Microscopy

Both popular electron microscopy techniques—scanning electron microscopy (SEM) and transmission electron microscopy (TEM)—and their hybrids or variants (Klein et al. 2011; Meli et al. 2012; Rades et al. 2014; Rice et al. 2013) implemented across a wide range of commercial instruments are considered to be the primary *Tier 2* techniques because they provide direct measurements of the size, morphology, and aggregation state of particles across a uniquely broad size range as well as of number-size distributions from direct counting (Babick et al. 2016; Rasmussen et al. 2018). The electron microscopy size measurements produced a consistent nanomaterial classification and the best reproducibility among the methods tested in the NanoDefine project, with results falling within a factor 1.2 for half of the materials and within a factor 1.5 for most, hence the use of the number-weighted medians $d_{EM}$ as reference values for other techniques (Babick et al. 2016).

The practical caveats of using electron microscopy for nanocharacterization are related primarily to the widely acknowledged uncertainties and ambiguities arising from the preparation of representative samples, especially from polydisperse materials (Babick et al. 2016; Rasmussen et al. 2018). Accordingly, the use of the appropriate *Tier 1* techniques is recommended to cross-check the general plausibility of results obtained from electron microscopy (Babick et al. 2016). The fundamentals of the measurements carried out under vacuum and via exposure to high-energy electron beams also intrinsically limit the use of SEM and TEM for broad classes of sensitive samples, including most of the organic, biological, and other soft materials (Section 7.3) relevant in the context of food (Linsinger et al. 2013; McClements and McClements 2016).

### 7.2.3 Concentration

The concentration of nanoparticles is a parameter conspicuously absent from general discussions of their physicochemical characterization, e.g., in the overview of the Organisation for Economic Co-operation and Development Testing Programme (Rasmussen et al. 2018). This may appear surprising, given the importance of quantifying the exposure or administered doses of nanomaterials in environmental (Hassellöv et al. 2008), food (Linsinger et al. 2013; McClements and McClements 2016), or biomedical (Grainger 2013; Wu et al. 2011) contexts. In a specific medical application of nanoparticles to produce magnetic hyperthermia, for example, the variations and ambiguity in specifying the concentration of nanoparticles lead to difficulties in comparing the effectiveness of treatment protocols reported by different groups (Vilas-Boas et al. 2018). For the purposes of risk assessment (EFSA et al. 2018; Linsinger et al. 2013), the dose of a nanomaterial in suspension is most commonly specified as a mass concentration (McClements and McClements 2016). But unlike in conventional toxicology or pharmacology where the known molecular weight of the specified compound allows for a trivial conversion between mass and molar concentrations, the typical heterogeneity of nanomaterials makes such nominal conversions unreliable (Hassellöv et al. 2008; Linsinger et al. 2013). Yet, the presumptive individual nature of typical nanoparticle–cell interaction events (EFSA et al. 2018; Grainger 2013; Westmeier et al. 2018; Wu et al. 2011) strongly advocates that molar concentrations or, in other words, *absolute* rather than only relative number concentrations of nanoparticles need to be considered in most applications (Shang and Gao 2014; Shard et al. 2018). Addressing the lack of a general technique for measuring concentrations of nanoparticles is the primary motivation for the Innanopart project (Table 7.1) supported by the European Metrology Programme for Innovation and Research.

The ensemble techniques used to measure particle concentrations in suspensions significantly overlap with those used for particle sizing (described in Section 7.2.2.2). The signal in the ensemble techniques based on light scattering or absorption, including DLS, ultraviolet-visible (UV-vis) absorption, and turbidimetry, fundamentally depends on both size and concentration of the particles, so the ability to reliably measure either of the two parameters strongly depends on having a monodisperse population of particles and always requires the particles to have additional properties (Shang and Gao 2014). For example, the UV-vis absorption can be used to measure particle concentration via Beer-Lambert law only for particles that exhibit specific/unique extinction peaks in UV-vis spectra and for which the molar extinction coefficient is known. Via a combination of theoretical calculations and empirical results, the molar extinction coefficients have been derived for nanoparticles composed of common materials, including gold (Liu et al. 2007; Navarro and Werts 2013), silver (Navarro and Werts 2013), and semiconductor quantum dots (Sun and Goldys 2008; Yu et al. 2003). These molar extinction coefficients, however, are based on multiple assumptions of idealized size, composition, and internal structure, so their accuracy, and hence that of the measured particle concentrations, typically needs to be verified using independent methods (Shang and Gao 2014; Shard et al. 2018). Similarly, particle concentration measurements by turbidimetry are limited to non-absorbing particles with known refractive index and scattering coefficient (Khlebtsov et al. 2008; Shang and Gao 2014). And DLS measurements of particle concentration, likewise, require the knowledge of refractive index and scattering coefficient for the particles being measured and for absolute concentration measurements, a calibration sample of a known concentration (Shang and Gao 2014; Vysotskii et al. 2009). For samples of nominally monomodal particles, the concentration measurements by any of the above techniques can be adjusted for the presence of dimers and multimers based on analytical centrifugation (Mehn et al. 2017a).

The single-particle techniques for measuring particle concentrations can be roughly divided in two categories: visualization and counting. The visualization techniques include PTA and electron microscopy, subject to the challenges with representative sampling analogous to those mentioned in Sections 7.2.2.3 and 7.2.2.4 (Shang and Gao 2014). The advanced counting techniques for nanoparticles in suspension typically rely on a transduction mechanism that produces a pulse for each individual particle passing by or into a detector. Resistive-pulse sensing, for example, is based on detecting a transient signal as a particle passes through a tightly constrained channel or pore (Kozak et al. 2011), but the small analysis volume and constrained flow paths raise the representative-sampling caveats, as mentioned above for the PTA, and require a standard calibration sample with a known concentration of nanoparticles for converting the pulse count into absolute concentration values (Shang and Gao 2014).

Inductively coupled plasma mass spectrometry (ICP-MS) and its variants are commonly used to analyze composition, contamination, and authenticity of food samples by detecting specific elements or atomic clusters (Taylor et al. 2018). In a standard ICP-MS measurement, a mass concentration of one or more elements can be established for nanoparticles. When analyzing a suspension of nanoparticles by ICP-MS with sufficient temporal resolution, instead of the conventional quasi-constant flow of ions, bunches of ions (peaks in ion intensity) corresponding to individual particles are detected, resulting in single-particle ICP-MS technique, for which applications to nanoparticles in complex media are being explored in the environmental and biomedical contexts (Montaño et al. 2016). While single-particle ICP-MS features an advantage of a signal proportional to the masses of individual particles (or aggregates), which helps to resolve some ambiguities associated with other counting techniques, accurate measurements of absolute number concentrations would require either a perfect transport and atomization/ionization in plasma or appropriate calibration standards to account for instrumental factors (Montaño et al. 2016; Shang and Gao 2014).

### 7.2.4 Composition

For nanoparticles in suspension, the most general techniques recommended for elemental analysis are inductively coupled plasma optical emission spectrophotometry (ICP-OES), ICP-MS, and their variants (Montaño et al. 2016; Rasmussen et al. 2018; Taylor et al. 2018). The specific variant optimal for characterization of a given nanomaterial needs to be selected based on the requirements, for example, ICP-MS is generally more sensitive than ICP-OES, but performs poorly for light elements, whereas

ICP-OES is suitable for both organic and inorganic nanomaterials, but may be difficult for complex samples due to the interference between emission lines of different elements (Rasmussen et al. 2018; Taylor et al. 2018). The single-particle ICP-MS variant can be used to statistically sample the elemental composition of individual nanoparticles (Montaño et al. 2016).

For samples of powder or dried nanoparticles, energy dispersive X-ray spectroscopy implemented in both SEM and TEM instruments can provide a detailed analysis of elemental composition, even for individual particles (Hassellöv et al. 2008; Rades et al. 2014; Rasmussen et al. 2018). Energy dispersive X-ray spectroscopy, in principle, is suitable for detecting elements with an atomic number >5, whereas for lighter elements and for resolving chemical states of some elements electron energy loss spectroscopy can be used as a complementary or alternative technique (Hassellöv et al. 2008; Rasmussen et al. 2018). For sufficiently small nanoparticles (ca. <10 nm), preferably of uniform composition, X-ray photoelectron spectroscopy (XPS) can provide detailed information about the elemental composition and the chemical states of those elements (Baer and Engelhard 2010; Baer et al. 2010), in many cases with high sensitivity to the presence of minor elements (Shard 2014; Shard and Clifford 2018). With the help of models and simulations, XPS data can be also interpreted to check the internal structure of core-shell nanoparticles (Cant et al. 2016; Chudzicki et al. 2015; Powell et al. 2016, 2018; Shard 2012).

### 7.2.5 Surface

The chemistry of the particle surface is regulatory relevant information for nanomaterials in general (Rasmussen et al. 2018) and is specifically of interest in the context of food (EFSA et al. 2018; McClements and McClements 2016) and biomedical (Grainger 2013; Lynch et al. 2007; Wu et al. 2011) applications. Nanomaterials inherently have a much larger specific surface area than do bulk materials, so surfaces play a critical role in the interactions of nanoparticles with their environment and with each other (Wu et al. 2011). Furthermore, surfaces of nanoparticles can be intentionally or unintentionally functionalized, whereby the intentional functionality may modify the stability of the particles or their affinity for the matrix or other objects, whereas the unintentional functionalization or modification typically occurs due to specific or non-specific interactions with the environment (Baer 2018).

The most common techniques for surface characterization of nanoparticles are XPS and time-of-flight secondary ion mass spectrometry (ToF-SIMS), both techniques are very sensitive and inherently surface-specific, with typical sampling depth of ca. 10 nm and 1–2 nm, respectively (Baer et al. 2008, 2010; Rafati et al. 2016; Rasmussen et al. 2018; Shard 2014). The shallow sampling depth makes XPS and ToF-SIMS particularly suitable for chemical analysis of monolayers of organic or biological molecules as well as a-few-nm-thin polymeric or inorganic surface layers that provide functionality (e.g., capping/passivation, electronic-structure confinement, etc.) or interact with the environment (e.g., via oxidation, protonation, or hydration). The combination of the sampling depth and angle-dependence of the photoelectron signal enable the use of XPS for characterization of shells in core-shell nanoparticles (Cant et al. 2016; Chudzicki et al. 2015; Powell et al. 2016, 2018; Shard 2012).

Adapting XPS to characterization of complex materials on nanoparticles typically starts with a detailed analysis of model (mono)layers on flat surfaces, e.g., for organic molecules (Techane et al. 2011), polymers (Lock et al. 2010), DNA (Petrovykh et al. 2004), peptides (Fears et al. 2013), or proteins (Ray and Shard 2011; Ray et al. 2015), followed by the extension and validation of the methodology to the analogous (mono) layers on nanoparticle surfaces (Belsey et al. 2015, 2016; Chudzicki et al. 2015; Minelli et al. 2014; Minelli and Shard 2016; Rafati et al. 2016; Shard 2012; Techane et al. 2011).

Notably, molecular adsorption or attachment onto surfaces of model nanoparticles can be followed quantitatively by a variety of individual or complementary sizing techniques, for example, by DLS, PTA, analytical centrifugation, and UV-vis spectroscopy (Bell et al. 2013; Belsey et al. 2015), by DLS, SAXS, and analytical centrifugation (Minelli et al. 2014), by DLS, SAXS, PTA, and analytical centrifugation (Gollwitzer et al. 2016), or by analytical centrifugation (Davidson et al. 2017). Effects of the environment and surface adsorption on the surface charge of nanoparticles can be also followed by several complementary techniques, including electrophoretic light scattering (Lamberty et al. 2011), PTA, and resistive-pulse sensing (Sikora et al. 2015). Quantitative measurements of surface adsorption onto more realistic particle populations and from more complex media, however, remain an important, but unresolved analytical challenge (Hassellöv et al. 2008; Linsinger et al. 2013; Lynch et al. 2007; McClements and McClements 2016; Wu et al. 2011; Zhang et al. 2011).

## 7.3 SOFT NANOPARTICLES

The regulatory consideration of soft nanoparticles to-date can be characterized as equivocal. The original EC Recommendation for a definition of a nanomaterial (EC 2011) refers to a particle as a minute piece of matter with defined physical boundaries. This terminology neither explicitly includes nor excludes soft particles, so amendments have been proposed to resolve this ambiguity, with one option specifying exclusively "solid matter" and another option that would include soft materials, such as micelles and liquid droplets (Rauscher et al. 2015). EFSA guidance resolves the regulatory ambiguity in the food context by including within the scope "[n]anoscale entities made of natural materials that have been deliberately produced to have nano-enabled/enhanced properties, or that have been modified for use in the development of other nanoscale materials, e.g. for encapsulating (bioactive) compounds" and "organic nanomaterial, such as encapsulates" (EFSA et al. 2018). The defining characteristic of this scope appears to be the deliberately produced or engineered nature of the nanomaterial, as it excludes "other 'natural' nanoscale entities [that] may be present in food/feed" (EFSA et al. 2018). This explicit consideration of the soft nanomaterials by EFSA is eminently justified in the food context because food-grade nanoparticles are commonly produced from soft materials, such as proteins, carbohydrates, and lipids, and by methods that inherently produce soft particles: homogenization, antisolvent precipitation, spontaneous emulsification, and coacervation (McClements and McClements 2016).

### 7.3.1 Visualization of Particle Morphology

Examples of TEM imaging of soft nanoparticles tend to be primarily from the biomedical rather than food context, but they provide good illustrations of the state-of-the-art implementations of TEM for this general class of samples. The first overarching conclusion from comparative studies of different preparation approaches of soft nanoparticles for TEM is that drying such samples produces a broad range of artifacts, for example, as illustrated by systematic imaging of liposomes (Franken et al. 2017) and polymeric micelles (Patterson et al. 2015) or by observing the destruction of vesicles in a mixed population of polymeric vesicles and micelles (Laan and Denkova 2017). Accordingly, dried samples of soft nanoparticles are not suitable for obtaining TEM images that are representative of the properties of the population being characterized. In contrast, cryogenic TEM (cryo-TEM) is considered to be much more reliable in preserving the morphology of soft particles and in protecting them from damage by the high-energy electron beam used during the imaging (Franken et al. 2017; Klang et al. 2012; Laan and Denkova 2017). The morphology and microstructure have been successfully imaged by cryo-TEM for different liposome variants (cubosomes, hexosomes, micellar cubosomes), transitional mesophases during formation of liposomes, vesicles, amphiphilic Janus dendrimers, spherical dendrimersomes, spherical and wormlike micelles, and microemulsions (Helvig et al. 2015). Nanomedicine drug carriers successfully imaged by cryo-TEM include liposomes, colloidal lipid emulsions, solid lipid nanoparticles, thermotropic and lyotropic liquid crystalline nanoparticles, as well as polymer-based colloids and delivery systems for nucleic acids (Kuntsche et al. 2011). While all of these examples used model systems exhibiting varying degrees of realistic features, the soft particles considered for food (McClements and McClements 2016) or biomedical (Klang et al. 2013) applications include many lipid and liquid-crystalline nanoparticles as well as microemulsions, the morphology and microstructure of which can be investigated following analogous cryo-TEM methodologies.

Among SEM variants, environmental SEM (ESEM) helps to avoid some of the drying artifacts by imaging soft particles under a humid atmosphere and thus in a partially hydrated state (and following the kinetics of dehydration) or even in emulsions (Stokes 2001) and liquid droplets (Méndez-Vilas et al. 2009). Cryogenic SEM can be used for morphological characterization of soft materials: compared to cryo-TEM, it reveals partial 3D information about the shapes of soft nanoparticles, e.g., cubosomes, hexosomes, or nanoemulsions, but does not provide details of their internal structure (Boyd et al. 2007; Klang et al. 2012, 2013).

### 7.3.2 Sizing of Soft Particles by Electron Microscopy

The fundamental importance of electron microscopy for characterization of solid nanoparticles is difficult to overstate: it is the most reliable method for sizing solid nanoparticles and provides reference data on sizes and size distribution for benchmarking and validation of other techniques (Section 7.2.2). In contrast, soft nanoparticles are not easily considered following the strict size-threshold approach to definition of solid nanoparticles because their sizes generally depend on the chemical and physical forces (and history of such forces) exerted by their environment (EFSA et al. 2018; Rauscher et al. 2015). The discretionary interpretation of the threshold size for nanomaterials in the EFSA guidance (EFSA et al. 2018) provides a more natural framework for incorporating the unique challenges encountered in characterization of soft particles.

An important insight into the size measurements for soft particles by electron microscopy is provided by considering another class of model systems: bacteria and other microorganisms. *Staphylococcus aureus* (*S. aureus*) bacteria are a particularly convenient model system for size measurements due to their nearly spherical shape (Monteiro et al. 2015; Zhou et al. 2015) and robust viability and mechanical stability under a wide range of physicochemical conditions (Monteiro et al. 2015; Sousa et al. 2015). As illustrated in Figure 7.1, different preparation protocols strongly affect the apparent sizes and size distributions of *S. aureus* cells imaged by cryo-TEM: images from either of the two preparations interpreted on their own would provide very different conclusions regarding both polydispersity and mean particle sizes in the typical *S. aureus* population.

By analogy with lipid nanoparticles (Boyd et al. 2007; Klang et al. 2013), ESEM should be a good choice of a complementary and self-consistent electron microscopy technique for cross-validation of cryo-TEM results. Furthermore, reported evidence indicates that under ESEM conditions microorganisms can even remain viable (Ahmad et al. 2011; Misirli et al. 2007; Ren et al. 2008), suggesting that the environmental (including physicochemical) stress induced under ESEM conditions is relatively mild and thus, hypothetically, may not strongly affect the size of the imaged soft particles.

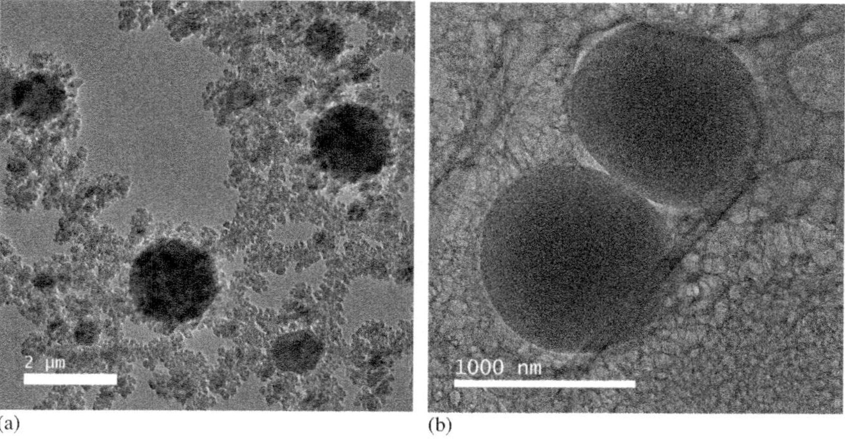


**FIGURE 7.1** *Staphylococcus aureus* bacterial cells imaged by cryo-TEM. Both samples have been prepared by robotic plunge-freezing in liquid ethane, the only difference in the preparation prior to freezing was the medium in which the live cells have been resuspended: deionized water (a) and 40% dextran in 0.01 M phosphate-buffered saline (PBS) (b).

The apparent size of the *S. aureus* cells imaged by ESEM (Figure 7.2) is ca. 1.1 μm, in good agreement with that in the cryo-TEM image prepared using the second method in Figure 7.1. When fixed and dried *S. aureus* cells are imaged by SEM under vacuum, their apparent sizes are typically in the 0.6–0.8 μm range (Monteiro et al. 2015; Sousa et al. 2015; Zhou et al. 2015), so at least some drying clearly can be avoided under both ESEM and cryo-TEM conditions. In high-resolution optical microscopy images, acquired in liquid using either phase-contrast or structured-illumination mode, the individual live *S. aureus* cells consistently appear to be larger than 1 μm and as large as 1.5 μm (Monteiro et al. 2015; Zhou et al. 2015). These variations clearly illustrate the strong dependence of the size of a soft particle on its environment, as postulated at the beginning of this section. The ca. 0.5–1.5 μm size range observed for *S. aureus* model also is close to the limit for a systematic comparison between the optical and electron microscopy techniques, as optical microscopies become resolution-limited (Yao and Carballido-López 2014) in the ca. 100 nm "nanoscale" range formally defined for nanomaterials (Section 7.2.1).

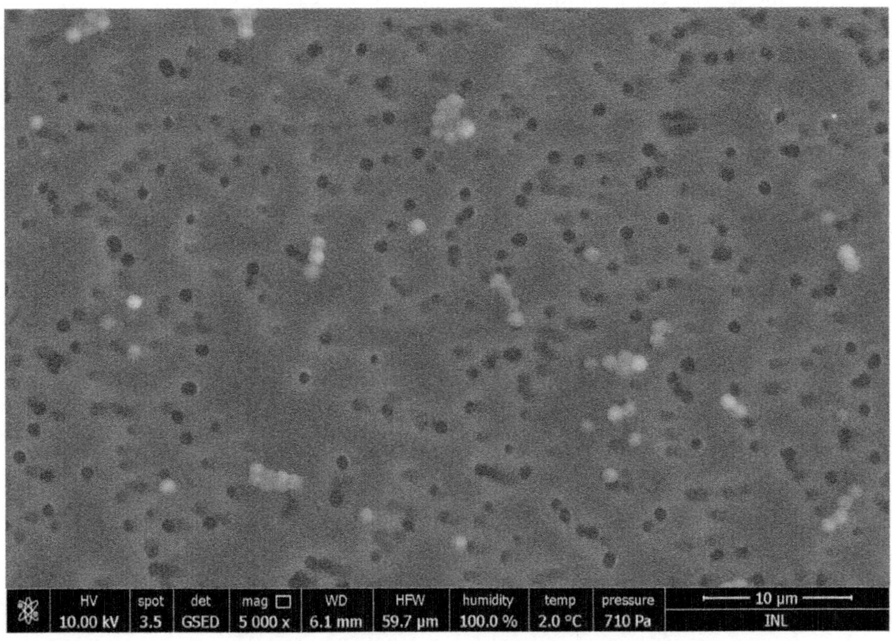


**FIGURE 7.2** *Staphylococcus aureus* bacterial cells imaged by ESEM. Live cells were filtered from suspension onto a polycarbonate filter with ca. 0.2 μm pores, which appear in the image as dark circular features. A piece of wet filter with cells was introduced into the ESEM chamber and imaged with a 10-kV beam and a gaseous secondary electron detector (GSED), on a Peltier stage at 2°C and 100% relative humidity at the background gas pressure of 710 Pa.

#### 7.3.2.1 Electron Microscopy in Liquid Environment

Considering the functional aspects of the nanomaterial definition in the EFSA guidance (EFSA et al. 2018), which suggests that the relevant size range or threshold can be established based on phenomena such as nanoparticle–cell interactions (Gioria et al. 2018; Grainger 2013; Westmeier et al. 2018), the most practically relevant size of a soft particle should be defined and measured under the conditions that are as close as possible to those of the intended use. For most of the soft particles in food (McClements and McClements 2016) or biomedical (Gioria et al. 2018; Grainger 2013) applications, the relevant environment is that of being a component in a mixed suspension of other particles in a complex media. Therefore, even the most reductionist version of the relevant environment would imply size measurements of soft particles in an aqueous solution. There are three major variants of TEM that are able to measure nanoparticles in solution, implementing each of them requires specialized sample cells and modifications of the standard instruments.

*In situ* liquid TEM is implemented using a liquid sample cell that can be introduced into a TEM instrument, in such a sample cell a thin (50–500 nm) layer of liquid is confined between ultra-thin (ca. 50 nm) membranes of "electron transparent" material, such as silicon nitride or graphene. For model platinum-core polymeric micelles, in which the platinum provided intrinsic staining, *in situ* liquid TEM imaging revealed a size distribution having a similar mean at ca. 90 nm and a somewhat narrower width compared to cryo-TEM imaging, in dry-state TEM the distribution was shifted to smaller sizes, while with uranyl acetate staining a distinct second population emerged, centered about 45 nm (Patterson et al. 2015). The frame rate in that implementation of *in situ* liquid TEM enabled real-time observation of particle agglomeration (Patterson et al. 2015).

Using a similar type of liquid sample cell, a scanning TEM (STEM) variant can be implemented to take advantage of the atomic number (Z) contrast intrinsic to STEM and to be able to measure, e.g., gold nanoparticles with diameter of ca. 1.4 nm, through water layers up to 3 μm in thickness (de Jonge et al. 2010). The intrinsically slower frame rate in STEM compared to TEM imaging limits the temporal resolution for dynamic measurements in this configuration, but "video rate" with 10 μs per pixel dwell time has been demonstrated for tracking the movement of 5-nm gold nanoparticles (Ring and de Jonge 2012).

Another implementation of STEM imaging takes advantage of ESEM instruments and their capability to operate at 100% relative humidity to perform STEM measurements through a drop of liquid placed on a conventional TEM grid (Bogner et al. 2005, 2007). These "wet STEM" measurements have demonstrated for gold and latex nanoparticles as well as for liquid emulsions of styrene or polystyrene-styrene in water, latex nanoparticles with different surface modification could be distinguished as well (Bogner et al. 2005).

All the above specialized variants of TEM for measurements in liquid are currently implemented on a limited number of instruments, so until a broader adoption and commercialization of these techniques, they would not be practical for routine characterization, even as the equivalent of *Tier 2* techniques for soft particles. In the meantime, one approach for amplifying the impact of the few existing instruments would be to use them to validate the methodology (both preparation and imaging of specific soft particle systems) for the more commonly available cryo-TEM.

### 7.3.3 Ensemble Techniques for Sizing Soft Particles

Among the ensemble techniques for characterizing suspensions of soft nanoparticles, flow field-flow fractionation (FFFF or F4) and its many variants are commonly used in the nanomedicine context (Qureshi and Kok 2011; Wagner et al. 2014; Zattoni et al. 2014). The FFFF fundamentally is a separation technique based on particle diffusion coefficients (Wagner et al. 2014), which makes it suitable for separation of particles in a broad size range from nanometers to micrometers, FFFF has been recently approved by the United States Food and Drug Administration for validation of protein drug samples (Zattoni et al. 2014). FFFF is often coupled to an optical detection technique, such as static multi-angle light-scattering (Zattoni et al. 2014) or DLS (Mehn et al. 2017b; Sitar et al. 2017), to measure size distribution analysis of soft particles and to investigate their aggregation in (native) solution conditions. In the context of drug-delivery soft nanoparticles, FFFF-multi-angle light-scattering has been successfully used for characterization of lipid and (bio)polymer particles (Wagner et al. 2014; Zattoni et al. 2014).

In a systematic comparison of different sizing techniques for monodisperse samples of empty and drug-loaded liposomes, both conventional DLS and FFFF-DLS measurements measured their mean sizes as 85 and 80 nm, respectively, both values agreed with those from analytical centrifugation (Mehn et al. 2017b) and PTA (Gioria et al. 2018) measurements. In contrast, average diameters of 63 and 57 nm, respectively, were determined for the empty and drug-loaded liposomes by cryo-TEM (Mehn et al. 2017b), indicating a strong bias between the values measured by electron microscopy and those obtained from the ensemble techniques in solution. After incubation with serum proteins, conventional DLS indicated a shift to a smaller size, however, essentially identical elution profiles in FFFF-DLS demonstrated that for these model particles protein adsorption from serum was negligible and the indication from conventional DLS was misleading (Mehn et al. 2017b). For polydisperse samples, DLS was found to be unable to resolve the complex particle size distributions that were successfully resolved by both PTA and FFFF-DLS (Mehn et al. 2017b).

## 7.4 REPRODUCIBILITY IN NANOCHARACTERIZATION

Reproducibility challenges associated with the characterization of nanoparticles arise directly from many of the same inherent characteristics that make them of interest in applications (Baer 2018). The multi-disciplinary nature of the communities involved in producing and characterizing nanoparticles further compounds the difficulties of communicating and understanding the underlying phenomena, best practices, nuanced interpretation of the characterization data, and particularly of any associated health or environmental risks (Baer 2018; Nel et al. 2015; Petersen et al. 2014). Outlined below are some of the major issues that have been identified by expert communities as contributing to the reproducibility challenges in nanocharacterization.

Reproducibility in the synthesis and production of nanomaterials is notoriously difficult to ensure. Nominally the same protocols, even when applied by the same practitioner, will often produce nanomaterials with batch-to-batch variations at both short- and long-term timescales (Baer 2018). In some cases, extensive characterization of the produced nanomaterial may reveal the factors that contribute to this variability, but the effort and expertise required for such comprehensive characterization make it impractical to be pursued routinely.

Nanomaterials are fundamentally dynamic systems, so over time they can be dramatically affected by internal thermodynamically driven processes and by the environmental conditions and other external interactions during storage, transport, handling, and even preparation for characterization (Baer 2018; Baer et al. 2018; McClements and McClements 2016; Petersen et al. 2014). Collecting and analyzing the detailed provenance information along with carefully designing and implementing appropriately timed characterization plans are the most important measures recommended to address this challenge (Baer 2018; Baer et al. 2016, 2018).

Both extraction from and dispersion in the matrix are critically important for handling and characterization of nanomaterials (Baer et al. 2018; McClements and McClements 2016; Petersen et al. 2014; Rasmussen et al. 2018). Some of the steps in such complex protocols may have different effects on nanomaterials compared to those assumed based on the standard procedures used for small molecules, polymers, or powders and microparticles.

Adapting the traditional toxicology and toxicity assays for assessment of health risks associated with nanoparticles requires a careful review and validation of the underlying principles and mechanisms, ranging from understanding the exposure dose, to chemical (e.g., impurities from synthesis) and biological (e.g., endotoxin) contamination, to the effects of nanoparticles on the assay read-out (e.g., interference or quenching in colorimetric assays) (Grainger 2013; McClements and McClements 2016; Nel et al. 2015; Petersen et al. 2014).

## 7.5 CONCLUDING REMARKS

The critical importance of physicochemical characterization of nanomaterials is emphasized in the regulatory guidelines and requirements for their food and medical applications (EFSA et al. 2018; Pita et al. 2016; Rasmussen et al. 2018). Since the EC issued the original recommended definition of a nanomaterial (EC 2011), a significant concerted effort by various European authorities, metrology organizations, international standards bodies, and major international projects resulted in a dramatically improved understanding of nanocharacterization needs and in the development and validation of characterization methods for nanomaterials. In particular, the importance of particle sizes and size distribution for classification of nanomaterials has generated a wave of metrological and analytical activity on improving and validating the sizing methods for solid nanoparticles (Babick et al. 2016; Rasmussen et al. 2018). The characterization of composition and surface properties of nanoparticles continues to improve in terms of speed, sensitivity, and reliability, based on adapting and extending analytical methods from the more traditional materials and surface analysis domains (Baer et al. 2010; Rasmussen et al. 2018). Measurement of absolute particle concentrations has received relatively less direct attention to-date, despite its practical importance for the current and future applications of nanoparticles, but it benefits indirectly from the development of new and improved particle sizing techniques that can be adapted for concentration measurements. Finally, characterization of soft particles is an area of recognized importance and the resulting growth in analytical techniques and capabilities.

## REFERENCES

Ahmad, M. R., Nakajima, M., Kojima, S., Homma, M. and Fukuda, T. 2011. "Buckling nanoneedle for characterizing single cells mechanics inside environmental SEM". *IEEE Transactions on Nanotechnology* 10:226–236.

Anderson, W., Kozak, D., Coleman, V. A., Jämting, Å. K. and Trau, M. 2013. "A comparative study of submicron particle sizing platforms: Accuracy, precision, and resolution analysis of polydisperse particle size distributions". *Journal of Colloid and Interface Science* 405:322–330.

Baalousha, M., Prasad, A. and Lead, J. R. 2014. "Quantitative measurement of the nanoparticle size and number concentration from liquid suspensions by atomic force microscopy". *Environmental Science: Processes and Impacts* 16:1338–1347.

Babick, F., Mielke, J., Wohlleben, W., Weigel, S. and Hodoroaba, V. D. 2016. "How reliably can a material be classified as a nanomaterial? Available particle-sizing techniques at work". *Journal of Nanoparticle Research* 18:158.

Baer, D. R. 2018. "The chameleon effect: Characterization challenges due to the variability of nanoparticles and their surfaces". *Frontiers in Chemistry* 6:145.

Baer, D. R. and Engelhard, M. H. 2010. "XPS analysis of nanostructured materials and biological surfaces". *Journal of Electron Spectroscopy and Related Phenomena* 178–179:415–432.

Baer, D. R., Amonette, J. E., Engelhard, M. H., Gaspar, D. J., Karakoti, A. S., Kuchibhatla, S., Nachimuthu, P., Nurmi, J. T., Qiang, Y., Sarathy, V. et al. 2008. "Characterization challenges for nanomaterials". *Surface and Interface Analysis* 40:529–537.

Baer, D. R., Engelhard, M. H., Johnson, G. E., Laskin, J., Lai, J., Mueller, K., Munusamy, P., Thevuthasan, S, Wang, H. and Washton, N. 2013. "Surface characterization of nanomaterials and nanoparticles: Important needs and challenging opportunities". *Journal of Vacuum Science and Technology A* 31:050820.

Baer, D. R., Gaspar, D. J., Nachimuthu, P., Techane, S. D. and Castner, D. G. 2010. "Application of surface chemical analysis tools for characterization of nanoparticles". *Analytical and Bioanalytical Chemistry* 396:983–1002.

Baer, D. R., Karakoti, A. S., Clifford, C. A., Minelli, C. and Unger, W. E. S. 2018. "Importance of sample preparation on reliable surface characterisation of nano-objects: ISO standard 20579-4". *Surface and Interface Analysis* 50:902–906.

Baer, D. R., Munusamy, P. and Thrall, B. D. 2016. "Provenance information as a tool for addressing engineered nanoparticle reproducibility challenges". *Biointerphases* 11:04B401

Bell, N. C., Minelli, C. and Shard, A. G. 2013. "Quantitation of IgG protein adsorption to gold nanoparticles using particle size measurement". *Analytical Methods* 5:4591–4601.

Belsey, N. A., Cant, D. J. H., Minelli, C., Araujo, J. R., Bock, B., Brüner, P., Castner, D. G. et al. 2016. "Versailles project on advanced materials and standards interlaboratory study on measuring the thickness and chemistry of nanoparticle coatings using XPS and LEIS". *Journal of Physical Chemistry C* 120:24070–24079.

Belsey, N. A., Shard, A. G. and Minelli, C. 2015. "Analysis of protein coatings on gold nanoparticles by XPS and liquid-based particle sizing techniques". *Biointerphases* 10:019012.

Bogner, A., Jouneau, P. H., Thollet, G., Basset, D. and Gauthier, C. 2007. "A history of scanning electron microscopy developments: Towards 'wet-STEM' imaging". *Micron* 38:390–401.

Bogner, A., Thollet, G., Basset, D., Jouneau, P. H. and Gauthier, C. 2005. "Wet STEM: A new development in environmental SEM for imaging nano-objects included in a liquid phase". *Ultramicroscopy* 104:290–301.

Bowen, P. 2002. "Particle size distribution measurement from millimeters to nanometers and from rods to platelets". *Journal of Dispersion Science and Technology* 23:631–662.

Boyd, B. J., Rizwan, S. B., Dong, Y.-D., Hook, S. and Rades, T. 2007. "Self-assembled geometric liquid-crystalline nanoparticles imaged in three dimensions: Hexosomes are not necessarily flat hexagonal prisms". *Langmuir* 23:12461–12464.

Cant, D. J. H., Wang, Y.-C., Castner, D. G. and Shard, A. G. 2016. "A technique for calculation of shell thicknesses for core-shell-shell nanoparticles from XPS data". *Surface and Interface Analysis* 48:274–282.

Chudzicki, M., Werner, W. S. M., Shard, A. G., Wang, Y. C., Castner, D. G. and Powell, C. J. 2015. "Evaluating the internal structure of core–shell nanoparticles using X-ray photoelectron intensities and simulated spectra". *Journal of Physical Chemistry C* 119:17687–17696.

Davidson, A. M., Brust, M., Cooper, D. L. and Volk, M. 2017. "Sensitive analysis of protein adsorption to colloidal gold by differential centrifugal sedimentation". *Analytical Chemistry* 89:6807–6814.

de Jonge, N., Poirier-Demers, N., Demers, H., Peckys, D. B. and Drouin, D. 2010. "Nanometer-resolution electron microscopy through micrometers-thick water layers". *Ultramicroscopy* 110:1114–1119.

Domingos, R. F., Baalousha, M. A., Ju-Nam, Y., Reid, M. M., Tufenkji, N., Lead, J. R., Leppard, G. G. and Wilkinson, K. J. 2009. "Characterizing manufactured nanoparticles in the environment: Multimethod determination of particle sizes". *Environmental Science and Technology* 43:7277–7284.

EC (European Commission). 2011. "Commission recommendation of October 18, 2011 on the definition of nanomaterial (2011/696/EU)". *Official Journal of the European Union* 54:38–40.

EFSA Scientific Committee, Hardy, A., Benford, D., Halldorsson, T., Jeger, M. J., Knutsen, H. K., More, S. et al. 2018. "Guidance on risk assessment of the application of nanoscience and nanotechnologies in the food and feed chain: Part 1, human and animal health". *EFSA Journal* 16:5327.

EFSA. 2018. "Technical report of the public consultation on the draft guidance on risk assessment of the application of nanoscience and nanotechnologies in the food and feed chain: Part 1, human and animal health". *EFSA Supporting Publications* 15:1430E.

Fears, K. P., Clark, T. D. and Petrovykh, D. Y. 2013. "Residue-dependent adsorption of model oligopeptides on gold". *Journal of the American Chemical Society* 135:15040–15052.

Franken, L. E., Boekema, E. J. and Stuart, M. C. A. 2017. "Transmission electron microscopy as a tool for the characterization of soft materials: Application and interpretation". *Advanced Science* 4:1600476.

Gioria, S., Caputo, F., Urbán, P., Maguire, C. M., Bremer-Hoffmann, S., Prina-Mello, A., Calzolai, L. and Mehn, D. 2018. "Are existing standard methods suitable for the evaluation of nanomedicines: Some case studies". *Nanomedicine* 13:539–554.

Gollwitzer, C., Bartczak, D., Goenaga-Infante, H., Kestens, V., Krumrey, M., Minelli, C., Pálmai, M. et al. 2016. "A comparison of techniques for size measurement of nanoparticles in cell culture medium". *Analytical Methods* 8:5272–5282.

Grainger, D. W. 2013. "Connecting drug delivery reality to smart materials design". *International Journal of Pharmaceutics* 454:521–524.

Hackley, V. A. and Stefaniak, A. B. 2013. "'Real-world' precision, bias, and between-laboratory variation for surface area measurement of a titanium dioxide nanomaterial in powder form". *Journal of Nanoparticle Research* 15:1742.

Harris, R. 2017. "Reproducibility issues". *Chemical & Engineering News* 95(47):2.

Hassellöv, M., Readman, J. W., Ranville, J. F. and Tiede, K. 2008. "Nanoparticle analysis and characterization methodologies in environmental risk assessment of engineered nanoparticles". *Ecotoxicology* 17:344–361.

Helvig, S., Azmi, I. D. M., Moghimi, S. M. and Yaghmur, A. 2015. "Recent advances in cryo-TEM imaging of soft lipid nanoparticles". *AIMS Biophysics* 2:116–130.

Hodoroaba, V. D., Motzkus, C., Macé, T. and Vaslin-Reimann, S. 2014. "Performance of high-resolution SEM/EDX systems equipped with transmission mode (TSEM) for imaging and measurement of size and size distribution of spherical nanoparticles". *Microscopy and Microanalysis* 20:602–612.

ISO (International Organization for Standardization). 2015. ISO/TS 80004-2:2015 Nanotechnologies—Vocabulary—Part 2: Nano-objects, Geneva: International Organization for Standardization.

Kato, H., Nakamura, A. and Noda, N. 2014. "Determination of size distribution of silica nanoparticles: A comparison of scanning electron microscopy, dynamic light scattering, and flow field-flow fractionation with multiangle light scattering methods". *Materials Express* 4:144–152.

Khlebtsov, B. N., Khanadeev, V. A. and Khlebtsov, N. G. 2008. "Determination of the size, concentration, and refractive index of silica nanoparticles from turbidity spectra". *Langmuir* 24:8964–8970.

Klang, V., Matsko, N. B., Valenta, C. and Hofer, F. 2012. "Electron microscopy of nanoemulsions: An essential tool for characterisation and stability assessment". *Micron* 43:85–103.

Klang, V., Valenta, C. and Matsko, N. B. 2013. "Electron microscopy of pharmaceutical systems". *Micron* 44:45–74.

Klein, T., Buhr, E., Johnsen, K.-P. and Frase, C. G. 2011. "Traceable measurement of nanoparticles size using a scanning electron microscope in transmission mode (TSEM)". *Measurement Science and Technology* 22:094002.

Kozak, D., Anderson, W., Vogel, R. and Trau, M. 2011. "Advances in resistive pulse sensors: Devices bridging the void between molecular and microscopic detection". *Nano Today* 6:531–545.

Kuchenbecker, P., Gemeinert, M. and Rabe, T. 2012. "Interlaboratory study of particle size distribution measurements by laser diffraction". *Particle and Particle Systems Characterization* 29:304–310.

Kuntsche, J., Horst, J. C. and Bunjes, H. 2011. "Cryogenic transmission electron microscopy (cryo-TEM) for studying the morphology of colloidal drug delivery systems". *International Journal of Pharmaceutics* 417:120–137.

Laan, A. C and Denkova, A. G. 2017. "Cryogenic transmission electron microscopy: The technique of choice for the characterization of polymeric nanocarriers". *EJNMMI Research* 7:44.

Lamberty, A., Franks, K., Braun, A., Kestens, V., Roebben, G. and Linsinger, T. P. J. 2011. "Interlaboratory comparison for the measurement of particle size and zeta potential of silica nanoparticles in an aqueous suspension". *Journal of Nanoparticle Research* 13:7317–7329.

Lecloux, A. J., Atluri, R., Kolen'ko, Y. V. and Deepak, F. L. 2017. "Discussion about the use of the volume specific surface area (VSSA) as a criterion to identify nanomaterials according to the EU definition. Part two: Experimental approach". *Nanoscale* 9:14952–14966.

Linsinger, T. P. J., Chaudhry, Q., Dehalu, V., Delahaut, P., Dudkiewicz, A., Grombe, R., von der Kammer, F. et al. 2013. "Validation of methods for the detection and quantification of engineered nanoparticles in food". *Food Chemistry* 138:1959–1966.

Liu, X., Atwater, M., Wang, J. and Huo, Q. 2007. "Extinction coefficient of gold nanoparticles with different sizes and different capping ligands". *Colloids and Surfaces B: Biointerfaces* 58:3–7.

Lock, E. H., Petrovykh, D. Y., Mack, P., Carney, T., White, R. G., Walton, S. G. and Fernsler, R. F. 2010. "Surface composition, chemistry, and structure of polystyrene modified by electron-beam-generated plasma". *Langmuir* 26:8857–8868.

Lynch, I., Cedervall, T., Lundqvist, M., Cabaleiro-Lago, C., Linse, S. and Dawson, K. A. 2007. "The nanoparticle–protein complex as a biological entity; a complex fluids and surface science challenge for the 21st century". *Advances in Colloid and Interface Science* 134–135:167–174.

McClements, J. and McClements, D. J. 2016. "Standardization of nanoparticle characterization: Methods for testing properties, stability, and functionality of edible nanoparticles". *Critical Reviews in Food Science and Nutrition* 56:1334–1362.

Mehn, D., Caputo, F., Rösslein, M., Calzolai, L., Saint-Antonin, F., Courant, T., Wick, P. and Gilliland, D. 2017a. "Larger or more? Nanoparticle characterisation methods for recognition of dimers". *RSC Advances* 7:27747–27754.

Mehn, D., Iavicoli, P., Cabaleiro, N., Borgos, S. E., Caputo, F., Geiss, O., Calzolai, L., Rossi, F. and Gilliland, D. 2017b. "Analytical ultracentrifugation for analysis of doxorubicin loaded liposomes". *International Journal of Pharmaceutics* 523:320–326.

Meli, F., Klein, T., Buhr, E., Frase, C. G., Gleber, G., Krumrey, M., Duta, A., Duta, S., Korpelainen, V. and Bellotti, R. 2012. "Traceable size determination of nanoparticles, a comparison among European metrology institutes". *Measurement Science and Technology* 23:125005.

Méndez-Vilas, A., Jódar-Reyes, A. B. and González-Martín, M. L. 2009. "Ultrasmall liquid droplets on solid surfaces: Production, imaging, and relevance for current wetting research". *Small* 5:1366–1390.

Minelli, C. and Shard, A. G. 2016. "Chemical measurements of polyethylene glycol shells on gold nanoparticles in the presence of aggregation". *Biointerphases* 11:04B306.

Minelli, C., Garcia-Diez, R., Sikora, A. E., Gollwitzer, C., Krumrey, M. and Shard, A. G. 2014. "Characterization of IgG-protein-coated polymeric nanoparticles using complementary particle sizing techniques". *Surface and Interface Analysis* 46:663–667.

Misirli, Z., Öner, E. T. and Kirdar, B. 2007. "Real imaging and size values of *Saccharomyces cerevisiae* cells with comparable contrast tuning to two environmental scanning electron microscopy modes". *Scanning* 29:11–19.

Montaño, M. D, Olesik, J. W., Barber, A. G., Challis, K. and Ranville, J. F. 2016. "Single particle ICP-MS: Advances toward routine analysis of nanomaterials". *Analytical and Bioanalytical Chemistry* 408:5053–5074.

Monteiro, J. M., Fernandes, P. B., Vaz, F., Pereira, A. R., Tavares, A. C., Ferreira, M. T., Pereira, P. M. et al. 2015. "Cell shape dynamics during the staphylococcal cell cycle". *Nature Communications* 6:8055.

Navarro, J. R. G. and Werts, M. H. V. 2013. "Resonant light scattering spectroscopy of gold, silver and gold–silver alloy nanoparticles and optical detection in microfluidic channels". *Analyst* 138:583–592.

Nel, A. E., Parak, W. J., Chan, W. C. W., Xia, T., Hersam, M. C., Brinker, C. J., Zink, J. I., Pinkerton, K. E., Baer, D. R. and Weiss, P. S. 2015. "Where are we heading in nanotechnology environmental health and safety and materials characterization?" *ACS Nano* 9:5627–5630.

Nurmi, J. T., Tratnyek, P. G., Sarathy, V., Baer, D. R., Amonette, J. E., Pecher, K., Wang, C. et al. 2005. "Characterization and properties of metallic iron nanoparticles: Spectroscopy, electrochemistry, and kinetics". *Environmental Science and Technology* 39:1221–1230.

Patterson, J. P., Proetto, M. T. and Gianneschi. N. C. 2015. "Soft nanomaterials analysed by *in situ* liquid TEM: Towards high resolution characterisation of nanoparticles in motion". *Perspectives in Science* 6:106–112.

Peters, R. J. B., Herrera Rivera, Z., Bouwmeester, H., Weigel, S. and Marvin, H. J. P. 2014. "Advanced analytical techniques for the measurement of nanomaterials in complex samples: A comparison". *Quality Assurance and Safety of Crops and Foods* 6:281–290.

Petersen, E. J., Henry, T. B., Zhao, J., MacCuspie, R. I., Kirschling, T. L., Dobrovolskaia, M. A., Hackley, V., Xing, B. and White, J. C. 2014. "Identification and avoidance of potential artifacts and misinterpretations in nanomaterial ecotoxicity measurements". *Environmental Science and Technology* 48:4226–4246.

Petrovykh, D. Y., Kimura-Suda, H., Tarlov, M. J. and Whitman, L. J. 2004. "Quantitative characterization of DNA films by x-ray photoelectron spectroscopy". *Langmuir* 20:429–440.

Pita, R., Ehmann, F. and Papaluca, M. 2016. "Nanomedicines in the EU—regulatory overview". *AAPS Journal* 18:1576–1582.

Powell, C. J., Werner, W. S. M., Kalbe, H., Shard, A. G. and Castner, D. G. 2018. "Comparisons of analytical approaches for determining shell thicknesses of core–shell nanoparticles by X-ray photoelectron spectroscopy". *Journal of Physical Chemistry C* 122:4073–4082.

Powell, C. J., Werner, W. S. M., Shard, A. G. and Castner, D. G. 2016. "Evaluation of two methods for determining shell thicknesses of core–shell nanoparticles by X-ray photoelectron spectroscopy". *Journal of Physical Chemistry C* 120:22730–22738.

Qureshi, R. N. and Kok, W. T. 2011. "Application of flow field-flow fractionation for the characterization of macromolecules of biological interest: A review". *Analytical and Bioanalytical Chemistry* 399:1401–1411.

Rades, S., Hodoroaba, V. D., Salge, T., Wirth, T., Lobera, M. P., Labrador, R. H., Natte, K., Behnke, T., Gross, T. and Unger W. E. S. 2014. "High-resolution imaging with SEM/T-SEM, EDX and SAM as a combined methodical approach for morphological and elemental analyses of single engineered nanoparticles". *RSC Advances* 4:49577–49587.

Rafati, A., Shard, A. G. and Castner, D. G. 2016. "Multitechnique characterization of oligo(ethylene glycol) functionalized gold nanoparticles". *Biointerphases* 11:04B304.

Rasmussen, K., Rauscher, H., Mech, A., Sintes, J. R., Gilliland, D., González, M., Kearns, P. et al. 2018. "Physico-chemical properties of manufactured nanomaterials—Characterisation and relevant methods. An outlook based on the OECD testing programme". *Regulatory Toxicology and Pharmacology* 92:8–28.

Rauscher, H., Roebben, G., Boix Sanfeliu, A., Emons, H., Gibson, N., Koeber, R., Linsinger, T. et al. 2015. "*Towards a Review of the EC Recommendation for a Definition of the Term 'Nanomaterial'—Part 3: Scientific-Technical Evaluation of Options to Clarify the Definition and to Facilitate Its Implementation*". Edited by Rauscher, H. and Roebben, G. Luxembourg: Publications Office of the European Union.

Ray, S. and Shard, A. G. 2011. "Quantitative analysis of adsorbed proteins by x-ray photoelectron spectroscopy". *Analytical Chemistry* 83:8659–8666.

Ray, S., Steven, R. T., Green, F. M., Höök, F., Taskinen, B., Hytönen, V. P. and Shard, A. G. 2015. "Neutralized chimeric Avidin binding at a reference biosensor surface". *Langmuir* 31:1921–1930.

Ren, Y., Donald, A. M. and Zhang, Z. 2008. "Investigation of the morphology, viability and mechanical properties of yeast cells in environmental SEM". *Scanning* 30:435–442.

Rice, S. B., Chan, C., Brown, S. C., Eschbach, P., Han, L., Ensor, D. S., Stefaniak, A. B., Bonevich, J., Vladár, A. E. and Walker, A. R. H. 2013. "Particle size distributions by transmission electron microscopy: An interlaboratory comparison case study". *Metrologia* 50:663–678.

Ring, E. A. and de Jonge, N. 2012. "Video-frequency scanning transmission electron microscopy of moving gold nanoparticles in liquid". *Micron* 43:1078–1084.

Saveyn, H., de Baets, B., Thas, O., Hole, P., Smith, J. and Van der Meeren, P. 2010. "Accurate particle size distribution determination by nanoparticle tracking analysis based on 2-D Brownian dynamics simulation". *Journal of Colloid and Interface Science* 352:593–600.

Shang, J. and Gao, X. 2014. "Nanoparticle counting: Towards accurate determination of the molar concentration". *Chemical Society Reviews* 43:7267–7278.

Shard, A. G. 2012. "A straightforward method for interpreting XPS data from core–shell nanoparticles". *Journal of Physical Chemistry C* 116:16806–16813.

Shard, A. G. 2014. "Detection limits in XPS for more than 6000 binary systems using Al and Mg Kα X-rays". *Surface and Interface Analysis* 46:175–185.

Shard, A. G. and Clifford, C. A. 2018. "Summary of ISO/TC 201 standard: ISO 19668–Surface chemical analysis–X-ray photoelectron spectroscopy–Estimating and reporting detection limits for elements in homogeneous materials". *Surface and Interface Analysis* 50:87–89.

Shard, A. G., Sparnacci, K., Sikora, A., Wright, L., Bartczak, D., Goenaga-Infante, H. and Minelli, C. 2018. "Measuring the relative concentration of particle populations using differential centrifugal sedimentation". *Analytical Methods* 10:2647–2657.

Sikora, A., Bartczak, D., Geißler, D., Kestens, V., Roebben, G., Ramaye, Y., Varga, Z. et al. 2015. "A systematic comparison of different techniques to determine the zeta potential of silica nanoparticles in biological medium". *Analytical Methods* 7:9835–9843.

Sitar, S., Vezočnik, V., Maček, P., Kogej, K., Pahovnik, D. and Žagar, E. 2017. "Pitfalls in size characterization of soft particles by dynamic light scattering online coupled to asymmetrical flow field-flow fractionation". *Analytical Chemistry* 89:11744–11752.

Sousa, C., Sequeira, D., Kolen'ko, Y. V., Pinto, I. M. and Petrovykh, D. Y. 2015. "Analytical protocols for separation and electron microscopy of nanoparticles interacting with bacterial cells". *Analytical Chemistry* 87:4641–4648.

Stokes, D. J. 2001. "Characterisation of soft condensed matter and delicate materials using environmental scanning electron microscopy (ESEM)". *Advanced Engineering Materials* 3:126–130.

Sun, J. and Goldys, E. M. 2008. "Linear absorption and molar extinction coefficients in direct semiconductor quantum dots". *Journal of Physical Chemistry C* 112:9261–9266.

Taylor, A., Barlow, N., Day, M. P., Hill, S., Martin, N. and Patriarca, M. 2018. "Atomic spectrometry update: Review of advances in the analysis of clinical and biological materials, foods and beverages". *Journal of Analytical Atomic Spectrometry* 33:338–382.

Techane, S., Baer, D. and Castner, D. G. 2011. "Simulation and modeling of self-assembled monolayers of carboxylic acid thiols on flat and nanoparticle gold surfaces". *Analytical Chemistry* 83:6704–6712.

Ullmann, C., Babick, F., Koeber, R. and Stintz, M., 2017. "Performance of analytical centrifugation for the particle size analysis of real-world materials". *Powder Technology* 319:261–270.

Vilas-Boas, V., Espiña, B., Kolen'ko, Y. V., Bañobre-Lopez, M., Duarte, J. A., Martins, V. C., Petrovykh, D. Y., Freitas, P. P. and Carvalho, F. D. 2018. "Combining CXCR4-targeted and nontargeted nanoparticles for effective unassisted *in vitro* magnetic hyperthermia". *Biointerphases* 13:011005.

Vysotskii, V. V., Uryupina, O. Ya., Gusel'nikova, A. V. and Roldugin, V. I. 2009. "On the feasibility of determining nanoparticle concentration by the dynamic light scattering method". *Colloid Journal* 71:739–744.

Wagner, M., Holzschuh, S., Traeger, A., Fahr, A. and Schubert, U. S. 2014. "Asymmetric flow field-flow fractionation in the field of nanomedicine". *Analytical Chemistry* 86:5201–5210.

Westmeier, D., Hahlbrock, A., Reinhardt, C., Fröhlich-Nowoisky, J., Wessler, S., Vallet, C., Pöschl, U., Knauer, S. K. and Stauber, R. H. 2018. "Nanomaterial–microbe cross-talk: Physicochemical principles and (patho)biological consequences". *Chemical Society Reviews* 47:5312–5337.

Wohlleben, W. 2012. "Validity range of centrifuges for the regulation of nanomaterials: From classification to as-tested coronas". *Journal of Nanoparticle Research* 14:1300.

Wohlleben, W., Mielke, J., Bianchin, A., Ghanem, A., Freiberger, H., Rauscher, H., Gemeinert, M. and Hodoroaba, V. D. 2017. "Reliable nanomaterial classification of powders using the volume-specific surface area method". *Journal of Nanoparticle Research* 19:61.

Wu, L., Zhang, J. and Watanabe, W. 2011. "Physical and chemical stability of drug nanoparticles". *Advanced Drug Delivery Reviews* 63:456–469.

Yao, Z. and Carballido-López, R. 2014. "Fluorescence imaging for bacterial cell biology: From localization to dynamics, from ensembles to single molecules". *Annual Review of Microbiology* 68:459–476.

Yu, W. W., Qu, L., Guo, W. and Peng, X. 2003. "Experimental determination of the extinction coefficient of CdTe, CdSe, and CdS nanocrystals". *Chemistry of Materials* 15:2854–2860.

Zattoni, A., Roda, B., Borghi, F., Marassi, V. and Reschiglian, P. 2014. "Flow field-flow fractionation for the analysis of nanoparticles used in drug delivery". *Journal of Pharmaceutical and Biomedical Analysis* 87:53–61.

Zhang, H., Burnum, K. E., Luna, M. L., Petritis, B. O., Kim, J.-S., Qian, W.-J., Moore R. J., Heredia-Langner, A. et al. 2011. "Quantitative proteomics analysis of adsorbed plasma proteins classifies nanoparticles with different surface properties and size". *Proteomics* 11:4569–4577.

Zhou, X., Halladin, D. K., Rojas, E. R., Koslover, E. F., Lee, T. K., Huang, K. C. and Theriot, J. A. 2015. "Mechanical crack propagation drives millisecond daughter cell separation in *Staphylococcus aureus*". *Science* 348(6234):574–578.

# *Section III*

## *Evaluation of Bio-nanosystems Behavior Containing Bioactive Compounds*

# 8 Delivery Systems
## *Improving Food Quality, Safety and Potential Health Benefits*

*Edgar Acosta and Mehdi Nouraei*

## CONTENTS



## 8.1 NANOSCALE DELIVERY SYSTEMS IN FOOD PRODUCTS

The introduction of nanotechnology-based delivery systems in food started to be the topic of academic and industrial research in the early 2000s (Acosta 2009; Chau et al. 2007; Garti 2005; Sanguansri et al. 2006). Various sources still put the "nanofood" potential market in the order 5–20 USD billions. However, there are no specifics as to the origin of those numbers, thus it is difficult to assess how well they represent that potential market. Perhaps the most objective "pulse" of the nanotechnology industry, including the food-related aspects of it, are third-party databases such as the Nanotechnology Consumer Products Inventory (CPI) (The Project on Emerging Nanotechnologies 2018; Vance et al. 2015), a United States-based database, and Nanodatabase, a European-based database (The Nanodatabase 2018). Table 8.1 includes a list of products (and companies) producing nanotechnology-based delivery

**TABLE 8.1**
**Products and Companies Listed in Nanotechnology Databases under the Food Category, Involving the Delivery of Nutraceuticals (Minerals Not Listed)**

| Product | Origin | Product Description | Claim Type |
|---|---|---|---|
| Aquanova® Novasol® | Germany | 30 nm micelle for delivery of lipophilic actives | 4s |
| Bionic Joint Support™ by Life Enhancements | USA | Liposomal phospholipid delivery material, "nanospheres" for the delivery of medium MW hyaluronic acid | 2 |
| Canola Active Oil by Shemen Industries | Israel | Nano-sized self-assembled structured liquids, reverse micelles containing water-soluble vitamins, minerals, and phytochemicals | 4 |
| Hydracel™ by Rbc Life Sciences® | USA | 5 nm "NanoCluster" colloids that reduce the surface tension of water to improve wettability after intake | 3 |
| Lypo-Spheric Vitamin C by Livon Labs | USA | Liposomal delivery of vitamin C | 4 |
| Nano Humic and Fulmic Acids by Nano Health Solutions | USA | Not described in website, but other sources claim to be dendritic-type structures | 4 |
| Nano-Sized Self-Assembled Liquid Structures by Nutralease | Israel | Nano-sized self-assembled Liquid Structures (NSSL), expanded micelles in the size of ~30 nm | 4 |
| Nanocoq10® | USA | Complex of CoQ10 with B-cyclodextrin | 4 |
| Nanocurcuminoids™ by Life Enhancement | USA | 1–1000 nm solid lipid nanoparticles of curcumin | 2 |
| Nanoresveratrol™ by Life Enhancement | USA | 1–50 nm "nanospheres" of oil and phospholipids | 2 |
| Nanoslim by Nanoslim | Canada | Jet-milled extract from various plants for weight loss purposes | 4 |
| Nutri-Nano™ Coq-10 3.1x Softgels by Solgar | USA | 1–30 nm preformed micelles containing CoQ10 to improve bioavailability | 4 |
| Spray For Life® Vitamin Supplements by Health Plus International®, Inc. | USA | 90 nm particles produced via microfluidization, patent no. 6861066 | 4 |
| Nanonutravitamin C, B12, Curcumin, and others by Nanonutrausa | USA | 200 nm liposomes | Nano-database |

*(Continued)*

**TABLE 8.1 (*Continued*)**
**Products and Companies Listed in Nanotechnology Databases under the Food Category, Involving the Delivery of Nutraceuticals (Minerals Not Listed)**

| Product | Origin | Product Description | Claim Type |
|---|---|---|---|
| Sunshine Mist Vitamin D Spray by Mercola Advanced Nutrition | USA | Unspecified nanodroplets | 5 |
| Summit Vitamins Vita-Sedds Multi-Packs by Summit Medical Group | USA | Self-emulsifying delivery systems for vitamin D3 and coQ10 | 4 |
| Vitamin D3 Vesisorb by Pure Encapsulation | USA | Self-assembled nanocolloids for the delivery of vitamin D | 4 |
| 24 hr Microactive® Coq10 Genceutic Naturals | USA | Beta cyclodextrin encapsulated coQ10 | 5 |
| Anabolic Vitakic | USA | Nanoparticulated vitamins | 5 |

systems for nutraceuticals, not including minerals. Nanotechnologies that involve nanoparticles of minerals are now ubiquitous and not relevant to the discussion on delivery systems (Vance et al. 2015).

After two decades of research into nanotechnology for food delivery systems, it is interesting to observe in Table 8.1 that the number of products is not as widespread as one could have expected it to be. In fact, all the products in Table 8.1 are classified as under the category of supplements in the CPI and the Nanodatabase. Searching the Nanodatabase for the category of food (not supplement), the nanotechnology-based products one finds are Kraft Jet Puffed Marshmallow because of its use of nano-titania as color additive, and in the same category one would find various M&M chocolates, mint gum products, and various Hershey's chocolate products also for the use of nano-titania.

The penetration of nanotechnology-based delivery systems in mainstream food has not happened yet. The reasons for the lack of disclosed nanotechnology-based delivery systems in everyday food products include: (a) consumer concerns about the long-term safety and potential environmental impact of nanotechnology-based products; (b) the manufacturers apprehension about potential unknown side-effects of nanotechnology-based products; (c) the fact that regulations on nanotechnologies incorporated in food products are still evolving; and (d) costs of incorporating nanotechnology-based delivery systems into food products.

Potential reasons "a" and "b" indicated above reflect the same problem, seen from the consumer and producer perspective. The fundamental problem is the lack of long-term safety data for products that introduce nanotechnology-based delivery systems. As a scientific community, we have concentrated on developing delivery systems either via novel chemistries or formulations or via novel processing methods. However, the concerns for safety, efficacy, and potential environmental impact, as reflected in the data of the CPI or the Nanodatabase, have remained largely unanswered.

The last column in Table 8.1 presents the claim type or category classification for each product on the CPI database. Claim type 1, not included in Table 8.1, is reserved for products with extensively verified claims. As of April of 2018, there are only 12 products in the entire CPI database (of approximately 3000 products) that meet this category, and none of the 12 are used in food products. According to Table 8.1, the products Bionic Joint Support™, Nanocurcuminoids™, and NanoResveratrol™ by Life Enhancement are classified as type 2 because the claims have been verified by data provided by the company and data provided by independent third-party entities. HydraCel™ by RBC Life Sciences has a type 3 classification because the company provided data sustaining their claims. The rest of the products in Table 8.1 are either type 4 (unsupported claim) or type 5 where the presence of nanotechnology-based delivery system is not claimed, but suspected from the description of the product. The Nanodatabase website does not have the category or claim type classification, but a pictographic description concentrated on safety, and for most of the products listed in Table 8.1 there are symbols depicting the unknown status for their safety and environmental impact. For most of the products in Table 8.1, the likelihood that they are effective and safe is very high, mainly because most of them use lipid-based systems with ingredients that are food grade. However, we all need to realize that this is not enough according to recent regulatory changes. As a field, we need data on people using these products, frequently, over an extended period to get consumers and manufacturers to understand the risks and benefits of nanotechnologies (even beyond delivery systems) in food. In some ways, the field of nanotechnology-based delivery systems is going through the valley of death in the technology transfer cycle. Institutional research funding covers the development of the technology and perhaps limited validation of prototypes. However, the large-scale testing of the technology requires substantial resources, which typically involves large companies that can afford this type of pre-market evaluation with selected groups of consumers.

The potential reason "c" for the delay on breakthrough "nanofoods," involves the uncertainty in the regulatory landscape, which has also been influenced by the lack of safety and efficacy on test subjects using the products long enough to get a better understanding of the risks. The recent reviews by Jain et al. (2018) and Kaphle et al. (2018) on the safety and regulatory aspects of nanotechnology in foods reveal that, to date, there is still a large degree of uncertainty on how to regulate nanotechnology in food. Both reviews cite the European regulation as the most developed thus far. The European Council regulation EC 1333/2008, in its article 12 states that "When a food additive is already included in a Community list and there is a significant change in its production methods or in the starting materials used, or there is a change in particle size, for example through nanotechnology, the food additive prepared by those new methods or materials shall be considered as a different additive and a new entry in the Community lists or a change in the specifications shall be required before it can be placed on the market". Although there are other regulations regarding smart materials and packaging, the regulation EC1333/2008 is the most relevant for delivery systems in food products. Based on a conservative interpretation of article 12, even when all the components of a delivery system are food-grade additives, the delivery system could still require a monograph if there is a *significant* change to the process.

In addition to safety and regulatory aspects, the cost/benefit for delivery systems in food should be considered, especially if the delivery system has nanoscale features. Nanoscale systems tend to have large surface area to volume ratio, which is excellent to improve mass transport, but it also represents energy costs to produce that area by comminution and costs of additives used to protect or stabilize that surface area. Because of these issues, one should question the value-added of nanoscale delivery systems for the specific application of interest. The next section summarizes the advantages and costs associated with various nanoscale delivery methods, along with a brief description of those methods. By a way of a case study, we will concentrate on the design of self-microemulsifying delivery systems (SMEDS). We believe that through this exercise would help serve as guideline for future studies. Overall, in our experience, the application of delivery systems in food is substantially more challenging than drug delivery because of the constrains on the type of ingredients that can be used, the safety and regulatory aspects, and the small profit margins in food products.

## 8.2 THE CASE FOR (OR AGAINST) NANOSCALE DELIVERY SYSTEM

Previously, Acosta (2009) indicated that "thermodynamic and mass transfer equations reveal that, in order to generate a broad-spectrum delivery system, nanoparticles with 100 nm diameter (or less) should be produced. However, experimental data reveal that, in some cases, even nanoparticles in the 100–1000 nm range are capable of producing substantial improvement in the bioavailability." More recently, McClements (2015) in an invited review of nanoscale food delivery systems concluded that "these delivery systems can be carefully controlled to tailor their functional properties for specific applications, such as improved dispersibility, enhanced chemical stability, increased bioavailability, or controlled release. Future research should focus on the development of nanoscale delivery systems that are commercially viable." The first quote summarized the state of the field a decade ago, with great expectations and a few lab-scale examples. The second quote establishes the current state, with many lab-scale examples but with very few commercial products, and the pressing need for understanding the value-added proposition for nanoscale delivery systems in a commercial product.

To get a better understanding of the potential benefits (case for) and costs (case against) nanoscale delivery systems, Figure 8.1 includes a summary of relative magnitudes of these benefits and costs (in relation to a 1 μm in diameter delivery system) as a function of the characteristic size of the delivery system. The following sections explain these costs and benefits in more detail.

### 8.2.1 Power (cost) Needs to Produce a Nanoscale Delivery System

To produce nanoscale delivery system there are two main types of processes: self-assembly or bottom-up approach, and the other is the comminution or top-down approach (Acosta 2009; McClements 2015). The power cost in Figure 8.1 refers to the top-down approach.

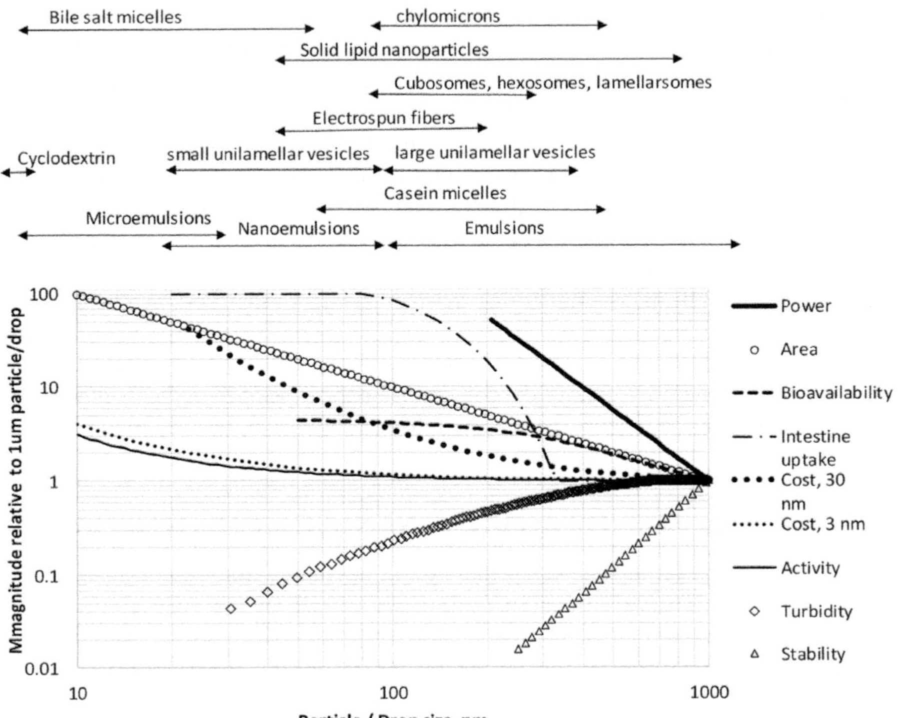


**FIGURE 8.1** Relative benefits and costs of nanoscale delivery systems compared to a 1 μm delivery system. Power refers to the power dissipation (W/kg) for high pressure homogenization. Area is the area to volume ratio. Bioavailability was obtained from a regression of the data in Figure 8.5 of Acosta (2009). Intestine uptake was calculated considering the diffusion into the intestine mucous layer. The cost of 30 and 3 nm coatings are compared based on coating/core volume ratios. Activity calculated using the Kelvin equation. The relative turbidity was calculated from Figure 8.3 of Hernandez and Baker (1991). The relative stability is based on the characteristic Brownian collision time.

#### 8.2.1.1 Comminution Approach (Top-Down)

The "power" trend in Figure 8.1 was obtained considering the correlation between the maximum drop diameter ($d_{max}$) of an emulsion and the power dissipation in valves, colloidal mills, or high pressure homogenizers. Hinze (1955) derived this relationship by considering the Weber number ($We = \rho V^2 d/\gamma$, $\rho$ being the density of the continuous phase, $V$ a characteristic velocity, $d$ the diameter of the drop, and $\gamma$ the interfacial tension between oil and water). The Weber number is the ratio between inertial forces that drive emulsification and interfacial tension forces that oppose it. The characteristic velocity $V$ is difficult to establish, and the power dissipation ($\varepsilon$, W/kg) is used instead, as a more appropriate indicator of the dissipation of the kinetic energy per unit of mass (m) of emulsion, during a time scale $\tau$, such that $\varepsilon \sim (mV^2/m)/\tau$. The time scale $\tau$ can be interpreted in terms of a length scale of dissipation (L), where $\tau \sim L/V$, leading to $\varepsilon \sim V^2/(L/V) = V^3/L$. Reconsidering the $V^2$ term in the Weber number, $V^2 \sim (\varepsilon L)^{2/3}$. The dissipation length scale, L, has a size similar to the smallest surviving eddies where the kinetic energy is dissipated in the form of viscous losses. The largest surviving drop, $d_{max}$, should have a size similar to that of the smaller surviving eddy, under this condition, $V^2 = c_1(\varepsilon d_{max})^{2/3}$. It has been proposed that $c_1$ has an approximate value of 2 (Hinze 1955). Under these conditions, $We_{critical} = 2\rho(\varepsilon d_{max})^{2/3} d_{max}/\gamma = 2(\rho\varepsilon^{2/3} d_{max}{}^{5/3})/\gamma$. Then,

$$\varepsilon\ (W/kg) = ((We_{critical})/2)^{(3/2)}\ (\gamma/\rho)^{(3/2)}\ d\_{max}{}^{(-5/2)} \tag{8.1}$$

According to Equation 8.1 (and as depicted in Figure 8.1), the smaller the desired drop size, the larger the energy dissipation required, and the slope of the power curve in Figure 8.1 is −2.5. For solids, there are various theories of comminution, but as the particle size approaches 1 μm or less, the general equation of Hukki is applicable, where the exponent (in the coordinates of Figure 8.1) would be $-3+d_H$, where "$d_H$" is Hukki's surface dimensionality factor, and it has to do as to how the energy is dissipated into the particle. A $d_H$ of 2 would mean that the energy is dissipated along the planes of cleavage (also known as Rittinger's law), but as the particle size approaches 1 μm, $d_H$ approaches 1.25 (slope of −1.75 in the coordinates of Figure 8.1) (Martins 2016). What this suggests is that either comminution of solids or emulsification of liquids by a top-down approach, reducing the size of the particles from 1 μm to 100 nm, it takes about 100 times more energy than it takes to form the 1 μm particle or emulsion drop in the first place. To get an idea of the absolute energy costs, Latta et al. (2018) calculated the power dissipation from the conditions reported by Raikar (2010) for 5% sunflower oil emulsion in water containing 0.1% pluronic surfactant F-68 (interfacial tension 18.7 mJ/m$^2$), finding that in order to produce an emulsion with Dv95 of 1.25 μm, a $10^7$ Watts/kg of emulsion was necessary. Luckily, the residence time in the homogenizer is a fraction of a second. Assuming a residence time in the homogenizer of 1 second (considering multiple passes), then the energy required is about 30 kWh/kg. Assuming a cost of USD 0.1/kWh, this means at least USD 3/kg of emulsion. This may not seem expensive for the 1.25 μm emulsion, but it would represent close to USD 300/kg to produce a 100 nm emulsion, based on the trends of Figure 8.1.

The estimates above were made based on a high-pressure homogenizer, where a coarse-sized emulsion (made by simple stirring) is fed to a microfluidizer chamber where the fluid typically bifurcate and then meets head-on at the end of the chamber, producing a high pressure drop at that point. High pressure homogenizers are currently the standard production method of emulsions and sub-micron emulsions in the pharmaceutical and food industries. However, there is increasing interest in the use of ultrasonic means to produce nanoemulsions. Ultrasonicators have been used at the lab scale, particularly because they can focus large amount of energy to be dissipated in a small space, thus avoiding the need for the infrastructure of pumps or compressors needed with high pressure homogenizers. However, the minimum power dissipation requirement for ultrasonicators is still of the same order of magnitude to that used in high pressure homogenizers (Abbas et al. 2013). Furthermore, the use of ultrasound at large (industrial) scale remains a challenge because of the difficulty in focusing the power and controlling the residence time in an industrial-scale flow chamber (Abbas et al. 2013).

#### 8.2.1.2 Solvency (Bottom-up + Top-down) Approach

There are other methods to produce nanoemulsions and nanoparticles that do not require large power demands. One of the main alternatives is the use of solvents that undergo some form of phase transition. For example, lipids or oils with melting point above room temperature can be dissolved in a supercritical solvent at high pressure (Türk et al. 2002). Carbon dioxide is often the solvent, and this supercritical solution is then forced through an expansion nozzle where the supercritical fluid flashes. This process leaves behind a mist of lipid particles in a glassy state. The size of the lipid particles can be controlled by the depressurization conditions and the concentration of the lipid in the supercritical fluid. This method has been used to produce 2–8 nm β-sitosterol primary particles that eventually form aggregates of 100–500 nm without the addition of an anionic surfactant to stabilize the particle and 10–100 nm when an anionic surfactant was included (Türk et al. 2002). This technique is known as rapid expansion in supercritical solution (RESS).

One can also use solvency swings, which basically means dissolving the solute of interest in solvent A, where the solute is fully soluble, and then dilute this solution with a solvent B, in which the solute is insoluble. This dilution then induces a precipitation of solid lipid particles (Horn and Rieger 2001; Sabliov and Astete 2008) with sizes that can be controlled by the concentration of lipid, mixing condition, and the addition of polymers and/or surfactants to prevent the aggregation of the precipitate. Using this solvency swing method, 20–80 nm β-carotene particles were synthesized using acetone as the hydrophilic solvent, poly-(lactic-co-glycolic) acid (PLGA) as the polymer, and Tween® 20 as emulsifier (Horn and Rieger 2001).

The methods of emulsification and solid lipid nanoparticle synthesis via solvent or solvent mixtures have also been applied to other systems such as dispersed liquid crystals (cubosomes, lamellarsomes, hexosomes in Figure 8.1). Compared to SLNs, however, liquid crystal dispersions have amphiphilic environments that can serve as dissolving media for a variety of actives (Larsson 1989; Yaghmur and Glatter 2009). Liquid crystals can coexist with an excess aqueous phase, which means they can be broken down in small domains (much like an emulsion) and dispersed in the excess aqueous phase. One can use high-pressure homogenizers at room temperature to break the suspension of the liquid crystal in water or increase the temperature to melt the liquid crystal phase, emulsify, and then cooled the dispersion to room temperature where the small drops of lipids turn back into liquid crystals. One can also use a co-solvent like ethanol to facilitate the dispersion with milder agitation. The co-solvent is then evaporated leaving the dispersed liquid crystal in the system. These methods are similar to those used to produce liposomes, and often the production of liquid crystal dispersions lead to some liposome production (Barauskas and Nylander 2008). As in the case of lipid nanoparticle synthesis, polymeric surfactants, such as pluronic F-127, are used to stabilize the dispersed liquid crystal.

#### 8.2.1.3 Self-Emulsification (Bottom-up + Top-down) Approach

The self-emulsification approach aims to reduce the work required for emulsification by introducing surfactants that can produce ultralow interfacial tensions ($\gamma$ in Equation 8.1) with the oil phase. To achieve this, the surfactant-oil-water (SOW) system is formulated around the phase inversion point of the emulsion, where the interfacial tension reaches low to ultralow values (0.001 mN/m or dyn/cm, up to 5 orders of magnitude lower than the oil-water interfacial tension in the absence of surfactants). When the formulation is taken to the phase inversion point, a simple overhead mixer can be enough to produce sub-micron drops in the emulsion. The only problem is that emulsions are also very unstable at the point of phase inversion. Once the emulsion is formed, the emulsion is quenched via the addition of more of the continuous phase of the emulsion (typically water) at conditions farther away from those of the inversion point in order to take the formulation to conditions far from those of the inversion point. For conditions far from the inversion point the emulsion becomes more stable, stabilizing the small drops produced at the inversion point. McClements (2011) presents a more detailed description and schematics of the production of food-grade nanoemulsions using this phase inversion method.

##### *8.2.1.3.1 Self-Emulsification and the Hydrophilic-Lipophilic-Difference*

The self-emulsification method is not prevalent in the food industry because of the difficulty in designing formulations that produce ultralow tensions. There are various methods to induce phase inversion (and the accompanying ultralow tensions), which have been summarized in the literature (Salager et al. 2005). Furthermore, there are empirical equations of states that can predict the location of the inversion point and the properties of those formulations (Acosta et al. 2003). The equations that predict the phase inversion point are known as the hydrophilic-lipophilic difference (HLD) equations (Acosta et al. 2008; Salager et al. 2000; Salager et al. 2005). Equation 8.2 presents the HLD for nonionic surfactant systems, and Equation 8.3 for ionic surfactants:

$$\mathrm{HLD} = \mathrm{Cc} - \mathrm{k}\cdot\mathrm{EACN} + \mathrm{b}\cdot\mathrm{S} + \alpha_{\mathrm{T}}\cdot(\mathrm{T} - 25^{\circ}\mathrm{C}) \tag{8.2}$$

$$\mathrm{HLD} = \mathrm{Cc} - \mathrm{k}\cdot\mathrm{EACN} + \ln(\mathrm{S}) - \alpha_{\mathrm{T}}\cdot(\mathrm{T} - 25^{\circ}\mathrm{C}). \tag{8.3}$$

Cc is the characteristic curvature of the surfactant (positive values correspond to hydrophobic surfactants, and negative ones to hydrophilic surfactants). EACN is the equivalent alkane carbon number of the oil. For normal alkanes, EACN is simply the number of carbons in the chain. For other oils, the EACN is estimated based on EACN calibration curves of phase inversion conditions versus the EACN of known oils (Zarate et al. 2016). The values of k, b, and $\alpha_T$ are constants that depend on the surfactant used. However, for most surfactants k = 0.16, b = 0.13, when S (the electrolyte concentration) is expressed in g NaCl/100 mL of solution. Finally, T is the temperature of the system in Celsius.

Figure 8.2 presents a general schematic on the production of nanoemulsions via the phase inversion method considering the use of HLD as the guiding principle.

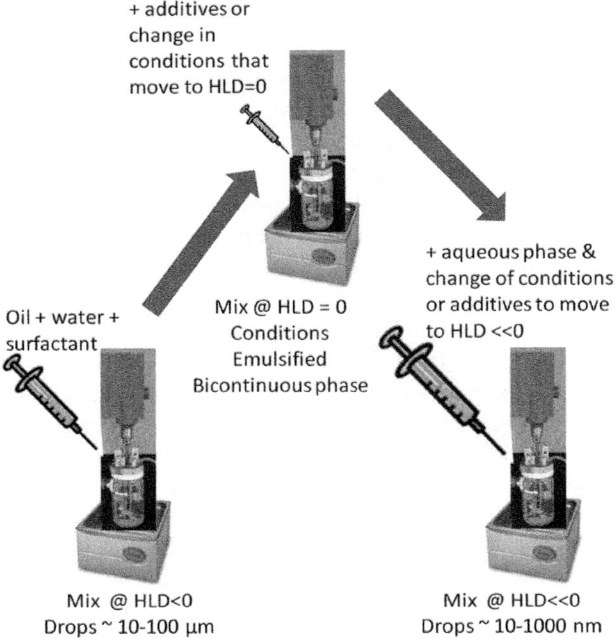


**FIGURE 8.2** Schematic of the phase inversion method to produce nanoemulsions.

The conditions to achieve HLD~0 in the middle step of the process can include an increase in temperature (T in Equations 8.2 and 8.3), also known as the phase inversion temperature method, or a change in surfactant composition (change in Cc in Equations 8.2 and 8.3) or electrolyte concentration (S in Equations 8.2 and 8.3), also known as the phase inversion composition method.

While the HLD values are used to understand the type of emulsions formed, and trends in emulsion stability (Salager et al. 1982), the origin of the HLD equations come from correlations of the conditions for the phase inversion of microemulsions. Microemulsions (μEs) are SOW systems that, different from emulsions, exist in thermodynamic equilibrium. The most common method to investigate the phase inversion of μEs is the phase scan, where equal volumes of oil and aqueous phase are added to a series of test tubes containing a low surfactant concentration (typically less than 5% v/v based on the total volume of the system). From one test tube to the next, a formulation variable is changed, for example, the salinity of the aqueous phase (in that case, the experiment is called a salinity scan). The test tubes where the surfactant resides in the aqueous phase (hydrophilic formulations), forming oil-swollen micelles are called Winsor Type I μEs, having a negative HLD. Systems where bicontinuous middle phase μEs form (phase inversion zone) are called Type III μEs, and it is in that region were ultralow interfacial tension is obtained, and HLD is close to zero. Systems where the surfactant resides in the oil phase (lipophilic formulations), forming water-swollen reverse micelles, are referred to as Type II μEs, having positive HLD values.

One challenge with the use of HLD to produce nanoemulsions via the phase inversion method is that databases of EACN and Cc values for surfactants are still limited (more so for Cc). Some values can be found in Abbott's practical surfactants website (Abbott 2018). For long chain (C14+) triglycerides, the EACN of the oil typically ranges from 16 to 20, depending on the fatty acid composition (Phan et al. 2010). For ethyl esters of fatty acid, the EACN ranges from 5 to about 10, and for medium chain triglycerides the EACN ranges from 10 to 14 (Ontiveros et al. 2013). Nouraei and Acosta (2017) used the HLD equation for nonionic surfactants (Equation 8.2) to design pharmaceutical and food grade self-emulsifying delivery systems using ethyl caprate as oil phase, having an EACN of 5. Using Equation 8.2, one can select an appropriate level of electrolyte (Nouraei and Acosta selected a fed-state simulated intestinal fluid formulation, with total sodium equivalent to 1.8 g NaCl/100 mL of solution, thus, $S = 1.8$). Nouraei and Acosta aimed at negative HLDs, but if one aimed at $HLD = 0$, at $T = 25°C$, then Equation 8.2 would have predicted the required $Cc = 0.16 \times 5 - 0.13 \times 1.8 = +0.6$. Nouraei and Acosta (2017) used mixtures of lecithin ($Cc = +4$), glycerol monooleate ($Cc = +7$), and polyglycerol caprylate ($Cc = -3$) to obtain the necessary Cc.

Nouraei and Acosta (2017) used lecithin as the main surfactant that brings together the hydrophilic linker, polyglycerol caprylate, and the lipophilic linker, glycerol monooleate. Linkers are surfactant-like molecules that segregate primarily to one of the sides of the oil/water interface and cannot form bicontinuous μEs on their own (at HLD~0), without the main surfactant (Sabatini et al. 2003). The linker combination not only improves the solubilization capacity, and reduces the interfacial tension of SOW systems, but linkers also help mitigating the formation of liquid crystals. Lecithin cannot form μEs on its own because it tends to form liquid crystals. However, introducing food-grade linkers makes it possible for lecithin to form μEs with a wide range of oils (Acosta et al. 2005).

One note on working with triglycerides is that these oils are extremely difficult to form μEs with and obtain ultralow interfacial tensions. The large molar volume of triglycerides and their tendency to form organized structures, in some cases compared to reverse micelles (Warren et al. 2009) and in others compared to layered (lamellar-like) structures (Sum et al. 2003), tend to reduce their solubilization capacity in μEs. Nevertheless, they can still reach interfacial tensions of the order of 0.1–1 mN/m at the phase inversion point of the surfactant in the system, which corresponds to $HLD = 0$ (Engelskirchen et al. 2007). One way in which one can work with triglycerides and still reach ultralow interfacial tension (~0.001 mN/m) is the use of extended surfactants. Extended surfactants have, between their hydrocarbon tail and their head group, a polypropylene glycol (PPG) group that is said to breakdown the local structure of triglycerides and facilitate their solubilization in μEs (Salager et al. 2005). Unfortunately, there are no food-grade extended surfactants in the market.

#### *8.2.1.3.2 Self-Emulsification and the Net-Average Curvature*

There is more to HLD than locating the conditions for emulsion or μE phase inversion. The HLD has been related to the difference in chemical potential of transferring the surfactant from the oil phase into the aqueous phase (Salager et al. 2000). More recently, the HLD has been related to the net curvature (Hn) of the interface, normalized by a length parameter "L" proportional to the extended tail length of the surfactant (Acosta et al. 2003):

$$Hn = -HLD/L = (1/Ro - 1/Rw) \tag{8.4}$$

Ro and Rw are the solubilization radii of oil and water, respectively, in the μE system. These solubilization radii are used in the net-average curvature (NAC) framework to track the solubilization of oil and water in all types of μE. The NAC assumes that any μE system can be statistically described as an average of two coexisting states, one where oil is solubilized as spheres of radius Ro in a continuous aqueous media, and a second one where water is solubilized as spheres of radius Rw in a continuous oil phase. The radius of solubilization of the dispersed phase ($R_{disp}$) is calculated as:

$$R_{disp} = 3 \cdot V_{disp}/A_S \tag{8.5}$$

$V_{disp}$ is the volume of the dispersed phase (oil or water) solubilized in the continuous phase, and $A_S$ is the interfacial area calculated on the basis of the number of molecules of surfactant "i" adsorbed ($n_{S,i}$) at the oil-water interface, and the area per molecule of that surfactant species "i" ($a_{S,i}$):

$$A_S = \Sigma n_{S,i} \cdot a_{S,i} \tag{8.6}$$

While Equation 8.4 uses Ro and Rw to describe the curvature of the interface, these solubilization radii can also be used to calculate the average curvature ($H_a$) curvature, which is interpreted as the area to volume ratio of the μE (Kiran and Acosta 2010):

$$H_a = (1/2) \cdot (1/Ro + 1/Rw) \tag{8.7}$$

The inverse of this average curvature cannot exceed the characteristic length (ξ) of the μE, which is interpreted as the maximum solubilization capacity of a given μE:

$$1/Ha < \xi = 6 \cdot \phi_O \cdot \phi_W \cdot V_m/A_S \tag{8.8}$$

To calculate ξ, the values of $\phi_O$ and $\phi_W$, the volume fractions of oil and water in the middle phase (Type III) μE are determined along with the volume of that middle phase microemulsion ($V_m$). The total area $A_S$ can be calculated using Equation 8.6.

An extremely important equation, that is also part of the HLD-NAC framework, is the equation used to predict the interfacial tension (γ) of SOW systems (the term SOW system is used instead of μE because it also applies to emulsions). This equation introduces the interfacial rigidity (Er) as the energy used by the surfactant assembly to maintain the μE in thermodynamic equilibrium (Acosta et al. 2003):

$$4\pi \cdot R_{disp}^{2} \cdot \gamma = Er \tag{8.9}$$

The value of interfacial rigidity (Er) for ionic surfactant systems typically ranges between 1 and 3 $K_BT$ ($K_B$ is the Boltzmann constant and T the absolute temperature) and for nonionic surfactants Er ~ 3 to 9 $K_BT$. The interfacial tension ($\gamma$) of the system obtained from Equation 8.9 has been used to predict the drop size of emulsions with equations similar to 8.1 that account for the power dissipation ($\varepsilon$) (Kiran and Acosta 2015).

Kiran and Acosta (2015) analyzed not only the formation of emulsion around the phase inversion point, but also the stability of those emulsions. The authors extended the hole nucleation theory of emulsion stability to estimate the activation energy ($E_{ac}$) for the formation of a liquid bridge of length $t_h$ across two approaching drops:

$$Eac = 4Er + 0.73(t_h^2)\cdot\gamma \tag{8.10}$$

Equation 8.10 predicts that at HLD~0 where the interfacial tension ($\gamma$) is ultralow, then the activation energy for coalescence reaches its minimum value, explaining why at the emulsion, stability reaches a minimum at the phase inversion point. According to Equation 8.4, extremely negative HLDs (assuming Rw>>Ro) would produce small Ro values. According to Equation 8.9, for a given Er, these low Ro values would turn into relatively high $\gamma$ (when compared to the ultralow $\gamma$ values at HLD~0). According to Equation 8.10, these high $\gamma$ would lead to high activation energies and therefore increased emulsion stability at extreme HLD values. This explains the purpose of the last dilution/HLD shift in Figure 8.2 as an emulsion quenching step.

Figure 8.3 further illustrates the dependence of emulsion properties on HLD and the use of the HLD-NAC equations to predict interfacial tension, and the emulsion drop size for the case of the anionic surfactant emulsion of Kiran and Acosta (2015).

In summary, self-emulsification methods, and specifically nanoemulsion preparation via phase inversion, are scalable methods with relatively low power cost. The HLD and HLD-NAC parameters, relevant to food delivery systems, have been

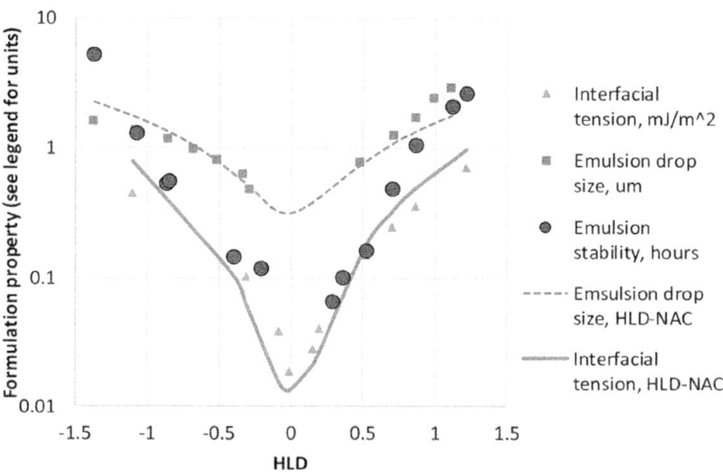


**FIGURE 8.3** Dependence of emulsion properties (interfacial tension, emulsion drop size, and emulsion stability) on HLD. Experimental data obtained from Kiran and Acosta (2015).

developed over the last decade, opening the door to use these principles to design of numerous nanoemulsion-based delivery systems.

#### 8.2.1.4 Solubilization Approach

The solubilization approach, different from emulsification, implies that the delivered active exists in thermodynamic equilibrium in the delivery system. It is important to clarify that because solubilization is a thermodynamically driven process, and low-power mixing is only used to speed up the solubilization process.

##### *8.2.1.4.1 Bile Salt Micelles*

Solubilization of lipids in the hydrophobic core of micelles is the premiere example of the solubilization approach. Bile salt micelles are nature's solubilization-based nanoscale delivery system, having an approximate hydrodynamic radius of 2 nm, but when swollen with solubilized lipids they can grow to 30–100 nm, depending on the cholesterol content (Staggers et al. 1990). The formation of bile salt micelles is a process that starts before the small intestine and ends with lipid delivery to the enterocytes. The enterocytes take the lipids in these micelles and repackage them into chylomicrons (another solubilization assembly) as described below.

During digestion, fats and oils hydrolyze in the stomach via gastric lipases. The free fatty acids, and the mono- and di-glycerides formed are surfactant-like species, much like the lipophilic linkers described earlier. As this colloidal suspension of particles and emulsified oil makes its way toward the small intestine, it mixes with the pancreatic juice (containing bicarbonate for pH neutralization, and enzymes for lipid and protein hydrolysis) and the discharge of bile salts and cholesterol from the bile duct. The lipases in the pancreatic juice react with triglycerides to produce additional free fatty acids and mono- and di-glycerides that mix with the bile to produce mixed bile salt-intestinal lipid micelles that solubilize the remaining oil or oil-soluble substances in the hydrophobic core of these bile salt micelles. These micelles and its solubilized oil interact with the enterocytes, leading to the uptake of these oils primarily via passive absorption. Oil solubilization in micelles improves the absorption of lipids because micelles enhance transport through the mucous layer lining of the intestines (Shen et al. 2001) and promote cholesterol-mediated active transport (Watt and Symmond 1976). However, cholesterol active transport has been linked to colon cancer (De Jong et al. 2003; Rao and Janezic 1992).

Once bile salt micelles are taken by the enterocytes, the absorbed lipids in the form of free fatty acids and mono- and di-glycerides are reassembled into triglycerides and incorporated into chylomicrons. Chylomicrons are large assemblies (70–600 nm) composed of apolipoproteins, phospholipids, cholesterol, and a core of triglycerides (Shen et al. 2001). The chylomicrons are released to the lymphatic system via the lacteals that discharge into the thoracic tube. The thoracic tube discharges into the left subclavian vein where the chylomicrons are distributed by the bloodstream. After the chylomicrons deliver the lipids to the various tissues, they become chylomicron remnants (De Jong et al. 2003) that disassemble in the liver and its components recycled via the bile juice.

Bile salts micelles have inspired the development of various solubilization-based methods, including cholate nanoparticles (solid-lipid-nanoparticles made with cholic acids and derivatives), mixed bile salt micelles (micellar delivery systems with composition similar to bile salts), bilosomes (liposomes of bile salts), and surface-modified (mostly pegylated) bilosomes (Elnaggar 2015). The efficacy of bilosomes in delivering hydrophilic and lipophilic actives is not yet clear and can be considered an emerging area. One practical problem, at least for food delivery systems, is the safety and cost of using cholic acids and cholesterols to produce bile salt-based delivery systems. However, the idea of producing oil-swollen micellar systems (i.e., Type I μEs) for the solubilization-based delivery of lipophilic actives is still relevant. This approach is best known as the self-microemulsifying delivery system delivery method.

#### 8.2.1.4.2 Self-Microemulsifying Delivery Systems

Self-microemulsifying drug delivery system (SMEDDS) was introduced by Pouton and Porter (Pouton 2000; Pouton and Porter 2008). They undertook the formulation of lipid mixtures that would produce μEs (SMEDS) upon dilution with an aqueous solution that simulates digestive fluids. In other words, SMEDS are formed if the formulation (oil + surfactant mixture) follows a dilution path that leads to μEs without phase separation.

The group of Garti at the Casali Institute introduced various advances in the field of μE-based delivery systems for food applications (Garti and Yuli-Amar 2008; Garti et al. 2001, 2004, and 2005). Garti's group introduced the concept of U-type dilutable μEs, which could be classified as SMEDS formulations, only that they did not use simulated intestinal fluid as diluting media.

There are blockbuster applications of SMEDS in the pharmaceutical industry, particularly Neoral® a SMEDS formulation for the delivery of cyclosporin A. Closer to food applications, Cui et al. (2009) formulated curcumin-loaded SMEDDS containing 57.5% of a 1:1 surfactant mixture of alkylphenol polyether 10 and Cremorphor EL (polyethoxylated castor oil), 30.0% polyethylene glycol (PEG 400), and 12.5% oil (ethyl oleate). The authors found that the formulation increased curcumin absorption by 4-fold when compared to curcumin suspension, however, the surfactants used were not food-grade surfactants. Liu et al. (2015) used Tween 80 (polyethylene glycol ester of sorbitan monooleate) as surfactant, polyethylene glycol 400 as co-solvent, and ethyl oleate as oil to deliver vitamins A and D, finding an increase of 1.5-fold in the absorption capacity of the vitamins as compared to the delivery in emulsions. In this case, Tween 80 is an acceptable surfactant in food applications, but with certain limitations. Many more examples can be found in the literature, but the ones presented above are representative of the current formulation approach, including the use of pegylated surfactants, polyethylene glycol (PEG) as co-solvent, and a fatty acid ester as oil. Sometimes the PEG co-solvent is changed to alcohols like ethanol. One problem with this co-solvent approach is that the progressive addition of aqueous phase would dilute the water-soluble PEG and ethanol, removing them from the lipid mixture, and causing the eventual precipitation of drugs, as it has been seen in various formulations (Dokania and Joshi 2015). Similarly, the use of ethoxylated (pegylated) surfactants represents a problem because the digestive system has not evolved to hydrolyze the ester bond of PEG groups. While this feature contributes to the stealth nature of PEG-functionalized nanoscale systems, it also prevents the nanoscale delivery system from being disassembled in the enterocytes and reassembled in the chylomicrons, thus missing out on the opportunity of lymphatic transport (Dokania and Joshi 2015; Tso et al. 1981; Watt and Simmonds 1976). PEG-based surfactants tend to inhibit lipase activity, interfering with lipid uptake (Christiansen et al. 2010). Because of these PEG-mediated interferences with the normal lipid transport cycle, it is undesirable to use PEG-based surfactants on a continuous basis, as it would be expected for the consumption of food products. This is where the difference between pharmaceutical-grade and food-grade formulas is important. A PEG-based formulation is acceptable in pharmaceutical applications because the risks associated with its use are typically outweighed by the potential benefits of the life-saving drug delivered. For food formulations, even the potential for lower lipid uptake due to the presence of PEG functionalities is a cause of concern if the formulation goes into staple foods such as vegetable oils, butter/margarine, and others that are continuously consumed and that are meant to deliver triglycerides for nutritional purposes.

Nouraei and Acosta (2017) set out to produce a SMEDS formulation that would not use co-solvents, nor PEG-based surfactants or co-surfactants, and that would simulate the bile salt micelles, without cholesterol or cholic acids (to prevent the risk of colon cancer). To this end, the authors used the HLD-NAC framework to guide the selection of additives that could work with lecithin as main surfactant. The other two additives were a lipophilic linker, glycerol monooleate (also found in bile salt micelles), and a hydrophilic linker, polyglycerol caprylate (food grade surfactant, amenable to hydrolysis by digestive enzymes). The use of the HLD for this system was discussed earlier. NAC was used to predict the 2-phase boundary of the formulation. The ternary phase diagram for one of the formulations of Acosta and Nouraei is presented in Figure 8.4, along with the vials obtained during the dilution with Fed State Simulated Intestinal Fluid (FeSSIF). The solid double line in the diagram is the 2-phase boundary predicted by NAC. According to the NAC, one would need at least 37% surfactant in mixture with the oil to obtain a path for the SMEDS. However, in this case a dilution path with 50% surfactant mixture (D50) was used. DLS-measured sizes along the dilution line revealed that although in most cases the structures tend to have a size close to 10 nm, the system passes through two transition regions, one near 12.5% FeSSIF where the system transitions from oil-continuous to bicontinuous, and then another transition at 75% FeSSIF where the system transitions from bicontinuous to FeSSIF-continuous. At these transition points the reverse micelles and micelles elongate, creating hydrodynamic radii close to 100 nm. *In vivo* studies carried out with these formulations are yet to be published, but the data have confirmed that this formulation can produce a substantial increase in bioavailability equal or greater than other SMEDS formulations.

#### *8.2.1.4.3 Solubilization in Protein-Based Delivery Systems*

As described earlier, lipoproteins are nature's delivery systems taking the lipids from the enterocytes to the blood stream. Caseins and whey proteins are often used as delivery systems (Livney 2010; Subirade and Chen 2008). The most abundant

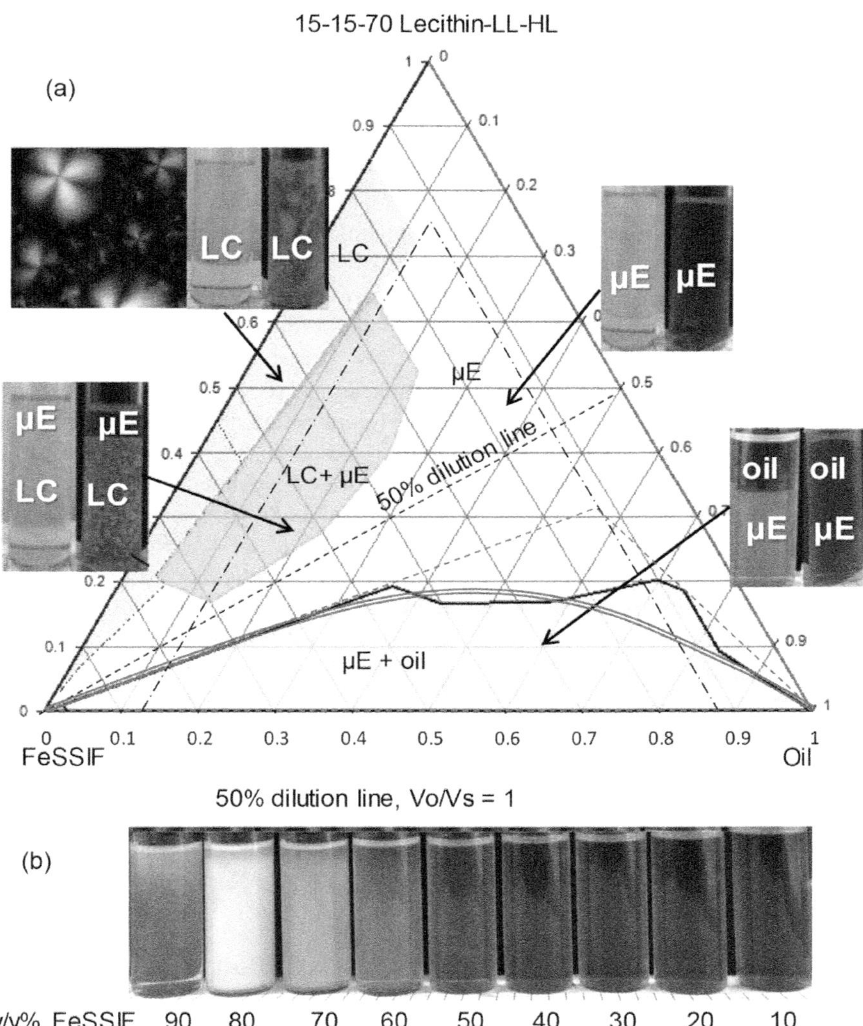


**FIGURE 8.4** (a) Ternary phase diagram for the system of Lecithin/Glycerol monooleate/Polyglycerol caprylate (15/15/70)—ethyl caprate as oil—and Fed State Simulated Intestinal Fluid (FeSSIF) as aqueous phase. (b) Vials showing the FeSSIF dilution of a SMEDS formulation containing 50% of surfactant and 50% ethyl caprate (D50 dilution). Figure Reprinted from Acosta and Nouraei (2017), with permission from Elsevier.

amino acid in casein is glutamic acid (~20% of the protein). Glutamic acid is anionic at neutral pH, producing a negatively charge crown for the micelle-like structure of casein. The negative charge of $\alpha_{s_1}$-, $\alpha_{s_2}$-, and β-casein micelles promote the binding of calcium and other multivalent cations, making casein micelles a suitable means to improve the permeability of these cations through the intestine (Livney 2010).

Whey proteins (β-lactoglobulin, α-lactalbumin, bovine serum albumin, immunoglobulins, lactoferrin) have a similar amino acid profile to casein, where a hydrophobic core can be used as delivery system for hydrophobic compounds. A limitation of milk proteins is that some digestive enzymes can degrade the assembly itself. In some cases, that limitation can be turned into an advantage for triggered release.

##### *8.2.1.4.4 Inclusion Complexation (Cyclodextrins)*

Inclusion complexation involves the thermodynamic-driven binding (thermodynamic equilibrium, no high mixing power required) between the active of interest and a molecule or a group of molecules that will serve as carriers for the transport of that active. The complexation involves the insertion of lipophilic molecules in the hydrophobic interior of cyclodextrin rings. Cyclodextrins (CDs) consist of six (alpha), seven (beta), or eight (gamma) glucopyranosyl monomers linked in a cyclic configuration by α-(1,4) bonds. This binding allows the glucopyranosyl units to orient its OH groups toward the external side of the ring, leaving the internal side of the ring with the more hydrophobic -CH- groups. The alpha, beta, and gamma CDs have inner diameters of 5, 6.2, and 8 Å. The height of the ring is 7.9 Å. The main use of CDs is similar to that of micelles, increase the solubilization of an otherwise water-insoluble component, which is inserted in the hydrophobic core of the CD. In food applications, CDs have been used to solubilize fragrances and flavors, particularly cinnamon oil, close oil, lemon oil, and other essential oils (Cheirsilp and Rakmai 2016). In addition to produce an increase in solubilization, the CD structure can also be used to improve the stability of the oils against oxidative agents. One disadvantage of CDs is the relatively small size of the hydrophobic cavity, meaning that they have a limited loading capacity, and they can only be used with molecules of certain size.

Other future inclusion complexation agents are dendrimers based on the polymerization of glycerol and succinic acid monomers (both food-grade monomers) (Frey and Haag 2002). However, these dendrimers have not received food grade status and are relatively early in the regulatory pipeline.

### 8.2.2 Area, Bioavailability, and Intestine Uptake (Benefit)

The term "Area" in Figure 8.1 was calculated based on the surface area to volume ratio, calculated 6/diameter and normalized by the area to volume ratio for a particle of 1 μm. Certainly, one of the main reasons for nanoscale delivery systems is to increase the exposed surface area per unit volume, which should result in an improved transport of the active. A central question with regards to area is... is the delivery of the active limited by the surface area of transport? To answer this question, one can look at the work of Oh et al. (1993) on the dissolution of actives from particles and permeation through the intestine, work that eventually led to the Biopharmaceutical Classification System (BCS). According to that work, the transport of actives depends on three transport numbers, the absorption number, the dissolution number (Dn), and the Dose number (Do). The absorption number can be interpreted as the ratio between the rate of absorption and the rate of convection. Do is the ratio between the dose concentration (mass of solute/volume of gastric fluid) and the solubility of the active. Finally, Dn is the only term influenced by the particle size as it represents the ratio between residence time ($t_{res}$) in the small intestine (~3 hours) and the time for all the content of the particle of radius ($r_p$) to dissolve. Considering the original definition of Dn, one can find the required particle size to guarantee adsorption ($d_{p\ max}$) as:

$$d_{p\ max} = (3 \cdot \mathfrak{D} \cdot C_s \cdot t_{res}/(\rho \cdot Dn_{min}))^{0.5} \quad (8.11)$$

The term $\mathfrak{D}$ is the diffusion coefficient of the species in the intestinal fluid, $C_s$ is the solubility of the active in the intestinal fluid, and ρ is the density of the active in the particle. If the active is extremely hydrophobic, it is most likely that the only dissolution is through bile salt micelles, thus the diffusion could be calculated on the basis of the size of those micelles using Einstein's diffusivity formula, assuming the bile salt micelles as spheres of 100 nm diameter, then $\mathfrak{D}$ ~ 3.7E-12 $m^2/s$. For the solubility ($C_s$), one can consider this concentration to be a fraction of the total concentration of bile salt micelle lipids. According to Jantratid et al. (2008), the total lipid concentration of fed state intestinal fluid can be as high as 60 mM. The value of $Dn_{min}$ is the minimum dissolution number to achieve complete absorption. This number depends on the absorption number and Do, but $Dn_{min}$ typically ranges between 1 and 14 (Oh et al. 1993) and for most cases is less than 4. One can assume, conservatively, a value of 14 to estimate $d_{p\ max}$. For an active with molecular weight of 500 g/mol and density of 1000 g/L (values close to β-carotene), then ρ(molar basis) ~ 2000 mM. Marisiddaiah and Baskaran (2009) evaluated the bioavailability of β-carotene using a 22 mM concentration of lipids and a $C_s$~ 0.2 mM concentration of beta-carotene in the intestinal fluid (a ~1/100 molar fraction or 10,000 ppm in the bile salt micelle). For that concentration, $d_{p\_max}$ ~ 1.4 μm, that means that even a 1 μm particle would have been enough to guarantee full dissolution in 3 hours, in the presence of the intestinal fluid. If the solubility in bile salt micelle in the bile salt micelle would have been 1000 ppm, then $d_{p\_max}$ ~ 400 nm, if the solubility would have been 100 ppm, then $d_{p\_max}$ ~ 130 nm, and if 10 ppm, then $d_{p\_max}$ ~ 40 nm. Considering that beta-carotene is one of the most hydrophobic nutrients, it is hard to imagine substances with solubility in bile salts micelles less than 100 ppm. Meaning that for most actives, sizes of 100 nm are small enough to guarantee full solubilization. According to the bioavailability trend in Figure 8.1 (obtained from a correlation of experimental values in Acosta 2009), then the improvement in bioavailability follows the trend of improvement in area up to about 300 nm. Sizes smaller than 300 nm did not yield a substantial improvement in bioavailability. The discussion above then would suggest that for most lipophilic drugs, that are insoluble in water, their solubility in bile salt micelles might range of 100–1000 ppm.

The dissolution analysis of Oh et al. (1993) assumes that the dissolution and permeability through the membrane are the potential limiting steps of the absorption process, and that the particle of the active dissolves in the continuous phase. However, when it comes to nanoscale delivery systems, the particle itself can be absorbed via passive or active absorption mechanisms. However, for that to happen, the particle must diffuse through the mucous layer lining the small intestine. The process of nanoparticle diffusion through hydrogels can be estimated using the concept of effective diffusivity in gels. There are various equations to calculate diffusivity in hydrogels, but the following can be used without fitting coefficients (Amsden 1998):

$$\mathfrak{D}_{eff} = \mathfrak{D}_o {}^*\exp(-(\pi/4)(r_s + r_f)^2/(\xi_{gel}/2 + r_f)^2) \tag{8.12}$$

The particle diffusion coefficient $\mathfrak{D}_o$ can be calculated from Einstein's equation for the diffusion coefficient of spheres, $r_s$ is the cross-sectional radius of the solute (the particle in this case), $r_f$ is the cross-sectional radius of the fibers that make up the hydrogel, and $\xi_{gel}$ is the mesh size of the hydrogel. For the mucous lining of the intestine, this $\xi_{gel}$ ~ 100 nm (Yildiz et al. 2015). Neglecting the cross-sectional radius of the fibers ($r_s$ ~ 0 nm), then the effective diffusion coefficient, $\mathfrak{D}_{eff}$, can be calculated for a given particle size ($r_s$). The diffusion time for a particle to find the surface of the enterocyte should be less than 1 hour, considering that the turn-over rate of the mucous layers ranges from 50–270 minutes (Yildiz et al. 2015). The thickness of the mucous layer can change depending on the composition of the intestinal fluid, but its thickness is in the order of 100 μm (Yildiz et al. 2015). Considering 60 min of diffusion time, one can estimate the length diffused into the gel as $L_{diff} \sim (\mathfrak{D}_{eff} \cdot 60 \text{ min})^{0.5}$ diffusion and estimate the percentage penetration as $L_{diff}$/100 μm this fraction, in the form of percentage is represented in Figure 8.1 as intestine uptake. According to that figure, one needs to have close to 100 nm of particle diameter to guarantee complete penetration of the particle through the mucous layer. This simple prediction is consistent with the experimental observations of Datta et al. (2016) that only particles with diameters close to 100 nm and smaller were able to penetrate through a colonic mucous hydrogel.

It must be clarified, however, that size is not the only factor affecting the transport of colloids through the mucous layer. The surface composition of the particle also plays a significant role. PEG-decorated surfaces are less prone to interact with the mucous layer, ensuring faster penetration. On the other hand, particles with carboxylic acid moieties tend to interact more strongly with the glycoproteins of the mucous layer, retarding their transport, even for small bile salt micelles (Yildiz et al. 2015).

The concepts behind the Biopharmaceutical Classification System and the discussion around the mechanisms of permeation through the mucous layer and uptake mechanisms have been revisited by McClements et al. (2015) to develop a Nutraceutical Bioavailability Classification (NuBCS). The NuBCS consists of three multiplying terms, namely, the bioaccessibility (B*), the absorption (A*), and the transformation (T*) factors. The bioaccessibility factor represents the fraction of the dose that can be fully dissolved in the intestinal fluid or solubilized (for the case of hydrophobic drugs) in the bile salt micelles of the intestinal fluid within a given time. The details of the method to evaluate bioaccessibility can change, in some cases it might involve the sequential action of mouth, gastric, and intestinal fluids. In some cases only the dissolution in intestinal fluids. The dissolution time can vary, but it is often in the order of 2 hours, at least in the intestinal fluid. Different from drugs, any nutraceutical or active food ingredient is likely co-delivered with food. Thus, the dissolution protocol used to assess bioaccessibility should consider the food matrix used to deliver the active.

The absorption term (A*), includes various aspects, starting with mucin layer transport, directly related to the earlier calculations on diffusivity in gels, and the surface interactions between the delivery system and the glycoproteins making up the mucous layer. Other elements include the permeability, related passive transport discussed earlier, active transport mechanisms (both for uptake or efflux), and direct translocation of the delivery system through tight junctions or Peyer's patches.

The transformation term (T*) relates to the chemical (e.g., oxidation) or metabolic (e.g., enzymatic hydrolysis) transformation of the active food ingredient being delivered. However, the concept could also be extended to the degradation of the delivery system components that could render the vehicle inefficient. For example, changes in surfactant (e.g., phospholipids) charge with changes in pH, particularly during gastric passage.

### 8.2.3 Cost of Nanoscale Delivery System Material (Coatings of 3 nm and 30 nm)

Figure 8.1 presents the relative cost of producing a delivery system of a given size (assumed spheres) with respect to that of producing a 1 μm delivery system. The two calculations assume that the material used to produce the delivery system can be represented as a coating layer that is placed on top of the carrier solvent or matrix. There could be an oil core (if the delivery system is an emulsion), an aqueous core (e.g., liposomes), or a solid-like particle if the delivery system is a solid-lipid-nanoparticle or a nanoparticle produced by comminution or other methods. The purpose of this coating material is to produce a thermodynamically or kinetically stabilized dispersion that can protect the active food ingredient against biological, chemical, and physical degradation (including colloidal aggregation) during storage and consumption. Under this core-shell assumption, the ratio presented in Figure 8.1 is simply a volume ratio that takes the form $[((d_p + 2r_{coat})^3 - d_p^3)/d_p^3]/[((1\ \mu m + 2r_{coat})^3 - 1\ \mu m^3)/1\ \mu m^3]$. According to Figure 8.1, reducing the size from 1 μm to 100 nm, one would need to increase the amount of coating material (thus its costs) by about 3 times if one uses a 30 nm coating. However, if one uses a 3 nm coating, one could reduce the size from 1 μm to 10 nm and still one would only need to increase the mass of coating agent by about 4 times.

The trends in Figure 8.1 would suggest one should strive to use thinner coatings to produce stable nanoscale delivery systems. While this is certainly an objective in the mind of formulators, the problem is that a thinner coating does not necessarily offer the necessary protection. In practice, the thickness of the applied coating is not expressed in nanometers, instead is often reported as surface load, in $mg/m^2$. However, considering that the density of most coating materials are in the order of $\sim 1\ g/cm^3 = 1\ g/(1E\text{-}6\ m^3)$. Therefore, $1\ mg = 1\ E\text{-}3g \sim 1\ E\text{-}9m^3$, then a $1\ mg/m^2$ surface load $\sim 1\ E\text{-}9\ m^3/m^2 \sim 1\ nm$.

McClements and Gumus (2016) summarized the surface load used with natural emulsifiers. For surfactant molecules such as pegylated sorbitan laurate (Tween 20), sodium dodecyl sulfate (SDS), and for saponins, the authors cite values of surface loads in the range of 1.5–3 $mg/m^2$, closer to the 3 nm curve in Figure 8.1. For hydrophobic proteins with molecular weights in the order fo 20 kDa such as β-lactoglobulin and β-casein, a surface load close to 2–3 mg/m$^2$ is still used. For larger molecules, such as gum arabic (~1000 kDa), the surface load needs to be greater, in the order of 30 mg/m$^2$ to maintain a sufficient number of molecules attached to the surface and able to protect the delivery system. One advantage of using gum arabic is that the resulting colloidal delivery system tends to be stable in a wide range of pHs and electrolyte concentrations. From a colloidal (physical) stability point of view, the surface load, molecular weight of the coating agent, its degree of hydration, the charge of the colloidal system (affected by the pH of the system), and the electrolyte composition and concentration are all factors that need to be considered when deciding the thickness of the coating agent. These aspects will be considered in the colloidal stability section.

For solubilization-based systems such as SMEDS, micellar delivery systems, and inclusion complexation (cyclodextrins), the sizes are typically small (often less than 30 nm), the coating levels are typically of the order of 3 nm (~3 mg/m$^2$). These systems, however, exist in thermodynamic equilibrium, meaning that they are completely stable, at least from the physical point of view. Micellar and microemulsion systems, and even cyclodextrin complexes can still be susceptible to chemical degradation. Oxidation is typically a concern for the case of micellar and microemulsion systems.

Typically, the biggest problem when it comes to cost is that most nanoscale delivery system have some sort of matrix or carrier media (the core discussed earlier) where the active food ingredient is dissolved or suspended and then this matrix is then incorporated into the nanoscale delivery system. This means that for some systems the loading of the active component can be relatively low. In most articles dealing with nanoscale delivery systems, the loading is not often discussed, simply reported. Some studies include an assessment of the solubility of the active in various matrices or solvents. However, no discussion is offered as to whether this level of solubility level achieved with the best matrix or solvent is enough to make the final formulation effective. In our experience, this is one of the most critical analysis that decides whether a delivery system is useful for a specific solute.

Whenever one would like to explore a nanoscale delivery system for an active food ingredient one should start by considering the required dose, and how soluble the active could be in the matrix of the delivery system. Table 8.2 has some values for required doses and solubility in lipids (mainly medium chain triglycerides or mixtures of triglycerides and monoglycerides) for some hydrophobic actives. If one considers a lipid-based nanoscale delivery system for vitamins A or E, then there is little concern about the loading of these vitamins in the lipid. The required amount of these vitamins for single dose is substantially smaller than 1 gram, and these vitamins are completely soluble with lipid mixtures. On the other end of the spectrum, between 1 and 8 grams of curcumin are required to have a noticeable (positive) health effect. Even if one would like to deliver 1 gram of curcumin, and considering a solubility of 2% in lipid mixtures, that means that 50 gram of lipid matrix (not even counting the amount of protective coating required) would be required. A 51g dose of active + delivery media is unreasonable and expensive.

One feature of Table 8.2 is that the doses cited for nutraceuticals tend to be much larger than those of vitamins. The problem with most nutraceuticals is that there is

**TABLE 8.2**
**Recommended Dose of Water-Insoluble Active Food Ingredients and Their Solubility in Lipid Mixtures**

| Nutrient | DRI[a] (grams) | References | Solubility in Lipids (wt%) | References |
|---|---|---|---|---|
| Vitamin A | 9E-4 | National Academy of Sciences (2011) | Soluble | |
| Vitamin D3 | 1.5E-5 | National Academy of Sciences (2011) | 0.1 | Ozturk et al. 2015 |
| Vitamin E | 1.5E-2 | National Academy of Sciences (2011) | Soluble | |
| Vitamin K2 | 1.2E-4 | National Academy of Sciences (2011) | 1–2 | Shah et al. 2018 |
| Nutraceutical | Dose[b] (grams) | | | |
| β-Carotene | 5.0E-3 | Diosady et al. 2013 | 0.1–0.5 | Salvia-Trujillo et al. 2013 |
| Omega 3-6-9 | 2–26 | EFSA 2012 | Soluble | |
| Phytosterols | 2 | Racette et al. 2010 | 2–5 | Vaikousi et al. 2007 |
| Curcumin | 1–8 | Gupta et al. 2013 | 0.3–2 | Ahmed et al. 2012 |
| CoQ10 | 0.2–0.9 | Hidaka et al. 2008 | 10–20 | Thanatuksorn et al. 2009 |
| Quercetin | 0.1–1 | Li et al. 2016 | 5–20 | Shah et al. 2018 |
| trans-resveratrol | 0.05 | Shah et al. 2018 | 5–20 | Shah et al. 2018 |

[a] Dietary reference intake (g/day for a 70 kg adult male).
[b] Dose or dose range based on health improvement effect or safe intake level (g/day for a 70 kg adult male).

no clear number for the minimum dose required to observe a given positive health effect. For curcumin, for example, some researchers have seen some health effects at doses lower than 1 gram, as referenced in the review of Gupta et al. 2013, but in the same review, no health effects were observed for doses lower than 5 grams. The reported range in Table 8.2 for curcumin dose corresponds to the range where there are more references citing positive health effects and no negative health effects. One problem with the values of doses evaluated in clinical studies is that they normally correspond to suspensions of the drugs, not formulated in nanoscale delivery systems. This means that future clinical studies to set the minimum dose of nutraceuticals should consider the delivery system used.

Reconsidering the SMEDS formulation of Figure 8.4, as a case study, one could use Table 8.2 to estimate the mass of a SMEDS + active dose. If one considers β-carotene, for example, the required dose is 0.005g, and assuming a solubility of 0.1% in the lipid mixture, this means one would need (100g SMEDS/0.1g β-carotene)* 0.005g β-carotene dose. Thus, 5 grams of SMEDS would be needed. This number looks large, but where should one set the limit? If the product is meant to be filled in gelatin capsules, the largest 000 size capsule can hold 1.37 ml of liquid (~1.2 gr of the SMEMDS, considering its density). One teaspoon is about 5 ml of liquid, and 1 tablespoon is about 15 ml of liquid. Evidently, only a teaspoon of product would provide the dietary reference intake (DRI) for β-carotene (calculated on the basis of vitamin A). However, the discussion about required dose and the way it is delivered should not end here. It was determined earlier, when considering Dn, that if we can guarantee that any insoluble portion of beta-carotene has a size smaller than 1 micron, then there will be a good chance that that fraction will be solubilized by bile salt micelles before 3 hours. This means, that one could still dose a smaller volume of SMEDS, but supersaturated with β-carotene, for as long as the insoluble portion has a particle size smaller than 1 μm.

Another important element in the discussion of the dose is that, especially for the case of vitamins and minerals, one does not need to provide all the dietary needs in a single dose. Part of the idea behind not providing the entire need is that it is likely that other foods in the diet could be providing the rest of the required dose. Considering the background intake of the active food ingredient is important to avoid over-dosing, particularly when there are toxic effects associated with over-dosing.

The earlier discussion about dose assumes that the product is consumed as a supplement in the form of capsules or as a bulk liquid or powder. However, the best chances for breakthrough products are ready to use food products such as vegetable oil, margarine, yogurts, fruit or vegetable juices, sport or soft drinks, rice, salt, pastas, flour, cereals, and baked products.

As a case study for the fortification of foods, let us consider the fortification of vitamin A in vegetable oil. According to Table 8.2, because vitamin A is soluble in oils, then we could incorporate vitamin A directly into vegetable oil without the need of a delivery system. Diosady and Venkatesh-Mannar (2013) explored this possibility. To start this exercise, they evaluated the typical vegetable oil consumption in various countries (often ranging from 10 to 30 grams per day). The authors conducted a careful review of the conditions of use of the oil, identifying that oxidation of vitamin A during cooking is the main source of concern. The use of antioxidants was considered. Even after the use of antioxidants (vitamin E among others) vitamin can still be oxidized. The authors assumed that only 60% of vitamin A was retained after production, storage, and cooking. To calculate the necessary concentration of vitamin A in the vegetable oil, they then conducted a simple calculation as {9E-4 g Retinol (DRI)*33% of the DRI (fortification level)/60%(retained fraction)}/30 g oil consumed ~17 μg retinol/g vegetable oil, or 17 mg retinol/kg of vegetable oil. The authors produced an estimation of costs and confirmed that the cost of fortification with vitamin A was less than 1% of the cost of the vegetable oil. This threshold of 1% of the cost was proposed by the authors based on their experience with fortification of staple foods for developing countries. Products marketed for niche markets may afford a greater fraction for the cost of incorporation of active food ingredients.

The type of detailed cost and production analysis undertaken by Diosady and Venkatesh-Mannar (2013) is not seen in research articles or even reviews about nanoscale delivery systems in foods. This should be part of the of the discussions of future studies regarding nanoscale delivery systems in food applications.

### 8.2.4 Activity and Turbidity

The potential benefits of improved bioavailability obtained with nanoscale delivery systems must consider the potential impact (positive or negative) on the organoleptic (taste, smell, texture, optical appearance) properties of the food product (if the actives are introduced in a food product instead of a supplement formula).

With regards to turbidity (optical appearance), the introduction of nanoscale systems can represent a benefit, as illustrated in Figure 8.1 by the relative turbidity curve. This curve was obtained dividing the turbidity calculated by Hernandez and Baker (1991) for citrus oil nanoemulsions of a given diameter by the turbidity obtained with a 1 μm emulsion. The turbidity was calculated using the van de Hulst approximation for Mie scattering. Mie scattering is the main mechanism of light scattering (causing turbidity) when the size of the particle is at least 1/10 of the wavelength used to determine the turbidity. Considering that Hernandez and Baker used a laser with wavelength of 650 nm, the threshold wavelength explains why the turbidity in Figure 8.1 decreases substantially for drops smaller than 65 nm, where the Rayleigh scattering (less intense than Mie scattering) is the dominant mechanism. Considering that the visible light starts at 390 nm, then drops smaller than 40 nm would not experience significant scattering (at least not milk-like turbidity). This is consistent with the observation that colloids smaller than 50 nm are needed for clear drinks (McClements 2015).

If the active food ingredient incorporated in the delivery system is a flavoring agent, then decreasing the size of the delivery system can aid accentuating hydrophobic flavoring agents for two reasons, first an increase in the dissolution rate in the mouth (larger surface areas for mass transfer), and second, an increase in activity ($a_i$). The relative activity for a saturated species (e.g., poorly soluble oil in water) in Figure 8.1 was calculated using the Kelvin equation (Butt et al. 2003):

$$a_i = \exp\left(2\gamma_i \cdot Vm_i/(RT \cdot r_p)\right) \tag{8.13}$$

The activity ($a_i$) is 1 at saturation conditions for a large particle, but it is higher for smaller particles with radius $r_p$. The calculations in Figure 8.1 were conducted for limonene with an interfacial tension ($\gamma_i$) of 45 mJ/m$^2$, and a molar volume ($Vm_i$) of 160 cm$^2$/mol, at a temperature (T) of 298 K (25°C). According to Figure 8.1, the activity can be increased by nearly 3 folds if one reduces the drop size to 10 nm. However, one can only realize that if one does not use any surface-active material to produce this size reduction. If one uses surfactants to reduce the interfacial tension to 1 mJ/m$^2$, for example, then the activity at 10 nm is only 1.02. Furthermore, if one introduces some form of solvent to mix with the active food ingredient, the activity of the ingredient will decrease because activity is proportional to the concentration of the ingredient in the mixture with the solvent. Overall, the idea of increasing the activity of active food ingredients via nanoscale delivery system is not a promising option because most systems require the use of surface active stabilizers (surfactants or polymers).

The use of nanoscale delivery system as part of controlled release strategies is possible when the nanoscale system is encapsulated within a gel matrix (hydrogel or organogel) that can respond to changes in the chemistry of the media. Zhang et al. (2015) produced hydrogel network microparticles with mixtures of casein and alginate that can encapsulate nanoemulsions and other nanoscale delivery systems. This casein-alginate complex can then release the encapsulated material in the mouth, delivering the flavors and aroma at that point. Those flavors and aroma components would have been protected from evaporation and oxidation during storage by the hydrogel network. The key factor in this formulation approach is the use of the ionic interaction between the positive groups in the caseinate protein and the negative charges in some polysaccharides. For example, Ilyasoglu and Nehir-El (2014) used caseinate and gum arabic to nano-encapsulate polyunsaturated fatty acids (PuFAs).

### 8.2.5 Stability

Various reviews on nanoscale delivery systems may appear contradictory, some indicating that getting smaller, nano-sized, particles would make the system more physically stable, and others (like this chapter) that indicate that physical stability decreases with decreasing particle size. The reason for this inconsistency is due to the differences in the definition of physical (colloidal) stability. For those who define physical stability as a macroscopic observation of the onset (or lack of) creaming or sedimentation of the colloidal system, then yes, decreasing the size of the particles would lead to smaller settling velocity (according to Stokes' law), thus hindering creaming or sedimentation. Kiran and Acosta (2015) showed that for particles smaller than 1 micron, settling is not an important driving force for the destabilization of nanoscale systems. Instead, Brownian motion is the important factor driving the collision among nanoemulsions and other nanoparticles. These collisions may lead to some form of aggregation that might not result in settling, but it will result in the growth of the particles. If one uses a definition of stability as a nearly constant particle size distribution as a function of time, then the stability of nanoscale delivery system tends to decrease with decreasing particle size. There are two reasons for this, first, that for a given volume fraction of dispersed nanoscale system, then the smaller the size means the more nanoscale particles in a given volume of suspension/emulsion. This means that the distance between the particles is smaller as the particle size reduces. Second, as particle size reduces, the Brownian velocity of the particle increases. If the distance between particles reduces and the velocity of the particles increases, then the average time between collisions reduces. From the equations for Brownian collisions listed by Kiran and Acosta (2015), the characteristic Brownian collision time ($t_b$) for spheres in a dilute media is:

$$t_b = \pi \cdot \eta \cdot d^3/(48K_B \cdot T \cdot \varphi^2) \tag{8.14}$$

This collision time ($t_b$) is then proportional to the viscosity ($\eta$) of the fluid, the diameter (d) of the nanoscale delivery system cube, inversely proportional to the temperature (T) of the system, the square of the volume fraction ($\varphi$) of the nanoscale delivery system, and the Boltzmann constant ($K_B$). The actual characteristic time for coalescence ($t_{coal}$) could be estimated as $t_{coal} \sim t_b/p_c$, where $p_c$ is the probability of coalescence for a given collision event. Assuming that the probability of coalescence ($p_c$) is the same for a 1 μm particle and a particle of smaller diameter, then $t_{coal\ @d}/t_{coal\ @1\mu m} \sim (d/1\ \mu m)^3$ can be used as an expression of relative stability, as shown in Figure 8.1.

For the case of nanoemulsions, the stability is often thought as being controlled by Ostwald ripening (Tadros et al. 2004), driven by the increase in activity with decreasing particle size (Equation 8.13 shown earlier). Using that approach (instead of collision time/probability), one obtains a linear relationship between the particle volume (proportional to $d^3$) and time, a similar trend to that predicted by Equation 8.14.

The assumption behind the stability trend in Figure 8.1 considered that the probability of flocculation/coalescence was the same for a 1 μm particle as for a nanoparticle. This assumption, however, needs to be reconsidered. According to Kiran and Acosta (2015), for the case of coalescence, this probability is a function of how close can approaching drops get before repulsion interactions push them apart. This distance, "$t_h$" plays an extremely important factor in the activation energy of coalescence (Equation 8.10). The best way to assess this "$t_h$" distance is to conduct a Derjaguin-Landau-Verwey-Overbeek (DLVO)-type analysis that, on top of the attractive van der Waals (vdW) interactions and the electrostatic repulsion, it would also account for the steric repulsion brought about by protective coatings (Butt et al. 2003; Israelachvili 2011):

$$W = -A_H \cdot d/(24D) + 64\pi\varepsilon_o\varepsilon_r(K_BT/e)^2\tanh^2(\psi_o/4K_BT)\cdot(d/4) \cdot e^{-\kappa D} + 4K_BT \cdot Nc\cdot e^{-(D/2Rg)^{\wedge}2} \quad (8.15)$$

The term W is the interaction energy between two approaching spheres of diameter "d," separated by a distance "D," each sphere is coated by polymers with a radius of gyration "Rg." The term "$A_H$" is the Hamaker constant for the material of the sphere across the medium that separate the two spheres. The term $\varepsilon_o$ is the vacuum permittivity, and $\varepsilon_r$ is the dielectric constant of the continuous media. $\Psi_o$ is the electrical surface potential on the particles, and κ is the inverse Debye length of the aqueous phase separating the particles. Nc is the number of polymer chains that enter in direct contact the other particle. This Nc can be estimated as a fraction of the total number of chains adsorbed on the particle. For the example interaction profiles in Figure 8.5, it is estimated that 10% of the chains enter in direct contact. Other assumptions in Equation 8.15 are that the separating media is an aqueous phase containing 1:1 electrolytes (assumed to be an isotonic 0.15 M solution of sodium chloride for the systems in Figure 8.5), that the Derjaguin approximation is valid for the electrostatic repulsion (Israelachvili 2011), and that the steric repulsion (last term of Equation 8.15) is valid for separation distances beyond 4 Rg (Butt et al. 2003).

The curves in Figure 8.5 were obtained assuming a zeta potential (an approximation for the surface potential $\psi_o$ in Equation 8.15) of −50 mV, which is considered high and often capable of stabilizing particles. However, even at this zeta potential, a negative "well" in interaction energy is observed with the original DLVO (solid lines only van der Waals and electrostatic) for the 10 nm particle ($-0.13K_BT$ well, at 6.2 nm), for the 100 nm particle ($-1.3\ K_BT$ well, at 6.5 nm), and for the 1000 nm

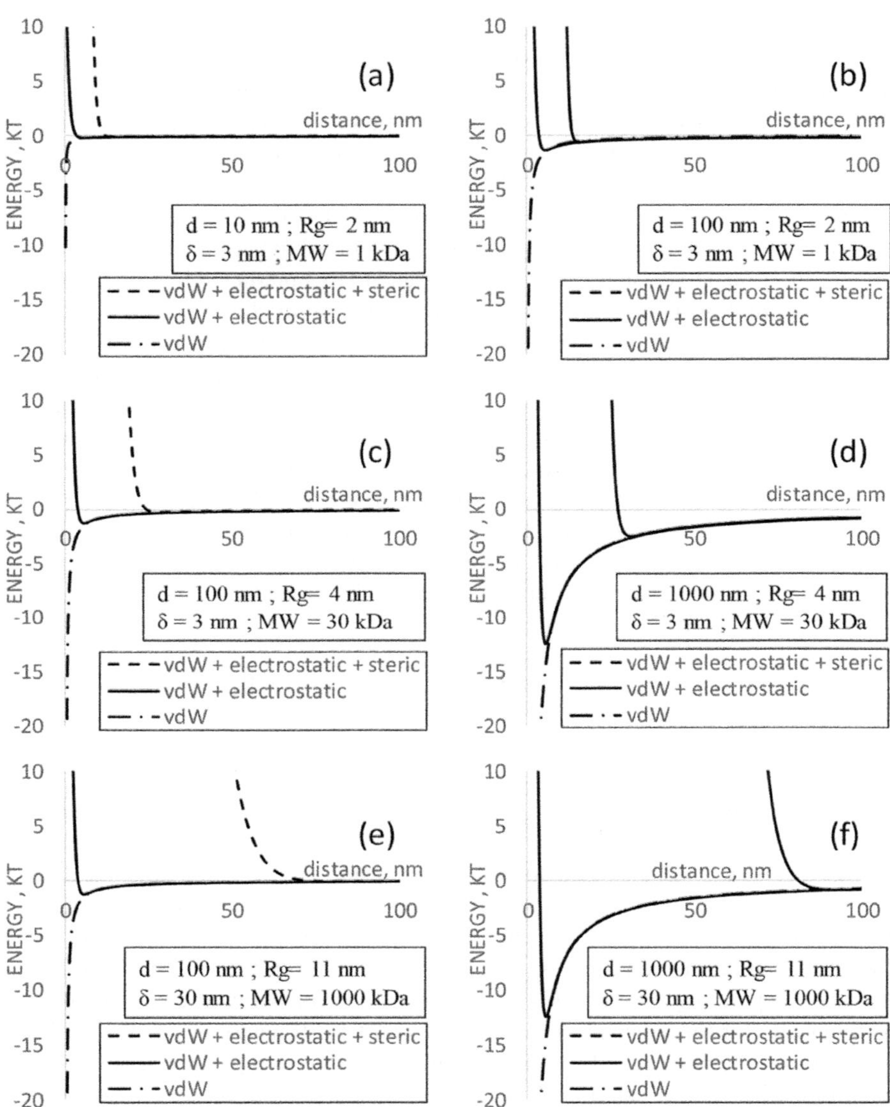


**FIGURE 8.5** Extended DLVO analysis for the interaction energy between two spheres of diameter "d" coating with a film of thickness "δ" containing a stabilizer with a given molecular weight (MW) and radius of gyration (Rg), as a function of their separation distance. Negative values of energy represent attractive interactions, leading to aggregation. The conditions for each figure a–f are indicated in the insert boxes.

particle (−13 $K_BT$ well, at 6.3 nm). These interaction energy wells are the product of the relative high electrolyte concentration (0.15 M NaCl) assumed for the calculations, however, most body fluids have total 1:1 ion concentrations close to this value. The calculations also use a Hamaker constant of $A_H = 4E-21$ J, typical for alkane-water-alkane (Israelachvili 2011). Under these typical, yet somewhat optimistic (high negative surface potential) conditions for body fluids, the presence of negative interaction energy wells for all the particle sizes considered mean that there is a risk of flocculation for all nanoscale systems, and a risk of coalescence for the case of emulsions. For the 10 nm particle well, the ambient thermal energy of 1 $K_BT$ might be enough to destabilize a pair of particles that have been locked in the −0.13 $K_BT$ interaction well. For the case of 100 nm, then the chance of the ambient thermal energy overcoming a −1.3 $K_BT$ is less optimistic. For the 1 μm particle (1000 nm), then ambient thermal energy is not enough to overcome a −13 $K_BT$ well and destabilize a flock of two particles that have come together. When it comes to coalescence, the DLVO theory (without steric hinderance), then would predict that all the drops can get as close as 6.2–6.5 nm… this would be "$t_h$" in the calculation of the activation energy for coalescence in Equation 8.10. This suggests that, at least when it comes to probability of coalescence, then the particle size of unprotected drops is not expected to make a big difference.

For coated spheres the situation is different, as shown in Figure 8.5. For the total extended DLVO, counting steric interactions (dashed lines), Figures 8.5a and b present the total interaction for spheres coated with a relatively high molecular weight surfactant (something like pegylated sorbitan laurate) with molecular weight (MW)~ 1 kDa, coated at 3 nm (~3 mg/m$^2$) and with a radius of gyration 2 nm. For the 10 nm spheres (Figure 8.5a), the introduction of this type of surfactant coating should reduce the interaction well to −0.06 $K_BT$ and 14 nm. This interaction well is extremely weak, and assuming the "$t_h$" term in Equation 8.10 dominates the activation energy, then an increase in $t_h$ from 6.3 to 14 nm would mean a 5-fold increase in activation energy, meaning a substantial reduction in the coalescence probability. For the 100 nm sphere (Figure 8.5b), the same surfactant would reduce the interaction well energy to −0.5 $K_BT$ and increase the separation distance to 17 nm. If one uses a medium molecular weight polymer (MW ~ 30 kDa), as in the case of Figures 8.5c, one could further reduce the well of the 100 nm sphere to −0.3 $K_BT$ and increase the separation distance to 28 nm. Under those conditions, those 100 nm particles or emulsions are, for practical purposes, colloidally stable (no aggregation should be expected). For the 1 μm spheres, one needs to coat them with the largest of polymers, 1000 kDa (Figure 8.5f) to reduce the interaction well to −1 $K_BT$ and increase the separation distance to 85 nm. The properties of the coating for Figure 8.5e and f are typical of coatings produced with gum arabic.

In addition to colloidal (physical) stability, the change in particle size would also affect chemical stability. The chemical stability is not illustrated in Figure 8.1, and frankly, this is a topic that is not covered by most researchers, perhaps because the mechanisms of degradation are specific to the active food ingredient of interest (Wu et al. 2011). However, we can still consider this effect in terms of the mass transfer of chemical agents such as dissolved oxygen ($O_2$), dissolved free radicals, or enzymes that could degrade the active in the nanoscale delivery system. To this end, the diffusion time scale is $t_{diff} = Lc^2/\mathfrak{D}$, where Lc is a characteristic diffusion length scale, and $\mathfrak{D}$ is the diffusivity of the degrading agent ($O_2$, free radicals, enzymes, etc.) in the matrix of the nanoscale delivery system. If one assumes the diffusion length scale Lc ~ volume/surface area, then for a sphere Lc ~ d/6. Then, the diffusion time scale should be of the order $t_{diff} \sim d^2/36\mathfrak{D}$. One could establish the ratio of stability with 1 μm particles as the radio of diffusion times, $t_{diff}/t_{diff@1\,\mu m} = (d/1\ \mu m)^2$. Therefore, particles smaller than 1 μm are less chemically stable than particles of 1 μm. Thus, chemical stability is really a reason against nanoscale delivery systems. Nevertheless, this cost can be managed by using polymeric coatings that would produce viscous or semi-solid layers around the nanoscale delivery system to reduce the diffusion coefficient of the degrading agent and increase the diffusion length scale. The matrix of the nanoscale delivery system can also be selected to minimize the solubility and diffusion coefficient of the degrading agent. On that front, solid-lipid-nanoparticles and dispersed liquid crystals tend to produce the best protection against chemical agents. Unfortunately, this often come at a cost of low loading capacity of the active. The co-addition of chemical protectants, such as vitamin E and butylated hydroxytoluene (BHT) (antioxidants) is a common practice in the manufacture of delivery systems (Diosady and Venkatesh-Mannar 2013).

## 8.3 SUMMARY AND OUTLOOK

Nanoscale delivery systems can improve the efficacy of active food ingredients by increasing the surface area for mass transfer (faster release), by increasing the bioavailability of the active, by facilitating its transport through mucous layers, by decreasing the turbidity of the dispersed system, and under special circumstances even increasing the activity of the food ingredient. However, these benefits normally come at a cost of higher power consumption to generate the nanoscale domains, higher costs of surfactants or polymers used as stabilizers, and lower chemical and physical stability as compared to larger particles.

A review of the current state-of-the-art, in terms of translating nanoscale delivery systems to food products, reveals a more important cost—uncertainty. The uncertainty around the safety of nanoscale delivery systems is likely the most important barrier to realizing the full potential of these delivery systems in food applications. As a community of scientists and engineers, we need to realize that simply producing delivery systems and testing their efficacy *in vitro* is not enough. It is good to see that more and more studies are obtaining pharmacokinetic data with food delivery systems (Oehlke et al. 2014), and it is a step forward, but there is still a big gap on safety *in vivo* studies. There is an even bigger gap in understanding the minimum dose required to achieve certain positive health benefits when the active food ingredient is formulated in a given delivery system. The current reference doses, at least for nutraceuticals, tend to be high, thus limiting the range of applicability of numerous delivery systems because restrictions in the level of active that can be loaded in those systems.

In some ways, the field of food delivery systems needs to be turned on its head. Currently, the approach is centered around the delivery system. The field needs to concentrate on active food ingredients instead, and then look for what alternative delivery systems could fit that active. It is our opinion that this may happen soon with the most unlikely of actives… cannabinoids. The legalization of these compounds in some countries has sparked the interest of large and small companies on delivery systems that could incorporate cannabinoids in beverages, chewing gums, baked products, and more. The relative low dose required to observe an effect, and the currently low oral bioavailability of these compounds, represent an ideal situation for various delivery systems to showcase their potential advantages.

This chapter presents various equations that are offered to facilitate the formulation process centered around a given active food ingredient. The concepts of HLD and NAC should help selecting the appropriate surfactant and formulation conditions to solubilize the active in micellar systems or to produce nanoemulsions with minimum energy input. Various transport equations and discussions were also introduced to get an idea of how small one needs to go when it comes to taking advantage of some of the benefits of nanoscale delivery systems.

Finally, the outlook of delivery system depends on the way the field evolves. Embracing the *in vivo* studies of safety and dose effects can represent the breakthrough that the field needs. However, if we all continue to concentrate on *in vitro* studies, the chances of realizing the full potential of delivery systems in food products is not as likely. That uncertainty cost still weighs heavily on the future of these technologies.

## REFERENCES


Abbas, S., Hayat, K., Karangwa, E., Bashari, M., Zhang, X. 2013. "An overview of ultrasound-assisted food-grade nanoemulsions". *Food Engineering Reviews*, 5: 139–157.

Abbott, S. 2018. "Practical Surfactants". Accessed September 9, 2018, https://www.stevenabbott.co.uk/practical-surfactants/.

Acosta, E., Szekeres, E., Sabatini, D.A., Harwell, J.H. 2003. "Net-average curvature model for solubilization and supersolubilization in surfactant μEs". *Langmuir*, 19: 186–195.

Acosta, E.J., Nguyen, T., Witthayapanyanon, A., Harwell, J.H., Sabatini, D.A. 2005. "Linker-based bio-compatible μEs". *Environmental Science and Technology*. 39: 1275–1282.

Acosta, E.J., Yuan, J.S., Bhakta, A.S. 2008. "The characteristic curvature of ionic surfactants". *Journal of Surfactants and Detergents*. 11: 145–158.

Acosta, E. 2009. "Bioavailability of nanoparticles in nutrient and nutraceutical delivery". *Current Opinion in Colloids and Interface Science*. 14: 3–15.

Ahmed, K., Li, Y., McClements, D.J., Xiao, H. 2012. "Nanoemulsion- and emulsion-based delivery systems for curcumin: Encapsulation and release properties". *Food Chemistry*.132: 799–807.

Amsden, B. 1998. "Solute diffusion within hydrogels. Mechanisms and models". *Macromolecules*. 31: 8382–8395.

Barauskas, J., Nylander, T. 2008. "Lyotropic liquid crystals as delivery vehicles for food ingredients". In N. Garti, ed. *Delivery and Controlled Release of Bioactives in Foods and nutraceuticals*. CRC Press, Boca Raton, FL, pp. 107–131.

Butt, H., Graf, K. and Kappl, M. 2003. "Physics and Chemistry of Interfaces". Wiley-VCH, Weinheim, p. 373.

Chau, C.F., Wu, S.H., Yen, G.C. 2007. "The development of regulations for food nanotechnology". *Trends in Food Science and Technology*. 18:269–280.

Cheirsilp, B., Rakmai, J. 2016. "Inclusion complex formation of cyclodextrin with its guest and their applications". *Biology, Engineering and Medicine*. 2:1–6.

Christiansen, A., Backensfeld, T., Weitschies, W. 2010. "Effects of non-ionic surfactants on in vitro triglyceride digestion and their susceptibility to digestion by pancreatic enzymes". *European Journal of Pharmaceutical Sciences*. 41: 376–382.

Cui, J., Yu, B., Zhao, Y., Zhu, W., Li, H., Lou, H., Zhai, G. 2009. "Enhancement of oral absorption of curcumin by self-microemulsifying drug delivery systems". *International Journal of Pharmaceutics*. 371:148–155.

Datta, S.S., Preska, S.A., Ismagilov, R.F. 2016. "Polymers in the gut compress the colonic mucus hydrogel". *Proceedings of the National Academy of Sciences of the United States of America*. 113:7041–7046.

De Jong, A., Plat, J., Mensink, R.P. 2003. "Metabolic effects of plant sterols and stanols". *Journal of Nutritional Biochemistry*. 14: 362–369.

Diosady, L.L., Venkatesh-Mannar, M.G. 2013. "Vitamin A fortification of cooking oils". In *Handbook of Food Fortification and Health: From Concepts to Public Health Applications*. Springer. New York, pp. 275–290.

Dokania, S., Joshi, A.K. 2015. "Self-microemulsifying drug delivery system (SMEDDS)—Challenges and road ahead". *Drug Delivery*. 22: 675–690.

EFSA (European Food Safety Authority). 2012. "Scientific opinion on the tolerable upper intake level of eicosapentaenoic acid (EPA), docosahexaenoic acid (DHA) and docosapentaenoic acid (DPA)". *EFSA Journal*. 10: 1831–4732.

Elnaggar, Y.S.R. 2015. "Multifaceted applications of bile salts in pharmacy: An emphasis on nanomedicine". *International Journal of Nanomedicine*. 10: 3955–3971.

Engelskirchen, S., Elsner, N., Sottmann, T., Strey, R. 2007. "Triacylglycerol microemulsions stabilized by alkyl ethoxylate surfactants-A basic study. Phase behavior, interfacial tension and microstructure". *Journal of Colloid and Interface Science*. 312: 114–121.

Frey, H., Haag, R. 2002. "Dendritic polyglycerol: A new versatile biocompatible material". *Reviews in Molecular Biotechnology*. 90: 257–267.

Garti, N. 2005. "Food goes nano". *INFORM* 6: 588–589.

Garti, N., Yaghmur, A., Leser, M.E., Clement, V., Watzke, H.J. 2001. "Improved oil solubilization in oil/water food grade μEs in the presence of polyols and ethanol". *Journal of Agricultural and Food Chemistry.*, 49: 2552–2562.

Garti, N., Zakharia, I., Spernath, A., Yaghmur, A., Aserin, A., Hoffman, R.E., Jacobs, L. 2004. "Solubilization of water-insoluble nutraceuticals in nonionic μEs for water-based use". *Progress in Colloid and Polymer Science*. 126: 184–189.

Garti, N., Spernath, A., Aserin, A., Lutz, R. 2005. "Nano-sized self-assemblies of nonionic surfactants as solubilization reservoirs and microreactors for food systems". *Soft Matter*. 1: 206–218.

Garti, N., Yuli-Amar, I. 2008. "Micro- and nano-emulsions for delivery of functional food ingredients". In N. Garti, ed. *Delivery and Controlled Release of Bioactives in Foods and Nutraceuticals*. CRC Press, Boca Raton, FL, pp. 149–183.

Gupta, S.C., Patchva, S., Aggarwal, B.B. 2013 "Therapeutic roles of curcumin: Lessons learned from clinical trials". *The AAPS Journal*. 15: 195–218.

Hernandez, E., Baker, R.A. 1991. "Turbidity of beverages with citrus oil clouding agent". *Journal of Food Science*. 56: 1024–1026.

Hidaka, T., Fujii, K., Funahashi, I., Fukutomi, N., Hosoe, K. 2008."Safety assessment of coenzyme Q10 (CoQ10)". *Biofactors*. 32: 199–208.

Hinze, J.O. 1955. "Fundamentals of the hydrodynamic mechanism of splitting in dispersion processes". *American Institute of Chemical Engineers Journal*. 1: 289–295.

Horn, D., Rieger, J. 2001. "Organic nanoparticles in the aqueous phase—Theory, experiment, and use". *Angewandte Chemie—International Edition*. 40: 4330–4361.

Ilyasoglu, H., Nehir El, S. 2014. "Nanoencapsulation of EPA/DHA with sodium caseinate–gum arabic complex and its usage in the enrichment of fruit juice". *LWT—Food Science and Technology*. 56: 461–468.

Israelachvili, J.N. 2011. *Intermolecular and Surface Forces*. 3rd ed. Academic Press, Burlington, MA, p. 704.

Jain, A., Ranjan, S., Dasgupta, N., Ramalingam, C. 2018. "Nanomaterials in food and agriculture: An overview on their safety concerns and regulatory issues". *Critical Reviews in Food Science and Nutrition*, 58: 297–317.

Jantratid, E., Janssen, N., Reppas, C., Dressman, J. 2008. "Dissolution media simulating conditions in the proximal human gastrointestinal tract: An update". *Pharmaceutical Research*. 25: 1663–1676.

Kaphle, A., Navya, P.N., Umapathi, A., Daima, H.K. 2018. "Nanomaterials for agriculture, food and environment: Applications, toxicity and regulation". *Environmental Chemistry Letters*. 16: 43–58.

Kiran, S.K., Acosta, E.J. 2010. "Predicting the morphology and viscosity of microemulsions using the HLD-NAC model". *Industrial and Engineering Chemistry Research*. 49: 3424–3432.

Kiran, S.K., Acosta, E.J. 2015. "HLD-NAC and the formation and stability of emulsions near the phase inversion point". *Industrial and Engineering Chemistry Research*. 54: 6467–6479.

Larsson, K. 1989. "Cubic lipid-water phases: Structures and biomembrane aspects". *Journal of Physical Chemistry*, 93: 7304–7314.

Latta, T.M., Acosta, E.J., van Teeffelen, N., Sveen, J.K., Tienhaara, M.K.S. 2018. "Design considerations to minimize hydrocarbon entrainment in the aqueous phase". *Proceedings of the Annual Offshore Technology Conference*. 1: 497–582.

Livney, Y.D. 2010. "Milk proteins as vehicles for bioactives". *Current Opinion in Colloid Interface Science*. 15: 73–83.

Liu, Y., Jiang, X., Wang, X. 2015. "Prescription design and bioavailability assessment of self-microemulsifying system of vitamin AD". *Latin American Journal of Pharmacy*. 34: 3853.

Li, Y., Yao, J., Han, C. Yang, J., Chaudhry, M.T., Wang, S., Liu, H., Yin, Y. 2016. "Quercetin, inflammation and immunity". *Nutrients*. 8: 167.

Marisiddaiah, R., Baskaran, V. 2009. "Bioefficacy of β-carotene is improved in rats after solubilized as equimolar dose of β-carotene and lutein in phospholipid-mixed micelles". *Nutrition Research*. 29: 588–595.

Martins, S. 2016. "Size-energy relationship in comminution, incorporating scaling laws and heat". *International Journal of Mineral Processing*. 153: 29–43.

McClements, D.J. 2011. "Edible nanoemulsions: Fabrication, properties, and functional performance". *Soft Matter*. 7: 2297–2316.

McClements, D.J. 2015. "Nanoscale nutrient delivery systems for food applications: Improving bioactive dispersibility, stability, and bioavailability". *Journal of Food Science*. 80: N1602–N1611.

McClements, D.J., Li, F., Xiao, H. 2015. "The nutraceutical bioavailability classification scheme: Classifying nutraceuticals according to factors limiting their oral bioavailability". *Annual Review of Food Science and Technology*. 6: 299–327.

McClements, D.J., Gumus, C.E. 2016. "Natural emulsifiers—Biosurfactants, phospholipids, biopolymers, and colloidal particles: Molecular and physicochemical basis of functional performance". *Advances in Colloid and Interface Science*. 234: 3–26.

National Academy of Sciences. 2011. "Dietary Reference Intakes (DRIs): Recommended dietary allowances and adequate intakes, vitamins". Accessed October 5, 2018, https://www.ncbi.nlm.nih.gov/books/NBK56068/table/summarytables.t2/?report=objectonly.

Nouraei, M., Acosta, E.J. 2017. "Predicting solubilisation features of ternary phase diagrams of fully dilutable lecithin linker microemulsions". *Journal of Colloid and Interface Science*. 495: 178–190.

Oehlke, K., Adamiuk, M., Behsnilian, D., Gräf, V., Mayer-Miebach, E., Walz, E., Greiner, R. 2014. Potential bioavailability enhancement of bioactive compounds using food-grade engineered nanomaterials: A review of the existing evidence. *Food & Function*. 5: 1341–1359.

Oh, D.-M., Curl, R.L., Amidon, G.L. 1993. "Estimating the fraction dose absorbed from suspensions of poorly soluble compounds in humans: A mathematical model". *Pharmaceutical research*. 10: 264–270.

Ontiveros, J.F., Pierlot, C., Catté, M., Molinier, V., Pizzino, A., Salager, J.-L., Aubry, J.-M. 2013. "Classification of ester oils according to their Equivalent Alkane Carbon Number (EACN) and asymmetry of fish diagrams of $C_{10}E_4$/ester oil/water systems". *Journal of Colloid and Interface Science*. 403: 67–76.

Ozturk, B., Argin, S., Ozilgen, M., McClements, D.J. 2015. "Nanoemulsion delivery systems for oil-soluble vitamins: Influence of carrier oil type on lipid digestion and vitamin D3 bioaccessibility". *Food Chemistry*. 187: 499–506.

Phan, T.T., Harwell, J.H., Sabatini, D.A. 2010. "Effects of triglyceride molecular structure on optimum formulation of surfactant-oil-water systems". *Journal of Surfactants and Detergents*. 13: 189–194.

Pouton, C.W. 2000. "Lipid formulations for oral administration of drugs: Non-emulsifying, self-emulsifying and 'self-microemulsifying' drug delivery systems". *European Journal of Pharmaceutical Sciences*. 11: S93–S98.

Pouton, C.W., Porter, C.J.H. 2008. "Formulation of lipid-based delivery systems for oral administration: Materials, methods and strategies". *Advanced Drug Delivery Reviews*. 60: 625–637.

Racette, S.B., Lin, X., Lefevre, M., Spearie, C.A., Most, M.M., Ma, L., Ostlund, R.E. 2010. "Dose effects of dietary phytosterols on cholesterol metabolism: A controlled feeding study". *The American Journal of Clinical Nutrition*. 91:32–38.

Raikar, N.B. 2010. "Prediction and manipulation of drop size distribution of emulsions using population balance equation models for high-pressure homogenization". PhD Thesis, University of Massachusetts, Amherst, MA.

Rao, A.V., Janezic, S.A. 1992. "The role of dietary phytosterols in colon carcinogenesis". *Nutrition and Cancer*. 18: 43–52.

Sabatini, D.A., Acosta, E., Harwell, J.H. 2003. "Linker molecules in surfactant mixtures". *Current Opinion in Colloid Interface Science*. 8: 316–326.

Sabliov, C.M., Astete C.E. 2008. "Encapsulation and controlled release of antioxidants and vitamins". In N. Garti, ed. *Delivery and Controlled Release of Bioactives in Foods and Nutraceuticals*. CRC Press, Boca Raton, FL, pp. 297–330.

Salager, J.L., Loaiza-Maldonado, I., Minana-Perez, M., Silva, F. 1982. "Surfactant-oil-water systems near the affinity inversion. Part I: Relationship between equilibrium phase behavior and emulsion type and stability". *Journal of Dispersion Science and Technology*. 3: 279–292.

Salager, J.L., Marquez, N., Graciaa, A., Lachaise, J. 2000. "Partitioning of ethoxylated octylphenol surfactants in μE-oil-water systems: influence of temperature and relation between partitioning coefficient and physicochemical formulation". *Langmuir*. 16: 5534–5539.

Salager, J.-L., Antón, R.E., Sabatini, D.A., Harwell, J.H., Acosta, E.J., Tolosa, L.I. 2005. "Enhancing solubilization in μEs—State of the art and current trends" *Journal of Surfactants and Detergents*, 8: 3–21.

Salvia-Trujillo, L., Qian, C., Martín-Belloso, O., McClements, D.J. 2013. "Influence of particle size on lipid digestion and β-carotene bioaccessibility in emulsions and nanoemulsions". *Food Chemistry*. 141: 1472–1480.

Sanguansri, P., Augustin, M.A. 2006. "Nanoscale materials development—A food industry perspective". *Trends in Food Science and Technology*. 17: 547–556.

Shah, A.V., Desai, H.H., Thool, P., Dalrymple, D., Serajuddin, A.T.M. 2018. "Development of self-microemulsifying drug delivery system for oral delivery of poorly water-soluble nutraceuticals". *Drug Development and Industrial Pharmacy*. 44: 895–901.

Shen, H., Howles, P., Tso, P. 2001. "From interaction of lipidic vehicles with intestinal epithelial cell membranes to the formation and secretion of chylomicrons". *Advanced Drug Delivery Reviews*. 50: S103–S125.

Staggers, J.E., Hernell, O., Stafford, R.J., Carey, M.C. 1990. "Physical-chemical behavior of dietary and biliary lipids during intestinal digestion and absorption. 1. Phase behavior and aggregation states of model lipid systems patterned after aqueous duodenal contents of healthy adult human beings". *Biochemistry.* 29: 2028–2040.

Subirade, M., Chen, L. 2008. "Food-protein-derived materials and their use in carriers and delivery systems for active food components". In N. Garti, ed. *Delivery and Controlled Release of Bioactives in Foods and Nutraceuticals.* CRC Press, Boca Raton, FL, pp. 251–278.

Sum, A.K., Biddy, M.J., De Pablo, J.J., Tupy, M.J. 2003. "Predictive molecular model for the thermodynamic and transport properties of triacylglycerols". *Journal of Physical Chemistry B*, 107: 14443–14451.

Tadros, T., Izquierdo, P., Esquena, J., Solans, C. 2004. "Formation and stability of nanoemulsions". *Advances in Colloid and Interface Science.* 108–109: 303–318

Thanatuksorn, P., Kawai, K., Hayakawa, M., Hayashi, M., Kajiwara, K. 2009. "Improvement of the oral bioavailability of coenzyme Q10 by emulsification with fats and emulsifiers used in the food industry". *Food Science and Technology.* 42: 385–390.

The Nanodatabase. 2018. Accessed April 7, 2018, http://nanodb.dk/en/.

The Project on Emerging Nanotechnologies. 2018. "Consumer products inventory". Accessed April 7, 2018, http://www.nanotechproject.org/cpi.

Tso, P., Balint, J.A., Bishop, M.B., Rodgers, J.B. 1981. "Acute inhibition of intestinal lipid transport by Pluronic L-81 in the rat". *American Journal of Physiology—Gastrointestinal and Liver Physiology.* 4: 487–497.

Türk, M., Hils, P., Helfgen, B., Schaber, K., Martin, H.-J., Wahl, M.A. 2002. "Micronization of pharmaceutical substances by the Rapid Expansion of Supercritical Solutions (RESS): A promising method to improve bioavailability of poorly soluble pharmaceutical agents". *Journal of Supercritical Fluids.* 22: 75–84.

Vaikousi, H., Lazaridou, A., Biliaderis, C.G., Zawistowski, J. 2007. "Phase transitions, solubility, and crystallization kinetics of phytosterols and phytosterol-oil blends". *Journal of Agricultural and Food Chemistry.* 55: 1790–1798.

Vance, M.E., Kuiken, T., Vejerano, E.P., McGinnis, S.P., Hochella, M.F., Hull, D.R. 2015. "Nanotechnology in the real world: Redeveloping the nanomaterial consumer products inventory". *Beilstein Journal of Nanotechnology*, 6: 1769–1780.

Warren, D.B., Chalmers, D.K., Pouton, C.W. 2009. "Structure and dynamics of glyceride lipid formulations, with propylene glycol and water". *Molecular Pharmaceutics.* 6: 604–614.

Watt, S.M., Simmonds, W.J. 1976. "The specificity of bile salts in the intestinal absorption of micellar cholesterol in the rat". *Clinical and Experimental Pharmacology and Physiology.* 3: 305–322.

Wu, L., Zhang, J., Watanabe, W. 2011. "Physical and chemical stability of drug nanoparticles". *Advanced Drug Delivery Reviews.* 63: 456–469.

Yaghmur, A., Glatter, O. 2009. "Characterization and potential applications of nanostructured aqueous dispersions". *Advances in Colloid Interface Science.* 147–148: 333–342.

Yildiz, H.M., McKelvey, C.A., Marsac, P.J., Carrier, R.L. 2015. "Size selectivity of intestinal mucus to diffusing particulates is dependent on surface chemistry and exposure to lipids". *Journal of Drug Targeting.* 23: 768–774.

Zarate-Muñoz, S., Texeira de Vasconcelos, F., Myint-Myat, K., Minchom, J., Acosta, E. 2016. "Simplified methodology to measure the characteristic curvature (Cc) of alkyl ethoxylate nonionic surfactants". *Journal of Surfactants and Detergents.* 19: 249–263.

Zhang, Z., Zhang, R., Decker, E.A., McClements, D.J. 2015. "Development of food-grade filled hydrogels for oral delivery of lipophilic active ingredients: pH-triggered release". *Food Hydrocolloids.* 44: 345–352.

# 9 Uptake and Digestion

*Amelia Torcello-Gómez and Alan R. Mackie*

## CONTENTS



## 9.1 INTRODUCTION

The term uptake refers to intestinal absorption and can be defined as the fraction of an oral dose that is absorbed through the intestinal walls. This differs from the term bioavailability, which refers to the fraction of a dose that is available at the site of action in the body, often interpreted as entering the bloodstream (Acosta 2009). Therefore, uptake precedes oral bioavailability, although not all the fraction absorbed in the intestine may become bioavailable since other processes are involved in the absorption of nutrients. Uptake also relates to the term bioaccessibility, which is the fraction of a dose that is potentially available for absorption or uptake after digestion. The gastrointestinal (GI) tract contains several major barriers that need to be overcome for optimal absorption (uptake) and bioavailability of bioactive compounds. These include the potentially low pH of the stomach, the sharply varying pH values, digestive enzymes, the mucus layer that lines the GI tract, and the intestinal epithelium (Kalantzi et al. 2006).

Encapsulation in nanoformulations improves the solubility and stability of bioactive compounds and may partially protect them from the degradative environment in the stomach and small intestine, and achieve controlled release at site of absorption, but GI motility significantly limits their retention. Therefore, the bioavailability of bioactive compounds loaded into nanosystems still requires improvement, requiring further research on the interactions between nanocarriers and GI tract to achieve optimized absorption of bioactive compounds in nutraceuticals (Katouzian and Jafari 2016).

## 9.2 GASTROINTESTINAL BARRIERS DURING DIGESTION AND ABSORPTION

The pH environment in the GI tract is indeed complicated. The normal pH range for the stomach under fasted conditions is between 1.0 and 2.5 due to the presence of hydrochloric acid. However, this can rise to above pH 5 in the fed state, depending on the properties of the meal. The pH value in the small intestine is between 6.0 and 7.0, whereas the mean pH in the distal ileum and in the body fluid at intercellular spaces between enterocytes is about 7.4 (Evans et al. 1988). This pH variation can be even more complex due to the buffering capacity of food in the fed state, making it difficult to keep nanocarrier integrity throughout the entirety of the GI tract. Furthermore, nanocarriers may be susceptible to degradation by digestive enzymes: proteases (mainly pepsin in the stomach, and trypsin, chymotrypsin, and elastase in the small intestine), lipases (mainly gastric lipase in the stomach, and pancreatic lipases in the small intestine), and amylases (salivary amylase in the mouth, and pancreatic amylase in the small intestine) (Figure 9.1). Along with pH variations and enzymes, there are endogenous surface-active components, such as low concentrations of phospholipids in the stomach or in greater concentrations in the small intestine where they are mixed with bile acids. Although these biosurfactants help to emulsify fats and oils and solubilize digestion products into mixed micelles (Maldonado-Valderrama et al. 2011), they can also contribute to the colloidal destabilization of nanocarriers within the GI tract (Jodar-Reyes et al. 2010).

Nanocarriers must retain their cargo of bioactive compounds and reach the small intestine to be absorbed. Once there, the nanocarriers must overcome the barrier of the mucus layer lining the surface of the GI tract. Mucus is secreted by goblet cells and submucosal glands and is composed of large anionic glycoproteins, predominantly of the mucin family, forming an entangled and cross-linked network. In the small intestine the primary secreted mucin is MUC2. However, the composition and average thickness of the mucus layer varies throughout the GI tract, being as thick as 170 μm in the stomach to 10 μm in the ileum (Lai et al. 2009) for optimized nutrient absorption. One major problem of this barrier is the quick mucus clearance and the high enterocyte turnover (from 2 to 5 days in human small intestine) that can also clear nanocarriers entrapped in the loosely adherent outer mucus layer (Ensign et al. 2012). In addition, extracellular DNA from shed epithelial cells can significantly contribute to the microrheological and permeability properties of small intestine mucus (Macierzanka et al. 2014). The mucus layer is a viscous hydrated matrix (Macierzanka et al. 2011) that reduces the shear effect from the movement of

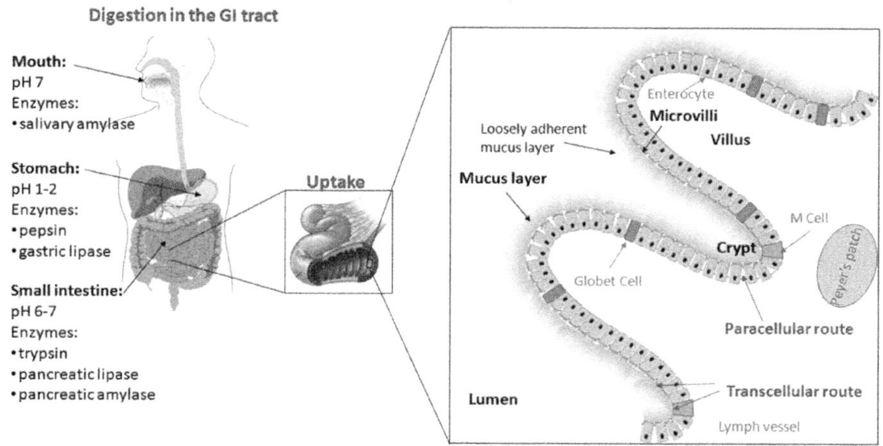


**FIGURE 9.1** Schematic representation of the main GI barriers for bio-nanosystems digestion and absorption.

GI fluids creating a so-called unstirred layer. Therefore, if the nanosystems exhibit mucoadhesive properties and can bind to the mucus layer, they will not diffuse to the enterocytes for absorption. However, if they are free to diffuse through the low-viscosity pores/channels in the mucus network, they can be absorbed. Negatively charged hydrophilic particle surfaces exhibit limited interactions with mucus, conferring rapid diffusion through the mucus layer, but is detrimental to membrane permeation and entry into the epithelial cell (Lundquist and Artursson 2016).

The secreted mucus layer is linked to the enterocytes through the membrane-bound mucins comprising the glycocalyx. The glycocalyx covers the microvilli that crenelate the upper surface of each epithelial cell providing a large area for nutrient absorption. Here, the transport through the cell membrane in the epithelial layer will depend on the size and chemical compatibilities between the surface of the nanocarriers and intestinal epithelium. The presence of tight junctions in the interstitial space between epithelial cells (0.3–1 nm) limits passive diffusion of nanocarriers via paracellular route (Pade and Stavchansky 1997). These are mostly transported by transcellular route, whereas hydrophilic, polar solutes diffuse through the paracellular route (Norris et al. 1998). The transcellular route involves the uptake by epithelial cells in a process called transcytosis, either by enterocytes, which represent 90%–95% of the intestinal epithelial cells, or by M cells (microfold cells) which are located in the Peyer's patches primarily in the distal intestine. M-cells are involved in endocytosis of macromolecules and microbes that can be potentially antigenic. Transcellular uptake can take place via two modes of transport: active and passive. Active transport occurs through specific transporter channels on the surface of the epithelial cell that use the cell's own energy and is regulated by the cell in such a way that a certain level of nutrients and minerals are maintained in the blood. Any excess of these substances is accumulated in tissue or excreted and additional doses are not absorbed via active mechanism. Passive transport occurs by simple diffusion and is controlled by differences in activity of the specific nutrient across the epithelial tissue, defined by the concentration multiplied of the activity coefficient. The activity coefficient is inversely proportional to the solubility of the nutrient. Therefore, more hydrophilic compounds tend to have low permeability and transport by means of active mechanism, whereas more hydrophobic compounds are very permeable and absorb via passive and active transport. Passive and active transport apply to both enterocyte and M cells. Although M cells are more permeable, they only represent less than 1% of the total intestinal area, making selective delivery to these cells more difficult (Hussain et al. 2001). If the direct uptake of the nanocarriers is not possible, then they should at least release the encapsulated bioactive compound in the small intestine in a sustained manner. This can be attained with the controlled degradation of the carrier by digestive enzymes or via pH-sensitive materials such as polymers [e.g., poly(meth)acrylates or alginates], otherwise the solubility (if the compound is hydrophobic) may be exceeded, with the consequent formation of crystals and decreased absorption (Acosta 2009).

Bearing in mind how the process of digestion and absorption occurs, we will now introduce the advantages that bio-nanosystems may offer, as oral delivery systems of bioactive compounds. Food-grade ingredients, such as polysaccharides, proteins, lipids, and low molecular weight surfactants are widely used in the fabrication of these nanosystems for oral delivery, being biodegradable and non-toxic. They protect the cargo from degradative GI environment, and the subcellular size improves not only sensorial aspects, but also solubility and bioavailability. This improvement in bioavailability seems, in most cases, to be related to the direct uptake of the nanocarriers (Acosta 2009). This may be linked to the larger surface area-to-volume ratio and physico-chemical interactions at the nanoscale (Cerqueira et al. 2014). These interactions include mucoadhesion and permeability enhancing properties, which potentially improve the absorption across intestinal epithelial cell membrane. All these attributes are related to a smaller size. Indeed, nanoparticles in the range of 100 nm can freely diffuse through intestinal mucus *ex vivo* as compared to larger particles (500 nm), which is consistent with the reported mucus pore size within the range of 200 nm (Bajka et al. 2015). This can also be explained by an increased retention, time, and degree of interaction between the nanocarriers and the mucus layer in the small intestine. In this sense, it is known that positively charged polysaccharides such as chitosan interact with negatively charged mucin and components in the intestinal epithelial membrane (Shukla et al. 2013). This suggests that electrostatic interactions can drive mucoadhesion, although physical entrapment by the mucus layer can also take place, as well as hydrophobic and van der Waals interactions and polymer chain penetration (Ensign et al. 2012). In fact, chitosan introduces hydrophilic groups on the surface of the nanocarriers, which promote the translocation across cellular cytoplasm. However, if the electrostatic interactions between the positively charged surface of nanocarriers and negatively charged mucin are too strong, the nanocarriers will be entrapped in the mucus without permeating through the epithelial tissue (Hussain et al. 2001). This may be ameliorated by the adsorption of bile salts and fatty acids, which can impart negative charge to the surface of nanocarriers and enhance the transport across the mucus network (Macierzanka et al. 2011).

When bio-nanosystems are incorporated into food or beverage products, they should be stable in the food formulation. Although they can influence its appearance, texture, stability, and flavor, they must avoid aggregation, undesirable release, and loss of activity of the encapsulated compound in the food matrix during storage before consumption. Therefore, interactions within the food matrix before and after intake need further understanding to unravel the fate during digestion and absorption.

Summarizing, the factors to take into account when designing an oral delivery nanosystem are as follows: compatibility between nanosystem materials and bioactive compound, biocompatibility of the synthesis procedure (such as organic solvent-free methods), and minimal processing of sensitive substances (avoid heat or vigorous agitation). In addition, solubility of bioactive compound in the nanosystem, high loading capacity, preservation, and protection during storage and behavior within the GI tract (susceptibility to chemical or enzymatic hydrolysis) (McClements et al. 2009) are all important, especially when targeting absorption at specific locations.

## 9.3 *IN VIVO* AND *IN VITRO* EXPERIMENTS FOR BIOACCESSIBILITY AND BIOAVAILABILITY EVALUATION

The process of evaluation of digestion and uptake of bio-nanosystems in food containing bioactive compounds starts with the modeling of *in vivo* characteristics by using *in vitro* methods. This is typically followed by *ex vivo*, *in situ*, and *in vivo* techniques for validation.

The simplest *in vitro* experiments involve the physico-chemical characterization of the nanosystems behavior in simulated GI fluids. There is a standardized static digestion model (Minekus et al. 2014) that allows direct comparison across different laboratories. This includes the appropriate average pH, ionic strength, and enzyme activity to mimic the physiological conditions of the gastric and intestinal fluids in sequence. This may serve as a preliminary test of the behavior of nanosystems containing bioactive compounds within the GI tract to screen colloidal and chemical stability, enzyme degradation, release of encapsulated compounds, and bioaccessibility. However, static models do not reproduce the dynamic aspects of GI physiology, such as progressive acidification and emptying from the stomach, gradual secretion of enzymes, or mixing profiles or peristaltic contractions, and since these can affect the kinetics of nutrient bioaccessibility, there is the need to develop a standardized dynamic model. There is currently a model that reproduces pH gradient in the stomach, stomach emptying, or gradual release of gastric enzymes, referred to as semi-dynamic method (Mulet-Cabero et al. 2017), since the dynamic aspects of the small intestine are not developed yet. Further, more sophisticated *in vitro* dynamic gastric simulators have been developed (Figure 9.2) and further details can be found elsewhere (Verhoeckx et al. 2015), but these models are often too complicated and costly to run on a daily basis.

In order to test the transport of nanocarriers or the encapsulated compound across the intestinal epithelium, membrane systems are often used like dialysis bags or tubing containing the nanosystems (Sessa et al. 2014) and suspended in simulated GI fluids for a more accurate approach. However, these do not mimic the epithelial cell behavior. To achieve a more realistic model of the human gut epithelium, human epithelial colorectal adenocarcinoma cell line (Caco)-2 monolayer cell cultures or

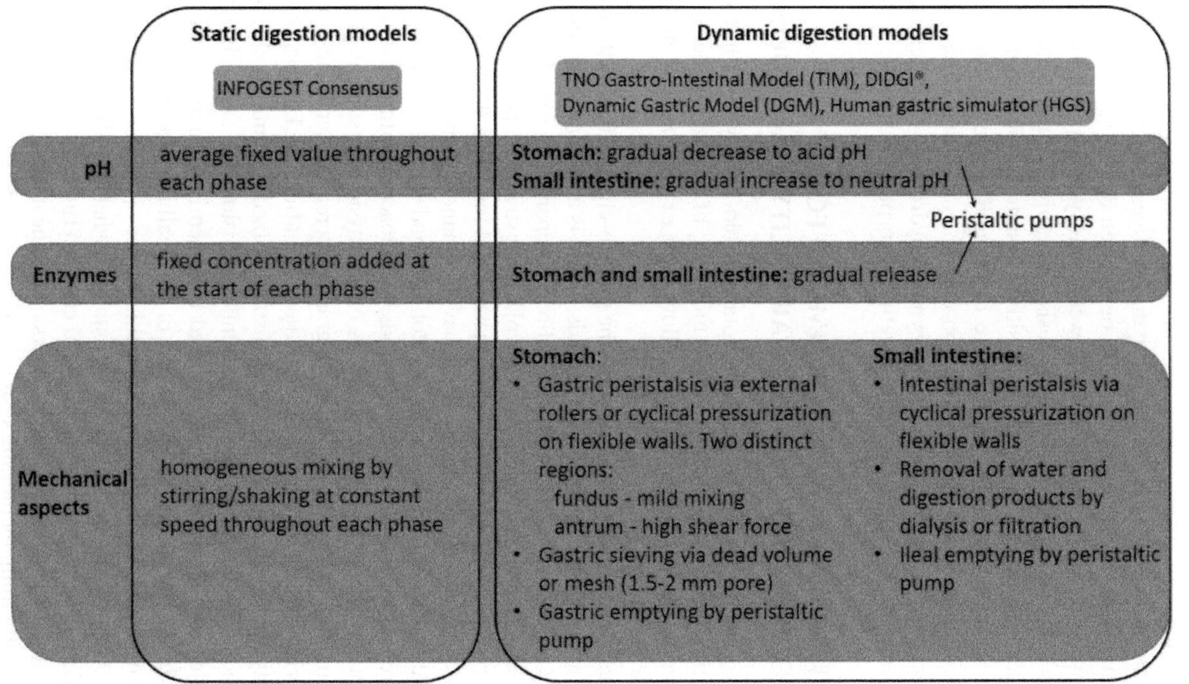


**FIGURE 9.2** Summary of the main features of static and dynamic *in vitro* digestion models with emphasis on stomach and small intestine.

co-cultures of Caco-2 can be grown in either a single cell culture well plate for uptake studies or in a membrane insert in a Transwell® system for transport studies (Gamboa and Leong 2013). Nevertheless, Caco-2 monolayer only reproduces enterocytes and is not an accurate model for small intestinal tissue, but rather colonic tissue instead. Co-cultures of Caco-2 and other cell lines may take into account aspects of the multicellular intestinal epithelium by including M cells (Caco-2 and RajiB or lymphocyte co-culture) and mucus secreting goblet cells (Caco-2 and HT29 co-culture). Good descriptions of the methods for these types of cell cultures are given elsewhere (Verhoeckx et al. 2015). A more advanced microdevice called gut-on-a-chip has upgraded the benefits of using Caco-2 cell cultures by implementing fluid flow and mechanical stress via vacuum microchambers alongside the microchannels that mimic the peristalsis in the GI tract (Kim et al. 2012). This increases the paracellular transport without compromising the integrity of the cell monolayer. In addition, human gut isolated microbial flora can be cultured on top of the Caco-2 monolayer. In all these techniques, sampling and composition analysis of the collected aliquots are required to measure the release/transport of bioactive compound from the nanocarriers.

*Ex vivo* studies usually involve working with segments of animal gut. This offers a better representation of the morphological and physiological features of the intestine, such as the presence of all the relevant cell types and architecture and the presence of a mucus layer (Gunness et al. 2016). These can be used to follow the transport of nanocarriers or nutrients across the intestinal epithelium, permeability, absorption, or interactions with the mucus layer (Norris and Sinko 1997). The simpler techniques are intestinal rings and intestinal segments, where these are isolated and immersed into highly oxygenated buffer containing the compound of interest. The tissues are viable for 1 to 2 hours depending whether the muscle layers are present or removed, respectively. The main disadvantage is that the exposure to luminal (apical) and serosal (basolateral) side is not made via individual compartments, therefore this procedure is mainly used to measure the accumulation of nanocarriers, in this case into the enterocytes rather than transport (Hillgren et al. 1995). The individualization of apical and basolateral compartments can be achieved with the everted sac model, whereby a segment of intestine can be sutured at one end, nanosystems introduced, and the open end also sutured, and immersed in physiological solution, such as Ringer's (Trapani et al. 2010). Another alternative is opening the intestinal segment so that the tissue can be mounted in an Ussing chamber, where the tissue is set on a frame dividing two semi-chambers, one facing the apical side, where the nanosystems are loaded, and the other facing the basolateral side (Lundquist and Artursson 2016). The electrophysiological properties: transepithelial electrical resistance, potential difference between the two chambers and short-circuit current of the tissue are monitored throughout the experiment as indicators of tissue integrity and viability. Most of these intestinal tissue models make use of an animal source, rats, rabbits, and pigs being the more common, due to the limited availability of healthy human intestinal tissue. Although pigs share more physiological and immunological similarities to human than rodents, the extrapolation of data to humans is complicated due to interspecies differences (Rowan et al. 1994), even the large inter-individual variability in humans make the interpretation of the results difficult in small studies. The use of human intestinal tissue in Ussing chambers has been discussed in a review by Lundquist and Artursson (2016), who include a limited number of studies of nanoparticle transport across human intestinal tissue. Once more, sampling is required from basolateral and luminal sides to determine the concentration of the bioactive compound and assess uptake across epithelial layer.

The most common *in situ* technique is the intestinal loop model. This method requires the animal to be under anesthesia during the procedure, in which a segment of the intestine is ligated to form a loop, the nanocarrier suspension injected into the loop, and this returned to the body cavity for up to 2 hours. Then the animal is sacrificed, and the loop or the entire intestine removed for analysis (Desai et al. 1996).

The most relevant information that can be obtained from *in vivo* studies includes compound release kinetics and biodistribution of the nanocarriers (Gamboa and Leong 2013). Non-invasive imaging techniques are usually preferred, although information is limited. These focus on stomach, small intestine, and the colon. Radiolabeling can enable monitoring and quantifying nanoparticles on their transit through the GI tract in real time. Nevertheless, it can be an invasive technique and involves radiation exposure. In addition, analysis of blood is performed to determine plasma level of the considered bioactive compound after oral delivery and organ analysis is carried out to quantify tissue concentration (Gamboa and Leong 2013).

## 9.4 EVALUATION OF BIO-NANOSYSTEMS CONTAINING BIOACTIVE COMPOUNDS WITHIN THE GI TRACT

Until 2014, most of the reviews on nanosystems for oral delivery and the behavior of these within the GI tract were largely focused on polymer-based micelles and lipid-based nanosystems such as nanoemulsions (Cerqueira et al. 2014) because of the scarce data on other nanosystems. The fact that most of the bioactive compounds such as fatty acids, carotenoids, and tocopherols, are lipophilic, justifies the relatively larger amount of studies on their encapsulation in lipid-based nanosystems (Tamjidi et al. 2013). In addition, the presence of digestible lipids facilitates the absorption of these bioactive compounds in the small intestine.

In this section, information will be provided about the behavior of these and other nanosystems encapsulating bioactive compounds within the GI tract in models where enzymes are included. Data regarding monitoring the rate and extent on digestion, and therefore the release and bioaccessibility of bioactive compounds as indicative of potential bioavailability will be also reviewed in a critical manner. In addition, we also highlight *in vivo* studies of uptake and bioavailability of bioactive compounds encapsulated in bio-based nanocarriers. Bioactive compound loading, encapsulation efficiency, and shelf life stability, as well as sensory properties or consumer acceptability are not part of the main discussion within the current chapter.

### 9.4.1 Nanohydrogels

Nanohydrogels are defined as nanosized hydrogel particles formed by physically or chemically cross-linked hydrophilic or amphiphilic polymer network

(Shin et al. 2015). The availability of the interior network for the incorporation of bioactive compounds can potentially increase uptake, absorption, and bioavailability (Cerqueira et al. 2014). The water holding capacity and permeability are the key features of these nanosystems in addition to responding to environmental stimuli for triggered delivery system (Shin et al. 2015).

Proteins and proteins-polysaccharides nanohydrogels have been developed. The main limitation of these systems under physiological conditions is that the labile bonds in the polymer backbone or in the cross-links can be hydrolyzed by enzymes. It has been reported that when comparing nanohydrogels comprising only protein or protein and polysaccharide, an external coating of polysaccharide, such as chitosan or alginate, offers better protection of the encapsulated bioactive compound under *in vitro* gastric conditions (Somchue et al. 2009). This is due to the slower rate of protein hydrolysis, greater particle stability (Bourbon et al. 2016), as well as prolonged release in the simulated intestinal phase (Somchue et al. 2009).

### 9.4.2 Nanocapsules/Nanoparticles

Nanocapsules or nanoparticles are formed by an external polymeric membrane and an internal part constituted by a liquid or polymeric matrix containing the bioactive compound. Three categories can be classified according to the material composing the nanoparticles: polysaccharide, protein, or both.

#### 9.4.2.1 Polysaccharide-Bioactive Compound Nanoparticles

Polysaccharides are considered beneficial for improving the intestinal absorption of active ingredients, above all those that are water-soluble, but have low permeability in the small intestine (Hu et al. 2017). Therefore, the development of nanoparticles with this type of food ingredient can be beneficial.

Nanocomplexes formed by amylose and lipids were proposed as delivery vehicles for polyunsaturated fatty acids within the small intestine. *In vitro* digestion in simulated stomach showed high retention of conjugated linoleic acid, however, a high rate of hydrolysis of amylase in simulated small intestine was observed with subsequent release of linoleic acid (Lalush et al. 2005). The high rate of hydrolysis of amylase might also potentially be an issue in the stomach if the pH is sufficiently high for the salivary amylase to remain active.

Water-soluble nanoparticles developed with low-molecular weight chitosan efficiently encapsulated lutein and improved the *in vitro* bioaccessibility, after simulated GI digestion and *in vivo* bioavailability in mice, according to higher concentration observed in plasma, liver, and eyes, as compared with lutein in mixed micelles of lipid, bile, and cholesterol as a control (Arunkumar et al. 2013). Nuclear magnetic resonance experiments showed that weak bonds were formed between lutein and cross-linked chains of chitosan in the presence of water molecules.

The inclusion of cyclodextrins in hybrid poly/oligosaccharides nanoparticles has been shown to improve the capacity of these nanocarriers not only to load poorly soluble drugs and hydrophilic molecules, but also to enhance their transport across intestinal mucosal barrier of frogs in *ex vivo* experiments (Trapani et al. 2010). The authors attributed this to particular interactions of the nanoparticles with the surrounding epithelium due to intrinsic physico-chemical properties of the nanoparticles added by the cyclodextrins (smaller size, potential chelating capacity).

Electrostatic interactions between oppositely charged polysaccharides, such as chitosan and gum arabic, were used to form a strong polysaccharide matrix to fabricate nanoparticles containing other emulsifying agents (Tween 80 and egg yolk phospholipids) carrying curcumin (Tan et al. 2016). These novel nanoparticles allowed a delayed and more effective release of curcumin into the simulated small intestine phase by increasing the stability of curcumin and nanoparticles under simulated gastric conditions, as compared to emulsion without polysaccharide coating.

#### 9.4.2.2 Protein-Bioactive Compound Nanoparticles

Food proteins have extraordinary binding capacity to drugs or nutraceuticals via hydrophobic interaction, electrostatic attraction, hydrogen bonding, and van der Waals force. Thus, protein nanoparticles can be used to encapsulate non-polar, polar, or charged compounds (Teng et al. 2014). They also have high nutritional value as a source of essential amino acids (Hu et al. 2017).

Bovine β-lactoglobulin (BLG) nanoparticles were developed by cross-linking with glutaraldehyde and reducing the cross-linker concentration by increasing the encapsulated curcumin that acts in turn as a physical cross-linker, due to the great protein binding affinity already mentioned. These nanoparticles show different curcumin release profile behavior under *in vitro* gastric conditions at either fed stated (gastric pH 5) or fasted state (gastric pH 2). Namely, nanoparticles were disintegrated in the fasted state and readily released the encapsulated curcumin, as opposed to the stability and controlled release displayed by nanoparticles in the fed state (Teng et al. 2014). Despite the known resistance of native BLG to pepsin digestion (Otte et al. 1997), which is largely active at pH 2, The authors attribute the behavior of nanoparticles in the fasted state to the susceptibility of intermolecular amide bonds produced by the glutaraldehyde to pepsin cleavage.

Casein micelles are also a potential nanodelivery system of bioactive compounds such as vitamin D. Reconstituted casein micelles loaded with vitamin D incorporated in low-fat milk and fat-free yogurt led to high stability of vitamin D under storage conditions, as well as *in vivo* bioavailability, as shown in human clinical trials (Haham et al. 2012, Levinson et al. 2016). This offers a natural alternative to synthetic emulsifiers, such as Tween 80, used in commercial dietary supplements of vitamin D, and better palatability of the product as confirmed by sensory evaluations. The *in vivo* human bioavailability of vitamin D encapsulated in casein micelles incorporated in fat-free yogurt is also as good as that of vitamin D dissolved within the fat of low-fat yogurt (Cohen et al. 2017a). A follow up study, under *in vitro* conditions, attributes these results to the protection of vitamin D conferred by the casein micelles under gastric conditions by means of protein-vitamin binding and curd formation, which allows an increase in vitamin retention as compared to free vitamin (Cohen et al. 2017b).

Complexation between native and pre-heated soy proteins with bioactive compounds like curcumin also leads to improved stability under *in vitro* GI conditions and bioaccessibility over the free bioactive compound. Pre-heated soy protein isolate (SPI) has been shown to bind to a larger extent to curcumin. However, protein hydrolysis during GI digestion induces nanoparticle aggregation to a larger extent in pre-heated protein nanoparticles that impairs bioaccessibility of the bioactive compound (Chen et al. 2015). On the other hand, complexation with curcumin improved protein digestibility for both native and pre-heated SPI.

The performance of different food proteins in the release of nanoencapsulated compounds has been compared. A recent study used whey protein isolate (WPI) nanoparticles showing that they were more resistant to *in vitro* pepsin digestion. This led to a very limited release of the incorporated β-carotene in the simulated stomach, as compared to sodium caseinate or SPI nanoparticles, followed by release after intestinal trypsin digestion (Yi et al. 2015). This was attributed to the lower digestibility of the native globular BLG, the predominant component in WPI, due to the stable conformation of the folded β-sheet-structure. All protein nanoparticles increased the cellular uptake of β-carotene in Caco-2 cells in relation to control (free β-carotene). However, the protective behavior of WPI in the stomach makes WPI nanoparticles a good candidate for a sustained release in the small intestine as the site of absorption.

#### 9.4.2.3 Protein-Polysaccharide-Bioactive Compound Nanoparticles

In order to overcome the drawback of protein digestibility in the gastric phase, complexation with polysaccharide offers better stability and protection against pepsin hydrolysis.

Self-assembly through electrostatic interactions between proteins and polysaccharides allows the formation of nanoparticles such as those composed by a zein or SPI core coated with carboxymethyl chitosan to encapsulate compounds like vitamin D (Luo et al. 2012, Teng et al. 2013). The chitosan coating provides better controlled release of vitamin D under *in vitro* GI conditions because carboxymethyl chitosan becomes insoluble and forms a gel-like barrier in the polymeric matrix at gastric pH (1.4–2.0) due to the protonation of the carboxylic group. Such feature allows carboxymethyl chitosan to delay significantly the decomposition of the protein matrix, thus minimizing the release of the embedded compounds in the stomach and maximizing their availability for intestinal absorption. In addition, the authors observed that the complex nanoparticles provided stronger interaction with vitamin D through hydrogen bonding in comparison to the ones formed with single ingredients.

Nevertheless, the combination of hydrophilic polysaccharide and protein creates mostly non-covalent interactions, which are sensitive to environmental conditions. Accordingly, aggregation or phase separation might take place arising from the binding at high biocompound loading. Maillard conjugation (non-enzymatic glycosylation by means of covalent bonds) between proteins (either milk or plant origin) and polysaccharides has allowed the development of nanocomplexes or nanoparticles to encapsulate polyphenols, to overcome the precipitation of protein caused by the strong binding affinity with polyphenols (Hu et al. 2017). These nanoparticles have been shown to be similar or better at retaining bioactive compounds as compared to complexes between native proteins and bioactive compounds, to have better compound stabilization under GI conditions, and more controlled release (Xue et al. 2014) also improving its *in vitro* bioaccessibility (Davidov-Pardo et al. 2015, Qiu et al. 2017). This is attributed to the greater steric hindrance provided by the polysaccharide molecules in the shell of the nanoparticles and less susceptibility to GI enzyme digestion of the glycosylated protein. In this sense, the polysaccharide coating may also improve the controlled release of the encapsulated compound as compared to the protein coating (Chen et al. 2016).

Cross-linking of peptide-polysaccharide nanoparticles with genipin is another alternative to improve stability under simulated GI conditions and sustained release (Hu et al. 2014). The advantages of this approach are not only the use of a natural and non-toxic cross-linker, but also the higher stability than chitosan-based nanoparticles in biological fluids.

## 9.4.3 Lipid-Based Nanosystems

### 9.4.3.1 Nanoemulsions

In general, nanoemulsions enhance lipid digestibility as compared to conventional emulsions due to the increased initial interfacial area exposed to lipase action, therefore a greater release of the encapsulated compound would be expected. Nevertheless, the rate and extent of lipid digestion also depends on other initial parameters, such as the emulsifier type, oil type and oil content used, and stability under GI conditions.

Salvia-Trujillo et al. showed under *in vitro* conditions that the rate and extent of lipid digestion increased with decreased initial droplet size of nanoemulsions, and therefore increased the bioaccessibility of β-carotene incorporated in the oil-phase (Salvia-Trujillo et al. 2013). In another study, the *in vivo* GI absorption of eicosapentaenoic and docosahexaenoic acids rich fish oils from nanoemulsion and conventional emulsion formulation was evaluated using a single pass perfusion rat model (Dey et al. 2012). The lipid absorption in the small intestine of the rats was increased by using a nanoemulsion formulation.

The emulsifier type can also have an impact on the interfacial stability upon digestion and permeability across the intestinal barrier. This will depend on the interactions with GI components and surface activity. Recent work reported on the effect of the surface charge of nanoemulsions on their physico-chemical stability, digestion, and release of encapsulated curcumin under *in vitro* GI conditions using a sophisticated human gastric simulator (Pinheiro et al. 2013). The authors showed that the cationic emulsifier induced greater destabilization of the nanoemulsions as compared to non-ionic or anionic emulsifiers, leading to larger droplet size, and hence poorer curcumin bioaccessibility. This was attributed to alterations in the bile and lipase adsorption. Li et al. showed recently that a protein-stabilized nanoemulsion is as good as protein complexation to improve stability under *in vitro* GI conditions and permeability of curcumin in Caco-2 cell monolayer model (Li et al. 2015). The proteins used were dairy proteins (BLG and WPI), which show resistance to pepsin digestion, but are more susceptible to trypsin digestion, which is necessary for the release of the encapsulated compound. Another study tested the capability of nanoemulsions, stabilized mainly by soy lecithin or glycerol monooleate combined with either Tween 20 or sugar esters, to encapsulate resveratrol and proved its stability and excellent antioxidant activity (>80%) in Caco-2 cells and by chemical assays under *in vitro* GI conditions (Sessa et al. 2011). This high antioxidant activity was related to better entrapment of resveratrol in the lipid phase due to the formation of reversed micelles of the more hydrophobic emulsifier within the lipid droplets stabilized by the more hydrophilic emulsifiers. This work suggests that nanoemulsions may improve the uptake of antioxidant compounds in their active form through the intestinal walls. In subsequent studies, the lecithin-based formulations of these nanoemulsions with encapsulated resveratrol were shown to enhance the transport of the antioxidant through Caco-2 cell monolayers in shorter times than those required for their metabolization (Sessa et al. 2014). This was attributed to the more similar composition of the interfacial layers in lecithin-based nanoemulsions to that of the phospholipid bilayer structure of the cellular membrane. Modified starches can also be efficient stabilizers of nanoemulsions that improved the bioaccessibility of β-carotene under *in vitro* GI conditions as compared to β-carotene dispersed in bulk oil (Liang et al. 2013). In addition, decreasing the dispersed molecular density of the modified starch significantly enhances the bioaccessibility of β-carotene, which might be related to the thickness of the modified starch layer stabilizing the oil droplets.

The effect of the oil type has also been studied in the *in vitro* intestinal digestion of nanoemulsions and release of encapsulated curcumin (Ahmed et al. 2012). Specifically, the length of triacylglycerol chains (long: LCT, medium: MCT, and short: SCT) had a marked effect on the rate and extend of release of free fatty acids and bioaccessibility of curcumin, the latter estimated as the curcumin incorporated into the micellar phase after digestion. Specifically, LCT nanoemulsions had a slower rate and lower extent of lipid digestion, due to the inhibitory effect on pancreatic lipase caused by the interfacial saturation with the more water-insoluble long chain fatty acids. Following the trend of nanoemulsion digestibility, one could also expect the lowest curcumin bioaccessibility in LCT nanoemulsions. However, SCT nanoemulsions showed the lowest curcumin bioaccessibility, despite the greater curcumin loading capacity, due to the high water-solubility of short chain fatty acids, which limits the capability for micelle formation. Similar trends were found for the rate and extent of lipid digestion of nanoemulsions and bioaccessbility of encapsulated vitamin D with varying oil type (MCT versus LCT) (Ozturk et al. 2015). The LCTs were found to improve the bioaccessibility of vitamin D due to better solubilization by long chain free fatty acids in mixed micelles.

The content of oil in the nanoemulsion formulations also plays a role in determining the rate of lipid digestibility, and hence bioaccessibility of encapsulated bioactive compounds under *in vitro* conditions. Xia et al. showed that nanoemulsions with lower fat content (4%) were digested at a faster rate and to a larger extent, and the bioaccessibility of the encapsulated β-carotene was accordingly higher than that from nanoemulsions with higher fat content (20%) (Xia et al. 2017).

#### 9.4.3.2 Solid Lipid Nanoparticles and Nanostructured Lipid Carriers

Lipidic nanoparticles can be produced from nanoemulsions by using a lipid phase that can fully (solid lipid nanoparticles [SLNs]) or partially (nanostructured lipid carriers [NLCs]) crystallize at room and body temperature. Solid crystalline phase is present in both, thus the effect of physical state of lipid can be crucial on its digestion and release of encapsulated compounds.

SLNs are formed by lipid droplets fully crystallized and have highly ordered crystalline structure. Some studies have shown the high efficiency of SLNs as compared to non-encapsulated compounds to stabilize and provide sustained and prolonged release under simulated GI conditions (Righeschi et al. 2016) and improve the oral bioavailability in animal studies (Pandita et al. 2014, Ramalingam et al. 2016). One could hypothesize that the solid matrix of SLNs will provide better stability to the encapsulated hydrophobic compounds against oxidation and display a slower rate of lipid digestion, and hence more controlled release of encapsulated bioactive compounds. However, a recent study showed that lipophilic molecules that are located within the lipid phase in emulsions are expelled from the core of the lipid droplet to the aqueous phase upon crystallization of the lipid phase in SLNs, and thus their chemical stability is greatly compromised (Berton-Carabin et al. 2013). The highly ordered structure formed by fat crystals leaves less space to accommodate the encapsulated compound (Tamjidi et al. 2013). In addition, the fat crystals present in SLNs promote partial coalescence, leading to a poorer physical stability as compared to liquid lipid nanoparticles (Qian et al. 2013). Hence, this may affect subsequent stability and degradation under GI conditions. It has been recently shown by means of *in vivo* live imaging that SLNs are efficiently digested in the mouse intestine, limiting the subsequent absorption of intact nanoparticles over the intestinal wall (Hu et al. 2016). This was also confirmed from results of *in situ* perfusion studies and transmembrane permeation across Caco-2 cell monolayers.

NLCs were developed to overcome the potential limitations related to SLNs, as explained above, in addition to providing higher loading capacity and slow release (Shin et al. 2015, Yang et al. 2017). NLCs are formed from lipid droplets that are partially crystallized and have a less-ordered crystalline structure. NLCs are a modification of SLNs in such a way that the liquid lipid phase is located in the core of the solid lipid, therefore the bioactive compound is better dissolved in the liquid core and simultaneously encapsulated by the solid shell. An *in vivo* study using bioluminescence imaging proved the prolonged retention of NLCs stabilized with lipophilic emulsifiers in the rat abdominal region (Chen et al. 2010). Fang and co-workers compared the oral bioavailability of curcumin in suspension or encapsulated in NLCs in rats after gastric administration and observed a significant increase in peak plasma concentration, which was also reached in shorter time, as well as an increase in area under the curve and tissue concentrations of curcumin when administered in the NLCs (Fang et al. 2012). This is hardly surprising given the limited solubility of curcumin in water. Similarly, cationic NLC increased the tissue concentration of quercetin after oral administration in mice as compared to quercetin suspension (Liu et al. 2014). Most of the studies so far tested the *in vitro* digestion of NLCs and release of encapsulated substances in NLCs prepared with one type of liquid lipid and solid lipid at a fixed ratio. These studies showed the stability of NLCs under GI conditions and increased solubility and release of encapsulated compounds in the simulated intestinal medium (Aditya et al. 2013, Park et al. 2017). A very recent study showed the effect of incorporating two different types of liquid lipids (MCT and LCT) at different ratios, in combination with one type of solid lipid in the NLCs formulation on the rate of lipid digestibility and release of encapsulated curcumin (Yang et al. 2017). The authors showed that the rate of lipid digestion and release of curcumin from

NLCs increased with increasing the ratio of MCT:LCT in the nanosystem formulation. This was due to the preference of the lipase to selectively digest the MCT in the lipid mixture, which as explained above are faster hydrolyzed as compared to LCT. The curcumin seems to better dissolve in the MCT phase, explaining the similar trend in the curcumin release profile as for the free fatty acid release.

#### 9.4.3.3 Nanoliposomes

Nanoliposomes consist of a vesicle made of a phospholipid bilayer enclosing a small volume of aqueous liquid and can contain both water-soluble and lipid-soluble compounds.

Nanoliposomes were reported to efficiently encapsulate curcumin increasing its absorption in the GI tract and bioavailability in rats after oral administration, as compared to non-encapsulated curcumin or the mixture of curcumin and lecithin (Takahashi et al. 2009). Liposomes are also promising delivery systems of substances like carotenoids, which may provide improved bioaccessibility, as compared to nanoemulsions delivery systems, due to the solubilization capacity of the digested products that contain greater absolute amount of mixed micelles and lipid bilayers (Tan et al. 2014). However, leakage and fast release of the encapsulated bioactive compound are still a major disadvantage of liposomes as delivery systems (Tamjidi et al. 2013), therefore other solutions have been proposed to enhance their nanocarrier performance.

Nanoliposomes that were coated by chitosan showed an increased mucoadhesion in comparison with bare nanoliposomes prepared by the same method (Shin et al. 2013). WPI-coated liposomes containing quercetin in a dairy drink showed better stability, in terms of particle size and lower release of free fatty acids, under simulated gastric conditions than uncoated liposomes. This was attributed to the reduced semi-permeability of the membrane by the protein coating, which hindered osmotic effects affecting the particle size of the liposomes in the dairy drink matrix. Next, the free fatty acid release profile was greater for coated liposomes under simulated intestinal conditions, which may be linked to an improved release of the encapsulated compound (Frenzel et al. 2015).

### 9.4.4 Nanolaminated Systems

Nanocomposites and nanolaminated coating with the layer-by-layer deposition can be designed so that their stability and properties change as a response to changes in environmental/physiological parameters (e.g., pH, temperature, and ionic strength) (McClements 2010).

Oil-in-water emulsions nanolaminated with oppositely charged proteins (β-lactoglobulin and lactoferrin) at neutral pH values have been shown to be stable under storage conditions. However, they all (mono-, bi-, or multi-layered) aggregated under *in vitro* GI conditions and did not have an impact on the digestion of triglycerides since protein was readily digested. The decreased bioaccessibility of β-carotene was attributed to binding with lactoferrin (Tokle et al. 2013).

A study reporting the *in vitro* digestibility of hybrid nanoparticles, fabricated with the layer-by-layer deposition of lactoferrin and bovine serum albumin onto liposomes, showed greater stability and more controlled and sustained release of the encapsulated compound from mono- and double-layered coated liposomes, as compared to bare liposomes under simulated intestinal conditions (Liu et al. 2017). The release under simulated conditions was similar and limited from all studied nanoliposomes. The nanolaminated coating in liposomes overcomes the drawbacks associated with the dynamic nature of the lipid bilayer, such as rapid fusion and aggregation between liposomes and substrates when incorporated in food matrices.

Layer-by-layer deposition of polysaccharides (chitosan and alginate) onto liposomes also showed similar trend of controlled lipid digestibility and release of encapsulated compound as compared to bare nanoliposomes (Liu et al. 2013). Complexation of polysaccharides can reduce the porosity and decrease the leakage of the encapsulated ingredients more effectively than either alone.

## 9.5 FUTURE TRENDS AND PERSPECTIVES

Further research should assess the safety and potential side effects, since the biological fate of biomaterials is altered due to the smaller size in nanosystems. Indeed, although these nanosystems are made with food-grade ingredients, they might cause undesired effects such as transporting or depositing active ingredients or excipients in tissue that they are not supposed to, or enhancing the absorption of substances that they are not meant to transport, but that are present in the food matrix. In addition, optimization of bioavailability of bioactive compounds encapsulated in these bio-nanosystems could be achieved by use of reverse engineering approach. The use of more realistic and standardized *in vitro* digestion models will allow easier comparison across research laboratories for bioaccessibility results. One recent research evidenced the differences in particle size and bioaccessibility of β-carotene from SLNs after applying static or dynamic *in vitro* digestion models (Gomes et al. 2017). The more realistic dynamic digestion model resulted in lower bioaccessibility of the encapsulated β-carotene, however, provided more reliable data related to release of free fatty acids, as compared to the simpler static digestion model.

The confluence of pharmaceutical, nutrition, and colloid sciences with food engineering will be the key to unlock the full potential of bio-nanosystems containing bioactive compounds in food applications. Future trends in nano-delivery systems should concentrate on the interactions between food components and nanoformulations in food systems, as well as their fate within the GI tract, since there is very scarce work of digestion and uptake of nanosystems incorporated in food products.

## REFERENCES

Acosta, E. 2009. "Bioavailability of nanoparticles in nutrient and nutraceutical delivery." *Current Opinion in Colloid & Interface Science* 14 (1):3–15. doi:10.1016/j.cocis.2008.01.002.

Aditya, N. P., M. Shim, I. Lee, Y. Lee, M. H. Im, and S. Ko. 2013. "Curcumin and genistein coloaded nanostructured lipid carriers: In vitro digestion and antiprostate cancer activity." *Journal of Agricultural and Food Chemistry* 61 (8):1878–1883. doi:10.1021/jf305143k.

Ahmed, K., Y. Li, D. J. McClements, and H. Xiao. 2012. "Nanoemulsion- and emulsion-based delivery systems for curcumin: Encapsulation and release properties." *Food Chemistry* 132 (2):799–807. doi:10.1016/j.foodchem.2011.11.039.

Arunkumar, R., K. V. H. Prashanth, and V. Baskaran. 2013. "Promising interaction between nanoencapsulated lutein with low molecular weight chitosan: Characterization and bioavailability of lutein in vitro and in vivo." *Food Chemistry* 141 (1):327–337. doi:10.1016/j.foodchem.2013.02.108.

Bajka, B. H., N. M. Rigby, K. L. Cross, A. Macierzanka, and A. R. Mackie. 2015. "The influence of small intestinal mucus structure on particle transport *ex vivo*." *Colloids and Surfaces B-Biointerfaces* 135:73–80. doi:10.1016/j.colsurfb.2015.07.038.

Berton-Carabin, C. C., J. N. Coupland, and R. J. Elias. 2013. "Effect of the lipophilicity of model ingredients on their location and reactivity in emulsions and solid lipid nanoparticles." *Colloids and Surfaces A-Physicochemical and Engineering Aspects* 431:9–17. doi:10.1016/j.colsurfa.2013.04.016.

Bourbon, A. I., A. C. Pinheiro, M. A. Cerqueira, and A. A. Vicente. 2016. "Influence of chitosan coating on protein-based nanohydrogels properties and in vitro gastric digestibility." *Food Hydrocolloids* 60:109–118. doi:10.1016/j.foodhyd.2016.03.002.

Cerqueira, M. A., A. C. Pinheiro, H. D. Silva, P. E. Ramos, M. A. Azevedo, M. L. Flores-Lopez, M. C. Rivera, A. I. Bourbon, O. L. Ramos, and A. A. Vicente. 2014. "Design of bio-nanosystems for oral delivery of functional compounds." *Food Engineering Reviews* 6 (1–2):1–19. doi:10.1007/s12393-013-9074-3.

Chen, C. C., T. H. Tsai, Z. R. Huang, and J. Y. Fang. 2010. "Effects of lipophilic emulsifiers on the oral administration of lovastatin from nanostructured lipid carriers: Physicochemical characterization and pharmacokinetics." *European Journal of Pharmaceutics and Biopharmaceutics* 74 (3):474–482. doi:10.1016/j.ejpb.2009.12.008.

Chen, F. P., B. S. Li, and C. H. Tang. 2015. "Nanocomplexation between curcumin and soy protein isolate: Influence on curcumin stability/bioaccessibility and in vitro protein digestibility." *Journal of Agricultural and Food Chemistry* 63 (13):3559–3569. doi:10.1021/acs.jafc.5b00448.

Chen, F. P., S. Y. Ou, and C. H. Tang. 2016. "Core-shell soy protein-soy polysaccharide complex (Nano)particles as carriers for improved stability and sustained release of curcumin." *Journal of Agricultural and Food Chemistry* 64 (24):5053–5059. doi:10.1021/acs.jafc.6b01176.

Cohen, Y., M. Levi, U. Lesmes, M. Margier, E. Reboul, and Y. D. Livney. 2017b. "Re-assembled casein micelles improve in vitro bioavailability of vitamin D in a Caco-2 cell model." *Food & Function* 8 (6):2133–2141. doi:10.1039/c7fo00323d.

Cohen, Y., S. Ish-Shalom, E. Segal, O. Nudelman, A. Shpigelman, and Y. D. Livney. 2017a. "The bioavailability of vitamin D-3, a model hydrophobic nutraceutical, in casein micelles, as model protein nanoparticles: Human clinical trial results." *Journal of Functional Foods* 30:321–325. doi:10.1016/j.jff.2017.01.019.

Davidov-Pardo, G., S. Perez-Ciordia, M. R. Marin-Arroyo, and D. J. McClements. 2015. "Improving resveratrol bioaccessibility using biopolymer nanoparticles and complexes: Impact of protein-carbohydrate Maillard conjugation." *Journal of Agricultural and Food Chemistry* 63 (15):3915–3923. doi:10.1021/acs.jafc.5b00777.

Desai, M. P., V. Labhasetwar, G. L. Amidon, and R. J. Levy. 1996. "Gastrointestinal uptake of biodegradable microparticles: Effect of particle size." *Pharmaceutical Research* 13 (12):1838–1845. doi:10.1023/a:1016085108889.

Dey, T. K., S. Ghosh, M. Ghosh, H. Koley, and P. Dhar. 2012. "Comparative study of gastrointestinal absorption of EPA & DHA rich fish oil from nano and conventional emulsion formulation in rats." *Food Research International* 49 (1):72–79. doi:10.1016/j.foodres.2012.07.056.

Ensign, L. M., R. Cone, and J. Hanes. 2012. "Oral drug delivery with polymeric nanoparticles: The gastrointestinal mucus barriers." *Advanced Drug Delivery Reviews* 64 (6):557–570. doi:10.1016/j.addr.2011.12.009.

Evans, D. F., G. Pye, R. Bramley, A. G. Clark, T. J. Dyson, and J. D. Hardcastle. 1988. "Measurement of gastrointestinal pH profiles in normal ambulant human-subjects." *Gut* 29 (8):1035–1041. doi:10.1136/gut.29.8.1035.

Fang, M., Y. L. Jin, W. Bao, H. Gao, M. J. Xu, D. Wang, X. Wang, P. Yao, and L. G. Liu. 2012. "In vitro characterization and in vivo evaluation of nanostructured lipid curcumin carriers for intragastric administration." *International Journal of Nanomedicine* 7:5395–5404. doi:10.2147/Ijn. S36257.

Frenzel, M., E. Krolak, A. E. Wagner, and A. Steffen-Heins. 2015. "Physicochemical properties of WPI coated liposomes serving as stable transporters in a real food matrix." *LWT-Food Science and Technology* 63 (1):527–534. doi:10.1016/j.lwt.2015.03.055.

Gamboa, J. M., and K. W. Leong. 2013. "In vitro and in vivo models for the study of oral delivery of nanoparticles." *Advanced Drug Delivery Reviews* 65 (6):800–810. doi:10.1016/j.addr.2013.01.003.

Gomes, G. V. L., M. R. Sola, L. F. P. Marostegan, C. G. Jange, C. P. S. Cazado, A. C. Pinheiro, A. A. Vicente, and S. C. Pinho. 2017. "Physico-chemical stability and in vitro digestibility of beta-carotene-loaded lipid nanoparticles of cupuacu butter (Theobroma grandiflorum) produced by the phase inversion temperature (PIT) method." *Journal of Food Engineering* 192:93–102. doi:10.1016/j.jfoodeng.2016.08.001.

Gunness, N., J. Michiels, S. De Smet, L. Vanhaecke, O. Kravchuk, and M. Gidley. 2016. "Blood lipids—Soluble dietary fibres: Study of bile salts diffusion across intestinal mucosa using the Ussing chamber system." *Journal of Nutrition & Intermediary Metabolism* 4:35. doi:10.1016/j.jnim.2015.12.281.

Haham, M., S. Ish-Shalom, M. Nodelman, I. Duek, E. Segal, M. Kustanovich, and Y. D. Livney. 2012. "Stability and bioavailability of vitamin D nanoencapsulated in casein micelles." *Food & Function* 3 (7):737–744. doi:10.1039/c2fo10249h.

Hillgren, K. M., A. Kato, and R. T. Borchardt. 1995. "In-vitro systems for studying intestinal drug absorption." *Medicinal Research Reviews* 15 (2):83–109. doi:10.1002/med.2610150202.

Hu, B., M. H. Xie, C. Zhang, and X. X. Zeng. 2014. "Genipin-structured peptide-polysaccharide nanoparticles with significantly improved resistance to harsh gastrointestinal environments and their potential for oral delivery of polyphenols." *Journal of Agricultural and Food Chemistry* 62 (51):12443–12452. doi:10.1021/jf5046766.

Hu, B., X. X. Liu, C. L. Zhang, and X. X. Zeng. 2017. "Food macromolecule based nanodelivery systems for enhancing the bioavailability of polyphenols." *Journal of Food and Drug Analysis* 25 (1):3–15. doi:10.1016/j.jfda.2016.11.004.

Hu, X. W., W. F. Fan, Z. Yu, Y. Lu, J. P. Qi, J. Zhang, X. C. Dong, W. L. Zhao, and W. Wu. 2016. "Evidence does not support absorption of intact solid lipid nanoparticles via oral delivery." *Nanoscale* 8 (13):7024–7035. doi:10.1039/c5nr07474f.

Hussain, N., V. Jaitley, and A. T. Florence. 2001. "Recent advances in the understanding of uptake of microparticulates across the gastrointestinal lymphatics." *Advanced Drug Delivery Reviews* 50 (1–2):107–142. doi:10.1016/S0169-409x(01)00152-1.

Jodar-Reyes, A. B., A. Torcello-Gomez, M. Wulff-Perez, M. J. Galvez-Ruiz, and A. Martin-Rodriguez. 2010. "Different stability regimes of oil-in-water emulsions in the presence of bile salts." *Food Research International* 43 (6):1634–1641. doi:10.1016/j.foodres.2010.05.005.

Kalantzi, L., K. Goumas, V. Kalioras, B. Abrahamsson, J. B. Dressman, and C. Reppas. 2006. "Characterization of the human upper gastrointestinal contents under conditions simulating bioavailability/bioequivalence studies." *Pharmaceutical Research* 23 (1):165–176. doi:10.1007/s11095-005-8476-1.

Katouzian, I., and S. M. Jafari. 2016. "Nano-encapsulation as a promising approach for targeted delivery and controlled release of vitamins." *Trends in Food Science & Technology* 53:34–48. doi:10.1016/j.tifs.2016.05.002.

Kim, H. J., D. Huh, G. Hamilton, and D. E. Ingber. 2012. "Human gut-on-a-chip inhabited by microbial flora that experiences intestinal peristalsis-like motions and flow." *Lab on a Chip* 12 (12):2165–2174. doi:10.1039/c2lc40074j.

Lai, S. K., Y. Y. Wang, and J. Hanes. 2009. "Mucus-penetrating nanoparticles for drug and gene delivery to mucosal tissues." *Advanced Drug Delivery Reviews* 61 (2):158–171. doi:10.1016/j.addr.2008.11.002.

Lalush, I., H. Bar, I. Zakaria, S. Eichler, and E. Shimoni. 2005. "Utilization of amylose-lipid complexes as molecular nanocapsules for conjugated linoleic Acid." *Biomacromolecules* 6 (1):121–130. doi:10.1021/bm049644f.

Levinson, Y., S. Ish-Shalom, E. Segal, and Y. D. Livney. 2016. "Bioavailability, rheology and sensory evaluation of fat-free yogurt enriched with VD3 encapsulated in re-assembled casein micelles." *Food & Function* 7 (3):1477–1482. doi:10.1039/c5fo01111f.

Li, M., J. Cui, M. O. Ngadi, and Y. Ma. 2015. "Absorption mechanism of whey-protein-delivered curcumin using Caco-2 cell monolayers." *Food Chemistry* 180:48–54. doi:10.1016/j.foodchem.2015.01.132.

Liang, R., C. F. Shoemaker, X. Q. Yang, F. Zhong, and Q. R. Huang. 2013. "Stability and bioaccessibility of beta-carotene in nanoemulsions stabilized by modified starches." *Journal of Agricultural and Food Chemistry* 61 (6):1249–1257. doi:10.1021/jf303967f.

Liu, L., Y. H. Tang, C. Gao, Y. Y. Li, S. D. Chen, T. Xiong, J. Li, M. Du, Z. Y. Gong, H. Chen, L. G. Liu, and P. Yao. 2014. "Characterization and biodistribution in vivo of quercetin-loaded cationic nanostructured lipid carriers." *Colloids and Surfaces B-Biointerfaces* 115:125–131. doi:10.1016/j.colsurfb.2013.11.029.

Liu, W. L., J. H. Liu, W. Liu, T. Li, and C. M. Liu. 2013. "Improved physical and in vitro digestion stability of a polyelectrolyte delivery system based on layer-by-layer self-assembly alginate-chitosan-coated nanoliposomes." *Journal of Agricultural and Food Chemistry* 61 (17):4133–4144. doi:10.1021/jf305329n.

Liu, W. L., Y. Y. Kong, P. H. Tu, J. M. Lu, C. M. Liu, W. Liu, J. Z. Han, and J. H. Liu. 2017. "Physical-chemical stability and in vitro digestibility of hybrid nanoparticles based on the layer-by-layer assembly of lactoferrin and BSA on liposomes." *Food & Function* 8 (4):1688–1697. doi:10.1039/c7fo00308k.

Lundquist, P., and P. Artursson. 2016. "Oral absorption of peptides and nanoparticles across the human intestine: Opportunities, limitations and studies in human tissues." *Advanced Drug Delivery Reviews* 106:256–276. doi:10.1016/j.addr.2016.07.007.

Luo, Y. C., Z. Teng, and Q. Wang. 2012. "Development of zein nanoparticles coated with carboxymethyl chitosan for encapsulation and controlled release of vitamin D3." *Journal of Agricultural and Food Chemistry* 60 (3):836–843. doi:10.1021/jf204194z.

Macierzanka, A., A. R. Mackie, B. H. Bajka, N. M. Rigby, F. Nau, and D. Dupont. 2014. "Transport of particles in intestinal mucus under simulated infant and adult physiological conditions: Impact of mucus structure and extracellular DNA." *PLoS One* 9 (4). doi:10.1371/journal.pone.0095274.

Macierzanka, A., N. M. Rigby, A. P. Corfield, N. Wellner, F. Bottger, E. N. C. Mills, and A. R. Mackie. 2011. "Adsorption of bile salts to particles allows penetration of intestinal mucus." *Soft Matter* 7 (18):8077–8084. doi:10.1039/c1sm05888f.

Maldonado-Valderrama, J., P. Wilde, A. Macierzanka, and A. Mackie. 2011. "The role of bile salts in digestion." *Advances in Colloid and Interface Science* 165 (1):36–46. doi:10.1016/j.cis.2010.12.002.

McClements, D. J. 2010. "Design of nano-laminated coatings to control bioavailability of lipophilic food components." *Journal of Food Science* 75 (1):R30–R42. doi:10.1111/j.1750-3841.2009.01452.x.

McClements, D. J., E. A. Decker, Y. Park, and J. Weiss. 2009. "Structural design principles for delivery of bioactive components in nutraceuticals and functional foods." *Critical Reviews in Food Science and Nutrition* 49 (6):577–606. doi:10.1080/10408390902841529.

Minekus, M., M. Alminger, P. Alvito, S. Ballance, T. Bohn, C. Bourlieu, F. Carriere et al. 2014. "A standardised static in vitro digestion method suitable for food—An international consensus." *Food & Function* 5 (6):1113–1124. doi:10.1039/c3fo60702j.

Mulet-Cabero, A. I., N. M. Rigby, A. Brodkorb, and A. R. Mackie. 2017. "Dairy food structures influence the rates of nutrient digestion through different *in vitro* gastric behaviour." *Food Hydrocolloids* 67:63–73. doi:10.1016/j.foodhyd.2016.12.039.

Norris, D. A., and P. J. Sinko. 1997. "Effect of size, surface charge, and hydrophobicity on the translocation of polystyrene microspheres through gastrointestinal mucin." *Journal of Applied Polymer Science* 63 (11):1481–1492. doi:10.1002/(sici)1097-4628(19970314)63:11<1481::aid-app10>3.0.co;2-5.

Norris, D. A., N. Puri, and P. J. Sinko. 1998. "The effect of physical barriers and properties on the oral absorption of particulates." *Advanced Drug Delivery Reviews* 34 (2–3):135–154. doi:10.1016/s0169-409x(98)00037-4.

Otte, J., M. Zakora, K. B. Qvist, C. E. Olsen, and V. Barkholt. 1997. "Hydrolysis of bovine beta-lactoglobulin by various proteases and identification of selected peptides." *International Dairy Journal* 7 (12):835–848. doi:10.1016/S0958-6946(98)00003-X.

Ozturk, B., S. Argin, M. Ozilgen, and D. J. McClements. 2015. "Nanoemulsion delivery systems for oil-soluble vitamins: Influence of carrier oil type on lipid digestion and vitamin D-3 bioaccessibility." *Food Chemistry* 187:499–506. doi:10.1016/goodchem.2015.04.065.

Pade, V., and S. Stavchansky. 1997. "Estimation of the relative contribution of the transcellular and paracellular pathway to the transport of passively absorbed drugs in the Caco-2 cell culture model." *Pharmaceutical Research* 14 (9):1210–1215. doi:10.1023/A:1012111008617.

Pandita, D., S. Kumar, N. Poonia, and V. Lather. 2014. "Solid lipid nanoparticles enhance oral bioavailability of resveratrol, a natural polyphenol." *Food Research International* 62:1165–1174. doi:10.1016/j.foodres.2014.05.059.

Park, S. J., C. V. Garcia, G. H. Shin, and J. T. Kim. 2017. "Development of nanostructured lipid carriers for the encapsulation and controlled release of vitamin D3." *Food Chemistry* 225:213–219. doi:10.1016/j.foodchem.2017.01.015.

Pinheiro, A. C., M. Lad, H. D. Silva, M. A. Coimbra, M. Boland, and A. A. Vicente. 2013. "Unravelling the behaviour of curcumin nanoemulsions during in vitro digestion: Effect of the surface charge." *Soft Matter* 9 (11):3147–3154. doi:10.1039/c3sm27527b.

Qian, C., E. A. Decker, H. Xiao, and D. J. McClements. 2013. "Impact of lipid nanoparticle physical state on particle aggregation and beta-carotene degradation: Potential limitations of solid lipid nanoparticles." *Food Research International* 52 (1):342–349. doi:10.1016/j.foodres.2013.03.035.

Qiu, C. Y., B. Wang, Y. Wang, and Y. L. Teng. 2017. "Effects of colloidal complexes formation between resveratrol and deamidated gliadin on the bioaccessibility and lipid oxidative stability." *Food Hydrocolloids* 69:466–472. doi:10.1016/j.foodhyd.2017.02.020.

Ramalingam, P., S. W. Yoo, and Y. T. Ko. 2016. "Nanodelivery systems based on mucoadhesive polymer coated solid lipid nanoparticles to improve the oral intake of food curcumin." *Food Research International* 84:113–119. doi:10.1016/j.foodres.2016.03.031.

Righeschi, C., M. C. Bergonzi, B. Isacchi, C. Bazzicalupi, P. Gratteri, and A. R. Bilia. 2016. "Enhanced curcumin permeability by SLN formulation: The PAMPA approach." *LWT-Food Science and Technology* 66:475–483. doi:10.1016/j.lwt.2015.11.008.

Rowan, A. M., P. J. Moughan, M. N. Wilson, K. Maher, and C. Tasmanjones. 1994. "Comparison of the ileal and fecal digestibility of dietary amino-acids in adult humans and evaluation of the pig as a model animal for digestion studies in man." *British Journal of Nutrition* 71 (1):29–42. doi:10.1079/bjn19940108.

Salvia-Trujillo, L., C. Qian, O. Martin-Belloso, and D. J. McClements. 2013. "Influence of particle size on lipid digestion and beta-carotene bioaccessibility in emulsions and nanoemulsions." *Food Chemistry* 141 (2):1472–1480. doi:10.1016/j.foodchem.2013.03.050.

Sessa, M., M. L. Balestrieri, G. Ferrari, L. Servillo, D. Castaldo, N. D'Onofrio, F. Donsi, and R. Tsao. 2014. "Bioavailability of encapsulated resveratrol into nanoemulsion-based delivery systems." *Food Chemistry* 147:42–50. doi:10.1016/j.foodchem.2013.09.088.

Sessa, M., R. Tsao, R. H. Liu, G. Ferrari, and F. Donsi. 2011. "Evaluation of the stability and antioxidant activity of nanoencapsulated resveratrol during in vitro digestion." *Journal of Agricultural and Food Chemistry* 59 (23):12352–12360. doi:10.1021/jf2031346.

Shin, G. H., J. T. Kim, and H. J. Park. 2015. "Recent developments in nanoformulations of lipophilic functional foods." *Trends in Food Science & Technology* 46 (1):144–157. doi:10.1016/j.tifs.2015.07.005.

Shin, G. H., S. K. Chung, J. T. Kim, H. J. Joung, and H. J. Park. 2013. "Preparation of chitosan-coated nanoliposomes for improving the mucoadhesive property of curcumin using the ethanol injection method." *Journal of Agricultural and Food Chemistry* 61 (46):11119–11126. doi:10.1021/jf4035404.

Shukla, S. K., A. K. Mishra, O. A. Arotiba, and B. B. Mamba. 2013. "Chitosan-based nanomaterials: A state-of-the-art review." *International Journal of Biological Macromolecules* 59:46–58. doi:10.1016/j.ijbiomac.2013.04.043.

Somchue, W., W. Sermsri, J. Shiowatana, and A. Siripinyanond. 2009. "Encapsulation of alpha-tocopherol in protein-based delivery particles." *Food Research International* 42 (8):909–914. doi:10.1016/j.foodres.2009.04.021.

Takahashi, M., S. Uechi, K. Takara, Y. Asikin, and K. Wada. 2009. "Evaluation of an oral carrier system in rats: Bioavailability and antioxidant properties of liposome-encapsulated curcumin." *Journal of Agricultural and Food Chemistry* 57 (19):9141–9146. doi:10.1021/jf9013923.

Tamjidi, F., M. Shahedi, J. Varshosaz, and A. Nasirpour. 2013. "Nanostructured lipid carriers (NLC): A potential delivery system for bioactive food molecules." *Innovative Food Science & Emerging Technologies* 19:29–43. doi:10.1016/j.ifset.2013.03.002.

Tan, C., J. H. Xie, X. M. Zhang, J. B. Cai, and S. Q. Xia. 2016. "Polysaccharide-based nanoparticles by chitosan and gum arabic polyelectrolyte complexation as carriers for curcumin." *Food Hydrocolloids* 57:236–245. doi:10.1016/j.foodhyd.2016.01.021.

Tan, C., Y. T. Zhang, S. Abbas, B. Feng, X. M. Zhang, and S. Q. Xia. 2014. "Modulation of the carotenoid bioaccessibility through liposomal encapsulation." *Colloids and Surfaces B-Biointerfaces* 123:692–700. doi:10.1016/j.colsurfb.2014.10.011.

Teng, Z., Y. C. Luo, and Q. Wang. 2013. "Carboxymethyl chitosan-soy protein complex nanoparticles for the encapsulation and controlled release of vitamin D-3." *Food Chemistry* 141 (1):524–532. doi:10.1016/j.foodchem.2013.03.043.

Teng, Z., Y. Li, and Q. Wang. 2014. "Insight into curcumin-loaded beta-lactoglobulin nanoparticles: Incorporation, particle disintegration, and releasing profiles." *Journal of Agricultural and Food Chemistry* 62 (35):8837–8847. doi:10.1021/jf503199g.

Tokle, T., Y. Y. Mao, and D. J. McClements. 2013. "Potential biological fate of emulsion-based delivery systems: Lipid particles nanolaminated with lactoferrin and beta-lactoglobulin coatings." *Pharmaceutical Research* 30 (12):3200–3213. doi:10.1007/s11095-013-1003-x.

Trapani, A., A. Lopedota, M. Franco, N. Cioffi, E. Ieva, M. Garcia-Fuentes, and M. J. Alonso. 2010. "A comparative study of chitosan and chitosan/cyclodextrin nanoparticles as potential carriers for the oral delivery of small peptides." *European Journal of Pharmaceutics and Biopharmaceutics* 75 (1):26–32. doi:10.1016/j.ejpb.2010.01.010.

Verhoeckx, K., P. Cotter, I. López-Expósito, C. Kleiveland, T. Lea, A. Mackie, T. Requena, D. Swiatecka, and H. Wichers, eds. 2015. *The Impact of Food Bioactives on Health: In Vitro and ex vivo Models*. Cham, Germany: Springer International Publishing.

Xia, Z. Y., D. J. McClements, and H. Xiao. 2017. "Influence of lipid content in a corn oil preparation on the bioaccessibility of beta-carotene: A comparison of low-fat and high-fat samples." *Journal of Food Science* 82 (2):373–379. doi:10.1111/1750-3841.13599.

Xue, J., C. Tan, X. M. Zhang, B. Feng, and S. Q. Xia. 2014. "Fabrication of epigallocatechin-3-gallate nanocarrier based on glycosylated casein: Stability and interaction mechanism." *Journal of Agricultural and Food Chemistry* 62 (20):4677–4684. doi:10.1021/jf405157x.

Yang, T. S., T. T. Liu, and H. I. Liu. 2017. "Effects of aroma compounds and lipid composition on release of functional substances encapsulated in nanostructured lipid carriers lipolyzed by lipase." *Food Hydrocolloids* 62:280–287. doi:10.1016/j.foodhyd.2016.08.019.

Yi, J., T. I. Lam, W. Yokoyama, L. W. Cheng, and F. Zhong. 2015. "Beta-carotene encapsulated in food protein nanoparticles reduces peroxyl radical oxidation in Caco-2 cells." *Food Hydrocolloids* 43:31–40. doi:10.1016/j.foodhyd.2014.04.028.

# 10 Mechanism of Action and Toxicological Profile of Essential Oils in Foodstuff

*Raquel Vieira, Ana C. Fortuna, Amélia M. Silva, Selma B. Souto, and Eliana B. Souto*

## CONTENTS



## 10.1 INTRODUCTION

Essential oils (EOs) played for a long time an important role in human history, since there are numerous documentations about their use in different locations, from India (5000 BC) to Mesopotamia or Greece (3000 BC), as food flavors and additives, medicines, aphrodisiacs, and cosmetics (Dima and Dima 2015).

An essential oil is defined by International Standards Organization as "a product obtained from vegetable raw material, either by distillation with water or steam, from the epicarp of citrus fruits by a mechanical process, or by dry distillation" (Dima and Dima 2015, Turek and Stintzing 2013). In turn, the European Pharmacopeia (7th edition) gives a more complete definition of an EO, defining it as an "odorant product, generally of a complex composition, obtained from a botanically defined plant raw material, either by driving by steam of water, by dry distillation or by a suitable mechanical method without heating; it is usually separated from the aqueous phase by a physical method that does not lead to significant change in its chemical composition" (El Asbahani et al. 2015).

EOs' constituents are highly volatile secondary plant metabolites, extracted either from flowers (rose, jasmine, lavender, and violet) or herbs (e.g., basil, cilantro, lemongrass), buds (e.g., clove), leaves (eucalyptus, thyme, salvia), fruits (e.g., star anise, anis), twigs, bark (cinnamon), zest (citrus), seeds (cardamom), wood (sandal), roots (ginger), and rhizome, by several different extraction methods (Dima and Dima 2015, El Asbahani et al. 2015, Turek and Stintzing 2013). There can be used either: (i) conventional or classical methods, such as hydrodistillation, entrainment by water steam (vapor-hydrodistillation and vapor-distillation/steam distillation), organic solvent extraction, and cold pressing—all of them based on water distillation by heating to recover EOs from plant matrix or (ii) advanced or innovative methods, such as supercritical fluid extraction, subcritical extraction liquids ($H_2$ and $CO_2$), extraction with subcritical $CO_2$, ultrasound assisted extraction of EOs, microwave assisted extraction, solvent free microwave extraction, microwave hydrodiffusion and gravity, microwave steam distillation, microwave steam diffusion, and instant control pressure drop—aiming to reduce extraction time, energy consumption, $CO_2$ emissions and solvent use, to increase the extraction yield, to improve EOs' quality, and finally to overcome EOs' components' inherent thermolability, thus trying to avoid chemical alterations, namely, hydrolysis, isomerization, and oxidation when applying high temperatures (Dima and Dima 2015, El Asbahani et al. 2015).

Representing a small portion of 5% of the vegetal plant dry matter after extraction, these oily aromatic liquids may contain more than 100 different constituents, in ratios ranging from 1% to 70% (Dima and Dima 2015, El Asbahani et al. 2015). The EOs' constituents may be grouped in two main families: (i) those from terpene origin, mainly monoterpenes (e.g., acyclic, monocyclic, or bicyclic terpenes, which are synthesized by monoterpene synthases using an intermediate of HMG-CoA reductase pathway, geranyl pyrophosphate, as substrate) and sesquiterpenes (e.g., acyclic, monocyclic, or bicyclic terpenes constituted by three isoprene units), which may suffer oxidation and/or rearrangement leading, respectively, to monoterpenoids and sesquiterpenoids formation, and thus comprising alcohols, aldehydes, carbures, ketones, esters, ethers, peroxides and phenols and (ii) aromatic compounds, which occur less frequently and comprise aldehydes, alcohol, phenols, methoxy derivatives, and ethylene dioxy compounds (Dima and Dima 2015, El Asbahani et al. 2015, Llana-Ruiz-Cabello et al. 2015, Patel and Gogna 2015). Terpene family members follow the isoprene rule which states that each terpenoid may be constituted by isoprene units ($C_5H_8$), mostly in a head-to-tail fashion, either directly or by means of cyclization, rearrangements, or further conversions from aliphatic isoprenoid precursors (Turek and Stintzing 2013). It is important to notice that EO composition depends on several factors, mainly, the species and subspecies of the extracted plant, its geographic location, cultivation method, vegetative stage, growing season, harvest time, extraction techniques, and processing methods (Dima and Dima 2015, Llana-Ruiz-Cabello et al. 2015).

The above-mentioned components of EOs are synthetized by means of three different pathways: (i) methyl-erythritol pathway, for both mono- and diterpenes, (ii) mevalonate pathway, for sesquiterpenes, and (iii) shikimic acid pathway, for aromatic phenylpropanoids (Dima and Dima 2015, El Asbahani et al. 2015, Turek and Stintzing 2013). After their biosynthesis in specialized secretory glandules—present either at plant surface and having an exogenous secretion or inside the plant and thus having an endogenous secretion—EOs are accumulated and stored, thus remaining protected against external factors (e.g., light, heat, moisture, and oxidation) until their release as consequence of a mechanical action or humidity variation, promoting their tearing (El Asbahani et al. 2015).

The major chemical components of EOs are responsible either for: (i) their physicochemical properties—low density compounds with an hydrophobic nature, soluble in organic solvents, and immiscible with water, (ii) their different biological properties (e.g., antibacterial, antifungal, anticancer, antiviral, antimutagenic, antiprotozoal, anti-inflammatory, antidiabetic, and antioxidant activities), which can be explored in order to use EOs for instance in pharmaceutical and food industries (e.g., active packaging to enhance foodstuff shelf life), and finally (iii) their toxicological profile, which may lead to undesirable side effects when using EOs for medical treatments or, on the other hand, lead to a desirable cytotoxicity in case of chemotherapeutic drugs (Dima and Dima 2015, Llana-Ruiz-Cabello et al. 2015).

Since EOs represent a "green" alternative to foodstuff, pharmaceutical, medical, cosmetic, perfume, and agriculture industries, there are great efforts in order to overcome some physicochemical and toxicological related issues, such as their high sensitivity to oxygen, light, temperature and pH, high lipophilicity, and some toxicity reported (Dima and Dima 2015, Turek and Stintzing 2013). Mechanisms are also being developed aiming to protect EOs during storage, transport, and processing, with encapsulation playing the major role in this new approach (Dima and Dima 2015, Turek and Stintzing 2013). EOs may thus be incorporated in several controlled delivery systems, namely, polymeric particles, liposomes, solid lipid nanoparticles (SLNs), nanostructured lipid carriers (NLCs), and nanoemulsions (El Asbahani et al. 2015).

In this chapter, special attention is given to the properties of essential oils and their increasing use in both food industry and medicine, to EOs toxicological profile, and to new controlled delivery systems developed to overcome some issues related to EOs physicochemical properties and reported toxicological effects.

## 10.2 *IN VIVO* AND *IN VITRO* ASSAYS

Essential oils have been increasingly integrated in numerous *in vitro* and *in vivo* assays in order to further investigate their physicochemical properties, biological activities, mechanisms of action, and toxicological profile. General toxicity assays intend to detect testing substance biological activity (Ekwall et al. 1990). While *in silico* and *in vitro* models are constantly being developed and refined, *in vivo* preclinical safety models remain the preferred assessing human risk assays, and they must: (i) use low compound concentrations, (ii) provide rapid results allowing decision-making and clinical efforts, and (iii) be flexible and provide relevant results to develop a plan for each target, drug class, or indication (Fielden and Kolaja 2008).

Since long ago that animal testing remains the gold standard method to assess toxicity of agrochemicals, cosmetics, industrial chemicals, and pharmaceuticals (Pereira and Tettamanti 2012). After identified specific organ or cell targets, there will be performed some *in vitro* studies, mostly in cell cultures and whose results may only be considered as exploratory, and then complementary *in vivo* studies must be performed, ideally either in animal models (most frequently rodents) and humans (rare) (Fischer and Chan 2007). The obtained results must not be assumed as a trustworthy transposal of the same cells behavior in the organ *in situ*, thus remaining a poor correlation between *in vivo* and *in vitro* events (Ekwall et al. 1990, Fischer and Chan 2007). As such, *in vitro* assays require an *in vivo* validation to be considered as reliable (Fischer and Chan 2007). Furthermore, some biological defense mechanisms, such as immunoregulatory events, only occur in their natural state, thus being difficult to replicate those biological processes in experimental models (Fischer and Chan 2007). Thus, no single test is capable to display all the possibilities of leading to genotoxic effects (Cartus and Schrenk 2017).

Although rarely performed, both *in vitro* and *in vivo* toxicological assays are extremely important for EOs evaluation before getting available to consumers. As such, standard regulatory genotoxicity tests, including two or three validated tests having at least one *in vitro* test in bacteria and one *in vitro* test on cell cultures, should be performed (Cartus and Schrenk 2017). Furthermore, being aware of the main mechanisms behind genotoxicity would allow a better understanding of the *in vivo* situation relevance level, as well as the assess to any gene point mutation and structural or numerical chromosomal aberrations induction (Cartus and Schrenk 2017). For example, food and feed safety assessment or human drugs current strategies recommend the achievement of both the Ames and an *in vitro* test on mammalian cells (e.g., micronucleus test) (Cartus and Schrenk 2017). Even when there is an evidence of assays complementarity, they still remain theoretical and limited at many levels, namely, deficiencies, lack of relevance, inadequacies, bias, and wrong interpretation (Cartus and Schrenk 2017).

After toxin exposure, there can be defined some toxicity index markers: morphological alterations (in cell layers or in monolayers shape), cell growth alterations, cellular viability (staining), lethality index (comparing the counted dead and vital cells with control), and biochemical or metabolic cell alterations measurement (enzyme release from cytosol, glycogen metabolism, beating rate in myocytes, phagocytosis, etc.) (Ekwall et al. 1990).

Hence, it is expected that these toxicological studies, both animal *in vivo* assays and clinical trials in humans, get increasingly performance and applied to the EOs recently thought to play a very important role in several health conditions management, foodstuff flavoring, and shelf life improvement, among many others.

## 10.3 TOXICOLOGICAL PROFILE AND SHELF LIFE

Since there has been observed an increasing interest of consumers in EOs' properties and their use as new natural approaches mostly in pharmacological and food industries, it is important to ensure their safety (Turek and Stintzing 2013). A tight regulatory legislation is thus currently in force: the Association Française de Normalisation, the European Federation of Essential Oils, and International Standards Organization are responsible for EOs' physical standards specification; the International Fragrance Association, the "Bundesinstitut für Risikobewertung," the Research Institute for Fragrance Materials, and the Scientific Committee on Consumer's Safety are, in turn, the regulators of the maximum quantities and uses of either EOs and their single constituents; the National or International Pharmacopoeias are responsible for the evaluation of medical usage of EOs; and finally, the United States Food and Drug Administration regulates the EOs dietary intake, defining which EOs are generally considered as safe (Turek and Stintzing 2013). A thorough evaluation of EOs' behavior during transport and storage (including their susceptibility to conversion and degradation, and the integrity of their constituents after exposure to several environment factors) is truly necessary (Dima and Dima 2015, Turek and Stintzing 2013).

Sharing a close structural relationship within the same chemical group, EOs' constituents may be rapidly converted into each other by means of several enzymatically or chemically triggered reactions, namely, oxidation, isomerization, cyclization, and dehydrogenation, once they are no longer on plant matrix protective compartments (Turek and Stintzing 2013). For instance, terpenoids are so volatile and thermolabile that easily suffer oxidation or hydrolysis, furthermore, there were also observed viscosity alterations and autoxidation processes (Turek and Stintzing 2013). The latter contribute to terpenoids deterioration, leading to the formation of: (i) primary autoxidation products, such as hydroperoxides, which are reported to suffer decomposition when exposed to light, heat, or low pH; and (ii) stable oxidized secondary products, namely, alcohols, aldehydes, ketones, epoxides, and peroxides (Turek and Stintzing 2013). Most frequently than imagined, secondary oxidation products share an unknown structure (Turek and Stintzing 2013).

Thus, there may be considered some determinant factors for essential oils' stability: (i) light—both ultraviolet and visible light accelerate autoxidation processes (by the production of alkyl radicals), promotes faster EOs' compositional changes (e.g., it accelerates monoterpenes degradation) and enhances photo-oxidation (a second-line oxidative pathway); (ii) temperature—while elevated temperatures promote chemical reactions acceleration (in such a way that a rise of 10°C doubles reactions rate), lower temperatures promote oxygen solubilization in liquids (negative effect on EOs' stability); (iii) oxygen availability—EO oxidation is accelerated by higher dissolved oxygen concentration (which is dependent on oxygen partial pressure and environmental temperature), and oxygen solubility is higher at lower temperatures; (iv) metal contaminants—resulting from distillation or storage in metallic containers, these metals (mostly copper and ferrous iron) enhance autoxidation reactions, especially in the presence of hydroperoxides; (v) water content—moisture is a possible cause of EO spoilage, and it is recommended to dry the oils after distillation (adding water-binding substances); and finally (vi) compound structure and chemical composition—e.g., allylic hydrogen-rich compounds are most frequently target of autoxidation (since hydrogen atom abstraction promotes resonance-stabilized radicals with lower activation energy), polyunsaturated terpenic hydrocarbons easily suffer oxidative deterioration (form radicals stabilized by either conjugated double-bonds or isomerization to tertiary radicals), and electron-donating groups, as well as alkyl substitution, promote strong carbon-peroxide bonds, thus increasing the stability of hydroperoxides (Turek and Stintzing 2013). It is important to note that these findings vary among plant species (Turek and Stintzing 2013). Terpenoids are particularly sensitive substances, since they are thermolabile and susceptible to high temperature-occurring rearrangement processes. For this reason, a four-group classification has been proposed for thermal oxidative reactions leading to terpenes degradation: double-bond cleavage, epoxidation, dehydrogenation (into aromatic compounds), and allylic oxidation (producing alcohols, ketones, and aldehydes) (Turek and Stintzing 2013). Furthermore, isolated terpenes have also demonstrated an increase in refractive index, relative density, viscosity, and oxygen consumption during the oxidation process evolution (Turek and Stintzing 2013). Several toxicological studies must be thus performed in order to evaluate mutagenicity and genotoxicity of essential oils or even their isolated constituents (Llana-Ruiz-Cabello et al. 2015, Raut and Karuppayil 2014).

When in contact with a cell, EOs may have several targets, being cytoplasmic membrane the first one: it can be disrupted and suffer permeabilization, thus leading to cellular function loss (such as ion homeostasis and electron transport chain) and also cell death by either necrosis and apoptosis (Raut and Karuppayil 2014). In this manner, EOs' constituents, mainly alcohols, aldehydes, and phenols, may be considered as responsible for several cytotoxic effects, which represent a new approach in chemotherapy drugs (Raut and Karuppayil 2014). On the other hand, these cytotoxicity promote undesirable side effects, such as corrosiveness, irritation, cellular sensitization, percutaneous absorption, phototoxicity, multiorgan acute toxicity, carcinogenicity, and teratogenicity, which lead to a limited use of these natural occurring compounds in medicine or food industry (Raut and Karuppayil 2014).

Although complicated taking into account the huge variability in EOs' composition and the affecting environmental factors, it remains relevant to do a toxicity profiling for each known EO or at least for selected major isolated constituents (Raut and Karuppayil 2014). Most of the available toxicity studies consist of case reports or animal studies where there was calculated LD50 for a particular EO or a specific isolated constituent (Raut and Karuppayil 2014). For example, it is known for a long time that ketone terpenoids share great toxic effects: estragole and methyl-isoeugenol have demonstrated carcinogenic effect (causing DNA mutation in mice); pulegone and menthofuran promoted hepatotoxicity in mice; limonene was responsible for hepatotoxicity in mice (after either oral and peritoneal administration); nephrotoxicity and carcinogenic effects in male rats; phototoxicity in both rats and rabbits; and finally teratogenic effects for rabbit and mouse (Raut and Karuppayil 2014). The obtained results from these toxicological studies cannot be linearly transposed to humans and also the dosages must be carefully studied, since there are several reported variations among different species and also within the same species and even a small error in concentrations calculation may be lethal (Raut and Karuppayil 2014). There have been observed toxicity in humans in cases of skin exposure to EOs, accidental ingestion, industrial products exposure, and controlled cutaneous toxicity clinical trials (Raut and Karuppayil 2014). Only a few of known EOs and their constituents had demonstrated human toxicity effects, when administrated in high concentration: citral caused necrosis and vacuolization of the eukaryotic cells; limonene promoted diarrhea and transient proteinuria; thujone, pulegone, β-asarone, and allylisocyanate have also reported toxic effects; 1,8-cineole, fenchone, pulegone, camphor, and thujone are lead to hepatic necrosis, convulsions, ataxia, dementia, and hallucinations; clove, coriander, melissa, origanum, summer savoury, tea tree, thyme, and turpentine oils acted as irritants; bergamot, cumin, grape fruit, lime, and orange oils demonstrated phototoxicity; calamus, croton, basil, nutmeg, and rose oils have proven to be carcinogenic either in humans and rodents; palmarosa, citronella, lemongrass, and vetiver oils demonstrated to induce both cytotoxicity and genotoxicity in human lymphocytes; and finally Spanish sage, dill seed, savin, worm wood, anise, fennel, nutmeg, and rosemary oils revealed to be toxic during pregnancy (thus contraindicated to fertile age women) (Raut and Karuppayil 2014). In contrast, if administered at low concentrations, no significant EOs' adverse effects were observed, and these oils may be considered as safe for human consumption (Raut and Karuppayil 2014). As such, it is recommended a careful evaluation of the dosage, route of administration, target consumer, major EOs' constituents, and their toxicological profile (Raut and Karuppayil 2014).

In food industry, for instance, the international organizations United States Food and Drug Administration, Codex Alimentarium, Food Chemical Codex, the Flavor and Extract Manufactures Association, the International Organization of Flavor Industries, and finally the Council of Europe not only tightly regulate which of the known existing EOs may be used by consumers as also guarantee that the norms are fulfilled (Dima and Dima 2015). Among the 160 essential oils generally recognized as safe by United States Food and Drug Administration, cinnamon, citrus, clove, coriander, lemongrass, oregano, pimento, rosemary, sage, and thyme oils are the most commonly used in food industry (Dima and Dima 2015). As flavoring agents, European countries have approved carvacrol, carvone, cinnamaldehyde, citral, eugenol, limonene, linalool, menthol, p-cymene, thymol, and vanillin oils and, on the other hand, removed estragole and methyl-eurenol from the safe list (Dima and Dima 2015, Llana-Ruiz-Cabello et al. 2015).

Furthermore, there were established three classes of toxic EOs' constituents: (i) class I—low toxicity compounds, that do not need special investigation since they belong to the fifth percentile of no-observed-effect levels of 3.0 mg/Kg/day; (ii) class II—less harmless compounds (compared to those from first class), that do not demonstrate major suspicious toxicity effects belonging to the fifth percentile of no-observed-effect levels of 0.91 mg/Kg/day; and (iii) class III—significant toxicity compounds, having reported a decreased safety of the EO, they are of the highest interest for further investigation studies and at the fifth percentile of no-observed-effect levels of 0.15 mg/Kg/day. The unidentified compounds belong to this last class (Baser and Buchbauer 2010, Dima and Dima 2015).

Because of the ongoing changes in worldwide market and consumer habits, one of the greatest concerns of food industry is the need to respond to daily demands in retail and distribution offering thereby long-term stable and improved products (Llana-Ruiz-Cabello et al. 2015). One of the possible approaches to improve the long-term stability of foodstuff is the development of the so-called "active packaging." Active food contact materials, which aim either to extend the foodstuff shelf life or to improve packaged food conditions, are designed as a packaging matrix that is able to incorporate components that will in turn release or absorb several substances into the food surrounding microenvironment (Llana-Ruiz-Cabello et al. 2015). These components may be either synthetic or natural compounds, but since consumers are increasingly interested in "biological products," there remains a current effort in integrating preferentially essential oils other than synthetic preservatives in packaging matrices (Llana-Ruiz-Cabello et al. 2015). The major problem is that, unlike Japan, United States, and Australia, which had already implemented this new technology, European countries have no currently published regulatory legislation about EOs' use in active packaging, while decisions are mainly guided by the European Food Safety Authority opinion about each and every substance (Llana-Ruiz-Cabello et al. 2015). Further research is still needed on food contact materials, especially the safety profile of EOs when loaded in nanoparticles (Llana-Ruiz-Cabello et al. 2015).

EOs may suffer degradation, resulting in unpleasant and pungent flavors, shifting colors, or changes in consistency (Turek and Stintzing 2013). This could be avoided or delayed by this "active packaging," since EOs demonstrated antimicrobial, antioxidant, and antimutagenic or antitoxinogenic properties (Llana-Ruiz-Cabello et al. 2015). As mentioned above, regarding EOs that reported mutagenicity or genotoxicity (even minimal), and having the consumers a higher exposure to these substances with "active packaging," further studies must be performed to: (i) establish the effective and safe concentrations of EOs; (ii) assess their mutagenic or genotoxic potential; (iii) identify possible toxic constituents; and (iv) develop a complete risk/benefit profile of EOs use in food industry (Llana-Ruiz-Cabello et al. 2015).

## 10.4 CLINICAL ADVANCES ON THE USE OF ESSENTIAL OILS

As mentioned in the previous sections, natural occurring essential oils and their constituents had become *gold standard* future approaches in several fields, especially in medicine, pharmaceutical, and food industries, regarding their below-mentioned great variety of biological properties (Raut and Karuppayil 2014).

### 10.4.1 Antibacterial Activity

Nowadays, a great number of infections are not properly eradicated since there has been observed an increase in resistant strains, drug-resistant microorganisms incidence, and number of immunodepressed individuals (Raut and Karuppayil 2014). Also, several adverse effects related to prolonged use of antibacterial agents have been increasingly reported (Raut and Karuppayil 2014). As such, novel antibacterial agents against infectious diseases must be developed (Raut and Karuppayil 2014). EOs extracted from plants seem to be a great and natural option, since they demonstrated large spectrum inhibitory activity against several Gram-positive and -negative pathogens (Raut and Karuppayil 2014). For instance, bay, cinnamon, clove, lemon grass, lemon-myrtle, oregano, rosewood, tea-tree, and thyme oils are considered the most potent antimicrobial agents, exerting their biological activity at concentrations <1% v/v; manuka, sandalwood, and vetiver oils are very potent in Gram-positive bacteria and almost no action on Gram-negative; bay, clove, lemongrass, oregano, and thyme are active against *Escherichia coli*; bay, clove, lemongrass, peppermint, rosemary, and thyme oils acted on *Staphylococcus aureus* at lower concentrations (≤0.05% v/v) than basil and eucalyptus oils (1 % v/v); and garlic, lemon myrtle, and tea-tree oils play an important role against methicillin resistant *Staphylococcus aureus* (Raut and Karuppayil 2014). Until now, *Pseudomonas aeruginosa* is the only microorganism tolerant to plant EOs' action (Raut and Karuppayil 2014). Although only in a few cases, it may be observed better antibacterial activity from major constituent molecule of the oils compared to the particular EO itself, as it happens either with carvacrol and eugenol from clove oil or terpinen-4-ol from tea-tree oil (Raut and Karuppayil 2014). Phenolics and aldehydes exhibited more potent antibacterial effects than other EOs' constituents or the particular EO (Raut and Karuppayil 2014).

To play their antimicrobial role, EOs or isolated compounds may act by several mechanisms: primarily, since they are highly lipophilic, EOs promote membrane destabilization, thus penetrating through the bacteria cell wall and membrane and then acting with their components, namely, phospholipids, polysaccharides, and free fatty acids. This increases the bacterial membrane permeability which, in turn, leads to several ion and cellular contents loss and, even to cell death. Simultaneously, EOs also decrease cellular viability when interfering with proton pumps activity, affecting membrane integrity and promoting cellular contents leakage. Moreover, they may act by denaturating cytoplasmic proteins and inactivating cellular enzymes, thus contributing to bacterial cell death (Raut and Karuppayil 2014). Nevertheless, it must be taken into account that this bactericidal effect may vary either among oils and bacterial family (Raut and Karuppayil 2014).

### 10.4.2 Antifungal Activity

Human pathogenic fungi (eukaryote) are very similar to their hosts at both molecular and cellular levels (Raut and Karuppayil 2014). Many opportunistic fungi, particularly *Aspergillus* spp., *Candida* spp., and *Cryptococcus* spp., became of a great concern, mainly to immunocompromised patients (Raut and Karuppayil 2014). Moreover, there are only a few antifungal successful agents, several drug resistant strains, associated biofilm infections, and adverse effects of those prescribed drugs, making it difficult to either prevent or treat these infections, thus contributing to elevated morbidity and mortality rates (Raut and Karuppayil 2014). Fortunately, it has been demonstrated that several plant and human pathogenic fungi (including yeasts) are sensitive to EOs' action, always depending on the target organisms and the tested oil (Raut and Karuppayil 2014). For instance, in a broad way, *Cymbopogon*. spp had demonstrated promising activities against yeasts; cinnamon, clove, geranium, gingergrass, Japanese mint, lemongrass, and mint oils act effectively against *Candida albicans*; phenylpropanoids-rich oils (such as eugenol) and monocyclic sesquiterpene alcohols (such as α-bisabolol) have demonstrated to inhibit dermatophytes growth and their spore development. EOs are able to reduce growth and aflatoxin production in molds (such as *Aspergillus flavus*); lemongrass oil is effective against filamentous fungi; grapefruit, lemon, mandarin, and orange oils inhibit *Aspergillus niger*, *Aspergillus flavus*, *Penicillium verrucosum*, and *Penicillium chrysogenum* fungi; while EOs rich in terpenoids are able to inhibit both drug resistant yeast and *Candida albicans*, the major fungi pathogen in humans (Raut and Karuppayil 2014).

All this above-mentioned EOs' antifungal activities are mediated by several possible mechanisms of action: (i) membrane ergosterol and signaling hyphae morphogenesis pathways inhibition in yeast; (ii) cell cycle inhibitory effects (e.g., citral, citronellol, geraniol, and geranylacetate have shown to block S phase of *Candida albicans* cell cycle; (iii) alteration of membrane fluidity, leading to cytoplasmic contents leakage and fungi loss of viability (e.g., tea tree oil prevention of membrane permeability and respiratory chain activity in *Candida albicans*, leading to cell death); (iv) apoptosis and necrosis when EOs enhance permeation of fungi mitochondrial membranes; (v) interfering in TOR signaling pathways, contributing to yeast loss of viability; and (vi) affecting $Ca^{2+}$ and $H^+$ homeostasis, thus promoting ion loss and fungi activity inhibition (e.g., carvacrol, eugenol and thymol oils action against *Saccharomyces cerevisiae*) (Raut and Karuppayil 2014).

### 10.4.3 Antiviral Activity

Antiviral properties of EOs are attributed to the presence of monoterpene, sesquiterpene, and phenylpropanoid constituents in plants (Raut and Karuppayil 2014). For example, eucalyptus and thyme oils play an inhibitory effect against herpes virus; tea tree oil (*Melaleuca alternifolia*) is very useful in recurrent herpetic infections, since it affects viral envelope structures, thus preventing both adsorption and entry of virus into the host cells. Oregano oil is active against yellow fever virus and also a good agent in disrupting viral envelope structures; German chamomile, isoborneol (viral proteins glycosylation inhibitor), lemon balm, manuka, pine, santolina, and tea tree oils have shown promising effects against HSV-1 (and some of them also against HSV-2, with lower $IC_{50}$ associated). Some EOs such as those from lignans, containing threo-4,4′-dihydroxy-3-methoxylignan, (–)-dihydroguaiaretic acid, talaumidin, 4′-hydroxy-3,3′,4-trimethoxylignan, 3,3′,4,4′-tetramethoxylignan, 4,4′-diacetyl-3,3′-dimethoxylignan, hinokinin, (–)-dihydrocubebin, and heliobuphthalmin, were reported to inhibit cytomegalovirus gene expression thus preventing viral activation (Pusztai et al. 2010, Raut and Karuppayil 2014).

### 10.4.4 Antiprotozoal Activity

Nowadays, protozoal infections still represent a major public health problem (Raut and Karuppayil 2014). Chagas disease (*Trypanosoma cruzi*), amoebiasis (*Entamoeba histolytica*), leishmaniasis (*Leishmania* spp.), giardiasis (*Giardia lamblia*), trichomoniasis (*Trichomonas vaginalis*), and malaria (*Plasmodium* spp.) are the most common (Raut and Karuppayil 2014). Since there are many reported adverse effects, drug resistance, and a current need for a prolonged use of the available antiprotozoal drugs, there remains a great need for an alternative therapy (Raut and Karuppayil 2014). Several EOs have been revealed as effective antiprotozoal agents (Raut and

Karuppayil 2014). Some recently performed studies showed that: *Lippia alba*, *Nepeta cataria*, and oregano oils promote cell lysis, thus inhibiting its growth; both *Thymus vulgaris* and its major component thymol destabilize trypanosomal plasma membrane; *Cymbopogon citratus* and *Ocimum gratissimum* exhibited the major antitrypanosomal activity; terpenoids from *Allium sativum* and *Timus vulgaris* oils, mostly carvacrol, linalool and thymol, inhibit *Entamoeba histolytica*; *Tillandsia capitata*, *Orthotylus virens*, *Thymus zygis* subsp. *Sylvestris*, *Ocimum basilicum*, and *Lippia graveolens* oils prevent *G. lamblia* growth and adherence; *Melaleuca alternifolia*, *Carum copticum*, and *Lavandula angustifolia* EOs and their phenolic constituents exhibit antiprotozoal effects; *C. citratus*, *Origanum* spp., *Lippia multiflora*, *Ocimum gratissimum*, and *S. thymbra* oils were effective against *Plasmodium* sp., thus demonstrating antimalarial activity; *Croton cajucara* oil, having linalool as its main constituent, was found to be the most effective anti-leishmanial EO; and *Achillea millefolium*, *Artemisia abrotanum*, *C. cajucara*, *C. citrates*, *O. gratissimum*, *Pinus caribaea*, *Piper* sp., and *Chenopodium ambrosioides* oils have demonstrated some anti-leishmanial activity, with the last one presenting the best activity (Raut and Karuppayil 2014).

### 10.4.5 Antioxidant Activity

Oxidative cellular damages due to free radicals and reactive oxygen species generation contribute either to physiological ageing process acceleration or to several health conditions, such as arteriosclerosis, cancer, Alzheimer's disease, Parkinson's disease, diabetes mellitus, and asthma (Raut and Karuppayil 2014). Natural occurring antioxidants presented in EOs, mainly terpenoids, flavonoids, and phenolic constituents, may be helpful as new antioxidant agents by ensuring a free radicals balance in cells (Raut and Karuppayil 2014). For instance, *Origanum majorana*, *Tillandsia filifolia*, *Bacopa monnieri*, and *Curcuma longa* oils have shown pronounced antioxidative effects; similarly, oils from *Achillea millefolium*, *Allium sativum*, *Allium cepa*, *Coriandrum sativum*, *Cuminum cyminum*, *Curcuma zedoaria*, *Magnolia officinalis*, *Melaleuca alternifolia*, *Mentha spicata*, *Ocimum* spp., *Pisum sativum*, *Sageraea cryptantha*, and *Salvia multicaulis* exhibit free radical scavenging activity, thus promoting an antioxidant action; and finally, thymol and carvacrol, from *Thymus* and *Origanum* EOs (respectively) proved to be strong antioxidants (Raut and Karuppayil 2014). Hence, EOs may be organized by their antioxidant activity: clove > cinnamon > nutmeg > basil > oregano > thyme (Miguel 2010, Raut and Karuppayil 2014, Tepe et al. 2004).

### 10.4.6 Anti-inflammatory Activity

For a long time that it is known EOs potent anti-inflammatory activity, having *Ocimum sanctum* oil as one of the most preeminent discoveries in this field (Raut and Karuppayil 2014). Furthermore, several others have demonstrated an effective anti-inflammatory activity: *Baphia nitida*, *clove*, *Eucalyptus* sp., *Lavandula angustifolia*, *lavender*, *Mentha* sp., *myrrh*, *pine*, and *rosemary* oils share a preventive effect on inflammation events mostly by reducing free radical scavenging efficacy during the oxidative burst of the inflammation, similarly, aloe vera, anise star, bergamot, cinnamon leaf, juniperus berry, lavender, thyme, and ylang-ylang oils also play an important anti-inflammatory activity (Raut and Karuppayil 2014).

These EOs' activity is mediated by several mechanisms, such as the inhibition of either lipoxygenase, COX-2, proinflammatory cytokines, interleukin-1$\beta$ and tumor necrosis factor-$\alpha$, leukotriene synthesis prevention, and proinflammatory genes repression (Raut and Karuppayil 2014).

### 10.4.7 Antidiabetic Activity

In diabetic patients, occasional hyperglycemic or hypoglycemic episodes may be recurrent if there is either an absence of insulin production or an insulin overproduction in normoglycemic patients (Raut and Karuppayil 2014). Although a great variety of plant derived substances have been studied, only a few information is available (Raut and Karuppayil 2014). Some *in vivo* studies were also performed, suggesting that EOs may prevent many systemic effects of diabetes (Raut and Karuppayil 2014). For example, rosemary oil showed an antidiabetic action in hyperglycemic rabbits, a combination of cinnamon, cumin, fennel, myrtle, and oregano oils exerted a synergistic effect enhancing insulin sensitivity in type 2 diabetic rats and have also demonstrated a blood glucose lowering effect, and *Satureja khuzestanica* oil leads to a significant fasting blood glucose levels decrease in diabetic rats (Raut and Karuppayil 2014). Unfortunately, the mechanisms inherent to these antidiabetic reported activity remain unknown and further studies must be performed (Raut and Karuppayil 2014).

### 10.4.8 Antimutagenic Activity

Several investigations have demonstrated a significant antimutagenic activity of EOs and their main constituents (Raut and Karuppayil 2014). For instance, *Matricaria chamomilla* oil was responsible for daunorubicine and methyl-methane sulfonate-induced mutagenic errors inhibition in bone marrow mouse cells; *Melaleuca. alternifolia* and *Lavandula angustifolia* oils showed to strongly attenuate-induced mutations in an *Escherichia coli* model; the sesquiterpene $\alpha$-Bisabolol exhibited an inhibitory effect on aflatoxin B1, benzopyrene, and 2-aminofluorene-induced mutagenesis; *Salmonella typhimurium*, *Escherichia. coli*, and *Saccharomyces cerevisiae* UV-light-induced mutations were prevented by *Salvia officinalis* oil; *Helichrysum. italicum*, *Ledum groenlandicum*, *Cinnamomum. camphora*, and *Orthophytum compactum* oils have shown to be active agents against urethane-induced mutations in a *Drosophila melanogaster* model; *Curcuma longa*, *Piper betel*, and *Areca catechu* extract mixture conferred protection to human lymphocytes against chromosomal damage; *Curcuma longa* revealed a chemopreventive effect on oral submucous cellular cytogenetic damage; and *Terminalia arjuna* constituents contributed to an antimutagenic action in *S. typhimurium* model (Raut and Karuppayil 2014).

This reported EOs' antimutagenic activity may reside on their inherent ability to: (i) act as inhibitors of the mutagenic agent's penetration inside the cells; (ii) promote free oxygen radical scavenging activity; (iii) either activate antioxidant enzymes or inhibit P450-mediated mutagens formation; (iv) interfere with mutations involving DNA repair systems; and (v) induce cellular necrosis or phenomena, thus leading to cell death (Raut and Karuppayil 2014).

### 10.4.9 Anticancer Activity

A greater prevalence of cancer has been observed worldwide, and there is a current need for novel chemotherapeutical approaches, preferentially able to treat the malignant cellular growth with less adverse effects associated (Raut and Karuppayil 2014). Some EOs and also some of their major constituents have evidenced great results in this field: taxol was active against cancerous cell proliferation; geraniol interfered with cellular membrane functions, ions homeostasis, and also cell signaling events in cancerous cells by inhibition of DNA synthesis; β-eudesmol contributed to prevent malignant tumors; terpenoids and polyphenols demonstrated to prevent tumor cell proliferation by necrosis or apoptosis induction; nutmeg oil has showed a significant hepatoprotective activity, possibly due to its major constituent myristicin, which it is believed to act through apoptosis induction such as in neuroblastoma cells; cital prevented the early phase of hepatocarcinogenesis in rat; garlic oil also presented anticancer properties by suppressing drug detoxifying enzymes; lemon balm oil inhibited several human cancer cells growth; and tea tree oil and terpinen-4-ol (its major monoterpene-alcohol) promoted apoptosis and are related to a lower incidence of human melanoma (Raut and Karuppayil 2014).

As great antioxidant and mitochondrial function-interfering agents, EOs may reduce metabolic events related to tumor development, such as increased cellular metabolism, mitochondrial overproduction, and permanent oxidative stress (Raut and Karuppayil 2014). As such, several malignancies, namely, glioma, digestive tract cancers (e.g., gastric and colon), hepatocellular carcinoma, pulmonary tumors, breast cancer, and leukemia were demonstrated to reduce after treatment with EOs (Raut and Karuppayil 2014).

Traditionally, essential oils may be administered to humans by several routes, namely: enteral (through the digestive tract), either oral (into the mouth) or gavage (esophageal, gastric, nasogastric, or orogastric); intravenous (into a blood vessel); epicutaneous (onto the skin); intradermal (into the skin); subcutaneous (under the skin); transdermal (across the skin); intramuscular (into a muscle); transcorneal (onto the eye); intraocular (into the eye); intracerebral (into the brain); epidural (into the duramater surrounding space); intrathecal (into distal spinal cord surrounding space); intraperitoneal (into the peritoneal cavity); intraosseous (into the marrow cavity); intranasal (sprayed into the nose and then absorbed by the nasal mucous membranes or into the lungs); intratracheal (into the lungs by direct tracheal instillation); or finally by inhalation (Turner et al. 2011).

Although there is a great variety of techniques available, there still remains an increasing need for new administration routes in order to overcome the physicochemical and toxicological issues related to EOs, namely, their inherent high lipophilicity, volatility, and susceptibility to degradation when exposed to abovementioned environmental factors. Some of these new approaches are addressed in the next section.

## 10.5 DELIVERY SYSTEMS

As mentioned above, there is an increasing need for novel delivery systems to overcome the disadvantages and optimize the traditional routes for the administration of bioactive compounds. Controlled delivery systems may represent such new approach, having several advantages that allow the transport of a lower dose of product to its site of action, where it performs its biological activity with minimal adverse effects, low toxicity, and maintaining its physicochemical properties (Wilczewska et al. 2012). Furthermore, cell-specific targeting may also be achieved by attaching drugs to carriers specially designed for drug delivery, such as liposomes, polymers, dendrimers, silicon or carbon materials, and nanoparticles (Wilczewska et al. 2012). The latter, nanoparticles (NPs), may be grouped into five categories: (i) carbon NPs, including carbon nanotubes, graphene and graphene oxide nanosheets, and nanodiamonds; (ii) inorganic NPs, namely, gold, silver, iron oxide, titanium oxide, silicon oxide, and mesoporous silica NPs; (iii) polymeric NPs, including products derived from natural polymers, such as chitosan, alginic, and hyaluronic acids, derived from synthetic polymers (mainly aliphatic polyesters), such as poly(lactic acid), poly(ε-caprolactone), and poly(lactic acid-co-glycolic acid); (iv) lipid NPs, including SLNs, NLCs, and lipid–drug conjugates (LDCs); and (v) dendrimers, such as poly(amido amide) (Wilczewska et al. 2012).

Lipid carriers, for instance, have been increasingly studied specially for EOs' delivery, thus representing a great and useful approach in phytotherapy (Turek and Stintzing 2013, Wilczewska et al. 2012). As mentioned in the previous sections, because essential oils are highly lipophilic, volatile, and sensitive to environmental factors, they may suffer oxidation reactions leading to production of free oxygen radical species and other oxidation products, thus losing their main biological activity or producing undesirable effects (El Asbahani et al. 2015, Rodríguez et al. 2016, Turek and Stintzing 2013). There remains an issue in delivering these agents to body tissues, situation that may be overcome by encapsulating these bioactive oils in controlled delivery systems (El Asbahani et al. 2015, Rodríguez et al. 2016, Turek and Stintzing 2013). Examples of promising lipid carriers that have been increasingly investigated as controlled delivery systems are mentioned below.

### 10.5.1 EMULSIONS

Microemulsions are thermodynamically stable (with a mean droplet size above 500 nm) and transparent dispersions consisting of two immiscible liquids which have their stability ensured by an interfacial film of surfactants (Donsi and Ferrari 2016). Among their advantages are the need for a very low energy to formulate these emulsions—since they are capable of spontaneously formulate when contacting with aqueous, oily, and amphiphilic components—and their low production cost (Donsi and Ferrari 2016). On the other hand, formulation requires high surfactant concentration which may be implicated in toxicity when applied in pharmaceutical industry (Donsi and Ferrari 2016).

In turn, nanoemulsions (NEs), also referred as miniemulsions, ultra-fine emulsions, or submicrometer emulsions, are non-equilibrium systems consisting of a fine oil-on-water dispersion with a constant need to separate into their constituent phases (Donsi and Ferrari 2016). Their major advantages may be the possibility of being prepared using lower surfactant concentrations than microemulsions, and a relatively high kinetic stability (even for several years) due to their steric stabilization between the droplets thus conferring a small size (10–500 nm) (Donsi and Ferrari 2016).

It is believed that emulsions' antimicrobial activity results from the small oil particles size, having a high surface tension, thus being able to fuse and disrupt prokaryotic cells, viruses, and fungal eukaryotic membranes (Donsi and Ferrari 2016). For instance, *in vitro* studies of nanoemulsion-encapsulated terpenes extracted from *Melaleuca alternifolia* and D-limonene showed an increased antimicrobial activity against *Lactobacillus delbrueckii*, *Escherichia coli*, and *Saccaromyces cerevisiae* (Donsi and Ferrari 2016). This can be proposed to food industry, since nanoemulsion encapsulation is proved to enhance EOs' dispersibility in food matrices, and thus improving their physicochemical stability and allowing their biological activities to occur (Donsi and Ferrari 2016). For example, several studies were performed applying nanoemulsion encapsulated EOs to: (i) liquid products: in milk of different fat content had a greater activity against inoculated microbial species, in fruit juices, tea tree oil, and cinnamaldehyde have showed to inhibit inoculated microbial load, and in orange juice eugenol proved to reduce heterotrophic bacterial population; (ii) food surface coating: oregano oil NEs played an enhanced antimicrobial activity in decontamination of fresh lettuce and spinach leaves, and chitosan NEs were proven to extend shelf life of green beans and broccoli florets by their antimicrobial activity; and finally (iii) porous food matrices: carvacrol NEs either in vegetable or animal tissues showed an enhanced diffusion rate which increased the antimicrobial activity, namely, against *Escherichia coli* (Donsi and Ferrari 2016).

### 10.5.2 Liposomes

Liposomes were the first lipid nanoparticles investigated to serve as drug delivery systems (Wilczewska et al. 2012). They consist of micro- or nanoparticles or colloidal carriers, arranged in spherical vesicles having 80–300 nm size range, which are composed by a phospholipids and steroids bilayer, and sometimes also a surfactant, dispersed in an aqueous media (Wilczewska et al. 2012). The drug suffers an encapsulation process to get incorporated into the liposome, which was found to increase its solubility, as well as to improve drug pharmacokinetic properties (Wilczewska et al. 2012). Guaranteed some conditions, namely, pH, surrounding environment, osmotic gradient, and liposome composition itself, the drug will reach its proper site of action where it will be released and exert its biological activity (Wilczewska et al. 2012). Several *in vitro* and *in vivo* studies have been performed for testing liposomes antioxidant activity. As example, leaf vegetables showed a high percentage of antioxidant activity reduction when 0.1 mg/ml concentration of liposomal rosemary oil in vegetables was used, offering the liposomes a safe and effective approach to prolong shelf-life of vegetables (Alikhani-Koupaei 2014).

### 10.5.3 Solid Lipid Nanoparticles, Nanostructured Lipid Carriers, and Lipid Drug Conjugates

All SLNs, NLCs, and LDCs are lipid nanoparticles that function as carrier systems based on a solid lipid matrix composed by lipids solid at body temperature (Souto and Müller 2010, Thassu et al. 2007, Wilczewska et al. 2012).

Both SLNs and NLCs are nanoparticles having pure lipids or a lipid compound mixture (including either triacylglycerols, fatty acids, steroids, waxes, or oils) and a single surfactant or an association of this with a co-surfactant, surrounding the particles, in its constitution (Figure 10.1). Depending on the chemical nature of the active agent and lipid, its solubility in the melted lipid, surfactants nature and concentration, production method, and production temperature, there may be distinguished several subtypes of these lipid nanoparticles with particular characteristics like particle size and distribution, yield of production, loading capacity, and encapsulation efficiency (Souto and Müller 2010, Thassu et al. 2007). SLNs, the first generation of lipid nanoparticles, are composed by solid lipids, either highly purified triglycerides, complex glyceride mixtures, or waxes, all stabilized by a surfactant (Geszke-Moritz and Moritz 2016, Souto and Müller 2010, Thassu et al. 2007, Wilczewska et al. 2012). There are three main subtypes: (i) type 1 SLN or homogeneous matrix model, which is derived from a solid solution of lipid and active compound, where this latter is molecularly dispersed in the lipid core or in the form of amorphous clusters; (ii) type 2 SLN or drug-enriched shell model, where a lipid core without drug is formed (by cooling after suffering hot high pressure homogenization) with a shell comprising both drug (at low concentration) and lipid surrounding it; and (iii) type 3 SLN or drug-enriched core model, which in contrast to type 2 has a shell of lipid and a core composed by both lipid and drug (at high concentration) (Souto and Müller 2010, Thassu et al. 2007). SLNs have

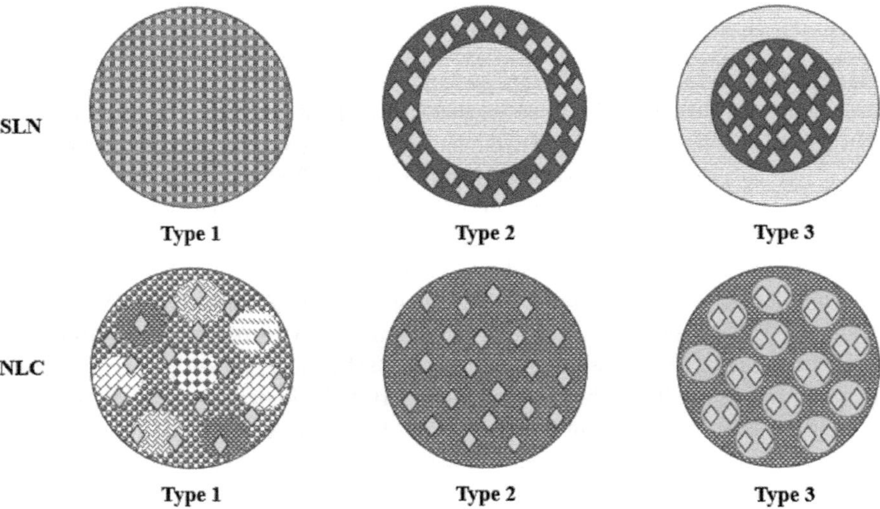


**FIGURE 10.1** Drug incorporation models into SLN and NLC.

reported great physical stability, incorporated drug protection against degradation, controlled release of the drug, and good tolerability (Geszke-Moritz and Moritz 2016, Souto and Müller 2010, Thassu et al. 2007, Wilczewska et al. 2012). On the other hand, there were also noticed some disadvantages, such as a reduced loading capacity, a relatively high-water content in the dispersion, and drug release after crystallization (Geszke-Moritz and Moritz 2016, Souto and Müller 2010, Thassu et al. 2007, Wilczewska et al. 2012). In order to overcome these issues, a second-generation of lipid nanoparticles were designed: NLCs and LDCs (Souto and Müller 2010, Thassu et al. 2007, Wilczewska et al. 2012). NLCs are lipid nanoparticles resulting from the mixture of solid and liquid lipids covered by a surfactant solution, a new nanostructure that prevents drug expulsion, a great improvement compared to SLNs (Souto and Müller 2010, Thassu et al. 2007, Wilczewska et al. 2012). Likewise, there are three main subtypes: (i) type 1 NLC or imperfect crystal model, which has many imperfections within the matrix, obtained by mixing together solid and liquid (oils) lipids, that allows the active molecules to be accommodated; (ii) type 2 NLC or amorphous model, where by mixing non-recrystallizing special lipids, after prior homogenization and cooling, these lipids create solid particles having an amorphous lipid structure, thus delaying or avoiding crystallization and reducing drug release; and (iii) type 3 or multiple model NLC, which consists of very small oil nanocompartments integrated into the solid-lipid matrix that was created by a phase-separation process when mixing together solid and liquid (oils) lipids in a ratio that exceeds the solubility of the oil molecules in the solid lipid; reached the miscibility gap, oil suffers a precipitation process thus giving rise to small oil droplets within the solid lipid (Souto and Müller 2010, Thassu et al. 2007).

In turn, LDCs are insoluble lipid-drug conjugates produced either by salt formation or covalent linking with subsequent homogenization, in order to expand the applicability of the lipid-based carriers to lipophilic drugs (Wilczewska et al. 2012).

Hence, all these particles have demonstrated to function as promising delivery systems, especially for EOs administration, and fortunately all of them may be administrated to body tissues by the above-mentioned routes, such as oral, endovenous, and parenteral, always considering the specific conditions that each procedure requires.

Food industry has been constantly demonstrating that EOs really remain an increasingly possibility in food "active packaging" and as antimicrobial agents thus leading to a prolonged foodstuff preservation. For instance, encapsulated thymol (in sodium caseinate) has proven to inhibit foodborne pathogens activity in milk more efficiently that the non-encapsulated thymol, once the first had both enhanced distribution and solubility; poly DL-lactide-co-glycolide NPs complex incorporating eugenol and cinnamaldehyde have demonstrated to act as a potential bactericidal agent against *Salmonella* spp. and *Listeria* spp.; and combining EOs and NPs was proven to be more effective as antibacterial agents against both Gram-positive and -negative bacteria (Rai et al. 2017). Furthermore, there are evidences that active packaging allowed to prevent browning and weight loss when compared to non-active paraffin-based packaging; when trays' bottom and walls are covered, foodstuff shelf life is much greater compared to the bottom alone; and active packaging with cinnamon oil was very effective on mushrooms postharvest deterioration (Calo et al. 2015, Rai et al. 2017).

Additionally, NLC encapsulation was proven to allow the delivery of the most important types of bioactive lipids within foods, namely, free omega-3 fatty acids (by decreasing their oxidation in enriched foods), carotenoids (by overcoming their poor hydro-solubility high melting point, chemical instability, and low bioavailability), phytosterols (by avoiding their oxidation and overcoming their high melting point), and oil-soluble vitamins (by inhibiting or delaying their oxidation avoiding their taste) (Tamjidi et al. 2013).

As such, food packaging sector may really benefit from antimicrobial nanocomposites, which reduce microbial growth on foodstuff surfaces, always considering some safety issues, such as the fact of nanosized materials frequently exhibit different properties than those of the corresponding starting materials; and the much larger nanoparticles surface area which allows a greater contact with cell membranes and a greater capacity for absorption and migration (Donsi and Ferrari 2016). Moreover, consumers minimal exposure to EOs-loaded nanoparticles may occur either through dermal contact, inhalation, or ingestion (if they have migrated to food) (Donsi and Ferrari 2016). Unfortunately, these antimicrobial nanostructure toxicity profiles cannot be extrapolated from those of EO itself, since they have more free movement through the body when compared to their higher scale counterparts, so they may eventually be released into the environment and indirectly enter the food chain (Donsi and Ferrari 2016). It is therefore necessary to be conscious of any eventual health effect from ingestion of nanoparticles, and it is even more important when regarding edible coatings, considered not only a food contact material, but part of the food itself (Donsi and Ferrari 2016). That is why further investigation must be performed in nanocomposite packaging industry, specially focusing on the nanotechnology products' potential toxicity and strategies to overcome these referred issues (Donsi and Ferrari 2016).

## 10.6 CONCLUSIONS AND FUTURE PERSPECTIVES

As natural plant constituents, EOs may be considered as a "green" approach to several industries, mainly food industry, with "active packaging" new approach, and pharmaceutical industry, regarding EOs' clinical application to several conditions treatment. As such, playing them an increasingly role at this level there remains an emergent need for both *vitro* and *in vivo* characterizing and toxicological and genotoxicity profiling studies to be performed in order to ensure consumers well-being. Since it is said that "the dosage makes the toxin," it is very important to dedicate some attention to EOs' chemical properties, mechanisms of biological action, and toxicological profile in further investigations.

## ACKNOWLEDGMENTS

The authors would like to acknowledge the financial support received through the project M-ERA-NET/0004/2015, from the Portuguese Science and Technology Foundation, Ministry of Science and Education through national funds, and co-financed by FEDER, under the Partnership Agreement PT2020.

## REFERENCES


Alikhani-Koupaei, M. 2014. "Liposome-entrapped essential oils on *in vitro* and *in vivo* antioxidant activity in leafy vegetables." *Quality Assurance and Safety of Crops & Foods* 7:369–373.

Baser, K. H. C., and G. Buchbauer. 2010. *Handbook of Essential Oils: Science, Technology and Applications*. 1st ed. Boca Raton, FL: CRC Press.

Calo, J. R., P. G. Crandall, C. A. O'Bryan, and S. C. Ricke. 2015. "Essential oils as antimicrobials in food systems—A review." *Food Control* 54:111–119. doi: 10.1016/j.foodcont.2014.12.040.

Cartus, A., and D. Schrenk. 2017. "Current methods in risk assessment of genotoxic chemicals." *Food and Chemical Toxicology* 106:574–582. doi:10.1016/j.fct.2016.09.012.

Dima, C., and S. Dima. 2015. "Essential oils in foods: Extraction, stabilization, and toxicity." *Current Opinion in Food Science* 5:29–35. doi:10.1016/j.cofs.2015.07.003.

Donsi, F., and G. Ferrari. 2016. "Essential oil nanoemulsions as antimicrobial agents in food." *Journal of Biotechnology* 233:106–120. doi:10.1016/j.jbiotec.2016.07.005.

Ekwall, B., V. Silano, A. Paganuzzi-Stammati, and F. Zucco. 1990. Toxicity tests with mammalian cell cultures. In *Short-Term Toxicity Tests for Non-genotoxic Effects*, P. Bourdeau, E. Somers, G. M. Richardson, and J. R. Hickman, eds. New York: John Wiley & Sons.

El Asbahani, A., K. Miladi, W. Badri, M. Sala, E. H. Ait Addi, H. Casabianca, A. El Mousadik et al. 2015. "Essential oils: From extraction to encapsulation." *International Journal of Pharmaceutics* 483 (1–2):220–243. doi:10.1016/j.ijpharm.2014.12.069.

Fielden, M. R., and K. L. Kolaja. 2008. "The role of early in vivo toxicity testing in drug discovery toxicology." *Expert Opinion on Drug Safety* 7 (2):107–110.

Fischer, H. C., and W. C. W. Chan. 2007. "Nanotoxicity: The growing need for in vivo study." *Current Opinion in Biotechnology* 18:565–571.

Geszke-Moritz, M., and M. Moritz. 2016. "Solid lipid nanoparticles as attractive drug vehicles: Composition, properties and therapeutic strategies." *Materials Science and Engineering* 68:982–994. doi:10.1016/j.msec.2016.05.119.

Llana-Ruiz-Cabello, M., S. Pichardo, S. Maisanaba, M. Puerto, A. I. Prieto, D. Gutierrez-Praena, A. Jos, and A. M. Camean. 2015. "In vitro toxicological evaluation of essential oils and their main compounds used in active food packaging: A review." *Food and Chemical Toxicology* 81:9–27. doi:10.1016/j.fct.2015.03.030.

Miguel, M. G. 2010. "Antioxidant and anti-inflammatory activities of essential oils: A short review." *Molecules* 15:9252–9287.

Patel, S., and P. Gogna. 2015. "Tapping botanicals for essential oils: Progress and hurdles in cancer mitigation." *Industrial Crops and Products* 76:1148–1163. doi:10.1016/j.indcrop.2015.08.024.

Pereira, S., and M. Tettamanti. 2012. "Testing times in toxicology—*In vitro* and *in vivo* testing." ALTEX Proceedings 2, 1/13, *Proceedings of Animal Alternatives in Teaching, Toxicity Testing and Medicine*, 99th Indian Science Congress, 3–7 January.

Pusztai, R., M. Abrantes, J. Sherly, N. Duarte, J. Molnar, and M. J. U. Ferreira. 2010. "Antitumor-promoting activity of lignans: Inhibition of human cytomegalovirus IE gene expression." *Anticancer Research* 30:451–454.

Rai, M., P. Paralikar, P. Jogee, G. Agarkar, A. P. Ingle, M. Derita, and S. Zacchino. 2017. "Synergistic antimicrobial potential of essential oils in combination with nanoparticles: Emerging trends and future perspectives." International Journal of Pharmaceutics 519 (1–2):67–78. doi:10.1016/j.ijpharm.2017.01.013.

Raut, J. S., and S. M. Karuppayil. 2014. "A status review on the medicinal properties of essential oils." *Industrial Crops and Products* 62:250–264. doi:10.1016/j.indcrop.2014.05.055.

Rodríguez, J., M. J. Martín, M. A. Ruiz, and B. Clares. 2016. "Current encapsulation strategies for bioactive oils: From alimentary to pharmaceutical perspectives." *Food Research International* 83:41–59. doi:10.1016/j.foodres.2016.01.032.

Souto, E. B., and R. H. Müller. 2010. "Lipid nanoparticles: Effect on bioavailability and pharmacokinetic changes." *Handbook of Experimental Pharmacology* 197:115–141. doi:10.1007/978-3-642-00477-3_4.

Tamjidi, F., M. Shahedi, J. Varshosaz, and A. Nasirpour. 2013. "Nanostructured lipid carriers (NLC): A potential delivery system for bioactive food molecules." *Innovative Food Science & Emerging Technologies* 19:29–43. doi:10.1016/j.ifset.2013.03.002.

Tepe, B., E. Donmez, M. Unlu, F. Candan, D. Daferera, G. Vardar-Unlu, M. Polissiou, A. Sokmen. 2004. "Anti microbial and antioxidative activities of the essential oils and methanol extracts of Salvia cryptantha (Montbret et Aucher ex Benth.) and Salvia multicaulis (Vahl)." *Food Chemistry* 84:519–525.

Thassu, D., M. Deleers, and Y. Pathak. 2007. Lipid nanoparticles (Solid lipid nanoparticles and nanostructured lipid carriers) for cosmetic, dermal, and transdermal applications. In *Nanoparticulate Drug Delivery Systems*, edited by D. Thassu, M. Deleers, and Y. Pathak. New York: Informa Healthcare.

Turek, C., and F. C. Stintzing. 2013. "Stability of essential oils: A review." *Comprehensive Reviews in Food Science and Food Safety* 12 (1):40–53. doi:10.1111/1541-4337.12006.

Turner, P. V., C. Pekow, M. A. Vasbinder, and T. Brabb. 2011. "Administration of substances to laboratory animals: Equipment considerations, vehicle selection, and solute preparation." *Journal of the American Association for Laboratory Animal Science* 50 (5):614–627.

Wilczewska, A. Z., K. Niemirowicz, K. H. Markiewicz, and H. Car. 2012. "Nanoparticles as drug delivery systems." *Pharmacological Reports* 64:1020–1037.

# Section IV

## Applications in Food Industries

# 11 Nanotechnology as a Way for Bio-based and Biodegradable Food Packaging with Enhanced Properties

*Miguel A. Cerqueira, Pablo Fuciños, and Lorenzo M. Pastrana*

**CONTENTS**

## 11.1 INTRODUCTION

The current food system is fully dependent on packaging because it plays different roles through the value chain: transportation, storage, food protection, safety, convenience, communication, or marketing among others. Food packaging allows preserving the quality and safety of raw and processed foods, thus increasing their shelf life and, in combination with new logistics solutions, allowing to reach new and farther markets.

On the other hand, packaging is a key factor for developing convenient food products in order to provide solutions for new customers' lifestyles (ready to go meals, microwavable, unit dose, and portion pack), but also for providing information about composition, nutritional facts, origin, or traceability. Food packaging is also an effective marketing tool. Customer choice is determined by the packaging design. For example, the color of packaging has conscious and subconscious influence in customers' decisions (Towal et al. 2013).

Different forms (e.g., bottles, bags, and trays) and materials (e.g., paper, wood, glass, metal, and plastic) have been used for food packaging purposes. Oil-based plastics are, by far, the most common material in food packaging, representing 26% of the total volume of plastics used as they are inexpensive, lightweight, versatile, durable and have a high strength-to-weight ratio, and high performance to keep food fresh. Production of plastic packaging is expected to continue its exponential growth quadrupling by 2050 at the current volume of production (Ellen MacArthur Foundation 2017). The main plastics based on oil (e.g., PET, HDPE, PVC, LDPE, PP, PS, EPS) are recyclable. However, only 14% of plastic packaging is collected for recycling, and at least 8 million tons of plastics leak into the ocean each year (Jambeck et al. 2015), constituting a very important environmental global issue. Thus, by 2050, it is expected that the ocean will contain more plastics than fish by weight (Ellen MacArthur Foundation 2017).

There are other drawbacks also related with the use of oil-based plastic packaging: they are produced from non-renewable sources, their production is associated with greenhouse gas emissions, and they contain additives (e.g., stabilizers, plasticisers, and pigments) with a potential risk for human health. For those reasons, nowadays there is a momentum greater than ever for rethinking the design and uses of plastics for packaging in order to make them reusable, recyclable, and eco-friendly. Thus, biodegradability and compostability are two properties, among others, that must be incorporated into the future plastic packaging materials, requiring further research and innovation efforts.

A promising alternative to oil-based plastics is the use of biopolymers (natural or synthetic) to develop biodegradable food packaging materials. Biopolymers can be obtained by synthesis (e.g., poly(lactic acid) [PLA], polycaprolactone, PGA, PVA, and PBS) or from natural sources, often food wastes, (e.g., starch, cellulose, chitosan, agar, alginate, gelatin, gluten, whey protein, collagen, xanthan, curdlan, and pullulan) using different strategies (extraction, fermentation). Biopolymers have several advantages for packaging purposes such as durability, flexibility, high gloss, clarity, ubiquity, low cost, and a broad range of chemical compositions (Othman 2014).

Biopolymers have been most frequently used to obtain edible films and coatings. In edible coatings, a film forming solution is applied directly on the food product by spraying, dipping, or fluidizing without impacting the sensory characteristics of the food. Edible films are formed by casting or extrusion. Some biodegradable polymers can also be industrially compostable. This bio-based packaging allows returning the nutrients to the soil. In spite of these advantages, films made of biopolymers also have some important disadvantages: they are often brittle, low stability under high temperatures, distortion temperature, low resistance to prolonged process operations, and poor mechanical and barrier properties. Due to these drawbacks, these materials have not been extensively used for food packaging purposes (Cerqueira et al. 2018).

Nanotechnology offers suitable solutions to overcome the above-mentioned inconveniences. It is possible to improve mechanical, thermal, and optical properties of biopolymers used to obtain biodegradable food packaging materials. For example, by adding nano-sized fillers such as silicate, clay, and titanium dioxide to nanostructured and self-assembled proteins, polysaccharides, or waxes, it is possible to obtain packaging materials with good performance. Additionally, those nanomaterials have antimicrobial and oxygen scavenging activity that can be used for active packaging purposes. Other antimicrobial compounds that could be used shortly are nano silver, nano magnesium oxide, nano copper oxide, and carbon nanotubes (Chaudhry et al. 2008). Nanocomposites for food packaging can also be designed to contain nanoparticles able to release functional compounds such as enzymes, flavors, and nutraceuticals. This is because in active food packaging, the packaging material is not a simple inert barrier: it can interact with the food in order to improve its quality and safety and extend its shelf life (Cerqueira et al. 2018).

Nanomaterials can also be used for sensing biochemical or microbial changes in the food. Smart packaging uses nanosensors and nanodevices to provide information to the customer about the freshness, the presence of contaminants in foods (chemical or microbial), or monitoring changes in packaging conditions (gas composition) or integrity. Some of these nanomaterials are able to change color acting as spoilage or oxygen indicators, or to be used for product identification and traceability (Kuswandi et al. 2011). Thus, embedding nanosensors into food packaging can empower customers, while providing a real-time status of food, thus avoiding wastage of suitable foods beyond the expiration date. Nanobarcodes and radio frequency identification active tags are also developed applications of nanotechnology in intelligent packaging to be used for tracking, product identification, and anticounterfeiting purposes (Abad et al. 2007).

This chapter reviews the role of nanotechnology in facing the main challenges of the bio-based and biodegradable food packaging industry in this century. The development of a new generation of food packaging solutions with enhanced properties based on nanostructured biodegradable materials is presented in the following lines. Additionally, the future of the active and intelligent packaging is discussed, and some examples based on nanotechnology are examined.

## 11.2 BIO-BASED AND BIODEGRADABLE MATERIALS FOR PACKAGING

Bio-based and biodegradable packaging materials are interesting materials to produce coatings, multilayers, and films by casting, however, their production in a similar way to the petroleum-based plastics is not trivial. In fact, several technological advances have allowed processing some of these types of materials using processing technologies such as extrusion, spinning, injection molding, and thermoforming (Lim et al. 2008; Mahalik and Nambiar 2010). Besides the use of a bio-based source, that is already an advantage, some of these materials are also biodegradable and edible, in some cases they can also be used as a vehicle for antioxidant and antimicrobial agents, improving packaging functionality (Abreu et al. 2015; Souza et al. 2015; Cerqueira et al. 2016). Bio-based materials can be divided in three main groups, such as presented on Figure 11.1. One of the groups is composed by those extracted from renewable resources, which include polysaccharides, proteins, lipids or waxes, and others such as lignin. Also being part of the bio-based materials are the biopolymers synthesized through chemical and biotechnological routes, which corresponds to the other two groups, which include, for example, the PLA and polyhydroxyalkanoates, respectively. On the group of the biopolymers synthesized by chemical routes, there are some polymers which are not biodegradable, such as PET and PE, that instead of being obtained from petroleum are synthesized from bio-derived monomers.

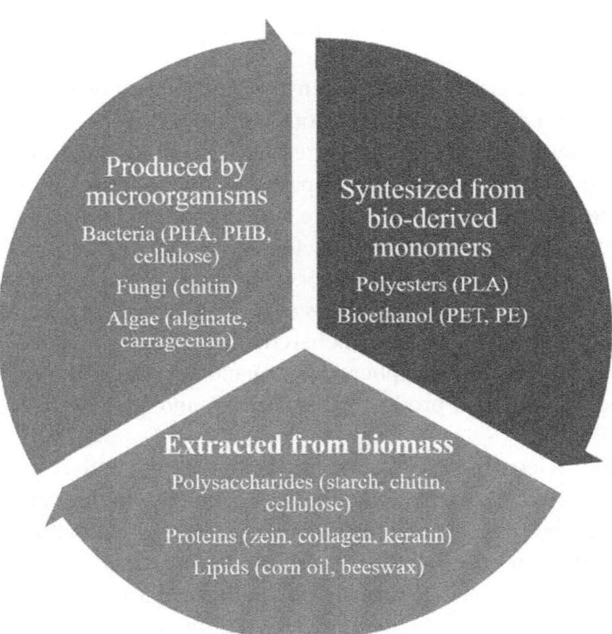


**FIGURE 11.1** Bio-based materials used in the packaging production.

## 11.2.1 Bio-based Packaging Materials Extracted from Biomass

### 11.2.1.1 Polysaccharides

Polysaccharides can be obtained from animals and plants, but also microorganisms can be used to produce a great variety of interesting polysaccharides. The variety of sources leads to a great number of possibilities, where it is possible to find polysaccharides with different structures and physicochemical characteristics (e.g., crystallinity and molecular weight). Among the ones obtained from plants, starch, cellulose, and pectin are the most used (Berezina and Martelli 2014). On the other hand, chitin is the main polysaccharide obtained from animals, being extracted from exoskeletons of arthropods such as crustaceans, crabs, lobsters, and shrimps, being also possible to obtain it from insects and fungi (Tang et al. 2015). Also, carrageenan and alginate gums, which can be obtained from algae, as well as from microorganisms (e.g., bacteria and fungi) are important polysaccharides that have been explored in the last years as main materials for films and coatings.

Starch can be obtained from different sources such as cereals, legumes, and tubers. At the moment starch is considered economically competitive with materials derived from petroleum, being used in several methods for preparing biodegradable and compostable plastics (López et al. 2015). Packaging materials obtained from starch are usually transparent and translucent and colorless. They have low permeability to oxygen at low and intermediate relative humidity (RH) values when compared with the commercial synthetic oxygen barrier materials such as ethylene vinyl alcohol copolymer (Lin and Zhao 2007). However, at high RH oxygen permeability can highly increase, and thus their application in high moisture products is compromised. One of the drawbacks are the mechanical properties, which are poor, being the films obtained from starch are normally brittle. One of the solutions is the production of composites and to blend starch with other hydrophilic materials such as plasticizers in order to improve the mechanical properties (Ghanbarzadeh et al. 2011; Arik Kibar and Us 2013). One of the ways to improve the processability and final properties of starch-based packaging is to subject starch to an extrusion process in order to obtain thermoplastic starch. Thermoplastic starches have been commercialized during the last several years and currently are used to produce several products, such as containers, films, bowls, plates, cups, and egg trays (Khan et al. 2017).

Cellulose is a low-cost raw material displaying a highly crystalline structure, hydrophilic nature, and low solubility. Its use as material for the production of packaging is a challenge and implies several pretreatments before being used. The packaging materials produced from cellulose normally present high moisture permeability and reduced flexibility and tensile strength (Tang et al. 2012). The most known packaging materials derived from cellulose are paper and cardboard, that result from its strong hydrogen bonded crystalline microfibrils and fibers. Most of the paper and cardboard are used as a secondary or tertiary packaging, in some cases, such as paper coated with wax and polyethylene, it can be used as primary food packaging (Robertson 2013). Other of the well-known packaging materials obtained from cellulose is cellophane films. They are produced by dissolving wood pulp in an aggressive mixture of sodium hydroxide and carbon disulfide. Afterwards, the obtained solution called viscose (xanthation) is extruded through a slit into a bath of dilute sulfuric acid and sodium sulfate to reconvert viscose into cellophane (Petersen et al. 1999). Cellophane is highly sensitive to moisture and presents good mechanical properties and can be coated with other materials (e.g., nitrocellulose wax, polyvinylidene chloride, and vinyl chloride-vinyl acetate copolymer) to improve their barrier properties. Cellophane packaging has been widely used in baked goods, processed meats, twist-wrapped confectionery packaging, cheeses and yeasts, as well as in the fabrication of ovenable and microwaveable packaging.

Cellulose derivatives, such as carboxymethylcellulose (CMC), hydroxypropylcellulose, methylcellulose (MC), hydroxypropylmethyl cellulose, and cellulose acetate, are cellulose ethers obtained by partial substitution of hydroxyl groups in cellulose by ether functions. These materials can be dissolved in aqueous solutions or in water-ethanol solutions in order to produce films and coatings with interesting oxygen and carbon dioxide barriers. CMC, that presents in its structure a hydrophobic polysaccharide backbone and hydrophilic carboxyl groups, is highly used in food applications as a thickener or viscosity modifier and also presents good film-forming properties and has been tested as a coating on fruits and vegetables, showing the capacity, when blend with other materials, to extend the shelf life of foods. Other of the cellulose derivatives that is used in food packaging is cellulose acetate, which presents good optical and mechanical properties, and relatively low gas and moisture barrier capacity, being used mainly to wrap baked goods and fresh products (Petersen et al. 1999; Puls et al. 2011).

Chitosan is, perhaps, one of the biopolymers that has been presented in the last years with high potential to be used in food packaging, but their industrialization for this application is still in its infancy. It is obtained from chitin, after deacetylation, and can be obtained from the sub-products of seafood processing industry (e.g., shells of crabs, shrimps, lobsters, and krill) or from the cell wall of some fungi. When compared to other polysaccharides, chitosan presents unique characteristics, due to its cationic nature, it is dissolved in acidic solutions, which leads to a positively charged solution. Also, it can present antimicrobial activity against some microorganisms that will also be influenced by the molecular weight and deacetylation degree (Kong et al. 2010).

#### 11.2.1.2 Proteins

Proteins can also be used for the production of packaging materials and have received great attention in the last 20 years. Several sources have been tested: protein from animal origins such as casein, collagen, gelatin, keratin, whey protein, and other from vegetal sources including wheat gluten, soy protein, corn-zein, cottonseed protein, and peanut protein are some examples of the most studied for food packaging. At low RH, protein-based packaging presents excellent barrier properties to oxygen, carbon dioxide, and lipids, however, when they are presented to high RH conditions, they can suffer relevant changes. The high hydrophilicity of most proteins (except corn zein and keratin) makes the packaging obtained from them very highly water sensitive (Krochta 2002; Guerrero and Caba 2016). This drawback can be overcome by covalent cross-linking agents such as glutaraldehyde, lactic acid, and tannic acid, which can be normally used to improve barrier and mechanical properties (Guerrero and Caba 2016). Proteins from animal origin such as collagen, whey protein, gelatin, and wheat gluten are some of the most studied materials. Collagen is perhaps one of the most studied for the production of films and coatings, and during several years it has been used for the production of sausage casings, that have been gradually replaced by cellulose-based casings. From vegetable sources, wheat gluten, soy protein, and corn zein have been the most used. Several studies showed the possibility to produce films by casting, but thermoprocessing showed that it is also possible to produce films by extrusion and compression molding (Vicente et al. 2011). Zein and keratin, due to their high hydrophobicity, are some of the most interesting proteins to be used for the production of packaging materials, achieving good barrier and mechanical properties (Reddy 2015; Huo et al. 2018).

#### 11.2.1.3 Lipids

Packaging materials based only on lipids and waxes are scarce, and they have been used mainly in blends or as coatings of foods or films. Waxes and oils, which include beeswax, candelilla, carnauba and paraffin waxes, vegetable oil, and shellac, are only some of the materials from this group that were used in the development of packaging materials. Their low polarity makes these materials excellent options to increase the barrier to moisture of packaging materials. Normally, they need to be blend with polysaccharides or proteins in order to be able to be processed or applied as thin coating on films (Callegarin et al. 1997; Debeaufort et al. 1998). The capacity of lipids and waxes to improve matrix hydrophobicity depends, mainly, on their chemical characteristics, such as physical state, degree of saturation, and fatty acid content. Also, the way that lipids or waxes are added to the matrix influences their final properties, such as in an emulsion or applied as a thin layer (Karbowiak et al. 2007). Among the waxes commercially available, beeswax, candelilla wax, and carnauba wax are the most used to manufacture edible coatings and films. They can also be applied as coating directly on fruits and vegetables, and several wax coatings are commercially available for apples, citrus, asparagus, beans, beets, carrots, sweet potatoes, and cassava (Alleyne and Hagenmaier 2000; Fallik et al. 2005; Aguirre-Joya et al. 2016).

### 11.2.2 Bio-based Packaging Materials Synthesized by Biotechnological or Chemical Routes

The use of biopolymers obtained from biomass has been extensively explored, but the use of new bio-based and biodegradable alternatives rose up in the last 20 years. Nowadays, biopolymers produced by classical chemical synthesis or through biopolymers produced by microorganisms or genetically modified bacteria have been shown to be sustainable and can result in packaging materials with interesting properties.

One of the examples is PLA, a biopolyester polymerized from lactic acid monomers, which can be derived from renewable resources such as corn starch, wheat, sugar cane, cassava roots, or chips (Okano et al. 2010). It is a biodegradable, thermoplastic, and aliphatic (non-aromatic and non-cyclic) polyester, being its properties related with the ratio between the two mesoforms (D or L) of the lactic acid monomer. If a 100% L-PLA is synthesized, it is possible to obtain a material with high melting point and high crystallinity, while a combination of D- and L-PLA can be needed if the aim is the production of packaging (Farah et al. 2016). PLA is one of most commonly used biopolymers in the world, being considered as one of the most promising bioplastics for the substitution of the petroleum-based polymers in packaging, and companies such as NatureWorks, invested by Cargill and PTT Global Chemicals, announced the production of high amounts of PLA per year (Vink et al. 2003). Other bio-based alternatives have been produced by companies such as Braskem (Brazil), being the production of polyethylene terephthalate by classical chemical synthesis using renewable bio-based monomers obtained from corn-starch and sugar cane as raw material. However, and despite being produced from a renewable source, it is not biodegradable.

Polyhydroxyalkanoate (PHA) and polyhydroxybutyrate (PHB), biopolymers obtained from microbial fermentation, emerge from the linear polyesters produced via fermentation and showed to be economic and technological alternatives for non-bio-based and non-biodegradable polymers. The final properties of the polymers are dependent on the monomer composition, as well as on the microorganism and the carbon source used during the fermentation process (Gumel et al. 2013). PHA- and PHB-based packaging materials are biodegradable, having relative low water vapor permeability and good mechanical properties. The main differences between both materials are the crystallinity and melting temperature, which is higher for PHB making it more suitable for industrial processes.

## 11.3 NANOSTRUCTURES FOR PACKAGING

Despite the great advances on the use of bio-based and biodegradable packaging on foods, there are several drawbacks that need to be overcome in order to present this type of packaging materials as a reliable solution for foods. These drawbacks are related with the price, which is expected to decrease when the demand increases and the technological barriers such as the use of production technologies normally applied for petroleum-based packaging, such as extrusion and co-extrusion, and their final properties, principally mechanical and barrier properties. Nanotechnology is pointed as a way to generate materials with unique properties and to produce innovative packaging materials, not only by the use of nanoparticles and nanocrystals, but also through the formation of layers or multilayers at nanoscale that can impart unique characteristics to the materials.

The advantages of nanoscale have led to a great interest by researchers from academy and industry on their use in packaging materials. Several advantages such as improved mechanical and barrier properties, thermal stability, and better optical properties were presented as enormous potential to improve the properties of packaging materials. Also, new functionalities, such as active and intelligent features are proposed by using nanotechnology. In this way, nanotechnology can be used in bio-based and biodegradable packaging materials to overcome some of the main drawbacks. The most studied nanomaterials have been inorganic and metallic nanoparticles such as clays and silver due to their capacity to improve barrier, thermal, and mechanical properties. Also, ZnO and $TiO_2$ nanoparticles showed to be interesting alternatives, even more if the aim is to obtain antimicrobial properties

(Cerqueira et al. 2018). Other of the options is to use bio-based and biodegradable materials for the production of nanostructures for food packaging applications, they can be divided in four main groups: nanoparticles, nanocrystals, nanofibers, and nanolayers. In this chapter, the metallic and inorganic nanoparticles will not be discussed, being focused on nanostructures obtained from bio-based and biodegradable materials.

### 11.3.1 Nanoparticles

Nanoparticles are zero-dimensional materials where all dimensions are at nanoscale. They can have several functionalities in packaging, and can be used to reinforce, add antimicrobial and antioxidant characteristics, or act as UV-blocking. Inorganic and metallic nanoparticles are the most used nanomaterials used in food packaging. The application of nanomaterials in food packaging was presented in 1993 (by the company AlliedSignal that joined Honeywell in 1999) by the production of extruded films and film laminates from a polymer nanocomposite (organo silanes) (Maxfield and Christiani 1993). In 1997, Mawatari et al. (Mawatari, Hamazaki and Furuyama, 1997) showed the possibility of using metal ions (e.g., silver) at nanoscale in a resin, to produce packaging materials with antibacterial properties. Since then, nanocomposites using silver, zinc oxide, and cloisite nanostructures have been tested on different packaging materials and discussed elsewhere (Cabedo and Gamez-Pérez 2018). Nowadays, some of the companies doing the commercialization of this kind of nanocomposites are Nanocor (Nanocor, Inc., USA) and PolyOne (PolyOne, Inc 2017).

The next stage on the development of nanoparticles for food packaging can be the use of bio-based and biodegradable nanoparticles. This can be done by the production of nanoparticles using polysaccharides, proteins, or compounds such as waxes or lignin. Several polysaccharides have been used for the production of nanoparticles, but only few were tested in packaging materials. Chitosan nanoparticles are one of the most studied in packaging materials. Based on the ionotropic gelation of chitosan, normally with sodium tripolyphosphate, this method comprises the crosslinking of chitosan by electrostatic interactions, resulting in chitosan nanoparticles which can be loaded with other bioactive molecules (Tsai et al. 2008; Chang et al. 2010a).

In 2009, De Moura et al. studied the effect of chitosan-based nanoparticles in hydroxypropyl methylcellulose-based films (De Moura et al. 2009). They evaluated mechanical properties, water vapor, oxygen permeability, and water solubility by evaluating the films structure by electron microscopy (SEM and TEM). Results showed that the incorporation of chitosan nanoparticles in the films improved their mechanical and barrier properties significantly (De Moura et al. 2009). Later on, the same authors evaluated the incorporation of chitosan nanoparticles in CMC-based films, which showed to be stable and uniform with sizes ranging between 80 and 110 nm. The incorporation of chitosan nanoparticles with higher sizes (around 100 nm) showed to improve thermal and mechanical properties of CMC-based films (De Moura et al. 2011).

One of the ways to produce bio-based nanostructures is by using acid hydrolysis, although it is mostly known for the production of nanocrystals (rod form), it is also possible to obtain spherical forms. This has been tested by consecutive acid hydrolysis and mechanical ultrasonication treatments of chitin, resulting in nanoparticles with sizes between 50 and 100 nm. In the same work, chitin nanoparticles were added to starch-based films in concentrations ranging between 1% and 5% and showed to decrease the water vapor permeability values of the films and increase tensile strength. Interestingly, it has been shown that higher loading concentrations (greater than 5 wt.%) lead to the aggregation of chitin nanoparticles thus having a negative effect on these properties (Chang et al. 2010b).

Starch is one of the materials employed in the production of nanoparticles frequently resorting to precipitation or cross-linking methodologies (Le Corre et al. 2010). Back in 2008, nanocomposites were prepared using starch nanoparticles in pea starch-based films. Different amounts of starch nanoparticles were used (between 0% and 4 wt.%) and showed to improve the barrier and mechanical properties of the films (Ma et al. 2008).

From proteins, zein is one of the most studied for the production of nanoparticles. Nanoprecipitation or antisolvent methods have been used to produce zein nanoparticles with diameters at nanoscale (Zhong and Jin 2009; Patel and Velikov 2014). Due to their thermal stability, they have been proposed as one of the ways to reinforce other bio-based films. In 2016, Oymaci and Altinkaya studied the effect of zein nanoparticles incorporation in WPI films, results showed that zein nanoparticles were able to improve the water vapor barrier and mechanical properties of the films and at the same time to decrease the fractional free volume and hydrophilicity of the WPI without changing the elongation-at-break of the films (Oymaci and Altinkaya 2016).

Other of the materials which have been tested for the production of nanoparticles is lignin. Yang et al. developed wheat gluten films with 0%, 1%, and 3% of lignin nanoparticles and showed that the incorporation of such nanoparticles in films led to a barrier to the ultraviolet spectrum and improved the water sensitivity of wheat gluten-based films. Results also showed that the mechanical properties and thermal stability was improved when lignin nanoparticles are added to the films (Yang et al. 2015).

### 11.3.2 Nanocrystals and Nanofibers

One-dimensional materials have a rod or tube shape, with lengths from 100 nm to few micrometers and thus one dimension can be outside the nanoscale. In the last years, several types of nanocrystals have be obtained from bio-based sources, cellulose, chitin and chitosan, and starch were some of the most explored materials. Cellulose-based nanostructures gained great attention due to mechanical, chemical, optical, and rheological characteristics, which increased the interest of researchers and companies. Cellulose at nanoscale shows many advantages, such as high specific strength and modulus, high surface area and unique optical properties, and absence of toxicity (Peng et al. 2011; Brinchi et al. 2013). The type or size of crystalline nanostructures affects their main properties and the corresponding applications of cellulose. Within this group, the best know nanostructures are microfibrillated cellulose and nanocrystalline cellulose (NCC), which present higher axial elastic modulus than the synthetic fiber Kevlar and mechanical properties similar to boron nanowhiskers, clay nanoplatelets, carbon fiber, and steel wire (Moon et al. 2011; Brinchi et al. 2013). Due to this, several studies were carried out on evaluating the incorporation of these nanostructured systems in bio-based and biodegradable packaging materials (Azeredo et al. 2017).

Wheat gluten-based films were reinforced with both cellulose nanofibrils microfibrillated cellulose and NCC extracted from sunflower stalks. This addition leads to better mechanical and barrier properties, especially in the case of films containing NCC (Fortunati et al. 2016). Also, bacterial cellulose has been used for this purpose (Fernandes et al. 2009). These authors evaluated the incorporation of micro- and nanofibrils of bacterial cellulose in chitosan films, as reinforcing agents. The resulting films showed better mechanical and moisture-barrier properties than those without this incorporation, and due to chitosan intrinsic properties, they also exhibited bacteriostatic and bactericidal activity (Fernandes et al. 2009). These results were confirmed by Velásquez-Cock et al. (2014), which showed that using bacterial cellulose nanoribbon, as reinforcing agent, improved the mechanical properties of chitosan-based films.

These evidences show the great potential of cellulose nanostructures that can be strategically used to overcome the limitation of several bio-based films such as the poor mechanical properties and water sensitivity that tremendously reduce the applications in some industrial sectors of packaging.

Also, nanocrystals from starch and chitin can be produced based on the same approach of NCC (Goodrich and Winter 2007; Le Corre et al. 2010) and used in packaging materials.

### 11.3.3 Nanolayers

Nanolayers, as a monolayer or as a multilayer, have been used in food packaging with different perspectives, as physical layer with barrier and mechanical properties, but also as an active layer, with antioxidant and/or antimicrobial properties. The nanolayers are two-dimensional exhibiting plate-like shape and can be films and coatings with nanometer thickness. The material used to produce the layer, the total number of layers, their sequence, and the process and conditions used to prepare each layer will determine the functionality of the final multilayer material.

In the packaging industry, it is possible to produce multilayer structures using three main technologies: co-extrusion, lamination, and coating. In co-extrusion, it is possible to produce up to more than nine layers of different materials, aiming at the combination of properties to form a unique final packaging material, however, only in few cases it is possible to produce layers at nanoscale. One of the ways is by multilayer co-extrusion which allows producing films with up to thousands of layers with layer thicknesses in the micro- and nanoscale, it is possible to combine in a multilayer structure, micro- and nanolayers, with up to 4096 layers, displaying each layer a thicknesses of less than 20 nm (Liu et al. 2003). An alternative is to use vacuum deposition technologies, such as thermal reactive evaporation, plasma-enhanced chemical vapor deposition, physical vapor deposition, electron-beam evaporation, and atomic layer deposition (Chatham 1996; Schneider et al. 2009; Struller et al. 2014) to form a thin inorganic layer on the film surface. Despite all the work performed using these technologies, their use on bio-based and biodegradable materials is still in its infancy (Hirvikorpi et al. 2010a, 2010b; Kääriäinen et al. 2011; Ramos et al. 2013).

One of the most used approaches to produce layers at nanoscale on films surface is the dipping process. In 2016, Slavutsky and Bertuzzi applied an oil phase by dipping on a starch-based film and observed the formation of a nanolayer (Slavutsky and Bertuzzi 2016). The formation of this layer allowed to improve the barrier properties and decreases the hydrophobicity of the starch-based film. Also by dipping, but based on the electrostatic interaction between materials, the layer-by-layer technique has been explored on the formation of multilayer structures in packaging materials. One of the materials tested was PLA, where the deposition of alternate layers of branched polyethyleneimine, hydrophobic fluorinated polymer (Nafion), and MMT allowed to obtain diverse multilayer conformations and characteristics, which decreased up to 98% and 78% the oxygen and water vapor permeability of the films, respectively (Carosio et al. 2014). It is also possible to use different bio-based and biodegradable materials to produce these nanolayers, and there are several works showing the possibility of using chitosan, alginate, and NCC (Carneiro-da-Cunha et al. 2010; Pillai and Renneckar 2016).

One of the techniques that have been recently explored was the electrohydrodynamic processing technology, through electrospinning and electrospraying. It can be used for the deposition of bio-based materials, such as proteins and polysaccharides on packaging materials as a way to improve their barrier properties or incorporate active compounds (Cerqueira et al. 2016a). One of the works that shows this possibilities was presented by Fabra et al. (2016), where α-tocopherol was mixed in three different hydrocolloid matrices, namely, whey protein isolate (WPI), zein, and soy protein isolate, which were directly electrospun or electrosprayed as coating layers on wheat gluten films. Results indicated that the antioxidant activity of the active compounds was preserved during the encapsulation process and storage time. This technique was also used on paper and cellulose-based films functionalization, not only to improve the barrier performance and mechanical properties, but also as a way to produce active films (Cherpinski et al. 2018).

One of the commercial applications of nanolayers was presented by Valentis Nanotech. They showed the possibility of coating different plastic films and improve their properties. Polyethylene (PE), biaxially oriented polypropylene (BOPP), and polyethylene terephthalate (PET) films showed better tensile properties (Valentis Nanotechn Ltd 2017).

## 11.4 ACTIVE PACKAGING

Active packaging provides functions that go beyond the simple passive barrier that separates food from the external environment in traditional packaging systems (Dainelli et al. 2008). In active packaging systems, materials are designed to interact with the product to maintain the quality, extend the shelf life, and improve safety (Biji et al. 2015). Various strategies have been developed to adapt the principles of active packaging to the specific needs of different food groups, mainly: humidity control, temperature and atmosphere composition (for example, concentration of $O_2$,

$CO_2$, and ethylene), release of antioxidant or antimicrobial compounds, or combinations of several of these strategies (Biji et al. 2015). The most common applications include controls of pathogen proliferation, microbiological deterioration, and oxidation (Brandelli et al. 2017). The use of bio-based materials for these cases is discussed in depth in this section.

### 11.4.1 Antimicrobial Active Packaging

Antimicrobial packaging is a form of active packaging designed to delay, reduce, or inhibit the growth of unwanted microorganisms in food (Appendini and Hotchkiss 2002). In general, two types of strategies can be distinguished in the production of antimicrobial active packaging systems: (i) incorporation of antimicrobial compounds that diffuse slowly from the container to the food and (ii) use of antimicrobial materials from which there is no migration of the active agent toward the food, but provide an antimicrobial barrier on the surface of the food product (Biji et al. 2015). Both strategies represent an advantage over the direct application of antimicrobials on the surface of the food or in bulk, which have limited effectiveness because the bioactive substances can be inactivated by reacting with other components of the food matrix (Quintavalla and Vicini 2002).

Several natural antimicrobial substances, including peptides, enzymes, essential oils, polysaccharides, and other metabolites of fungal and bacterial origin, have been used to develop materials for active packaging (de Azeredo 2013; Biji et al. 2015). In many cases, the active compounds are encapsulated in nanostructures as described in Section 11.3 (e.g., capsules and fibers). Encapsulation is performed with three objectives: (i) protect the bioactive compound itself, (ii) avoid unwanted reactions with components of the food matrix that can lead to changes in the sensory or nutritional properties of the food, and (iii) promote a controlled release of the active compound to extend the protective effect (Gómez-Mascaraque et al. 2015). The selection of the type of nanostructure (e.g., particle, capsule, emulsion, fiber, and film) and method of encapsulation depend on the characteristics of the bioactive compound (e.g., size, hydrophilic/lipophilic balance, and load) and the food product (e.g., composition and storage conditions). In any case, the size of the nanostructures usually has a strong effect on the release kinetics of the bioactive compounds (Brandelli et al. 2017).

Regarding peptide antimicrobials, the bacteriocin nisin has been incorporated, in free form, into biodegradable films of poly(butylene adipate-co-terephthalate), showing efficient inhibition of *Listeria monocytogenes* (Zehetmeyer et al. 2015). Nisin incorporated in starch-halloysite nanocomposite films inhibited *L. monocytogenes*, *Clostridium perfringens*, and *Staphylococcus aureus* in *in vitro* tests, and was successfully tested to inhibit *L. monocytogenes* in soft cheese (Meira et al. 2016). Correa et al. (2017) have incorporated nisin in nanocomposite-films made with PHB/polycaprolactone and organo-clays. Nisin-adsorbed PHB/polycaprolactone films were effective against *Lactobacillus plantarum* on sliced ham. Also, nisin-loaded chitosan/poly(L-lactic acid) films were reported to inhibit *Staphylococcus aureus* (Wang et al. 2015). Nisin encapsulated in different nanostructures has also been used in several antimicrobial active packaging applications. For example, polyethylene oxide nanofibers loaded with poly-$\gamma$-glutamate/chitosan nanoparticles containing nisin inhibited the growth of *L. monocytogenes* on cheese, without noticeable impact on the sensorial properties (Cui et al. 2017). Wang et al. (2015) used electrospinning to prepare nisin-loaded polyvinyl alcohol/wheat-gluten/zirconia nanofibrous membranes. These authors reported a well-controlled release and good antimicrobial activity against *S. aureus*. Nisin-loaded phosphatidylcholine liposomes were used to develop nanocomposite films made with gelatin and casein. The films presented antimicrobial activity against *L. monocytogenes*, *C. perfringens* and *Bacillus cereus*. Also, the incorporation of halloysite improved the barrier properties of the films providing a better controlled release of nisin (Boelter and Brandelli 2016). Other antimicrobial peptides such as lactocin 705 and lactocin AL705 from *L. curvatus* were also incorporated into gluten-based films and showed antimicrobial activity against spoilage lactic acid bacteria and *Listeria* in packed Wiener sausages (Blanco Massani et al. 2014). Some authors have even tested the entrapment of living bacteriocin-producing bacteria (*Enterococcus casseliflavus*) in polyvinyl alcohol coatings applied to the surface of poly(ethylene terephthalate) (PET) films, showing effectiveness in the control of *L. monocytogenes* on precooked chicken fillets stored at 4°C and 22°C and under simulated cold chain conditions (1 day at 30°C) (Degli Esposti et al. 2018).

The use of antimicrobial enzymes such as lysozyme has also been evaluated in the development of antimicrobial active packaging. Arcan and Yemenicioğlu (2014) developed zein-fatty acid films for the controlled release of lysozyme that were effective against *Listeria innocua* in *in vitro* tests. Silva et al. used the solvent casting technique to prepare nanocomposite films of pullulan and lysozyme nanofibers. They found that the nanocomposite films had antibacterial activity against *S. aureus*, which is a bacterium resistant to lysozyme in free form (Silva et al. 2018). Peptides or enzymes with antimicrobial activity have also been immobilized or covalently bound to the packaging materials. This strategy has been found to improve the stability to pH and temperature and resistance to proteolytic enzymes or denaturing agents (Brandelli et al. 2017). For instance, nisin grafted on carboxylated cellulose nanofibers designed for food packaging caused a 3.5-log reduction in the counts of *Bacillus subtilis* and *S. aureus* in *in vitro* tests (Saini et al. 2016). Wu et al. (2018) also immobilized nisin in oxidized cellulose films. In this case, the nisin was anchored using a Schiff base reaction between the amino groups of nisin and the aldehyde groups of oxidized cellulose. The nisin-grafted film had good antimicrobial activity against *Alicyclobacillus acidoterrestris*, a spoilage bacterium common in fruit juices, and the antimicrobial activity of the film was maintained for over 3 months.

An alternative strategy consists in obtaining antimicrobial surfaces without migration of the active agents by using polymers with intrinsic antimicrobial activity. Chitosan is an excellent example. This polysaccharide has demonstrated antimicrobial activity against Gram-positive and Gram-negative bacteria and filamentous fungi and yeasts (Kong et al. 2010). It has been used alone in the production of nano-structured antimicrobial films and in combination with other bio-based polymers and antimicrobial agents such as lysozyme in fresh egg coatings (Yuceer and Caner 2014) or in the production of chitosan-based nanocapsules and nanocomposite films for the encapsulation and controlled release of essential oils with strong antimicrobial activity, which have demonstrated activity against bacteria such as *Escherichia coli*, *L. monocytogenes*, *Salmonella enteritidis*, and *S. aureus* (Higueras et al. 2014; Kurek et al. 2014; Hosseini et al. 2016).

Packaging systems that release volatile antimicrobial compounds, such as plant essential oils, have the advantage that the active compound does not need to be in direct contact with the food. In these systems, antimicrobial agents can be incorporated directly into mixtures of film-forming polymers or can be previously encapsulated in compatible nanostructures from where they diffuse into the food or the surrounding internal atmosphere. In any case, the external packaging material must have high barrier properties to avoid the loss of the bioactive compound (Appendini and Hotchkiss 2002). Cinnamon, clove bud, and oregano oils are some examples of essential oils that have been tested in active antimicrobial packaging. Cinnamaldehyde was incorporated into ethyl cellulose-based active bi-layer films prepared by solvent casting and electrospinning. The obtained films presented a hydrophobic surface and high antimicrobial activity against *L. monocytogenes* and *S. typhimurium* (Martins et al. 2018). Cinnamon essential oil was also loaded into β-cyclodextrins and incorporated into a biodegradable polyvinyl alcohol electrospun film, exhibiting excellent antimicrobial activity on strawberries contaminated with *S. aureus* and *E. coli* (the minimum inhibitory and bactericidal concentrations were ca. 8.9–9.9 μg/mL and 69.3–79.2 μg/mL, respectively) (Wen et al. 2016). Otoni et al. tested the antimicrobial activity of methylcellulose films containing nanoemulsions of clove bud and oregano essential oils, observing a reduction in yeasts and molds in sliced bread stored in sealed bags at 25°C during 15 days (Otoni et al. 2014).

### 11.4.2 Packaging Systems for Preventing Oxidation

Oxygen can spoil many different food products, such as fatty fish, cooked meats, cheese, herbs, fruit juices, coffee, tea, and beer, in which oxidative reactions can result in off-favors, color modifications, and nutritional losses (Day and Potter 2011; Biji et al. 2015). Also, oxygen promotes the growth of aerobic microorganisms that can also reduce the product's shelf life. Modified atmosphere packaging or vacuum packaging is frequently used to reduce the oxygen content in packaged goods. However, these technologies do not remove oxygen completely, and there is always a fraction of oxygen that diffuses through the packaging materials. Additionally, vacuum packaging can damage the structure of some food products, limiting its application (Day and Potter 2011; Biji et al. 2015).

Oxygen scavengers can be used in combination with modified atmosphere packaging or vacuum packaging and nanocomposite films (for selective control of oxygen diffusion) to reduce the oxygen concentration in the package atmosphere to less than 100 ppm (Biji et al. 2015). The most common oxygen scavengers are based on the oxidation of iron powders, usually in the presence of sodium chloride, which acts as an activator, allowing the iron powder to oxidize at a higher rate (Rooney 2005). Nonetheless, some alternatives based on the oxidation of biomaterials, such as ascorbic acid, tocopherol, or gallic acid, have also been explored (Janjarasskul et al. 2013; Scarfato et al. 2015; Pant et al. 2017). Also, enzymatic systems have been proposed, such as those based on the combined use of glucose oxidase, glucose, and catalase. In this case, glucose oxidase catalyzes the oxidation of glucose to glucono-delta-lactone with the consequent production of hydrogen peroxide, which is degraded to water and oxygen by the catalase. Although oxygen is produced in the last reaction, there is an overall reduction in the oxygen level inside the package (Day and Potter 2011).

Most oxygen scavengers are commercialized in the form of small sachets. However, there is a current trend to incorporate the oxygen scavengers directly in the packaging materials to avoid contamination by accidental rupture of the sachets (Janjarasskul et al. 2013; Biji et al. 2015; Pant et al. 2017).

A different strategy to increase the shelf life of oxygen-sensitive foods is to use packaging materials for the controlled release of antioxidants, thus reducing the need for high concentration of preservatives in the food formulation. Incorporation of natural antioxidants such as vitamins, polyphenols, and essential oils in food packaging films has been shown to reduce oxidative reactions in different food products. For instance, Fabra et al. (2016) used electro-hydrodynamic processing to encapsulate $\alpha$-tocopherol in different biopolymers such as whey protein isolate, zein, and soy protein isolate. The $\alpha$-tocopherol-containing fibers were produced directly on the surface of a thermoplastic wheat gluten film, which demonstrated antioxidant activity in *in vitro* tests. Chitosan films loaded with polyphenols such as quercetin have also demonstrated strong free-radical scavenging activity (Souza et al. 2015), and many works have been reported on the use of essential oils, which combine antioxidant and antimicrobial activities (Ramos et al. 2014; Martins et al. 2018).

## 11.5 INTELLIGENT PACKAGING

Unlike active packaging, intelligent packaging is not designed to interact directly with packaged products to increase their shelf life. The objective of intelligent packaging is to monitor the condition of packaged foods or their surrounding environment (e.g., temperature, pH, gaseous composition, presence of specific molecules, or microorganisms) during storage and transport. This information is communicated in real-time to users (consumers or distributors) to facilitate market decisions or alert about possible stability problems (Yam et al. 2005; Realini and Marcos 2014). Intelligent packaging can eliminate the need for inaccurate expiration dates, thus improving the food safety and reducing food waste (Silvestre et al. 2011). In addition, as intelligent packaging does not require the migration of active compounds toward the food, its use finds fewer legal restrictions than that of active packaging in areas such as Europe or North America, where food packaging regulations are very restrictive. The most common intelligent packaging devices are indicators, biosensors, and data carrier systems (such as, radio frequency identification) (Vanderroost et al. 2014).

### 11.5.1 INDICATORS

Indicator systems usually provide information through colorimetric changes visible to the naked eye. These devices can be incorporated into the packaging materials or later printed or attached as an adhesive label (Brody et al. 2008). One of the most frequent applications are the indicators of time and temperature. These devices can record the thermal history of a food product (from the factory to the consumer home) and inform if the temperature has exceeded a certain threshold (Wang et al. 2015).

New types of time and temperature indicator devices based on biomaterials of natural origin have recently been described. Maciel et al. (2012) developed a time and temperature indicator prototype using chitosan films doped with anthocyanins, which undergo an irreversible color change from violet to yellow after a specific temperature range exposure (40°C–70°C). Other authors have reported the use of gold-nanoparticles/gelatin bionanocomposites, which show a color change after 6 hours at 30°C, and the color intensity is proportional to the duration of the temperature over exposure (Wang et al. 2015). Indirect methods have also been described to detect temperature changes based on the activity of microorganisms such as yeasts and lactic bacteria that remain inactive at low temperatures (<5°C) and grow progressively in certain temperature ranges, generating acids, resulting in the color change of a pH indicator (Wang et al. 2015). Another type of indicators are the freshness indicators, which detect changes in the quality of packaged foods through pH alterations or by detecting the presence of volatile or non-volatile compounds produced as a consequence of the food. For example, Pourjavaher et al. (2017) have developed an indicator label for pH changes (in the range of 2–10) based on a film composed of bacterial cellulose nanofibers and red cabbage anthocyanins. Xiaowei et al. (2014) have developed a sensor for the evaluation of meat quality based on the detection of biogenic amines (10–30 ppm) that induced color changes in an array made by printing nine natural pigments on a hydrophobic nanoporous film.

### 11.5.2 Biomaterials for Sensors and Data Carriers

Biosensors are devices that combine a process of recognition of biocompounds (e.g., microorganisms and organic metabolites) and a transducer capable of converting the biological response into an electrical signal (Maftoonazad and Ramaswamy 2018). Biorecognition is generally carried out by the incorporation of oligonucleotides, enzymes, aptamers, or antigen/antibody systems immobilized in nanocomposites (Shrivastava et al. 2016). On the other hand, transducers require conductive materials. For this purpose, the most used bio-materials in electroanalytical sensors are nanocomposites of polymers with conjugated double bonds such as polyaniline, polypyrrole, or polythiophene (Bagheri et al. 2013). Also, in recent years, greener biosensors are being developed based on bionanocomposites of carbon compounds and natural compounds such as graphite-peptide (Wang et al. 2017) and carbon nanotube-chitosan (Zhang et al. 2018).

Biosensors allow integration with the Internet of things (IoT) and Blockchain platforms. IoT provides a link between the physical food product and the information channels that consumers or retailers can access at any stage of the supply chain, while Blockchain provides a shared immutable record of all the transactions between all the different stakeholders involved in the supply chain, ensuring traceability and helping to identify potential safety risks (Deloitte 2017). Among the biggest challenges to overcome for the massive integration of biosensors in food packaging are the production costs and the biocompatibility of the required materials for the electronic elements. Nonetheless, big advances are being made in this direction. For instance, Salvatore et al. (2017) have developed a set of low-cost biodegradable materials that can be used in biodegradable sensors. The authors reported the fabrication of an ultra-thin temperature sensor, suitable for food applications, prepared from silicon dioxide and nitride on a substrate made out of a compostable polymer derived from starch. The sensor was connected, using water-soluble zinc wires to a Bluetooth module, demonstrating application in food tracking and potential integration in IoT/Blockchain platforms.

## 11.6 CONCLUSION AND FUTURE PERSPECTIVES

The role of the food packaging industry has to be redefined to face the challenges of the food system in this new century. Sustainability, reduction of food waste and petrol dependence, improvement of the quality and safety of foods, and traceability and authenticity are some of the issues not well solved yet (or generated) by the current traditional packaging technologies.

Food packaging is by far the most attractive, commercial, accepted by consumers, and fast-growing application of nanotechnology in the food system. Scientists have demonstrated that nanotechnology allows improving the performance of conventional food packaging materials and also to provide them new functionalities in order to extend the shelf life, quality, and safety of foods. Combination of biodegradable bio-based polymers with different nanofillers or by using nanotechnologies offers the possibility to obtain new eco-friendly food packaging materials suitable to face the new customer demands. These bionanocomposite materials not only are sustainable and allow replacing those petrol-based plastics, but also improve the performance (e.g., mechanical, thermal, and barrier properties) of biopolymers, while exhibiting other functions for active packaging (e.g., antimicrobial, antioxidant, and oxygen scavengers). These new food packaging solutions will not only allow saving no renewable resources, but also prevent food spoilage, making fresher, tastier, healthier, more nutritious, and safer foods.

Nanotechnology will empower consumers. By using intelligent packaging solutions, it will be possible to extract data about the state of the food inside the package, making the food chain supply more transparent and trustworthy. Thus, consumers will have information to make responsible purchase decisions. The nanosensors embedded into the food packages will alert consumers about the quality and safety of food, but also about its origin and authenticity. That implies a very broad type of sensors based in a wide range of technologies (e.g., DNA, optic, and electrochemical). Together with the sensorization of food packages, it will be necessary to design and produce labels and devices to avoid fraud and falsification. These systems should be based in the IoT concept and readable in all the steps of the food value chain. These devices and labels will be able to store and share information about the food and their history.

Combination of intelligent packaging with IoT and Big data will change the fabrication of the entire packaging industry. Food applications of the Blockchain technology will be the first step of this industrial transformation allowing the integration of all attributes of the food value chain: safety, authenticity, ethics, and quality of foods. This relates new food packaging to a new concept called *food integrity*. Food integrity connects the food value chains both at physical and digital layers, where the digital layer should provide reliable and trustworthy information on the origin and provenance of food products in the physical layer. Nanotechnology will support food integrity avoiding fraud and adulteration (also label imitation) and undesirable changes in the certification, safety, quality, and nutritional characteristics, as well as sensorial properties of foods.

However, many of the above-mentioned solutions still have a long way to be commercial. In order to reduce the time to the market of the bionanocomposite materials and to explore their maximum potential for active and smart food packaging applications, further studies to assess the potential dangers and ethical questions raising about the novel applications are still needed. For example, migration tests, evaluation of the toxicological effects of nanomaterials upon ingestion, the interaction of bionanocomposites with food components, and other safety studies have to be performed using standardized approaches, methods, and test procedures.

Nanotechnology opens a promising future in food packaging. The success of these new applications also passes by setting up proper communication strategies involving regulatory bodies, scientists, companies, and consumers associations. The objective of these communication plans is to generate trust in the food system avoiding misunderstandings and fake information. For that purpose, scientific facts should be presented in a consistent way explaining both the advantages and potential risks of new packaging materials.

## ACKNOWLEDGMENTS

This work was funded by the projects "Nanotechnology based functional solutions" (Norte 2020 Program, Ref. NORTE-01-0145-FEDER-000019), "CVMar+i: Industrial innovation through specific collaborations between companies and research centers in the context of marine biotechnological valorization" (INTERREG V-A España – Portugal – POCTEP 2014–2020, Ref. 0302_CVMAR_I_1_P), "MOBFOOD: Mobilizing scientific and technological knowledge in response to the challenges of the agri-food market" (COMPETE2020; LISBOA2020; PORTUGAL2020, Ref. POCI-01-0247-FEDER-024524), "YPack: High performance polyhydroxyalkanoates (PHB) based packaging to minimize food waste" (H2020, Ref. 773872), and "PACKTERIOPHAGE: Bacteriophage-releasing nanostructured smart packaging materials for the control of food-borne *Campylobacter*" (FCT, COMPETE2020, PORTUGAL2020, ERDF, Ref. POCI-01-0145-FEDER-032594).

## REFERENCES

Abad, E., S. Zampolli, S. Marco, A. Scorzoni, B. Mazzolai, A. Juarros, D. Gómez et al. 2007. "Flexible Tag Microlab Development: Gas Sensors Integration in RFID Flexible Tags for Food Logistic." *Sensors and Actuators, B: Chemical* 127: 2.

Abreu, A. S., M. Oliveira, A. D. Sá, R. M. Rodrigues, M. A. Cerqueira, A. A. Vicente, and A. V. Machado. 2015. "Antimicrobial Nanostructured Starch Based Films for Packaging." *Carbohydrate Polymers* 129: 127–134.

Aguirre-Joya, J. A., B. Álvarez, J. M. Ventura, J. O. García-Galindo, M. A. D. León-Zapata, R. Rojas, S. Saucedo, and C. N. Aguilar. 2016. "Edible Coatings and Films from Lipids, Waxes, and Resins." In *Edible Food Packaging*, edited by M. A. Cerqueira, R. N. Pereira, O. L. Ramos, J. A. Teixeira, and A. A. Vicente, pp. 121–152. Contemporary Food Engineering. Boca Raton, FL: CRC Press.

Alleyne, V., and R. D. Hagenmaier. 2000. "Candelilla-Shellac: An Alternative Formulation for Coating Apples." *HortScience* 35: 691–693.

Appendini, P., and J. H. Hotchkiss. 2002. "Review of Antimicrobial Food Packaging." *Innovative Food Science and Emerging Technologies* 3 (2): 113–126.

Arcan, I., and A. Yemenicioğlu. 2014. "Controlled Release Properties of Zein–Fatty Acid Blend Films for Multiple Bioactive Compounds." *Journal of Agricultural and Food Chemistry* 62 (32): 8238–8246.

Arik Kibar, E. A., and F. Us. 2013. "Thermal, Mechanical and Water Adsorption Properties of Corn Starch-Carboxymethylcellulose/Methylcellulose Biodegradable Films." *Journal of Food Engineering* 114: 123–131.

Azeredo, H. M. C., M. F. Rosa, and L. H. C. Mattoso. 2017. "Nanocellulose in Bio-based Food Packaging Applications." *Industrial Crops and Products* 97: 664–671.

Bagheri, H., Z. Ayazi, and M. Naderi. 2013. "Conductive Polymer-Based Microextraction Methods: A Review." *Analytica Chimica Acta* 767: 1–13.

Berezina, N., and S. M. Martelli. 2014. "Bio-based Polymers and Materials." In *Renewable Resources for Biorefineries*, edited by C. Lin and R. Luque, *RSC Green Chemistry Series*.

Biji, K. B., C. N. Ravishankar, C. O. Mohan, and T. K. S. Gopal. 2015. "Smart Packaging Systems for Food Applications: A Review." *Journal of Food Science and Technology* 52 (10): 6125–6135.

Blanco Massani, M., V. Molina, M. Sanchez, V. Renaud, P. Eisenberg, and G. Vignolo. 2014. "Active Polymers Containing Lactobacillus Curvatus CRL705 Bacteriocins: Effectiveness Assessment in Wieners." *International Journal of Food Microbiology* 178 (May): 7–12.

Boelter, J. F., and A. Brandelli. 2016. "Innovative Bionanocomposite Films of Edible Proteins Containing Liposome-Encapsulated Nisin and Halloysite Nanoclay." *Colloids and Surfaces. B, Biointerfaces* 145 (September): 740–747.

Brandelli, A., L. F. W. Brum, and J. H. Z. dos Santos. 2017. "Nanostructured Bioactive Compounds for Ecological Food Packaging." *Environmental Chemistry Letters* 15 (2): 193–204.

Brinchi, L., F. Cotana, E. Fortunati, and J. M. Kenny. 2013. "Production of Nanocrystalline Cellulose from Lignocellulosic Biomass: Technology and Applications." *Carbohydrate Polymers* 94: 154–169.

Brody, A. L., B. Bugusu, J. H. Han, C. K. Sand, and T. H. McHugh. 2008. "Scientific Status Summary. Innovative Food Packaging Solutions." *Journal of Food Science* 73 (8): R107–R116.

Cabedo, L., and J. Gamez-Pérez. 2018. "Chapter 2—Inorganic-Based Nanostructures and Their Use in Food Packaging." In *Micro and Nano Technologies*, edited by M. Â. P. R. Cerqueira, J. M. Lagaron, L. M. P. Castro, and A. A. de Oliveira Soares Vicente, pp. 13–45. Amsterdam, Netherlands: Elsevier.

Callegarin, F., J-A. Q. Gallo, F. Debeaufort, and A. Voilley. 1997. "Lipids and biopackaging." *Journal of the American Oil Chemists' Society*. 74(10): 1183–1192.

Carneiro-da-Cunha, M. G., M. A. Cerqueira, B. W. S. Souza, S. Carvalho, M. A. C. Quintas, J. A. Teixeira, and A. A. Vicente. 2010. "Physical and Thermal Properties of a Chitosan/Alginate Nanolayered PET Film." *Carbohydrate Polymers* 82 (1): 153–159.

Carosio, F., S. Colonna, A. Fina, G. Rydzek, J. Hemmerlé, L. Jierry, P. Schaaf, and F. Boulmedais. 2014. "Efficient Gas and Water Vapor Barrier Properties of Thin Poly(Lactic Acid) Packaging Films: Functionalization with Moisture Resistant Nafion and Clay Multilayers." *Chemistry of Materials* 26 (19): 5459–5466.

Cerqueira, M. A., M. J. Fabra, J. L. Castro-Mayorga, A. I. Bourbon, L. M. Pastrana, A. A. Vicente, and J. M. Lagaron. 2016. "Use of Electrospinning to Develop Antimicrobial Biodegradable Multilayer Systems: Encapsulation of Cinnamaldehyde and Their Physicochemical Characterization." *Food and Bioprocess Technology* 9 (11): 1874–1884.

Cerqueira, M. A., A. A. Vicente, and L. M. Pastrana. 2018. "Chapter 1—Nanotechnology in Food Packaging: Opportunities and Challenges." In *Micro and Nano Technologies*, edited by Miguel Ângelo Parente Ribeiro Cerqueira, Jose Maria Lagaron, Lorenzo Miguel Pastrana Castro, and António Augusto Martins B T—Nanomaterials for Food Packaging de Oliveira Soares Vicente, pp. 1–11. Elsevier.

Chang, P. R., R. Jian, J. Yu, and X. Ma. 2010a. "Fabrication and Characterisation of Chitosan Nanoparticles/Plasticised-Starch Composites." *Food Chemistry* 120: 736–740.

Chang, P. R., R. Jian, J. Yu, and X. Ma. 2010b. "Starch-Based Composites Reinforced with Novel Chitin Nanoparticles." *Carbohydrate Polymers* 80: 421–426.

Chatham, H. 1996. "Oxygen Diffusion Barrier Properties of Transparent Oxide Coatings on Polymeric Substrates." *Surface and Coatings Technology* 78 (1–3): 1–9.

Chaudhry, Q., M. Scotter, J. Blackburn, B. Ross, A. Boxall, L. Castle, R. Aitken, and R. Watkins. 2008. "Applications and Implications of Nanotechnologies for the Food Sector." *Food Additives and Contaminants—Part A Chemistry, Analysis, Control, Exposure and Risk Assessment* 25: 241–258.

Cherpinski, A., S. Torres-Giner, J. Vartiainen, M. S. Peresin, P. Lahtinen, and J. M. Lagaron. 2018. "Improving the Water Resistance of Nanocellulose-Based Films with Polyhydroxyalkanoates Processed by the Electrospinning Coating Technique." *Cellulose* 25: 1291–1307.

Corre, D. L., J. Bras, and A. Dufresne. 2010. "Starch Nanoparticles: A Review." *Biomacromolecules* 11: 1139–1153.

Correa, J. P., V. Molina, M. Sanchez, C. Kainz, P. Eisenberg, and M. B. Massani. 2017. "Improving Ham Shelf Life with a Polyhydroxybutyrate/Polycaprolactone Biodegradable Film Activated with Nisin." *Food Packaging and Shelf Life* 11 (March): 31–39.

Cui, H., J. Wu, C. Li, and L. Lin. 2017. "Improving Anti-Listeria Activity of Cheese Packaging via Nanofiber Containing Nisin-Loaded Nanoparticles." *LWT—Food Science and Technology* 81 (January): 233–242.

Dainelli, D., N. Gontard, D. Spyropoulos, E. Zondervan-van den Beuken, and P. Tobback. 2008. "Active and Intelligent Food Packaging: Legal Aspects and Safety Concerns." *Trends in Food Science & Technology* 19 (November): S103–S112.

Day, B. P. F., and L. Potter. 2011. "Active Packaging" In *Food and Beverage Packaging Technology*, edited by R. Coles and M. J. Kirwan, 1:251–262. Oxford, UK: Wiley-Blackwell.

De Azeredo, H. M. C. 2013. "Antimicrobial Nanostructures in Food Packaging." *Trends in Food Science & Technology* 30 (1): 56–69.

De Moura, M. R., F. A. Aouada, R. J. Avena-Bustillos, T. H. McHugh, J. M. Krochta, and L. H. C. Mattoso. 2009. "Improved Barrier and Mechanical Properties of Novel Hydroxypropyl Methylcellulose Edible Films with Chitosan/Tripolyphosphate Nanoparticles." *Journal of Food Engineering* 92 (4): 448–453.

De Moura, M. R., M. V. Lorevice, L. H. C. Mattoso, and V. Zucolotto. 2011. "Highly Stable, Edible Cellulose Films Incorporating Chitosan Nanoparticles." *Journal of Food Science* 76: N25–N29.

Degli Esposti, M., M. Toselli, C. Sabia, P. Messi, S. de Niederhäusern, M. Bondi, and R. Iseppi. 2018. "Effectiveness of Polymeric Coated Films Containing Bacteriocin-Producer Living Bacteria for Listeria Monocytogenes Control under Simulated Cold Chain Break." *Food Microbiology* 76 (January): 173–179.

Deloitte. 2017. "Continuous Interconnected Supply Chain: Using Blockchain & Internet-of-Things in Supply Chain Traceability." *Deloitte Tax and Consulting* 24: 1–24.

Ellen MacArthur Foundation. 2017. The New Plastics Economy: Catalysing Action. Ellen MacArthur Foundation.

Fabra, M. J., A. López-Rubio, and J. M. Lagaron. 2016. "Use of the Electrohydrodynamic Process to Develop Active/Bioactive Bilayer Films for Food Packaging Applications." *Food Hydrocolloids* 55: 11–18.

Fallik, E., Y. Shalom, S. Alkalai-Tuvia, O. Larkov, E. Brandeis, and U. Ravid. 2005. "External, Internal and Sensory Traits in Galia-Type Melon Treated with Different Waxes." *Postharvest Biology and Technology* 36, 69–75.

Farah, S., D. G. Anderson, and R. Langer. 2016. "Physical and Mechanical Properties of PLA, and Their Functions in Widespread Applications—A Comprehensive Review." *Advanced Drug Delivery Reviews* 107, 367–392.

Fernandes, S. C. M., L. Oliveira, C. S. R. Freire, A. J. D. Silvestre, C. P. Neto, A. Gandini, and J. Desbriéres. 2009. "Novel Transparent Nanocomposite Films Based on Chitosan and Bacterial Cellulose." *Green Chemistry* 11: 2023–2029.

Fortunati, E., F. Luzi, A. Jiménez, D. A. Gopakumar, D. Puglia, S. Thomas, J. M. Kenny, A. Chiralt, and L. Torre. 2016. "Revalorization of Sunflower Stalks as Novel Sources of Cellulose Nanofibrils and Nanocrystals and Their Effect on Wheat Gluten Bionanocomposite Properties." *Carbohydrate Polymers* 149: 357–368.

Ghanbarzadeh, B., H. Almasi, and A. A. Entezami. 2011. "Improving the Barrier and Mechanical Properties of Corn Starch-Based Edible Films: Effect of Citric Acid and Carboxymethyl Cellulose." *Industrial Crops and Products* 33, 229–235.

Gómez-Mascaraque, L. G., J. M. Lagaron, and A. López-Rubio. 2015. "Electrosprayed Gelatin Submicroparticles as Edible Carriers for the Encapsulation of Polyphenols of Interest in Functional Foods." *Food Hydrocolloids* 49 (July): 42–52.

Goodrich, J. D., and W. T. Winter. 2007. "Alpha-Chitin Nanocrystals Prepared from Shrimp Shells and Their Specific Surface Area Measurement." *Biomacromolecules* 8: 252–257.

Guerrero, P., and K. De la Caba. 2016. "Protein-Based Films and Coatings." In *Edible Food Packaging*, edited by M. A. Cerqueira, R. N. Pereira, Ó. L. Ramos, J. A. Teixeira, and A. A. Vicente, pp. 81–120, Boca Raton, FL: CRC Press.

Gumel, A. M., M. S. M. Annuar, and Y. Chisti. 2013. "Recent Advances in the Production, Recovery and Applications of Polyhydroxyalkanoates." *Journal of Polymers and the Environment* 21: 580–605.

Higueras, L., G. López-Carballo, P. Hernández-Muñoz, R. Catalá, and R. Gavara. 2014. "Antimicrobial Packaging of Chicken Fillets Based on the Release of Carvacrol from Chitosan/Cyclodextrin Films." *International Journal of Food Microbiology* 188 (January): 53–59.

Hirvikorpi, T., M. Vähä-Nissi, A. Harlin, and M. Karppinen. 2010a. "Comparison of Some Coating Techniques to Fabricate Barrier Layers on Packaging Materials." *Thin Solid Films* 518 (19): 5463–5466.

Hirvikorpi, T., M. Vähä-Nissi, T. Mustonen, E. Iiskola, and M. Karppinen. 2010b. "Atomic Layer Deposited Aluminum Oxide Barrier Coatings for Packaging Materials." *Thin Solid Films* 518 (10): 2654–2658.

Hosseini, S. F., M. Rezaei, M. Zandi, and F. Farahmandghavi. 2016. "Development of Bioactive Fish Gelatin/Chitosan Nanoparticles Composite Films with Antimicrobial Properties." *Food Chemistry* 194 (January): 1266–1274.

Huo, W., D. Wei, W. Zhu, Z. Li, and Y. Jiang. 2018. "High-Elongation Zein Films for Flexible Packaging by Synergistic Plasticization: Preparation, Structure and Properties." *Journal of Cereal Science* 79: 354–361.

Jambeck, J. R., R. Geyer, C. Wilcox, T. R. Siegler, M. Perryman, A. Andrady, R. Narayan, and K. L. Law. 2015. "Plastic Waste Inputs from Land into the Ocean." *Science* 347: 768–771.

Janjarasskul, T., S. C. Min, and J. M. Krochta. 2013. "Triggering Mechanisms for Oxygen-Scavenging Function of Ascorbic Acid-Incorporated Whey Protein Isolate Films." *Journal of the Science of Food and Agriculture* 93 (12): 2939–2944.

Kääriäinen, T. O., P. Maydannik, D. C. Cameron, K. Lahtinen, P. Johansson, and J. Kuusipalo. 2011. "Atomic Layer Deposition on Polymer Based Flexible Packaging Materials: Growth Characteristics and Diffusion Barrier Properties." *Thin Solid Films* 519 (10): 3146–3154.

Karbowiak, T., F. Debeaufort, and A. Voilley. 2007. "Influence of thermal process on structure and functional properties of emulsion-based edible films." *Food Hydrocolloids*. 21(5–6): 879–888.

Khan, B., M. B. K. Niazi, G. Samin, and Z. Jahan. 2017. "Thermoplastic Starch: A Possible Biodegradable Food Packaging Material—A Review." *Journal of Food Process Engineering* 40: e12447.

Kong, M., X. G. Chen, K. Xing, and H. J. Park. 2010. "Antimicrobial Properties of Chitosan and Mode of Action: A State of the Art Review." *International Journal of Food Microbiology* 144: 51–63.

Krochta, J. 2002. "Proteins as Raw Materials for Films and Coatings: Definitions, Current Status, and Opportunities." In *Protein-Based Films and Coatings*, edited by A. Gennadios, pp. 1–42. Boca Raton, FL: CRC Press.

Kurek, M., A. Guinault, A. Voilley, K. Galić, and F. Debeaufort. 2014. "Effect of Relative Humidity on Carvacrol Release and Permeation Properties of Chitosan Based Films and Coatings." *Food Chemistry* 144 (January): 9–17.

Kuswandi, B., Y. Wicaksono, Jayus, A. Abdullah, L. Y. Heng, and M. Ahmad. 2011. "Smart Packaging: Sensors for Monitoring of Food Quality and Safety." *Sensing and Instrumentation for Food Quality and Safety* 5: 137–146.

Lim, L.-T., R. Auras, and M. Rubino. 2008. "Processing Technologies for Poly(Lactic Acid)." *Progress in Polymer Science* 33: 820–852.

Lin, D., and Y. Zhao. 2007. "Innovations in the Development and Application of Edible Coating for Fresh and Minimally Processed Fruits and Vegetables." *Comprehensive Reviews in Food Science and Food Safety* 6: 60–75.

Liu, R. Y. F., Y. Jin, A. Hiltner, and E. Baer. 2003. "Probing Nanoscale Polymer Interactions by Forced-Assembly." *Macromolecular Rapid Communications* 24 (16): 943–948.

López, O. V., L. A. Castillo, M. A. García, M. A. Villar, and S. E. Barbosa. 2015. "Food Packaging Bags Based on Thermoplastic Corn Starch Reinforced with Talc Nanoparticles." *Food Hydrocolloids* 43: 18–24.

Ma, X., R. Jian, P. R. Chang, and J. Yu. 2008. "Fabrication and Characterization of Citric Acid-Modified Starch Nanoparticles/Plasticized-Starch Composites." *Biomacromolecules* 9 (11): 3314–3320.

Mawatari, M., C. Hamazaki, and T. Furuyama. 1997. "Antibacterial resin composition." US patent. Japan Synthetic Rubber Co., Ltd.

Maciel, V. B. V., C. M. P. Yoshida, and T. T. Franco. 2012. "Development of a Prototype of a Colourimetric Temperature Indicator for Monitoring Food Quality." *Journal of Food Engineering* 111 (1): 21–27.

Maftoonazad, N., and H. Ramaswamy. 2018. "Novel Techniques in Food Processing: Bionanocomposites." *Current Opinion in Food Science* 23 (October): 49–56.

Mahalik, N. P., and A. N. Nambiar. 2010. "Trends in Food Packaging and Manufacturing Systems and Technology." *Trends in Food Science & Technology* 21: 117–128.

Martins, V. D. F., M. A. Cerqueira, P. Fuciños, A. Garrido-Maestu, J. M. R. Curto, and L. M. Pastrana. 2018. "Active Bi-Layer Cellulose-Based Films: Development and Characterization." *Cellulose* 25 (11): 6361–6375.

Maxfield, M., and B. R. Christiani. 1993. Polymer Nanocomposites Formed by Melt Processing of a Polymer and an Exfoliated Layered Material Derivatized with Reactive Organo Silanes, Issued 1993.

Meira, S. M. M., G. Zehetmeyer, J. M. Scheibel, J. O. Werner, and A. Brandelli. 2016. "Starch-Halloysite Nanocomposites Containing Nisin: Characterization and Inhibition of Listeria Monocytogenes in Soft Cheese." *LWT—Food Science and Technology* 68 (May): 226–234.

Moon, R. J., A. Martini, J. Nairn, J. Simonsen, and J. Youngblood. 2011. "Cellulose Nanomaterials Review: Structure, Properties and Nanocomposites." *Chemical Society Reviews* 40: 3941–3994.

Nanocor Inc. IMPERM. http://www.nanocor.com/tech_sheets/i103.pdf (accessed 1 August 2017).

Okano, K., T. Tanaka, C. Ogino, H. Fukuda, and A. Kondo. 2010. "Biotechnological Production of Enantiomeric Pure Lactic Acid from Renewable Resources: Recent Achievements, Perspectives, and Limits." *Applied Microbiology and Biotechnology* 85: 413–423.

Othman, S. H. 2014. "Bio-nanocomposite Materials for Food Packaging Applications: Types of Biopolymer and Nano-Sized Filler." *Agriculture and Agricultural Science Procedia* 2: 296–303.

Otoni, C. G., S. F. O. Pontes, E. A. A. Medeiros, and N. de F. F. Soares. 2014. "Edible Films from Methylcellulose and Nanoemulsions of Clove Bud (Syzygium Aromaticum) and Oregano (Origanum Vulgare) Essential Oils as Shelf Life Extenders for Sliced Bread." *Journal of Agricultural and Food Chemistry* 62 (22): 5214–5219.

Oymaci, P., and S. A. Altinkaya. 2016. "Improvement of Barrier and Mechanical Properties of Whey Protein Isolate Based Food Packaging Films by Incorporation of Zein Nanoparticles as a Novel Bionanocomposite." *Food Hydrocolloids* 54: 1–9.

Pant, A. F., S. Sängerlaub, and K. Müller. 2017. "Gallic Acid as an Oxygen Scavenger in Bio-based Multilayer Packaging Films." *Materials* 10 (5): 489.

Patel, A. R., and K. P. Velikov. 2014. "Zein as a Source of Functional Colloidal Nano- and Microstructures." *Current Opinion in Colloid and Interface Science* 19: 450–458.

Peng, B. L., N. Dhar, H. L. Liu, and K. C. Tam. 2011. "Chemistry and Applications of Nanocrystalline Cellulose and Its Derivatives: A Nanotechnology Perspective." *Canadian Journal of Chemical Engineering* 89: 1191–1206.

Petersen, K., P. V. Nielsen, G. Bertelsen, M. Lawther, M. B. Olsen, N. H. Nilsson, and G. Mortensen. 1999. "Potential of Biobased Materials for Food Packaging." *Trends in Food Science and Technology* 10: 52–68.

Pillai, K. V., and S. Renneckar. 2016. "Dynamic Mechanical Analysis of Layer-by-Layer Cellulose Nanocomposites." *Industrial Crops and Products* 93: 267–275.

PolyOne Inc. Nanoblend MB 1201. http://www.matweb.com/search/datasheettext.aspx?matguid=fa221f13369841dfb1b8a876955d0535 (accessed 1 August 2017).

Pourjavaher, S., H. Almasi, S. Meshkini, S. Pirsa, and E. Parandi. 2017. "Development of a Colorimetric PH Indicator Based on Bacterial Cellulose Nanofibers and Red Cabbage (Brassica Oleraceae) Extract." *Carbohydrate Polymers* 156 (January): 193–201.

Puls, J., S. A. Wilson, and D. Hölter. 2011. "Degradation of Cellulose Acetate-Based Materials: A Review." *Journal of Polymers and the Environment* 19: 152–165.

Quintavalla, S., and L. Vicini. 2002. "Antimicrobial Food Packaging in Meat Industry." *Meat Science* 62 (3): 373–380.

Ramos, M., A. Beltrán, M. Peltzer, A. J. M. Valente, and M. D. C. Garrigós. 2014. "Release and Antioxidant Activity of Carvacrol and Thymol from Polypropylene Active Packaging Films." *LWT—Food Science and Technology* 58 (2): 470–477.

Ramos, Ó. L., I. Reinas, S. I. Silva, J. C. Fernandes, M. A. Cerqueira, R. N. Pereira, A. A. Vicente, M. F. Poças, M. E. Pintado, and F. X. Malcata. 2013. "Effect of Whey Protein Purity and Glycerol Content upon Physical Properties of Edible Films Manufactured Therefrom." *Food Hydrocolloids* 30 (1): 110–122.

Realini, C. E., and B. Marcos. 2014. "Active and Intelligent Packaging Systems for a Modern Society." *Meat Science* 98 (3): 404–419.

Reddy, N. 2015. "Non-food Industrial Applications of Poultry Feathers." *Waste Management* 45: 91–107.

Robertson, G. L. 2013. "Paper and Paper-Based Packaging Materials." In *Food Packaging: Principles and Practice*, edited by G. L. Robertson, 3rd ed., pp. 167–187. Boca Raton, FL: CRC Press/Taylor & Francis Group.

Rooney, M. L. 2005. "Oxygen-Scavenging Packaging BT—Innovations in Food Packaging." In *Innovations in Food Packaging*, edited by Jung H. Han, pp. 123–137. Amsterdam, Netherlands: Elsevier.

Saini, S., C. Sillard, M. N. Belgacem, and J. Bras. 2016. "Nisin Anchored Cellulose Nanofibers for Long Term Antimicrobial Active Food Packaging." *RSC Advances* 6 (15): 12422–12430.

Salvatore, G. A., J. Sülzle, F. D. Valle, G. Cantarella, F. Robotti, P. Jokic, S. Knobelspies et al. 2017. "Biodegradable and Highly Deformable Temperature Sensors for the Internet of Things." *Advanced Functional Materials* 27 (35): 1702390.

Scarfato, P., E. Avallone, M. R. Galdi, L. Di Maio, and L. Incarnato. 2015. "Preparation, Characterization, and Oxygen Scavenging Capacity of Biodegradable α-Tocopherol/PLA Microparticles for Active Food Packaging Applications." *Polymer Composites* 38 (5): 981–986.

Schneider, J., M. I. Akbar, J. Dutroncy, D. Kiesler, M. Leins, A. Schulz, M. Walker, U. Schumacher, and U. Stroth. 2009. "Silicon Oxide Barrier Coatings Deposited on Polymer Materials for Applications in Food Packaging Industry." *Plasma Processes and Polymers* 6: S700–S704.

Shrivastava, S., N. Jadon, and R. Jain. 2016. "Next-Generation Polymer Nanocomposite-Based Electrochemical Sensors and Biosensors: A Review." *TrAC Trends in Analytical Chemistry* 82 (September): 55–67.

Silva, N. H. C. S., C. Vilela, A. Almeida, I. M. Marrucho, and C. S. R. Freire. 2018. "Pullulan-based Nanocomposite Films for Functional Food Packaging: Exploiting Lysozyme Nanofibers as Antibacterial and Antioxidant Reinforcing Additives." *Food Hydrocolloids* 77 (January): 921–930.

Silvestre, C., D. Duraccio, and S. Cimmino. 2011. "Food Packaging Based on Polymer Nanomaterials." *Progress in Polymer Science* 36 (12): 1766–1782.

Slavutsky, A. M., and M. A. Bertuzzi. 2016. "Improvement of Water Barrier Properties of Starch Films by Lipid Nanolamination." *Food Packaging and Shelf Life* 7: 41–46.

Souza, M. P., A. F. M. Vaz, H. D. Silva, M. A. Cerqueira, A. A. Vicente, and M. G. Carneiro-da-Cunha. 2015. "Development and Characterization of an Active Chitosan-Based Film Containing Quercetin." *Food and Bioprocess Technology* 8 (11): 2183–2191.

Struller, C. F., P. J. Kelly, and N. J. Copeland. 2014. "Aluminum Oxide Barrier Coatings on Polymer Films for Food Packaging Applications." *Surface and Coatings Technology* 241: 130–137.

Tang, W. J., J. G. Fernandez, J. J. Sohn, and C. T. Amemiya. 2015. "Chitin Is Endogenously Produced in Vertebrates." *Current Biology* 25: 897–900.

Tang, X. Z., P. Kumar, S. Alavi, and K. P. Sandeep. 2012. "Recent Advances in Biopolymers and Biopolymer-based Nanocomposites for Food Packaging Materials." *Critical Reviews in Food Science and Nutrition* 52: 426–442.

Towal, R. B., M. Mormann, and C. Koch. 2013. "Simultaneous Modeling of Visual Saliency and Value Computation Improves Predictions of Economic Choice." *Proceedings of the National Academy of Sciences* 110: E3858–E3867.

Tsai, M. L., S. W. Bai, and R. H. Chen. 2008. "Cavitation Effects Versus Stretch Effects Resulted in Different Size and Polydispersity of Ionotropic Gelation Chitosan-Sodium Tripolyphosphate Nanoparticle." *Carbohydrate Polymers* 71: 448–457.

Valentis Nanotech Ltd. http://valentis-nano.com/wp-content/uploads/2014/12/Valentis-Nanotech-Coating-Charateristics.pdf (accessed 2 August 2017).

Vanderroost, M., P. Ragaert, F. Devlieghere, and B. De Meulenaer. 2014. "Intelligent Food Packaging: The Next Generation." *Trends in Food Science & Technology* 39 (1): 47–62.

Velásquez-Cock, J., E. Ramírez, S. Betancourt, J. L. Putaux, M. Osorio, C. Castro, P. Gañán, and R. Zuluaga. 2014. "Influence of the Acid Type in the Production of Chitosan Films Reinforced with Bacterial Nanocellulose." *International Journal of Biological Macromolecules* 69, 208–213.

Vicente, A. A., M. A. Cerqueira, L. Hilliou, and C. M. R. Rocha. 2011. *Protein-Based Resins for Food Packaging. Multifunctional and Nanoreinforced Polymers for Food Packaging*. Cambridge, Reino Unido: Woodhead Publishing.

Vink, E. T. H., K. R. Rábago, D. A. Glassner, and P. R. Gruber. 2003. "Applications of Life Cycle Assessment to NatureWorks™ Polylactide (PLA) Production." *Polymer Degradation and Stability* 80: 403–419.

Wang, H., H. Liu, C. Chu, Y. She, S. Jiang, L. Zhai, S. Jiang, and X. Li. 2015. "Diffusion and Antibacterial Properties of Nisin-Loaded Chitosan/Poly (L-Lactic Acid) Towards Development of Active Food Packaging Film." *Food and Bioprocess Technology* 8 (8): 1657–1667.

Wang, H., Y. She, C. Chu, H. Liu, S. Jiang, M. Sun, and S. Jiang. 2015. "Preparation, Antimicrobial and Release Behaviors of Nisin-Poly (Vinyl Alcohol)/Wheat Gluten/ZrO2 Nanofibrous Membranes." *Journal of Materials Science* 50 (14): 5068–5078.

Wang, L., Y. Zhang, A. Wu, and G. Wei. 2017. "Designed Graphene-Peptide Nanocomposites for Biosensor Applications: A Review." *Analytica Chimica Acta* 985 (September): 24–40.

Wang, S., X. Liu, M. Yang, Y. Zhang, K. Xiang, and R. Tang. 2015. "Review of Time Temperature Indicators as Quality Monitors in Food Packaging." *Packaging Technology and Science* 28 (10): 839–867.

Wen, P., D. H. Zhu, H. Wu, M. H. Zong, Y. R. Jing, and S.-Y. Han. 2016. "Encapsulation of Cinnamon Essential Oil in Electrospun Nanofibrous Film for Active Food Packaging." *Food Control* 59 (January): 366–376.

Wu, H., C. Teng, B. Liu, H. Tian, and J. Wang. 2018. "Characterization and Long Term Antimicrobial Activity of the Nisin Anchored Cellulose Films." *International Journal of Biological Macromolecules* 113 (January): 487–493.

Xiaowei, H., Z. Xiaobo, Z. Jiewen, S. Jiyong, L. Zhihua, and S. Tingting. 2014. "Monitoring the Biogenic Amines in Chinese Traditional Salted Pork in Jelly (Yao-Meat) by Colorimetric Sensor Array Based on Nine Natural Pigments." *International Journal of Food Science And Technology* 50 (1): 203–209.

Yam, K. L., P. T. Takhistov, and J. Miltz. 2005. "Intelligent Packaging: Concepts and Applications." *Journal of Food Science* 70 (1): R1–R10.

Yang, W., J. M. Kenny, and D. Puglia. 2015. "Structure and Properties of Biodegradable Wheat Gluten Bionanocomposites Containing Lignin Nanoparticles." *Industrial Crops and Products* 74: 348–356.

Yuceer, M., and C. Caner. 2014. "Antimicrobial Lysozyme-Chitosan Coatings Affect Functional Properties and Shelf Life of Chicken Eggs during Storage." *Journal of the Science of Food and Agriculture* 94 (1): 153–162.

Zehetmeyer, G., S. M. M. Meira, J. M. Scheibel, R. V. B. de Oliveira, A. Brandelli, and R. M. D. Soares. 2015. "Influence of Melt Processing on Biodegradable Nisin-PBAT Films Intended for Active Food Packaging Applications." *Journal of Applied Polymer Science* 133 (13).

Zhang, Q., Y. Qing, X. Huang, C. Li, and J. Xue. 2018. "Synthesis of Single-Walled Carbon Nanotubes–Chitosan Nanocomposites for the Development of an Electrochemical Biosensor for Serum Leptin Detection." *Materials Letters* 211 (January): 348–351.

Zhong, Q., and M. Jin. 2009. "Zein Nanoparticles Produced by Liquid-Liquid Dispersion." *Food Hydrocolloids* 23: 2380–2387.

# 12 Nanotechnology in Food Processing

*S. García-Pinilla, J.C. Villalobos-Espinosa, M. Cornejo-Mazón, and G.F. Gutiérrez-López*

## CONTENTS



## 12.1 INTRODUCTION: NANOTECHNOLOGY AND FOOD PROCESSING

Food processing is one of the various activities that derives from food engineering. The need to address the ever-growing and wider range of consumption needs requires novel approaches to product development, engineering, equipment design, and management, as well as its interaction with advanced disciplines such as nanoscience and nanotechnology, genomics, metabolomics, and nutrigenomics among others for developing new products with enhanced physical, chemical and biological properties, and increased shelf life as well as to aid in the handling of products and easiness to prepare (He and Hwang 2016).

Moreover, nanotechnology (which integrated with traditional physical, biological, and chemical backgrounds), has provided commercially successful foodstuffs through innovation in food processing. In the late 1980s, the food industry directed its attention to increase production, whereas at present much attention has been given to the manufacture of healthy, *close to natural*, fresher, easier to use, and tastier products with declared beneficial attributes and properly labelled (Gutiérrez-López et al. 2008).

The nanotechnology is defined as "the manipulation or self-assembly of very small particles (typically 1–100 nm) including individual atoms, molecules, or molecular clusters, to create materials, systems, devices, and therefore processes with new or vastly different properties" (Bhushan 2017) and is based on the unique properties of materials with at least one dimension that provides functionality within the $10^{-7}$ and $10^{-9}$ m range, although the upper limit of 100 nm has been a matter of discussion (EFSA 2009; Su-Waterhouse and Waterhouse 2016), since it is acknowledged that food particles sized between several hundred nanometers up to 20 mm possess size-dependent reactivity and bioavailability (Garnett and Kallinteri 2006) as well as, in cases, health risks that have to be overcome (Gatti and Rivasi 2002). Nano-sized materials have novel physicochemical characteristics (such as color, solubility, texture, diffusivity, material strength, and toxicity) in such a way that biological as well as physicochemical properties of structures and systems at nanoscale are substantially different than the macroscale counterparts owing to the interactions of individual atoms and molecules, thus offering unique and novel functional applications, many of which may be useful in food processing applications (Neethirajan and Jayas 2011; Tamjidi et al. 2013).

Nanotechnology in the agricultural and food industries was introduced by the United States Department of Agriculture (USDA) in 2003 and expanded across the world as a novel tool for the development of packing materials, ingredients, processing tools, foods, and other consumer products. Nanomaterials often display vastly novel characteristics in their physicochemical properties compared with their respective bulk materials. These novel features include improved optical response, mechanical strength, electrical conductance, magnetism, solubility, and chemical reactivity (Su-Waterhouse and Waterhouse 2016). It is foresighted that, nanotechnology in the food industry, will have more importance in applied engineering and food processing fields in the years to come (Hamad et al. 2017).

Introduction of nanotechnology in food processing opens opportunities for the use of nanomaterials as a base in manufacturing. Engineering teams find a continuous gap between the nano-application and the generation of novel developments and basic knowledge in the food industry (Jha et al. 2014). Relatively new processing equipment to produce nanofoods have been developed such as the ULTRA-TURRAX®s, Nano-spray driers (Büchi®), and microfluidizers (Microfluidics®), these pieces of equipment are derived from the widely used pressure homogenizers, the traditional spray driers, and mixers.

## 12.2 IMPORTANCE OF FOOD STRUCTURE IN NANOTECHNOLOGY

Considerations on the application of nanotechnology in food science and technology are classified by considering the functionality and the applicability of the nanomaterials involved. Nanomaterials used in food preparations can be naturally occurring or designed and produced by various techniques, and then added to a food preparation or actually be the main end consumed product as in the case of nanoemulsions (Magnuson et al. 2011). The functionality is, for instance, established given the desired role of the nanomaterial against biological deterioration when used as antimicrobial agent and in the increase of bioavailability of substances, the enhancement of physical properties as in color additives, anticaking agents, increased tensile strength, increased gas permeability-selectivity, increase of water and flame resistance, as well as in the protection of chemical ingredients such as antioxidants, vitamins, and flavors. Regarding the applicability of nanotechnology-based materials, they are used mainly for the following purposes: (i) in packaging technology as in active and intelligent packaging materials; (ii) the development of edible coatings; (iii) nanoencapsulation for target-delivery of functions, such as flavor nutrient delivery; and (iv) design of nanosensors as for those for pesticides, pathogens, and toxins detection (Pathakoti et. al. 2017). However, safety related topics in food nanotechnology are extremely important, being crucial to detecting unintended exposure of food additives as in the addition of nanoencapsulates and edible coatings which may release larger than desired amounts of substances that may have allergenic—or others—toxic effects. Toxicity problems with nanoparticles is one of the main difficulties that nanotechnology must deal with (Zare-Zardini et al. 2015; Jiang et al. 2017; Al-Mubaddel et al. 2017) as, for example, in the case of the agglomerates of titanium dioxide nanoparticles (Freyre-Fonseca et al. 2016), which have shown toxicity in cells cultivated in different culture media and may induce an adaptive inflammatory response and invasion and proliferation of lung epithelial cells (Medina-Reyes et al. 2015). With undefined toxicity level of nanoparticles, the lack of knowledge on human health effects and risk assessments programs may restrict the number of nanomaterial consumption in food-related applications. At this point, safety assessments of (*in vitro* and *in vivo*) its characterization (*in silico*) and legislation are extremely important and help defining the practical applications of a variety of new food products (He and Hwang 2016).

A wide range of procedures have been developed for making nanoparticles and nanostructures, but these can generally be sub-divided into two categories which are often described as the "top-down" and "bottom-up" approaches (Kirby 2011). The "top-down," attrition-based procedures commence with a macroscale material and then break it down to smaller units (Duncan 2011; Cushen et al. 2012). This may involve processes with high input of mechanical energy such as high-pressure homogenization or ball milling or the use of ultrasonic radiation. In the "bottom-up" approach, atomic or molecular building blocks are used which are encouraged to self-assemble to form nanostructures. For example, individual atoms or molecules can be made to crystallize under controlled conditions which prevent them from forming larger crystals (Shurin et al. 2012).

During processing and formulation, food structure is modified which can imply biopolymer transformations, phase creations, biochemical reactions, stabilization as in vitrification, crystallization, network formation, among others (Institute of Medicine 2009). These phenomena may occur, or not, in a simultaneous manner, sometimes giving place to metastable structures (Berk 2018). With the application of the nanotechnology in food processing, foods might be structured from single molecules as a starting component. These components can then be modified to induce interactions in the matrix and give place to the desired function of the final formed structure which has then to be stabilized. Food engineers often apply the uncoupled "matrix precursors/structural elements" paradigm (Institute of Medicine 2009), in which microstructural elements are engineered separately and then dispersed into a matrix precursor independently developed, so that the final product will have enhanced function. This process can be applied in the preparation of nanoemulsions which involves manipulating structural elements from different magnitudes and integrated into a matrix stabilized at a magnitude of $10^{-7}$–$10^{-9}$ m (Elnashaie et at. 2015). Nano-structuration is also a relatively new trend in nanotechnology processing that consists in creating nano-pores or nano-cracks into which small molecules are trapped and then may be delivered for a specific purpose (Viveros-Contreras et al. 2013; Acosta-Domínguez et al. 2016; Flores-Andrade et al. 2017).

Modifications of the original structure of polymers such as carbohydrates, can be reached by using them as nanoparticles to provide different physicochemical properties including stability of an oil phase as in the case of the Pickering emulsions (Leal-Castañeda et. al. 2018), that have been recently applied in food related fields given their potential applications (Rayner et al. 2014). Many food products are formed of immiscible phases, so that an emulsifier makes it possible to form a homogeneous and stable system, i.e., an emulsion which may be a suitable option for the delivering of several compounds, including vitamins such as α-tocopherol that is the most active form of vitamin E which has a potent antioxidant capacity (Wysota et al. 2017), and the preparation of emulsions containing this vitamin as well as vitamin D has been reported using different polymers as wall materials (Quintanilla et al. 2011; Granillo et al. 2017).

Figure 12.1 depicts native and modified (laurolyated) starch granules which in turn stabilized Pickering emulsions (Leal-Castañeda et al. 2018). Granule size plays

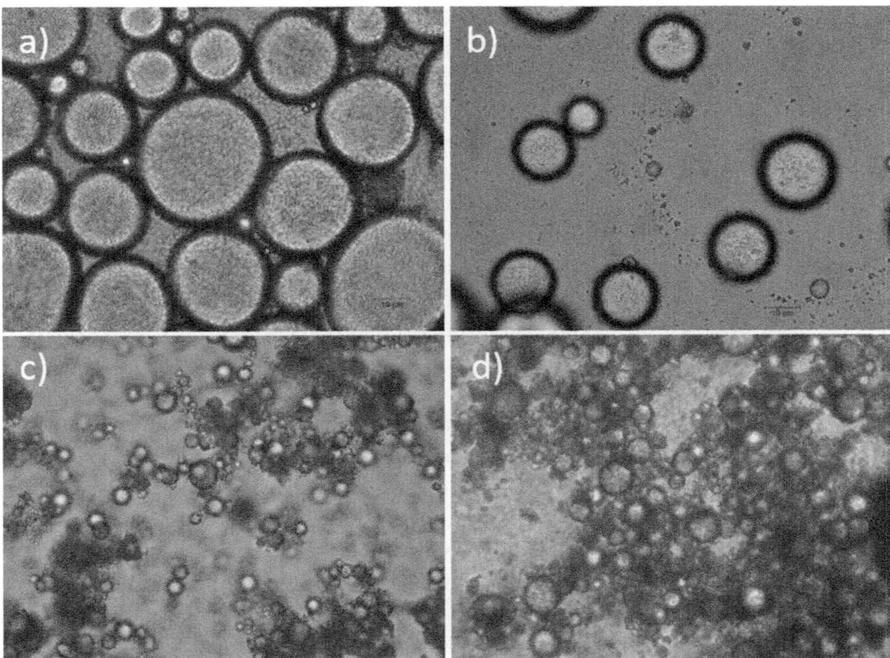


**FIGURE 12.1** Amaranth starch granule stabilized Pickering emulsions (optic microscopy image 40× magnification) at different concentrations (a) 2% wt of NS, (b) 2% wt of MS, (c) 30% wt of NS and (d) 30% wt of MS. Scale bar = 10 μm. In these emulsions, nanoscale starch particles act as stabilizers of micro droplets forming the emulsions.

an important role in the formation and stability of a Pickering emulsion, and it has been reported that small granules (particles around 600 nm) with smooth surfaces (Figure 12.1d), have a better contact in the oil-water interface (Saari et al. 2016). In this work, it was concluded that, food grade Pickering emulsions stabilized by native (Figure 12.1a and c) and laurolyated (Figure 12.1b and d) amaranth starches acted as good stabilizers of Pickering emulsions. In this case, the starch concentration had an influence on the droplet size of the emulsion and modified starch generated smaller droplet sizes and a greater emulsion stability attributed to the increased affinity of the modified starch with the oil phase as compared with the native granules (Leal-Castañeda et al. 2018).

## 12.3 FOOD NANOSTRUCTURE AND THE HEALTH-NUTRITION INTERACTIONS

The main goal of nanotechnology in food processing is the design of new products or to modify existing ones to accomplishing an optimal size, structure, and function while maintaining or improving health so contributing to well-being properties of the produced foods. For example, the bioavailability of phenolic compounds in black, green, and white tea leaves was compared with that of beads of jellified starch containing extracts of the different leaves. The availability of phenolic compounds was higher in black tea leaves, whereas in the beads, the white tea extract tea had the highest availability (although phenolic compounds content is lower in white than in black tea), thus showing the effects of the structure of the matrix and confirming its role in the bioavailability of active compounds (Sanna et al. 2015). However, in this case attention should be put to the relation between availability of trapped substances and glycemic index with the degree of gelatinization of the starch (Parada and Aguilera 2009).

Most polysaccharides (carbohydrates) and lipids (fats) are linear polymers with thicknesses less than nanometers, the functionality of many raw materials and the successful processing of foods can be achieved by the presence, modification, and generation of forms of self-assembled nanostructures (Huang et al. 2010; Neethirajan and Jayas 2011). Understanding the nature of nanostructures in foods (Figure 12.2) allows for a better selection of raw materials and enhanced food quality through processing. Techniques such as electron microscopy and the newer probe microscopies, such as atomic force microscopy (AFM), have started to reveal the nature of these structures, allowing rational selection, modification, and processing of raw materials (Vijayalakshmi et al. 2017).

Another role of nanotechnology in health/nutrition aspects is in the design of structures. Processing helps to maintaining the nutritional quality of the food or to modify the food matrix, according to the consumer demands. Functional ingredients added for food fortification (including vitamins, antimicrobials, antioxidants, probiotics, prebiotics, peptides and proteins, carotenoids, omega fatty acids, flavorings, colorants, and preservatives) are not administrated directly in their pure form, but are sometimes incorporated into the delivery system (e.g., nanostructures) (Elliott and

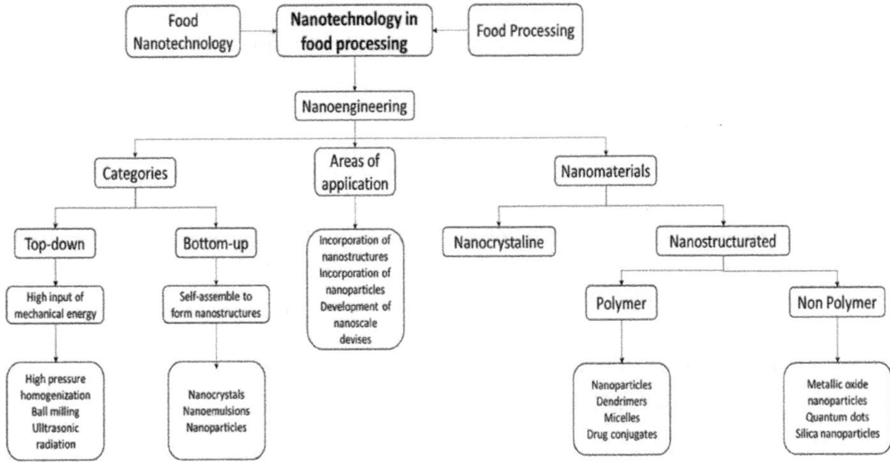


**FIGURE 12.2** Food nanotechnology and nanoengineering main categories, areas of application and nanomaterials in the food processing.

Ong 2002; Dasgupta et al. 2015). For example, the calorie reduction of food matrices by nanotechnology can be achieved by increasing the water and/or air content as in nanoemulsions, such as ice cream, in which it has been possible to lower sugar and oil contents by reducing the air bubble size which also increases creaminess. In general, the development of nutritious and sensory acceptable food products requires the use of specific food micro and nanoparticles within a tailored (or known) structure (Acosta 2009; Palzer 2009; Rosenthal 1998; Nehir and Simsek 2012). Applications include nano-sized feed supplements and feed additives, such as nano-forms of a biopolymer derived from the yeast cell walls that can bind mycotoxins to protect animals against mycotoxicosis and an aflatoxin-binding nano-additive for animal feed derived from modified nanoclay (Yinghua et al. 2005; Chaudhry and Castle 2011).

## 12.4 FOOD PROCESSING

Modern food processing technology makes use of a diverse range of individual operation or processes, for example, heat treatment, fermentation, filtration, curing, and drying. Food nanotechnology is a rapidly developing field which promises to revolutionize many aspects of food science, ranging from the improvements in safety and quality of foodstuffs, to enhanced rheological and organoleptic properties and increased bioavailability of essential nutrients (Kirby 2011). It has been proposed that by 2010, the overall market for food-related nanotechnologies would be worth US$20.4 billion (Helmut Kaiser 2008) (there have not been published more recent figures on this aspect). Moreover, factors such as climate change, population growth, and the need for cost efficiencies are expected to make significant contributions to the rate and direction of development of these technologies (Helmut Kaiser 2008).

Nanotechnology is being applied in a multitude of different manners in the food processing sector, some of them are shown in the Figure 12.2. The different areas of application can be divided into three main categories (Kirby 2011):

1. Incorporation of nanostructures comprising food compatible materials, or of food components themselves, where the intention is that those nanostructures will be consumed as a part of the food product. These "in vivo" approaches generally make use of "delivery systems". This category can also include formulations for administrating micronutrients and nutraceuticals
2. Use of nanoparticulates in food packaging or for incorporation into other food contact surfaces
3. Development of nanoscale devices for use as biosensors, processing tools, nanotracking devices, nanocatalysts, and so on. In this respect, these applications can be described as "in vitro" since many will not be part of the marketed food product.

Nutraceutical and functional foods are typical examples of products obtained with the aid of nanotechnology (Keller 2007). The basis for smart delivery is the selection of nanocarriers with appropriate surface properties which gives place to accumulation at some predetermined microscopic locations within a complex, multiphase food. When the encapsulated functional ingredient is eventually released, it will then be able to exert its intended action more selectively and effectively rather than when dispersed non-specifically throughout the food matrix. Novel tools, techniques, and processes allow to understand the mechanisms of targeted delivery that will potentially lead to smart delivery products used for improving well-being and of human health and to provide novel physical, visual, and sensory attributes to the original (no-nano) product (Paull and Lyons 2008).

Table 12.1, shows the potential applications of nanotechnology in food processing related areas and includes products whose physicochemical properties can be modified such as color, flavor, or nutrients to suit industrial requirements, as in the case of nano-filters that can remove toxins or modify flavors by shape instead of by size selection (Mognuson 2009). Foods can be enriched with fruit and vegetable compounds through nanotechnology by encapsulating nanocomponents to deliver higher nutrient densities foods (Chaudhary et al. 2005). Also, nano-processing can be used in dissolving additives, such as vitamins and phytochemicals, that are not normally soluble in water media (Ross et al. 2004) and to produce clear materials from opaque ones by preparing nanoparticles (Bhattacharya and Gupta 2005). Nanotechnology by reducing particle size can contribute to improve the properties of bioactive compounds, such as delivery, solubility, prolonged residence time in the gastrointestinal tract, and giving a place to efficient absorption of a variety of compounds by cells by means of nanoencapsulates (Chen 2006).

The advantages of encapsulation systems also include extended shelf life, protection of the encapsulated ingredients from the surrounding media and undesired interaction during processing, as well as the delivery of certain substances to specific targeted sites in the body (Augustin and Sanguansri 2009; Ravichandran 2010). Although such opportunities appear to be very promising with the inclusion of nanotechnology, new risks arise in food processing and food consumption that must be addressed.

**TABLE 12.1**
**Potential Applications of Nanotechnology in Food Processing Related Areas That Are Being Investigated, Experimentally Tested, and in Some Cases Already Applied in the Food Industry**

| Agriculture | Food Packaging | Supplements |
|---|---|---|
| • Single molecule detection to determine enzymes<br>• Nanocapsules for delivery of pesticides, fertilizer, and other agrochemicals more efficiently<br>• Delivery of growth hormones in a controlled fashion<br>• Nanosensors for monitoring soil conditions and crop growth<br>• Nanochips for identify preservation and tracking<br>• Nanosensors for detection of animal and plant pathogens<br>• Nanocapsules to deliver vaccines<br>• Nanoparticles to deliver DNA to plants (targeted genetic engineering)<br>• Nanoclays for water or agrochemicals retention for their slow release<br>• Nanomaterials for water purification and pollutant remediation | • Antibodies attached to fluorescent nanoparticles to detect chemicals or foodborne pathogens<br>• Biodegradable nanosensors for temperature, moisture, and time monitoring<br>• Nanoclays and nanofilms as barriers materials to prevent spoilage and prevent oxygen absorption<br>• Electrochemical nanosensors to detect ethylene<br>• Antimicrobial and antifungal surface coatings with nanoparticles (silver, magnesium, zinc)<br>• Lighter, stronger, and more heat-resistant films with silicate nanoparticles<br>• Modified permeation behaviour of foils<br>• Safeguarding food deterioration<br>• Enhancing mechanical properties of packaging (tensile strength, rigidity, gas permeability, water resistance, flame properties, polymer nanocomposites) | • Nanosize powders to increase absorption of nutrients<br>• Cellulose nanocrystal composite as drug carrier<br>• Nanoencapsulation of nutraceuticals for better adsorption and stability of targeted delivery<br>• Nanocochleates (coiled nanoparticles) to deliver nutrients more efficiently to cells without affecting color or taste of food<br>• Vitamin sprays dispersing active molecules into nanodroplets for better adsorption<br>• Protection against chemicals ingredients (antioxidants, flavors) |

*Source:* He, X. and Hwang, H.M., *J. Food Drug Anal.*, 24, 671–681, 2016; Youssef, A.M. *Polym. Plast. Technol. Eng.*, 52, 635–660, 2013; Ravichandran, R. *Int. J. Green Nanotechnol. Phys. Chem.*, 1, 72–96, 2010; Yada, R., *Nanotechnology: A New Frontier in Foods, Food Packaging, and Nutrient Delivery*, Nanotechnology in food products, National Academies, Washington, DC, 2009.

Food processing is the conversion of raw materials and ingredients into foods or other intermediate products in the food chain, making them marketable (Neethirajan and Jayas 2011; Pradhan 2015). Processing includes toxin removal, prevention of contamination from pathogens, preservation, improving the sensorial attributes, aids to achieve enhanced marketing, and efficient post-production and distribution (Chellaram 2014). Among the first deliberate uses for nanotechnology in food processing was the development of delivery systems for functional food ingredients. Also, it was introduced the idea that the principles underlying the drug delivery concept, for example, stabilization, targeting, and controlled release, might also be used to enhance the performance of functional ingredients in the food sector (McClements 2012; Tamjidi et. al. 2013).

Nanotechnology is applied in food processing in four main stages: materials, food safety and biosecurity, final products, and processing (Ravichandran 2010). All steps (Figure 12.3) provide added value to the final product, and as the food is developed and processed, nanotechnology provides different added values as in the products formulated by using nanoparticles, nanoemulsions, nanocomposites, and nanostructured materials (Figure 12.2). Once formulation is carried out, processing may involve heat/mass transfer operations, nanoscale reaction engineering, nanobiotechnology, and molecular synthesis which need to consider the various aspects related to preserve the functionality at the nanoscale. Food safety and biosecurity can be monitored with nanosensors and nanotracers (Pradhan et al. 2015).

Nanocapsules delivery systems play an important role in the processing sector, and their functional properties are maintained by entrapping a great number of compounds into matrixes and finally introduced in various foods (Abbas et al. 2009). Nanocapsules are nanovesicular systems that exhibit a typical core-shell structure in which the active component is confined to a reservoir or within a pore, cavity, or cracking and surrounded by a polymer membrane or coating which contain the active substance in liquid or solid form or as a molecular dispersion agent (Sekhon 2010). There are six basic forms for preparing nanocapsules: nanoprecipitation, emulsion-diffusion, double emulsification, emulsion-coacervation, polymer coating, and layer-by-layer (Maynard et al. 2006), and after the preparation of the emulsion, the diluent must be removed.

Nano-sized self-assembled structural lipids serve as liquid carriers of water insoluble healthy lipids in the form of nanodrops and are used to inhibit transport of cholesterol from the digestive system into the bloodstream (Dingman 2008). Other potential benefits include protection of vulnerable materials from heat, light

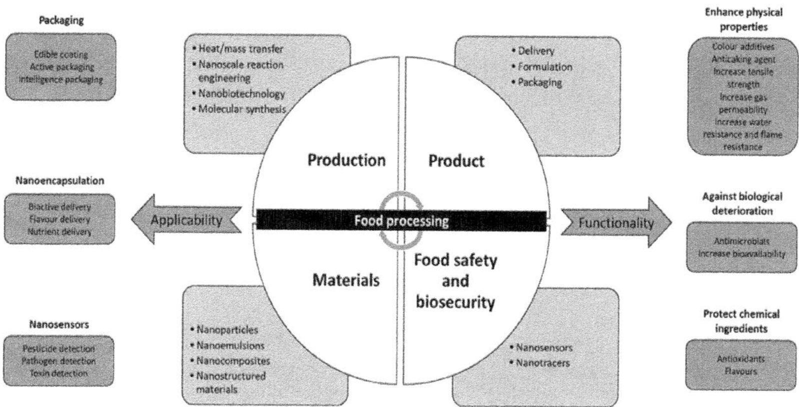


**FIGURE 12.3** A summarized version of the various steps of food management and the contribution of nanotechnology toward each one of such steps. (Adapted from nanoisrael.org, 2017; Pradhan, N. et al., *BioMed. Res. Int.*, Article ID 365672, 17, 2015; Ravichandran, R., *Int. J. Green Nanotechnol.: Phys. Chem.*, 1, 72–96.)

or oxidation, and masking of unpleasant tastes and odors, for example, in the case of fish oils. Nanoparticles, have been applied to improve nutritional quality, flow properties, flavor, color, and stability or to increase the shelf life of otherwise degradable compounds (Augustin and Hemar 2009). The incorporation of nutraceuticals, gelation and thickening agents, minerals, and vitamins as well as flavoring compounds into nanocapsules is a relatively frequent practice (Weiss et al. 2006; Huang et al. 2010).

Nano-sized carrier systems or nanocapsules, in the form of liposomes, micelles, or protein-based carriers have been used as nano-food additives, nutritional supplements, undesirable taste masking agents, enhancers of bioavailability and functional properties of the encapsulated compounds, and allow for better dispersion of insoluble additives without surfactants or emulsifiers (Morris et al. 2011; Cushen et al. 2012; Duran and Marcato 2013; Robles-García et al. 2016; Prasad et al. 2017). During nanoencapsulation, the food additive substances are enclosed in nanocomposite polymers for controlled release (Yu et al. 2009; Sekhon 2010). Furthermore, the use of lipid-based nanoencapsulation such as nanoliposomes, nanocochleates, and archaeosomes as nanodelivery system of nutraceuticals, enzymes, food additives, and antimicrobials has also been reported (Mozafari et al. 2006; Mozafari et al. 2008). Nanoencapsulation of probiotics to be targeted to specific regions in the gastrointestinal tract has been also achieved by this technique (Vidhyalakshmi et al. 2009). Easiness of handling, enhanced stability, protection against oxidation, retention of volatile ingredients, moisture and/or pH triggered controlled release, consecutive delivery of multiple active ingredients, change of flavor, long lasting organoleptic perception, and enhanced bioavailability and efficacy are other advantages of nanocapsules (Marsh and Bugusu 2007; Chaudhry et al. 2008).

### 12.4.1 Nanoemulsions

A frequently found difference between a conventional emulsion and a nanoemulsion is that a nanoemulsion does not change the appearance of the food when added (Pradhan et al. 2015). Nanoemulsions, with 500 nm or less, can entrap functional ingredients, which can facilitate a reduction in chemical degradation (McClements and Decker 2000; McClements and Rao 2011). These systems are created by two main approaches (Figure 12.4): the high energy approach which includes high-pressure

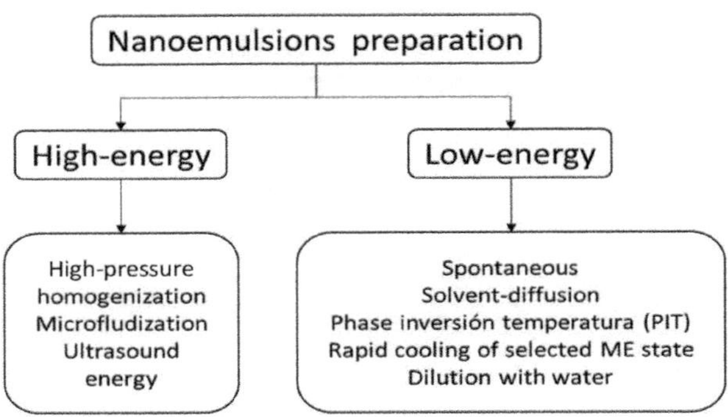


**FIGURE 12.4** High and low energy preparing methods used to produce nanoemulsions.

homogenization, ultrasound, high-speed liquid coaxial jets, and high-speed rotating shear methods (Letchford and Burt 2007), whereas the low energy approach involves membrane emulsification, spontaneous emulsification, solvent displacement, emulsion inversion point, and phase inversion point (Moore 1999; Preziosi et. al. 2013; Sen and Pathak 2016). The entrapment of the lipophilic component within the wall material in an oil in water emulsion depends on several factors such as molecular and physicochemical properties including hydrophobicity, surface activity, oil-water partition coefficient, solubility, presence of surfactant, and melting point (Ray and Okamoto 2003; Oberdorster et al. 2007).

Currently, nanoemulsions are preferred over conventional emulsions given the large contact area per unit weight of emulsion and the easiness of transportation across the epithelium enhancing the absorption of several bioactive compounds (Pradhan et al. 2015). More recently, nanoemulsions have being used to enable solubilization and delivery of poorly soluble drugs into the body. In the same way, they can be used in food applications for delivery of lipophilic ingredients such as flavor components. A work was done on encapsulation of carotenoids by using a nanostructured material prepared with alginate/zeolite valfor and another that was non-nanostructured prepared with alginate (Pascual-Pineda et al., 2014). The nanostructured material retained more carotenoids than the non-nanostructured one and protected the carotenoids at higher water activities due to the protection of the biomolecules into the nanostructured structure.

### 12.4.2 Nanoparticles

The procedures for preparing nanoparticles are not very complex and, be scaled up, and such methods make use of rather mild preparing conditions, and the materials involved are normally food compatible and are generally recognized as safe (GRAS). Inclusion of nanoparticles in the food industry has several purposes such as improving food's flow properties, color, and stability (Coma 2008; Fang et al. 2017). Hence, they are used in delivery systems such as plastic films, containing silicates, zinc oxide, and titanium dioxide which are used to reduce the flow of oxygen and for protection from light (Horner et al. 2006; Fuciños et al. 2016). They also help in reducing the loss of moisture and keeping the food fresh for a longer time acting as nano-sized preservatives (Horner et al. 2006; Zhang et al. 2016). There are nanoparticles that aid in the selective binding and hence lead to the removal of the pathogens or chemicals from food products (Nam et al. 2003; Kundu et al. 2017). Bottom-up or top-down approaches for preparing nanoparticles are, as in other systems, widely used. The main processes involved are mentioned in Figure 12.5 and include various techniques that are commonly used in chemical and mechanical engineering fields, including modern physicochemical processes (Iravani 2011).

The toxicity of carbon nanotubes is considerably high, and their use in food applications is limited (Madani et al. 2013). Polymeric nanoparticles are prepared by using polymers and surfactants, alginic acid, poly lactic-co-glycolic acid, and chitosan which are known to be efficient delivery compounds (Acosta 2009; Bush et al. 2017). Several nanoparticles have been reported to cause cellular damage to biological systems when they accumulate within the system. Sometimes they also disrupt the normal function of the cellular components since it has been reported that they

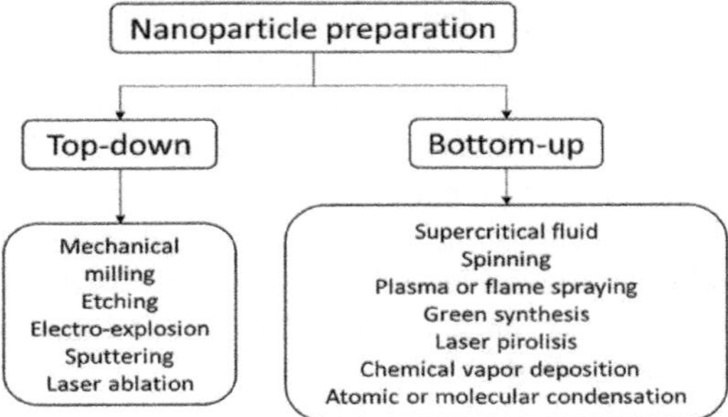


**FIGURE 12.5** Some manufacturing methods used to produce nanoparticles.

bind to cellular receptors of the immune system so causing its malfunction (Jordan et al. 2005; Pikhurov et al. 2017).

The use of organisms in this area is rapidly developing due to their growing success and ease of formation of nanoparticles. Moreover, biosynthesis of metal nanoparticles is an environmentally friendly method without use of toxic and expensive chemicals (Iravani 2011; Shah et al. 2015). For instance, production of silver nanoparticles by chemical reduction (e.g., hydrazine hydrate, sodium borohydride, N, N-dimethylformamide [DMF], and ethylene glycol) may lead to absorption of undesired chemicals on the surfaces of nanoparticles raising toxicity and legislation issues (Iravani et al. 2014; Akbarian et al. 2018).

## 12.5 CONCLUSIONS AND FUTURE PERSPECTIVES

Nanotechnology is becoming increasingly important for food processing. Promising results and applications are already being applied and others are being developed in areas such as heat/mass transfer, nanoscale reaction engineering, nanobiotechnology, and molecular synthesis, as well as packaging and food safety. It seems to exist no limit to food engineers on the applications of nanotechnology considering the whole new set of tools available to design new applications which in turn give place other challenges. However, to take fully advantage of the beneficial effects of nanotechnology in innovation and on improvement of consumer's well-being, it is advisable the inclusion of multidisciplinary teams for solving food product engineering situations. One of the most important problems facing the process engineer is the large amount of time consumed for achieving practical results. This issue can be solved by the inclusion of nano-ingredients or by creating (or degrading) nanostructures. Innovative devices and techniques are being developed that can facilitate the preparation of food samples and their precise and relatively low-cost analysis. Therefore, the main goal within this context nowadays is to be prepared to design nanofoods and processes for delivering predesigned food commodities (food product engineering) that are directed towards very demanding consumer needs within strongly globalized and highly competitive markets, always looking after the health risks associated and their legislation.

## ACKNOWLEDGMENTS

Authors thank IPN-Mexico and CONACYT-Mexico for financial support. Also, they are grateful to Dr. E. J. Leal-Castañeda, who kindly allowed authors to use unpublished images of Pickering emulsions.

## REFERENCES

Abbas, K. A., Saleh, A. M., Mohamed, A., & MohdAzhan, N. 2009. The recent advances in the nanotechnology and its applications in food processing: A review. *Journal of Food, Agriculture & Environment*. 7 (3&4), 14–17.

Acosta, E. 2009. Bioavailability of nanoparticles in nutrient and nutraceutical delivery. *Current Opinions in Colloid and Interface Science*. 14, 3–15.

Acosta-Domínguez, L., Hernández-Sánchez, H., Gutiérrez-López, G. F., Alamilla-Beltran, L., & Azuara, E. 2016. Modification of the soy protein isolate surface at nanometric scale and its effect on physicochemical properties. *Journal of Food Engineering*. 168, 105–112.

Akbarian, M., Mahjoub, S., Elahi, S. M., Zabihi, E., & Tashakkorian, H. 2018. Urtica dioica L. extracts as a green catalysis for the biosynthesis of zinc oxide nanoparticles: Characterization and cytotoxicity effects on fibroblast and Mcf-7 cell lines. *New Journal of Chemistry*. 42, 5822–5833.

Al-Mubaddel, F. S., Haider, S., Al-Masry, W. A., Al-Zeghayer, Y., Imran, M., Haider, A., & Ullah, Z. 2017. Engineered nanostructures: A review of their synthesis, characterization and toxic hazard considerations. *Arabian Journal of Chemistry*. 10, S376–S388.

Augustin, M. A., & Sanguansri, P. 2009. Nanostructured materials in the food industry. *Advances in. Food Nutritional Research*. 58, 183–213.

Augustin, M. A., & Hemar, Y. 2009. Nano- and micro-structured assemblies for encapsulation of food ingredients. *Chemical Society Reviews*. 38, 902–912.

Berk, Z. 2018. *Food Process Engineering and Technology*. Academic Press, Cambridge, MA.

Bhattacharya, D., & Gupta, R. K. 2005. Nanotechnology and potential of microorganisms. *Critical Reviews in Biotechnology*. 25, 199–204.

Bhushan, B. (Ed.). 2017. *Springer Handbook of Nanotechnology*. Springer, Berlin, Germany.

Bush, L., Stevenson, L., & Lane, K. E. 2017. The oxidative stability of omega-3 oil-in-water nanoemulsion systems suitable for functional food enrichment: A systematic review of the literature. *Critical Reviews in Food Science and Nutrition*. doi:10.1080/10408398.2017.1394268.

Chaudhry, Q., & Castle, L. 2011. Food applications of nanotechnologies: An overview of opportunities and challenges for developing countries. *Trends in Food Science & Technology*. 22(11), 595–603.

Chaudhry, Q., Scotter, M., Blackburn, J. et al. 2008. Applications and implications of nanotechnologies for the food sector. *Food Additives and Contaminants*. 25(3), 241–258.

Chellaram, C., Murugaboopathi, G., John, A. A., Sivakumar, R., Ganesan, S., Krithika, S., Priya, G. 2014. Significance of nanotechnology in food industry. *APCBEE Procedia*. 8, 109–113.

Chen, L. 2006. Food protein based materials as nutraceuticals delivery systems. *Trends in Food Science and. Technology*. 17, 272–283.

Coma, V. 2008. Bioactive packaging technologies for extended shelf life of meat-based products. *Meat Science*. 2, 90–103.

Cushen, M., Kerry, J., Morris, M., Cruz-Romero, M., Cummins, E. 2012. Nanotechnologies in the food industry—Recent developments, risks and regulation. *Trends in Food Science and Technology*. 24, 30–46.

Dasgupta, N., Ranjan, S., Mundekkad, D., Ramalingam, C., Shanker, R., & Kumar, A. 2015. Nanotechnology in agro-food: From field to plate. *Food Research International*, 69, 381–400.

Dingman, J. 2008. Nanotechnology, its impact on food safety. *Journal of Environmental Health*. 70, 47–50.

Duncan, T. V. 2011. Applications of nanotechnology in food packaging and food safety: Barrier materials, antimicrobials and sensors. *Journal of Colloid and Interface Science*. 363, 1–24.

Duran, N., & Marcato, P. D. 2013. Nanobiotechnology perspectives. Role of nanotechnology in the food industry: A review. *International Journal of Food Science and Technology*. 48, 1127.

EFSA (European Food Safety Authority). 2009. The potential risks arising from nanoscience and nanotechnologies on food and feed safety, Scientific Opinion of the Scientific Committee. *EFSA J*. 958, 1–39.

Elliott, R., & Ong, T. J. 2002. Science, medicine, and the future: Nutritional genomics. *British Medical Journal*. 324, 1438.

Elnashaie, S. S., Danafar, F., & Rafsanjani, H. H. 2015. From nanotechnology to nanoengineering. In *Nanotechnology for Chemical Engineers*, pp. 79–178. Springer, Singapore.

Fang, Z., Zhao, Y., Warner, R. D., & Johnson, S. K. 2017. Active and intelligent packaging in meat industry. *Trends in Food Science & Technology*. doi:10.1016/j.tifs.2017.01.002.

Flores-Andrade, E., Pascual-Pineda, L. A., Quintanilla-Carvajal, M. X., Gutiérrez-López, G. F., Beristain, C. I., & Azuara, E. 2017. Fractal surface analysis and thermodynamic properties of moisture sorption of calcium–sucrose powders. *Drying Technology*. 36, 1128–1141.

Freyre-Fonseca, V., Téllez-Medina, D. I., Medina-Reyes, E. I. et al. 2016. Morphological and physicochemical characterization of agglomerates of titanium dioxide nanoparticles in cell culture media. *Journal of Nanomaterials*. 36.

Fuciños, C., Fuciños, P., Amado, I. R., Míguez, M., Fajardo, P., Pastrana, L. M., & Rúa, M. L. 2016. Smart nanohydrogels for controlled release of food preservatives. *Antimicrobial Food Packaging*, pp. 349–362.

Garnett, M., & Kallinteri, P. 2006. Nanomedicines and nanotoxicology: Some physiological principles. *Occupational Medicine*. 56, 307–311.

Gatti, A., & Rivasi, F. 2002. Biocompatibility of micro- and nanoparticles. Part I: In liver and kidney. *Biomaterials*. 23, 2381–2387.

Granillo, V., Villalobos, J., Alamilla, L. et al. 2017. Optimization of the formulation of emulsions prepared with a mixture of vitamins D and E by means of an experimental design simplex centroid and analysis of a colocalization of its components. *Revista Mexicana de Ingeniería Química*. 1e7.

Gutiérrez-López, G. F., Alamilla-Beltrán, L., Chanona-Pérez, J., Parada-Arias, E., Ordorica-Vargas, C. 2008. Towards an integrated approach to food engineering: Structure-function relationships and convective drying. In Gutiérrez-López, G. F., Barbosa-Cánovas, G., Welti-Chanes, H., Parada-Arias, E (Eds.). *Food Engineering: Integrated Approaches*, Springer, Berlin, Germany, pp. 255–263.

Hamad, A. F., Jong-Hun, H. A. N., Kim, B. C., & Rather, I. A. 2017. The intertwine of nanotechnology with the food industry the intertwine of nanotechnology with the food industry. *Saudi Journal of Biological Sciences*. 25, 27–30.

He, X., & Hwang, H. M. 2016. Nanotechnology in food science: Functionality, applicability, and safety assessment. *Journal of Food and Drug Analysis*. 24(4), 671–681.

Helmut Kaiser Consultancy Report. 2008. Nanotechnology in food and food processing industry worldwide 2008-2010-2015. http://www.hkc22.com/nanofood.html (accessed February 27, 2018).

Horner, S. R., Mace, C. R., Rothberg, L. J., & Miller, B. L. 2006. A proteomic biosensor for enteropathogenic *E. coli*. *Biosensors and Bioelectronics*. 21(8), 1659–1663.

Huang, Q., Yu, H., & Ru, Q. 2010. Bioavailability and delivery of nutraceuticals using nanotechnology. *Journal of Food Science*. 75(1), R50–R56.

Institute of Medicine. 2009. Nanotechnology in food products: Workshop summary. Washington, DC: *The National Academies Press*. doi:10.17226/12633.

Iravani, S. 2011. Green synthesis of metal nanoparticles using plants. *Green Chemistry*. 13(10), 2638–2650.

Iravani, S., Korbekandi, H., Mirmohammadi, S. V., & Zolfaghari, B. 2014. Synthesis of silver nanoparticles: Chemical, physical and biological methods. *Research in Pharmaceutical Sciences*. 9(6), 385.

Jordan, J., Jacob, K. I., Tannenbaum, R., Sharaf., M. A., & Jasiuk, I. 2005. Experimental trends in polymer nanocomposites—A review. *Materials Science and Engineering* A, 393(1–2), 1–11.

Jha, R. K., Jha, P. K., Chaudhury, K., Rana, S. V., & Guha, S. K. 2014. An emerging interface between life science and nanotechnology: Present status and prospects of reproductive healthcare aided by nano-biotechnology. *Nano Reviews*. 5(1), 22762.

Jiang, X., Wang, L., Ji, Y. et al. 2017. Interference of steroidogenesis by gold nanorod core/silver shell nanostructures: Implications for reproductive toxicity of silver nanomaterials. *Small*. 13(10), 1602855.

Keller K. H. 2007. Nanotechnology and society. *Journal of Nanoparticle Research*. 9, 5–10.

Kirby, C. J. 2011. Nanotechnology in the food sector. *Food Processing Handbook*, 2nd ed., 693–726.

Kundu, A., Nandi, S., & Nandi, A. K. 2017. Nucleic acid based polymer and nanoparticle conjugates: Synthesis, properties and applications. *Progress in Materials Science*. 88, 136–185.

Leal-Castañeda, E. J., García-Tejeda, Y., Hernández-Sánchez, H. et al. 2018. Pickering emulsions stabilized with native and lauroylated amaranth starch. *Food Hydrocolloids*. 80, 177–185.

Letchford, K., & Burt, H. 2007 A review of the formation and classification of amphiphilic block copolymer nanoparticulate structures: Micelles, nanospheres, nanocapsules and polymersomes. *European Journal of Pharmaceutics and Biopharmaceutics*. 65(3), 259–269.

Madani, S. Y., Mandel, A., & Seifalian, A. M. 2013. A concise review of carbon nanotube's toxicology. *Nano Reviews*. 4(1), 21521.

Magnuson, B. A., Jonaitis, T. S., & Card, J. W. 2011. A brief review of the occurrence, use, and safety of food-related nanomaterials. *Journal of Food Science*, 76(6), R126–R133.

Chaudhary, M., Pandey, M. C., Radhakrishna, K., & Bawa, A. S. 2005. Nano-technology: Applications in food industry. *Indian Food Industry*. 24, 19–31.

Marsh, K., & Bugusu, B. 2007. Food packaging—Roles, materials, and environmental issues: Scientific status summary. *Journal of Food Science*. 72(3), R39–R55.

Maynard, A. D., Aitken, R. J., Butz, T. et al. 2006. Safe handling of nanotechnology. *Nature*. 444(7117), 267–269.

McClements, D. J. 2012. Crystals and crystallization in oil-in-water emulsions: Implications for emulsion-based delivery systems. *Advances in Colloid and Interface Science*. 174, 1–30.

McClements, D. J., & Rao, J. 2011. Food-grade nanoemulsions: Formulation, fabrication, properties, performance, biological fate, and potential toxicity. *Critical Reviews in Food Science and Nutrition*. 51(4), 285–330.

McClements, D. J., & Decker, E. A. 2000. Lipid oxidation in oil-in-water emulsions: Impact of molecular environment on chemical reactions in heterogeneous food systems. *Journal of Food Science*. 65, 1270–1282.

Medina-Reyes, E. I., Déciga-Alcaraz, A., Freyre-Fonseca, V. et al. 2015. Titanium dioxide nanoparticles induce an adaptive inflammatory response and invasion and proliferation of lung epithelial cells in chorioallantoic membrane. *Environmental Research*. 136, 424–434.

Mognuson, B. A. 2009. Nanoscale materials in foods: Existing and potential sources. ACS Symposium Series. *American Chemical Society*. 1020.

Moore, S. 1999. Nanocomposite achieves exceptional barrier in films. *Modern Plastics*. 76. 31–32.

Morris, V. J., Woodward, N. C., & Gunning, A. P. 2011. Atomic force microscopy as a nano-science tool in rational food design. *Journal of the Science of Food and Agriculture*. 91. 2117–2125.

Mozafari, M. R., Flanagan, J., & Matia-Merino, L. 2006. Recent trends in the lipid-based nanoencapsulation of antioxidants and their role in foods. *Journal of the Science of Food and Agriculture*. 86, 2038–2045.

Mozafari, M. R., Johnson, C., Hatziantoniou, S., & Demetzos, C. 2008. Nanoliposomes and their applications in food nanotechnology. *Journal of Liposome Res*earch. 18, 309–327.

Nanoisrael.org. 2017. http://www.nanoisrael.org/category.aspx?id=1277 (accessed August 24, 2017).

Nam, J. M., Thaxton, C. S., & Mirkin, C. A. 2003. Nanoparticle-based bio-bar codes for the ultrasensitive detection of proteins. *Science*. 301, 1884–1886.

Neethirajan, S., Jayas, D. S. 2011. Nanotechnology for the food and bioprocessing industries. *Food and Bioprocess Technology*. 4, 39–47.

Nehir, El. S., & Simsek, S. 2012. Food technological applications for optimal nutrition: An overview of opportunities for the food industry. *Comprehensive Reviews in Food Science and Food Safety*. 11, 2–12.

Oberdorster, G., Stone, V., & Donaldson, K. 2007. Toxicology of nanoparticles: A historical perspective. *Nanotoxicology*. 1, 2–25.

Palzer, S. 2009. Food structures for nutrition, health and wellness. *Trends in Food Science and Technology*. 20, 194–200.

Parada, J., Aguilera, J. M. 2009. In vitro digestibility and glycemic response of potato starch is related to granule size and degree of gelatinization. *Journal of Food Science*. 74, E34–E38.

Pascual-Pineda, L. A., Flores-Andrade, E., Alamilla-Beltrán, L., Chanona-Pérez, J. J., Beristain, C. I., Gutiérrez-López, G. F., & Azuara, E. 2014. Micropores and their relationship with carotenoids stability: A new tool to study preservation of solid foods. *Food and Bioprocess Technology*. 7(4), 1160–1170.

Pathakoti, K., Manubolu, M., & Hwang, H. M. 2017. Nanostructures: Current uses and future applications in food science. *Journal of Food and Drug Analysis*. 25(2), 245–253.

Paull, J., & Lyons, K. 2008. Nanotechnology: The next challenge for organics. *Journal of Organic Systems*. 3, 3–22.

Pikhurov, D. V., Sakhatskii, A. S., & Zuev, V. V. 2017. Rigid polyurethane foams with infused hydrophilic/hydrophobic nanoparticles: Relationship between cellular structure and physical properties. *European Polymer Journal*. 99, 403–414.

Pradhan, N., Singh, S., Ojha, N., Shrivastava, A., Barla, A., Rai, V., & Bose, S. 2015. Facets of nanotechnology as seen in food processing, packaging, and preservation industry. *BioMedical Research International*. Article ID 365672, 17p.

Prasad, R., Bhattacharyya, A., & Nguyen, Q. D. 2017. Nanotechnology in sustainable agriculture: Recent developments, challenges, and perspectives. *Frontiers in Microbiology*. 8, 1014.

Preziosi, V., Perazzo, A., Caserta, S., Tomaiuolo, G., & Guido, S. 2013. Phase inversion emulsification. *Chemical Engineering*. 32.

Quintanilla, M., Meraz, L., Alamilla, L., Chanona, J., Terres, E., Hernandez, H. et al. 2011. Morphometric characterization of spray-dried microcapsules before and after a-tocopherol extraction. *Revista Mexicana de Ingeniería Química*, 10, 301–312.

Ravichandran, R. 2010. Nanotechnology applications in food and food processing: Innovative green approaches, opportunities and uncertainties for global market. *International Journal of Green Nanotechnology: Physics and Chemistry*. 1, 72–96.

Ray, S.S., & Okamoto, M., 2003. Polymer/layered silicate nanocomposites: A review from preparation to processing. *Progress in Polymer Science*. 28, 1539–1641.

Rayner, M., Marku, D., Eriksson, M., Sjöö, M., Dejmek, P., & Wahlgren, M. 2014. Biomass-based particles for the formulation of Pickering type emulsions in food and topical applications. *Colloids and Surfaces A: Physicochemical and Engineering Aspects*, 458, 48–62.

Robles-García, M. A., Rodríguez-Félix, F., Márquez-Ríos, E., Aguilar, J. A., Barrera-Rodríguez, A., Aguilar, J., & Del-Toro-Sánchez, C. L. 2016. Applications of nanotechnology in the agriculture, food, and pharmaceuticals. *Journal of Nanoscience and Nanotechnology*, 16(8), 8188–8207.

Rosenthal, A. J. 1998. Technological factors in the development of low-calorie foods. In: Henry, C. J. K., Heppell, N. J. (Eds). *Nutritional Aspects of Food Processing and Ingredients*. Aspen Publication, Oxford, UK, pp. 24–41.

Ross, S. A., Srinivas, P. R., Clifford, A. J., Lee, S. C., Philbert, M. A., & Hettich, R. L. 2004. New technologies for nutrition research. *Journal of Nutrition*. 134, 681–685.

Saari, H., Heravifar, K., Rayner, M., Wahlgren, M., & Sjöö, M. 2016. Preparation and characterization of starch particles for use in Pickering emulsions. *Cereal Chemistry Journal*. 93, 116–124.

Sanna, V., Lubinu, G., Madau, P., Pala, N., Nurra, S., Mariani, A., & Sechi, M. 2015. Polymeric nanoparticles encapsulating white tea extract for nutraceutical application *Journal of Agriculture and Food Chemistry*. 63, 2026–2032.

Sekhon, B. S. 2010. Food nanotechnology—An overview. *Nanotechnology, Science and Applications*. 3, 1–15.

Sen, S., & Pathak, Y. (Eds.). 2016. *Nanotechnology in Nutraceuticals: Production to Consumption*. CRC Press, Boca Raton, FL.

Shah, M., Fawcett, D., Sharma, S., Tripathy, S. K., & Poinern, G. E. J. 2015. Green synthesis of metallic nanoparticles via biological entities. *Materials*. 8, 7278–7308.

Shurin, J. B., Clasen, J. L., Greig, H. S., Kratina, P., & Thompson, P. L. 2012. Warming shifts top-down and bottom-up control of pond food web structure and function. *Philosophical Transactions of the Royal Society B: Biological Sciences*. 367, 3008–3017.

Sun-Waterhouse, D., & Waterhouse G. I. 2016. Recent advances in the application of nanomaterials and nanotechnology in food research, In *Novel Approaches of Nanotechnology in Food*, Grumezescu, A. M. Editor. Academic Press, pp. 21–66, Novel Approaches of Nanotechnology in Food.

Tamjidi, F., Shahedi, M., Varshosaz, J., & Nasirpour, A. 2013. Nanostructured lipid carriers (NLC): A potential delivery system for bioactive food molecules. *Innovative Food Science & Emerging Technologies*. 19, 29–43.

Vidhyalakshmi, R., Bhakyaraj, R., & Subhasree, R. S. 2009. Encapsulation the future of probiotics: A review. *Advances in Biological Research*. 3, 96–103.

Vijayalakshmi, S., Sachin, C., & Kirtan, T. 2017. Nanotechnology: A growing need for agriculture and food sectors. *Integrated Ferroelectrics*. 185, 73–81.

Viveros-Contreras, R., Téllez-Medina, D., Perea-Flores, M., Alamilla-Beltrán, L., Cornejo-Mazón, M., Beristain-Guevara, C.I., Azuara-Nieto, E., & Gutiérrez-López, G. 2013. Encapsulation of ascorbic acid into calcium alginate matrices through coacervation coupled to freeze-drying. *Revista Mexicana de Ingeniería Química*. 12, 29–39.

Weiss, J., Takhistov, P., & McClements, D. J. 2006. Functional materials in food nanotechnology. *Journal of Food Science*. 71, R107–R116.

Wysota, B., Michael, S., Hiew, F. L., Dawson, C., & Rajabally, Y. A. 2017. Severe but reversible neuropathy and encephalopathy due to vitamin E deficiency. *Clinical Neurology and Neurosurgery*. 160, 19–20.

Yada, R. 2009. Nanotechnology: A new frontier in foods, food packaging, and nutrient delivery. *Nanotechnology in Food Products*. National Academies, Washington, DC.

Yinghua, S., Zirong, X., & Jianlei, F. (2005). In vitro adsorption of aflatoxin adsorbing nano-additive for aflatoxin B1, B2, G1, G2. *Scientia Agricultura Sinica*.

Youssef, A. M. 2013. Polymer nanocomposites as a new trend for packaging applications. *Polymer Plastic Technology and Engineering*. 52, 635–660.

Yu, H., Huang, Y., & Huang, Q. 2009. Synthesis and characterization of novel antimicrobial emulsifiers from—polylysine. *Journal of Agriculture and Food Chemistry*. 58, 1290–1295.

Zare-Zardini, H., Amiri, A., Shanbedi, M., Taheri-Kafrani, A., Kazi, S. N., Chew, B. T., & Razmjou, A. 2015. *In vitro* and *in vivo* study of hazardous effects of Ag nanoparticles and arginine-treated multi walled carbon nanotubes on blood cells: Application in hemodialysis membranes. *Journal of Biomedical Materials Research Part A*, 103, 2959–2965.

Zhang, H., Dunand, C. H., Wilson, P., & Miller, B. L. 2016. A label-free optical biosensor for serotyping unknown influenza viruses. In *SPIE Defense + Security*, pp. 982405–982405. International Society for Optics and Photonics.

# 13 Nanotechnology in Food Preservation

*Adriano Brandelli, Cristian M.B. Pinilla, and Nathalie A. Lopes*

## CONTENTS



## 13.1 INTRODUCTION

The maintenance of food quality and safety has always been a matter of great concern, therefore food preservation technologies are classified as a topic of utmost relevance. The food industry is constantly challenged to avoid the dissemination of microbial pathogens along the food chain and to reduce the economic losses caused by spoilage microorganisms. The increasing demand of the consumers for more natural foods and ready-to-eat products stimulates the development of novel products and processing technologies. Currently, most food preservation methods continue based on thermal processing, but increased attention has been devoted to innovative technologies in the last decades. Some emerging technologies include high hydrostatic pressure, pulsed-electric field, ultrasound, ohmic heating, infrared processing, among others (Sun 2014). These technologies have been proposed to produce more "fresh-tasting" foods with the assurance of microbiological safety as well.

In this context, the nanotechnology arose as an interesting alternative to provide solutions to these multi-faceted challenges necessary to improve the food chain. Nanotechnology is related with the fabrication, characterization, and/or manipulation of structures with at least one dimension in the nanometer length scale. The physical, chemical, and biological properties of nanostructured systems are significantly different to their micro- or macro-scale counterparts, thereby offering unique properties, better performance, and novel functional applications (Brandelli 2015; Brandelli and Taylor 2015). A diversity of techniques has been explored to fabricate nanostructures and nanomaterials, comprising nanosensors, new packaging materials, and encapsulated food components. Thereby, the connection between nanotechnology and the food industry is enhancing food security and extending storage life of foods, besides improving flavor and nutrient delivery, allowing the detection of food contaminants (e.g., pathogens, toxins, or pesticides), as can be seen in Figure 13.1 (He and Hwang 2016; Pathakoti et al. 2017).

Nanotechnology may present some advantages in food preservation, including the protection and controlled release of active substances in the food matrix, preventing their premature inactivation. Thus, nanotechnology has enormous potential for improvement of food safety, as a powerful tool for delivery and controlled release of natural antimicrobials and other bioactive substances (Pradhan et al. 2015). In this chapter, examples of nanomaterials and nanodevices potentially useful for food preservation are presented and the use of nanotechnology for improvement of food safety is discussed.

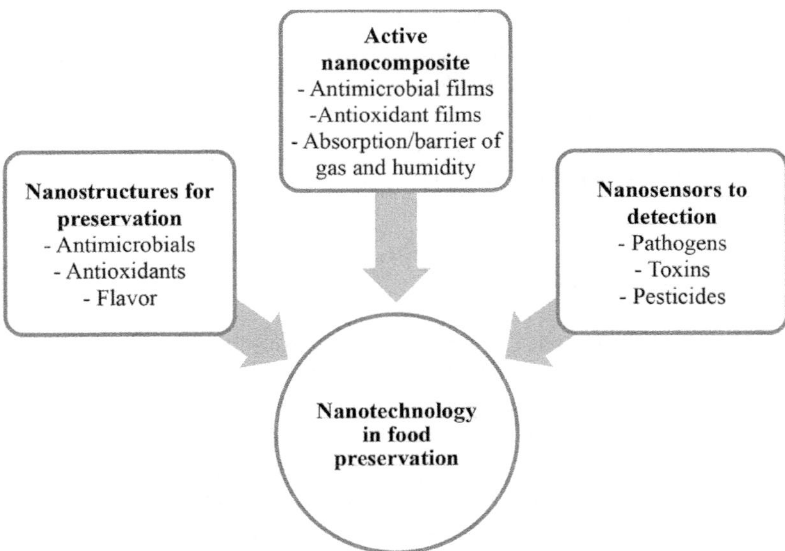


**FIGURE 13.1** Overview of the development of nanotechnology in food preservation and their applications in food science.

## 13.2 NANOSTRUCTURES FOR FOOD PRESERVATION

Nanostructured systems have intermediate size between a nanodimension and a microdimension that can be developed as various forms, including liposomes, polymeric nanoparticles (nanospheres and nanocapsules), nanofibers, nanotubes, among others. The characteristics of the nanomaterial are often associated with the aptness of the nanostructured system, facilitating controlled release and protecting bioactive components during manufacture and storage (Lopes and Brandelli 2017; Pathakoti et al. 2017). A number of nanostructures have been developed looking for the preservation of foods, often including active molecules like antimicrobials, antioxidants, or flavors.

### 13.2.1 Nanostructured Antimicrobials

The use of nanostructures for delivery of natural antimicrobials, such as antimicrobial peptides, plant-derived substances, and enzymes is an interesting alternative to protect antimicrobials against undesirable interactions in the food matrix. In addition, nanostructured systems can provide controlled release of antimicrobials, improving the control of spoilage and the prevention of pathogenic microorganism growth (Lopes and Brandelli 2017). Some examples of nanostructures for delivery of antimicrobials with interest in the food preservation are presented in Table 13.1.

Antimicrobial peptides and proteins, such as nisin, pediocin, lysozyme, and other antimicrobial enzymes present a great interest to the food-processing industry, due to the fact that they are potential substitutes for chemical preservatives. Although several antimicrobial peptides are described, only a few of them are allowed to be used as preservative in the food industry (Imran et al. 2015).

Nisin is the most widely used bacteriocin due to its generally recognized as safe (GRAS) approval by the United States Food and Drug Administration. It is a polypeptide produced by *Lactococcus lactis* subsp. *lactis* that shows antimicrobial activity against Gram-positive bacteria (Salmieri et al. 2014). The mode of application of antimicrobials is often by direct introduction into food products. However, this might result in a decrease of their efficacy against pathogens due to a possible interaction between different food components (Ibarguren et al. 2014). The antimicrobial activity of nisin encapsulated into different nanostructures has been described (Table 13.1), showing antibacterial activity against foodborne pathogens, such as *Listeria monocytogenes* and *Staphylococcus aureus*.

Another bioactive peptide that attracts research interest is pediocin, produced by *Pediococcus acidilactici*. The use of pediocin associated to nanotechnology allowed the development of liposomes prepared from partially purified soybean phosphatidylcholine by the film hydration method. The efficiency of encapsulation was 80%, and the stability of liposomes showed potential for application in foods (Mello et al. 2013).

Lysozyme is also a safe food preservative that has been extensively studied as a model protein for structural, physicochemical, and enzymatic research. The antimicrobial enzyme lysozyme has antibacterial activity against both Gram-positive and Gram-negative bacteria. However, when exposed to adverse environmental

**TABLE 13.1**
**Nanostructures for Delivery of Antimicrobials in Food Preservation**

| Nanostructure | Antimicrobial | Target Microorganisms | References |
|---|---|---|---|
| Solid lipid nanoparticles | Nisin | *L. monocytogenes* DMST 2871 and *Lactobacillus plantarum* TISTR 850 | Prombutara et al. (2012) |
| Chitosan/carrageenan nanocapsules | Nisin | *Micrococcus luteus*, *P. aeruginosa*, *S. enterica*, and *Enterobacter Aerogenes* | Chopra et al. (2014) |
| Nanoliposomes containing chitosan or chondroitin sulfate | Nisin | *L. monocytogenes* | Silva et al. (2014) |
| Nanoliposomes | Pediocin | *L. monocytogenes*, *Listeria innocua*, and *Listeria ivanovii* | Mello et al. (2013) |
| Nanoparticles coated with poly-γ-glutamic acid and chitosan | Lysozyme | *S. aureus*, *P. aeruginosa*, *B. subtilis*, and *E. coli* | Liu et al. (2013) |
| Nanocapsules | Tragacanth gum | *E. coli*, *S. aureus*, and *Candida albicans* | Ghayempour et al. (2015) |
| Liposomes | Apigenin | Gram-positive and Gram-negative bacteria | Banerjee et al. (2015) |
| PLGA nanoparticles | Anethole and carvone essential oils | Gram-positive and Gram-negative bacteria | Esfandyari-Manesh et al. (2013) |
| PLGA nanoparticles | Trans-cinnamaldehyde and eugenol | *Salmonella* spp. and *Listeria* spp. | Gomes et al. (2011) |
| Chitosan-based silver nanoparticles | Silver | *E. coli* | Wei et al. (2009) |
| Nanoparticles | Copper | *B. subtilis*, *S. aureus*, and *E. coli* | Chatterjee et al. (2012) |
| Nanoparticles dispersed on zeolites | Gold | *E. coli* and *S. typhimurium* | Lima et al. (2013) |

*Note:* PLGA—poly(D, L-lactic-co-glycolic) acid; DMST - Department of Medical Sciences Thailand; TISTR - Thailand Institute of Scientific and Technological Research.

conditions easily lose their antibacterial activity. Application of lysozymes can be enhanced by protective coatings and broadening of the antibacterial spectrum by adding other bactericides (Liu et al. 2013).

Properties of inorganic nanostructures have been investigated in food applications. A small number of metals and metal-based composites (silver, gold, iron, zinc oxide, titanium dioxide, copper oxide, among others) have been exploited in the food industry to improve the properties of food packaging (Hannon et al. 2015). Silver is well known to have antimicrobial activity against Gram-negative and Gram-positive bacteria, fungi, protozoa, and certain viruses, showing important processing-related advantages such as high temperature stability and low volatility, to be used in packaging and products storage for extending the shelf life of food (Azeredo 2013; Rai et al. 2015).

Other metallic nanoparticles have also shown antimicrobial properties. Copper (Cu) is present in most food in the form of ions and is considered as being relatively safe since it is not concentrated by animals, probably as a result of the homeostatic mechanisms controlling Cu absorption and excretion (Bost et al. 2016). At low concentrations, Cu is a cofactor for metalloproteins and enzymes, and it shows remarkable antimicrobial properties (Rhim et al. 2013). A method for preparation of Cu nanoparticles (CuNPs) that remains stable in ambient condition for about a month was developed by Chatterjee et al. (2012). The antibacterial effects of the CuNPs occurred on Gram-positive bacteria *Bacillus subtilis* and *S. aureus*, besides the Gram-negative *Escherichia coli.* Gold nanoparticles (AuNPs) exhibit interesting properties, such as the chemical inertness and resistance to surface oxidation, revealing good antibacterial activity against pathogens such as *S. aureus* and *Pseudomonas aeruginosa* (Bindhu and Umadevi 2014).

Nanoparticles based on metal oxides have been also investigated for their antimicrobial properties. A great advantage of metal oxides over organic antimicrobial agents is their higher stability (Azeredo 2013). Azam et al. (2012) demonstrated the antimicrobial activity of nanoparticles of three metal oxides (zinc oxide, copper oxide, and iron oxide, ZnO, CuO, and $Fe_2O_3$, respectively) against Gram-negative (*E. coli* and *P. aeruginosa*) and Gram-positive (*S. aureus* and *B. subtilis*) bacteria. The results indicated that ZnO nanoparticles had excellent antimicrobial potential, while $Fe_2O_3$ nanoparticles exhibited the least antimicrobial activity. Moreover, it was observed that nanomaterials were most effective against Gram-positive bacterial strains than to Gram-negative ones. Chorianopoulos et al. (2011) studied the photocatalytic activity of titanium dioxide ($TiO_2$) against *L. monocytogenes* bacterial biofilm, showing that the use of nanostructured $TiO_2$ combined with ultraviolet A (UVA) irradiation is an effective way to eliminate pathogenic microorganisms in food contacting surfaces, thus reducing the disinfection time.

The encapsulation of plant-derived antimicrobials has attracted the interest of many researchers as natural compounds that display a wide array of modes of action. Essential oils are complex mixtures of volatile constituent's biosynthesized by plants and are widely used in the food industry due to their antibacterial, antifungal, and antioxidant properties. The antimicrobial activity of essential oils is generally found in the oxygenated terpenoids, such as alcohols and phenolic terpenes (Bassolé and Juliani 2012). Nanoencapsulation of active compounds using poly-(D, L-lactide-co-glycolide) (PLGA) may have important applications in the food industry. PLGA nanoparticles containing cinnamon bark extract proved to be inhibitors of *Salmonella enterica* and *L. monocytogenes* after 24 and 72 hours for concentrations ranging from 225 to 550 μg/mL. The study suggests that these nanoparticles can be successfully used to deliver natural antimicrobials to pathogens in food products (Hill et al. 2013). Spinach samples were treated with eugenol-containing micelles against *E. coli* O157:H7 and *S. enterica* serotype Saintpaul, showing reduction on spinach surfaces. Data suggest that eugenol in micelles may be useful to produce surface decontamination from bacterial pathogens during postharvest washing

(Ruengvisesh et al. 2015). Thymol encapsulated in nanoparticles prepared with sodium caseinate and chitosan showed to be more effective against Gram-positive bacteria than non-encapsulated thymol for a longer time period (Zhang et al. 2014). Eugenol nanoliposomes were prepared by combining the ethanol injection method with dynamic high-pressure microfluidization exhibiting good storage stability and lower antibacterial activities (Peng et al. 2015).

### 13.2.2 Nanostructured Antioxidants

The lipid oxidation is the main deterioration process of fats, oils, and lipid-based foods, resulting in decreased nutritional value and sensory quality. The employment of compounds that possess antioxidant properties is a choice method for protection against oxidation. Nanostructured antioxidants such as vitamin E (tocopherols), vitamin C (ascorbic acid), carotenoids, and phenolic compounds may be utilized to protect the sensory and nutritive quality of food, also protecting the body against several chronic age-related disorders (Mozafari et al. 2006).

The antioxidants are able to delay the chain reaction caused by free radicals, being a powerful tool to reduce oxidative stress in the body (Oroian and Escriche 2015). The natural antioxidants are present in foods such as vegetables, fruits, and grains, therefore, the appearance of various common diseases may be prevented by a regular consume of these foods (Yashin et al. 2013). While the body has its own antioxidant defense mechanisms, consumption of foods alone may not be enough to obtain the necessary intake of antioxidants. Thus, antioxidants added to foods, as fortified functional foods, have the potential to augment these natural mechanisms, thus preventing the appearance of health disorders (Aguiar et al. 2016).

An antioxidant may be defined as any substance added to the food showing the capability of retarding or preventing the deterioration caused by oxidation (Mozafari et al. 2006). Synthetic or natural food antioxidants are generally acids and their salts and esters, such as citric and ascorbic acid or phenolic compounds, such as butylated hydroxyanisole (BHA) and tocopherols. The acids are used to prevent oxidative discoloration in fruit, meat, and other foods, whereas the phenolic compounds are employed to prevent oxidation of fats and lipids present in foods. Synthetic antioxidants have been used in food preservation for decades due to their low cost and mild flavor. However, safety concerns have been raised about synthetic antioxidants, and their use is limited by regulatory agencies. Furthermore, due to consumers demand for "clean label," the search for effective antioxidants from natural sources is required (Shahidi and Zhong 2015).

The control of oxidation reactions for extending shelf life has been studied through techniques involving encapsulation to protect the antioxidant activity from degradation. Chitosan nanoparticles loaded with jujube pulp and seed extracts were studied by Han et al. (2015), aiming to optimize extraction conditions to obtain maximum active ingredient yield and antioxidant activity. According to this study, the nanoencapsulation effectively improved the stability of jujube pulp and seed extract in terms of total phenolic content and antioxidant activity, being useful as a natural functional food ingredient with antioxidant activity.

A recent study highlighted guabiroba fruit for its high content of phenolic compounds (Pereira et al. 2018). To improve stability, bioavailability, and bioactivity of compounds, PLGA nanoparticles containing phenolic extracts of guabiroba were synthesized. The encapsulation into PLGA nanoparticles was effective in preserving the phenolic content for a prolonged time, protecting its active components and enhancing its functional properties. The results suggest that PLGA nanoparticles can be used as a delivery system for phenolic compounds at levels lower than originally required for non-encapsulated phenolics.

Gallic acid is an important polyphenol compound presenting biological activities. It is found in several fruits, nuts, green tea, and red wine, and presents a potent antioxidant capability, with the ability to scavenge the DPPH (2,2-diphenyl-1-picrylhydrazyl) radical. PLGA nanoparticles coated or not with polysorbate 80 were used to encapsulate gallic acid (Alves et al. 2016). Nanoparticle formulations were stable during storage, demonstrating sustained gallic acid release from nanoparticles. PLGA uncoated nanoparticles presented greater antioxidant potential than polysorbate 80-coated PLGA nanoparticles.

Among essential oils, thymol and carvacrol are predominant in oregano and thyme oils, respectively, and are recognized by their antioxidant properties. These two essential oils are listed by the Food and Drug Administration, but they have poor solubility in water, which limits their application as food additives. Wu et al. (2012) used zein to form nanoparticles encapsulating thymol and carvacrol, which can be dispersed in water while maintaining the antioxidant properties. The study demonstrated that encapsulating essential oils in zein nanoparticles can enhance their solubility up to 14-fold without hindering their ability to scavenge free radicals.

Lipid nanostructures have been also described to encapsulate natural antioxidants. Shah et al. (2016) studied the influence of different lipid-based formulations in the encapsulation of curcumin, and their antioxidant activity was investigated. As compared to free curcumin, the encapsulated curcumin showed higher radical scavenging activity, confirming the protective effect of the nanoemulsion systems on antioxidant activity of curcumin. An antioxidant peptide fraction isolated from rainbow trout (*Oncorhynchus mykiss*) skin gelatin hydrolysates was encapsulated in chitosan-coated nanoliposomes. Biopolymer-coated liposomes demonstrated more sustained peptide release behavior *in vitro* and maintained the antioxidant activity of the peptide fraction (Ramezanzade et al. 2017). The bioactive peptide fraction from sea bream scales showing antioxidant activity was encapsulated into phosphatidylcholine nanoliposomes. The encapsulation preserved the biological activity and could be an alternative to improve the stability of bioactive peptides for application in food matrices (Mosquera et al. 2014).

### 13.2.3 Nanostructured Flavor

Flavor is an important component of food systems, being essential to the appeal of food. Humans recognize the quality and condition of a food from the flavor or off-flavor. For instance, aroma, taste, and texture properties are parameters that determine the quality of foodstuffs, affecting the perception of flavor during food consumption. Nanoencapsulation techniques can provide structures that retain a sufficient amount of flavor and release the flavors at the desired rate when consumed, thus protecting from degradation, stabilizing, and prolonging the shelf life of products. Encapsulated flavors enable a high sensory impact, providing flavors and/or flavor combinations that are not yet known (Nakagawa 2014).

The use of flavoring compounds preserved through nanoencapsulation, such as essential oils extracted from leaves, fruits, and seeds can bring major innovations in the food industry. Food products such as ice creams, confectionery, bakery, chewing gum, and fast foods use essential oils in their formulations. The soft drink industry is a major consumer of essential oils, especially those of citrus origin, such as orange, lime, and lemon, have been used as flavoring agents. Besides providing flavor and aroma, they have several biological properties such as anticancer, antimicrobial, anti-inflammatory, antioxidant, and antiviral activities (Baser and Buchbauer 2009; Osorio-Tobón et al. 2016).

On the other hand, essential oils are susceptible to extreme environmental conditions (e.g., oxygen, light, and temperature), besides being poorly soluble in water, which limits their application in many foods. The strong flavor of the essential oils can change the original taste of food, however, to overcome this limitation, it is possible to entrap the compound into a capsule in order to mask their undesirable flavor (Osorio-Tobón et al. 2016). Jemaa et al. (2017) studied the effect of *Thymus capitatus* essential oil or its nanoemulsion on the quality of milk contaminated by bacteria. The results obtained improved the oxidative and fermentative stability of semi-skimmed ultra-high temperature (UHT) milk. However, the strong aroma and flavor of essential oils like thyme must be considered. In this way, it is important to evaluate the consumer acceptability of improved food products, namely, when some essential oils (such as thyme) are incorporated.

Nanoliposomes have been used to encapsulate fish oil to be utilized in fortifying yogurt (Ghorbanzade et al. 2017). Although fish oil has many benefits, its strong odor and rapid deterioration limits it application in food formulations. The results obtained by Ghorbanzade et al. (2017) demonstrated that fish oil can be effectively encapsulated by nanoliposomes and added into yogurt, showing similar characteristics in relation to control (without fish oil) in terms of sensory properties. In addition, the encapsulation resulted in a significant reduction in acidity, syneresis, and peroxide value, while increasing polyunsaturated fatty acids (docosahexaenoic acid [DHA] and eicosapentaenoic acid [EPA]) stability. The effects of carvacrol-loaded chitosan-tripolyphosphate nanoparticles to maintain the quality of carrot slices were studied by Martínez-Hernández et al. (2017). The carrot slices treated with nanoparticles achieved the best sensory scores avoiding carvacrol-related off-flavors, which was in turn, obtained for carrot slices with free carvacrol. The study suggests that nanoencapsulation of essential oils may increase the antimicrobial properties of carvacrol, which can be a suitable alternative to conventional sodium hypochlorite (NaOCl) sanitation procedure, without affecting the sensory attributes of carrots.

In another study conducted by Khoshakhlagh et al. (2017), *Alyssum homolocarpum* seed gum nanocapsules were developed for encapsulation of D-limonene. The nanocapsules loaded with D-limonene showed fully amorphous structure with no molecular interactions established between the encapsulated flavor and matrix materials (Khoshakhlagh et al. 2017). Moreover, the incorporation of D-limonene in nanoparticles enhanced the thermostability of flavor up to 230°C, demonstrated through the thermogravimetric analysis. This is a desirable property because its degradation temperature is far from the usual temperatures used for thermally processed food.

## 13.3 FOOD PRESERVATION: BIOACTIVE NANOCOMPOSITES

Coatings made of edible material have been used to protect foods long before their associated chemistries were understood. In the 12th century, in China, some records indicate that citrus fruits were waxed, and later lard or fats were used to prolong shelf life of meat products in England (Salgado et al. 2015). Recently, increasing consumer concerns led to development of edible films and coatings suitable as alternative for food packaging applications, offering extra advantages such as biocompatibility, esthetical appearance, barrier to gas, besides non-toxicity, non-polluting due its biodegradable behavior, and low cost (Elsabee and Abdou 2013; Tavassoli-Kafrani et al. 2016).

The use of packaging films or coatings containing antimicrobial or antioxidant agents is an alternative way to active packaging. This edible coating or films are defined as a thin and continuous layer of edible material formed or placed on or between foods or food components, acting as protective barriers. Edible films can include nanostructured additives for improved performance as carriers of bioactive compounds, thus enhancing the functional properties and quality of the food product, resulting in health benefits. The active packaging has components that release, absorb, or modify substances into or from the packaged food or the environment surrounding the food. Thus, the nanotechnology offers major developments on active nanocomposite packaging, such as antimicrobial films, radical scavenging systems, enzyme immobilization, and protective barrier systems (Ranjan et al. 2014; Brandelli et al. 2017), as showed in Figure 13.2. Because of their very high surface area to volume ratio, strong interfacial adhesion would potentially exist between nanoparticle

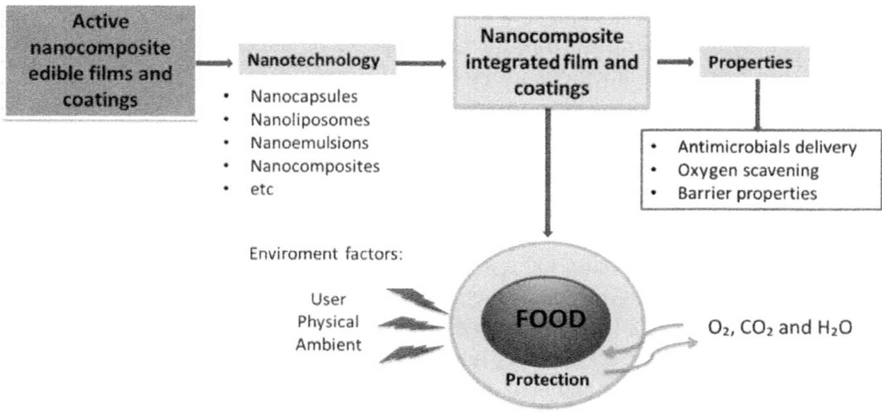


**FIGURE 13.2** Schematic illustration of nanotechnology applications in edible films and coatings.

and matrix, which, in turn, may lead to the formation of composites with unique outstanding characteristics, such as higher mechanical, thermal, and barrier properties (Ghanbarzadeh et al. 2015; Brandelli and Meira 2016).

### 13.3.1 Antimicrobial Films

The development of antimicrobial food packaging has increased over the last decade in order to provide suitable solutions for problems related with the microbial growth in food. These developments have included the use of both new polymeric materials and the application of antimicrobial agents (Appendini and Hotchkiss 2002). Several bioactive substances, including natural products like bacteriocins, essential oils, isothiocyanates and organic acids (e.g., sorbic acid), antimicrobial enzymes, metallic nanoparticles, and some modified clay minerals have been used to develop antimicrobial nanocomposite packaging materials (Azeredo 2013; Rhim et al. 2013; Brandelli and Meira 2016).

Recently, the effect of essential oil incorporation in nanoemulsions has been investigated with different combinations of polymers aiming to develop antimicrobial films and coatings against foodborne pathogens. These studies include modified chitosan and carvacrol nanoemulsion (Tastan et al. 2016), chitosan films and cinnamaldehyde (Chen et al. 2016a), gelatin films and ginger essential oil (Alexandre et al. 2016), alginate films and thyme (Acevedo-Fani et al. 2015), among others. As expected, nanoemulsification of essential oil has significant effect on the functional properties of films as it increased physicochemical activity and stability and improved biological properties, due to the higher surface area of the added particles at nanoscale that increase the bioactive compounds bioavailability (McClements 2011). Gahruie et al. (2017) recently prepared nanoemulsions of *Zataria multiflora* essential oil to be added into basil seed gum films with the aim of increase the efficacy of biopolymer-based antimicrobial films against *E. coli* and *Bacillus cereus*. The incorporation of essential oils into biopolymer-based films change their microstructure and barrier properties that may prolong the shelf life of food products such as fruits and vegetables through retarding the release of oxygen that disrupt the production of ethylene and minimized the loss of water. Thus, the fruits and vegetables remain firm, fresh, and nutritious for more time (Dhall 2013).

Diverse film systems based in proteins and biopolymers incorporated with inorganic nanoparticles have been described (Jafarzadeh et al. 2017; Xu et al. 2017). Some particles can have multiple applications, such as titanium dioxide that can act as reinforcing and antimicrobial agent (Sozer and Kokini 2008; Zhou et al. 2009). The incorporation of silver nanoparticles in biopolymer films such as cellulose, starch, chitosan, and alginate, exhibited a consistent antimicrobial activity against both Gram-positive and Gram-negative bacteria (Unalan et al. 2014). Moreover, the addition of essential oils from spices (i.e., rosemary and oregano) already known as antibacterial agents, as well as silver nanoparticles, may further improve the safety and the quality of foods. Khalaf et al. (2013) studied the antimicrobial activity of edible pullulan films incorporated with both nanoparticles (AgO and ZnO) and essential oils against *L. monocytogenes* and *S. aureus*. The pullulan films with silver nanoparticles and oregano oil caused a significant decrease in the population of both bacteria.

Other nanostructures such as nanoclays (Campos-Requena et al. 2016), halloysite nanotubes (Biddeci et al. 2016), and ZnO nanorods (Jafarzadeh et al. 2017) were used in films and coatings to improve their mechanical and microbiological properties. In addition, organic starch nanoparticles were used to prepare films containing modified montmorillonite and silver nanoparticles with antimicrobial activity (Abreu et al. 2015). In that work, the addition of silver nanoparticles improved the mechanical and gas barrier properties of the film and showed antimicrobial activity against *S. aureus*, *E. coli*, and *Candida albicans*. In addition, nano-crystalline cellulose was also used as organic reinforcement for antimicrobial films (Liu et al. 2017a; Salmieri et al. 2014).

### 13.3.2 Antioxidant Films

Oxidation is one of the most important deteriorative processes that affect the nutritional and sensorial properties of the foods containing oils and fats. Therefore, the oxidation process in packed foods must be prevented (Anbinder et al. 2015). Biodegradable active packaging containing active compounds such as antioxidants has been considered recently to enhance the shelf life of fresh-cut fruits. Further addition of antioxidants to the formulation of films and coatings can improve the preservative function, inhibit browning, and reduce the undesirable effects of nutrient oxidation (Bonilla et al. 2013). Several works focus in the reduction of hydrophilicity and improvement of physical and antioxidant properties of gelatin films by blending with other biopolymers, such as chitosan and sodium caseinate loaded with nanoemulsified active compounds (Alexandre et al. 2016; Dammak et al. 2017). In a recent work, Córdoba and Sobral (2017) evaluated the antioxidant activity of different nanoemulsified essential oils prepared by microfluidization method for application in active films-based biopolymers. According to the authors, the blend gelatin-chitosan exhibited good compatibility and showed a good distribution of the nanoemulsions, but the blend gelatin-sodium caseinate exhibited the highest antioxidant activity, when prepared with the nanoemulsified active compound (Córdoba and Sobral 2017).

The use of antioxidant compounds in association with edible coatings may act in the freshness of fresh-cut fruits, protecting from the undesirable conversion of phenolic compounds in dark-colored pigments in the presence of $O_2$ during storage and marketing (Zawistowski et al. 1991). However, there are only few applications reported of nanostructured films as antibrowning agents. Li et al. (2017) evaluated the effects of poly-lactic acid film incorporated with ZnO nanoparticles on the physical and biochemical properties of fresh-cut apples, measuring the changes in polyphenol oxidase, total phenolic content, and browning index. The results indicated that the nanostructured film provided a better retention of firmness, total phenolic content, color, and sensory quality, when compared to the pure poly-lactic acid film. In another work, Zambrano-Zaragoza et al. (2014) reported the application of a coating based on poly-$\varepsilon$-caprolactone as biopolymer matrix-incorporated nanocapsules containing DL-$\alpha$-tocopherol to fresh-cut Red Delicious apples. This coating decreased the browning index and preserved the firmness of the fresh-cut apples for longer time periods, when compared with the control (without coating application), both evaluated in the same conditions.

### 13.3.3 Nanoreinforcement of Films

Significant improvements in mechanical and barrier properties, dimensional stability, and solvent resistance can be achieved by including some nanofillers into biopolymer matrixes intended for packaging purposes. These active barrier films incorporate nanoadditives in the form of oxygen scavengers and/or moisture controllers to regulate the flow of these components to the primary product (Gokhale and Lee 2014; Brandelli and Meira 2016). The nanocomposites often exhibit increased barrier properties (solvent or gas resistance), increased mechanical strength, and improved modulus, dimensional stability, and heat resistance (e.g., melting points, degradation, and glass transition temperatures) compared to their neat polymers and conventional composites (Ghanbarzadeh et al. 2015). Nanoreinforcement materials can include clays and silicate nanoplatelets, silica nanoparticles, carbon nanotubes, cellulose nanofibers or nanowhiskers, organic (chitin, chitosan and starch), and metallic nanoparticles (Sorrentino et al. 2007).

The inorganic clays have attracted attention by the packaging industry, due to their physical properties and low cost. Mineral clays are considered environmentally friendly, naturally abundant, and inexpensive, besides being considered safe food additives under the established limits according to Food and Drug Administration and European Food Safety Authority (Ibarguren et al. 2014). When nanoclays are used in films, the clay forms layers intercalating the core of the polymer, thus increasing the interlayer spacing. Some degree of order is maintained in the parallel clay layers, which are separated by repeated polymer layers, this conformation creates a smaller space between the layers, which reduce the gas permeability (Ghanbarzadeh et al. 2015). Montmorillonite and halloysite, the natural clays most used as nanoadditives, are widely available, biodegradable, cost effective, and have been shown to improve the properties of several polymer materials (Azeredo 2013; Sadegh-Hassani and Mohammadi Nafchi 2014). Montmorillonite layers were uniformly dispersed in the hemicellulose matrix with polyvinyl alcohol to obtain homogeneous and smooth composite films, leading to enhanced tensile strength, thermal stability, transparency, mechanical resistance, and oxygen barrier permeability (Chen et al. 2015). The incorporation of halloysite improved surface hydrophobicity and mechanical properties of the films made from soluble soybean polysaccharide. However, the oxygen and water vapor permeability, moisture uptake, and water solubility of the films decreased significantly (Alipoormazandarani et al. 2015).

Cellulose nanocrystals are described as a multi-performance material with potential for application in nanostructured food packaging, showing promising properties such as biodegradability, enhanced tensile properties, optimal transparency, and improved oxygen and water barrier (Arrieta et al. 2014). The homogeneous dispersion of high-polarity cellulose nanocrystals into the hydrophobic polymer matrices could be favored by modifying the nanocrystal surfaces to produce flexible films with reduction in the water permeability and oxygen transmission rate (Arrieta et al. 2015; Fortunati et al. 2014). The cellulose nanocrystal obtained from the paper-mulberry pulp was tested as a reinforcing for the preparation of agar-based films (Reddy and Rhim 2014). Mechanical and water vapor barrier properties of the films were significantly improved by blending with cellulose nanocrystals. Recently, Liu et al. (2017b) developed sandwiched starch/cellulose nanowhiskers layers (CNW). The authors observed that the thickness of such layers increased with an increase in the CNW content due to the good interaction between the CNW dispersion in the starch matrix, creating layers structures in the core of the film. The obtained composite films showed self-assembled multi-layer structures with improved mechanical and gas barrier properties.

The incorporation into biopolymers of inorganic nano-sized materials, such as nano-$SiO_2$, nano-$TiO_2$, and nano-ZnO, have been proven to be an effective strategy to improve their mechanical and barrier properties (Jafarzadeh et al. 2017; Yang et al. 2016; Zhang et al. 2016a). $TiO_2$-protein/polysaccharide nanocomposite edible films were developed by Zhang et al. (2017) presenting reduced water vapor permeability, enhanced mechanical properties, thermal stability, and antimicrobial activity.

## 13.4 FOOD SAFETY AND PRESERVATION: NANOSENSORS

Food safety is an important problem that draws attention around the world. At the present, the most common food detection technologies include methods based on chemical, instrumental, enzymatic, and/or immunologic detection. However, these tests are often expensive and involve time-consuming processes for analysis and detection. Such disadvantages limit their use in routine analysis and monitoring. In this context, the development of nanotechnology can offer new alternatives to improve the performance and feasibility in food detection (Mohanty et al. 2009). A biosensor is recognized as a sensing element for selective and specific detection of different compounds in food, coupled to a method to transduce the interaction as a qualitative or quantitative signal, in easy and quick manner (Warriner et al. 2014). This emerging technology has great potential and is receiving growing interest because nanotechnology-based sensors have the potential to detect pathogens, gases, freshness of processed food, flavors, and food contaminants such as toxins and heavy metals (Ranjan et al. 2016).

The nanomaterial-based sensors used in production, quality, and safety control, include bioreceptors as recognition elements, i.e., nanobiosensors. Biosensors use nanostructured materials such as magnetic nanoparticles, carbon nanotubes, nanorods, quantum dots, nanowires, and nanochannels (Ranjan et al. 2016). These materials have remarkable properties such as high capacity for charge transfer, large active surface for immobilization of bioaffinity agents, high quantum yield, resistance to photo-degradation, and excellent optical properties (Gao and Nie 2003). The active surface and the affinity for biomolecules make possible the development of enzyme-based sensors, immunosensors, and microbial sensors (bacteria as bioreceptors). These properties of nanomaterials make them suitable to reach lower detection limits and higher sensitivity values, allowing the development of high-performance biosensors (Pérez-Lopez and Mercoçi 2011). With the benefits afforded to miniaturization, reduced sample volume, and detection time, the modern nanosensors are an efficient class of detection systems that can give a fast qualitative "yes-no" response or offer information to the end-user that reflects the actual food quality in real time (Ranjan et al. 2016; Brandelli et al. 2017).

### 13.4.1 Detection of Pathogens

The development of on-site and sensitive techniques for detection of pathogenic microorganisms is of critical importance to the prevention, surveillance, and control of infectious diseases and their outbreak (Mothershed and Whitney 2006; Rohde et al. 2015). Significant efforts have been made to improve the limitations associated with conventional techniques, such as plate culturing, polymerase chain reaction (PCR), and enzyme-linked immunosorbent assay (ELISA), which are limited by either time or high cost of each analysis (Lauri and Mariani 2009; Maurer 2011). The nanobiosensors can provide rapid detection of microbial cells, toxins, or DNA by converting affinity binding of target bacteria into a measurable physical output via various signal transduction methods (Velusamy et al. 2010). Detection of foodborne pathogens is usually achieved by exploiting the optical or electronic properties of nanomaterials, like metal nanoparticles (Gong-Jun et al. 2009), nanorods (Norman et al. 2008), or carbon nanotubes (So et al. 2008), to detect the microorganisms with high sensitivity.

The recognition element in the detection of specific bacteria relies on the binding of specific molecular receptors (antibodies/aptamers) to bacteria antigens (proteins and lipopolysaccharide on cell walls) immobilized on the nanoparticle or sensor surface. This platform is typically bound to the surface of the nanomaterial, and the interaction of this hybrid with the target bacteria is monitored through a signal transduction mechanism, which detects the interaction between the pathogen and the recognition element (Sutarlie et al. 2017). Currently, five signal transduction methods are used to generate the bacteria cell detection signals: (i) colorimetric; (ii) fluorometric or Förster resonance energy transfer (FRET); (iii) surface enhanced Raman scattering (SERS); (iv) electrochemical; and (v) magnetic relaxometry, typically through magnetic nanoparticles (MNPs) aggregation.

In colorimetric methods, metal nanoparticles conjugated with antibodies or aptamers are mixed directly with samples and in the sequence, selective binding of the bacteria cells to the particles induce the nanoparticle aggregation, leading to color change or absorbance change (Cho and Ku 2017; Wu et al. 2015). Multiple detection of bacteria (for example *E. coli* and *Salmonella typhimurium* at 10 and $10^8$ colony forming units [CFU]/mL in 30 min) can be achieved by using two nanoparticles with distinct absorbance signatures such as gold nanorods with different aspect ratios (Wang et al. 2011a). In the recent years, AuNPs have emerged as an excellent candidate for biosensor design because colloidal solutions containing AuNPs exhibit distinct colors and strong absorption bands, in the visible range of the electromagnetic spectrum, that are not present in the bulk metal. Therefore, the plasmonic properties of AuNPs can be used to produce a red-to-blue colorimetric response, thus the signal can be visibly detected by the naked eye. In the immunologic technique for colorimetric detection of pathogens such as *S. typhimurium*, a specific oligonucleotide DNA sequence of *S. typhimurium* was used as the target (McVey et al. 2017). In another work, two complementary sequences of target DNA were combined to magnetic nanoparticles and AuNPs, respectively, to fabricate capture probes and signal probes for detection of *S. typhimurium*. Sandwich-like structures were formed, where the presence of the target DNA could result in the changes of polymerization degree for AuNPs and the color of the solution change from red, purple, to blue (Ma et al. 2017).

In fluorometric methods, specific antibodies or aptamers are conjugated to photoluminescent nanomaterials such as quantum dots, single-walled carbon nanotubes, carbon nanodots, graphene quantum dots, fluorophores encapsulated in silica nanoparticles, among others. These conjugated nanoparticles are used as fluorescent probes to detect target bacteria cells. Zhao et al. (2009) demonstrated the ability of the combination of magnetic microbeads and quantum dots to detect simultaneously *E. coli* O157:H7, *S. typhimurium*, and *Shigella flexneri*. The conjugated antibody molecules were able to recognize their specific target bacteria in complex mixtures with a low detection limit. This method was extended to detect multiple species of bacteria such as *E. coli, Salmonella*, and *Listeria* simultaneously (Wang et al. 2011b). Recently, the photoluminescence of $TiO_2$ nanoparticles deposited on glass substrate was applied for the detection of *S. typhimurium*. A direct immobilization of antibodies into glass/$TiO_2$ sensitive layer resulted in an optical biosensor with a detection range from $10^3$ to $10^5$ CFU/mL (Viter et al. 2017).

In a FRET assay, as showed in Figure 13.3, a FRET donor (molecular receptors labeled with fluorophores) is initially bound to a FRET acceptor (graphene or AuNPs), and its fluorescence intensity is quenched. In the presence of bacterial cells, the FRET donor binds specifically to bacteria, and thus dissociates from the FRET acceptor, causing fluorescence recovery (Shi et al. 2015a). This method was used for detection of *S. typhimurium* with fluorescence "light on" signals in FRET-based assays, using aptamers labeled with fluorophores as FRET donor and graphene oxide as FRET acceptor, to obtain a detection limit (LOD) of 100 CFU/mL (Duan et al. 2014).

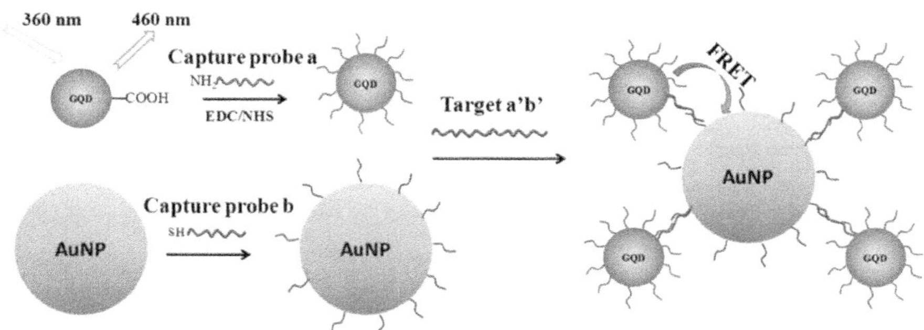


**FIGURE 13.3** Graphene quantum dots (GQDs) and AuNPs act as donor and acceptor of FRET pairs, respectively. Initially, amine modified capture probes **a** are immobilized on the GQDs surface while AuNPs were conjugated with reporter probes **b**. The added target *Staphylococcus aureus* gene oligo (a'b') cohybridizes with capture probes **a** on GQDs and reporter probes **b** on AuNPs, which bring GQDs and AuNPs into close proximity. Under 365 nm light excitation, the emission of GQDs is absorbed by AuNPs. By measuring the fluorescence intensity change of the solution, *S. aureus* target oligos can be detected. (Reproduced from Shi, J. et al., *Biosens. Bioelectron.*, 67, 595–600, 2015a.)

SERS method has been used in various biological applications due to its high sensitivity and specificity sensing molecules in trace amounts. In this technique, bacterial cells are detected based on Raman signals from SERS probes that bind the bacteria. The SERS probes are usually metallic nanoparticles (AuNPs or AgNPs) in various core-shell nanostructures (spheres, rods, stars, or popcorns) conjugated with specific antibodies or aptamers as molecular receptors (Sutarlie et al. 2017). The coupling of AuNPs and magnetic nanoparticles has been also demonstrated for multiplex detection of *S. typhimurium* and *S. aureus* with LOD of 15 and 35 CFU/mL, respectively, by conjugating the AuNPs with the use of different Raman reporter and specific aptamer to each bacterial species (Zhang et al. 2016b).

Electrochemical method utilizes nanomaterials conjugated to antibodies/aptamers to bind bacterial cells and reports the bacteria detection signal as electrical changes (electrical potential, current, conductance, or impedance). Various nanomaterials including metallic and magnetic nanoparticles, graphene, and carbon nanotubes have been used with this purpose. Bacteria were detected with stripping current changes when AuNPs or AgNPs were bound to the cells and release $Au^{3+}$ or $Ag^{+}$ ions upon acid treatment. This approach has been used to detect *Shewanella oneidensis* with a LOD of 12 CFU/mL (Wen et al. 2014), *E. coli* with a LOD of 3 CFU/mL (Eksi et al. 2015), and *S. aureus* with a LOD of 1 CFU/mL (Abbaspour et al. 2015). Table 13.2 summarizes some of the nanomaterial-based biosensors for pathogen detection and the bacterial target.

**TABLE 13.2**
**Examples of Nanoparticles-Based Detection of Food Pathogenic Bacteria**

| Nanoparticles (NPs) | Microorganism | Method/Technique | References |
|---|---|---|---|
| Gold NPs | *Salmonella* spp. | Electrochemical | Afonso et al. (2013) |
| Magnetic NPs/gold NPs | *S. typhimurium* | Colorimetric | Duan et al. (2016) |
| Magnetic NPs/gold NPs | *Vibrio parahemolyticus* | Colorimetric | Wu et al. (2015) |
| Gold NPs/quantum dots | *E. coli, L. monocytogenes, S. enterica* | Chromatographic strip | Bruno (2014) |
| Gold NPs/magnetic beads | *S. aureus* | Electrochemical | Abbaspour et al. (2015) |
| Magnetic NPs/quantum dots | *E. coli O157 and S. enterica* | Fluorescence bioassay | Bruno et al. (2016) |
| Upconverting nanoparticles (UCNPs) and $Fe_3O_4$ magnetic NPs | *S. aureus, V. parahemolyticus*, and *S. typhi* | Luminescence sensors | Wu et al. (2014) |
| Carboxymethyl chitosan/CdS quantum dots | *S. aureus* | Fluorescence bioassay | Wang et al. (2011) |
| Graphene quantum dots and gold NPs | *S. aureus* | Fluorescence FRET | Shi et al. (2015a) |
| Oligonucleotide microarray combined with quantum dots | Food-borne pathogenic bacteria | Fluorescent labels | Huang et al. (2014) |
| $Fe_3O_4$ magnetic gold NPs | *S. typhi* and *S. aureus* | SERS | Zhang et al. (2016b) |

### 13.4.2 Detection of Mycotoxins and Bacterial Toxins

Due to improper storage, agricultural products and animal feedstuffs are easily contaminated with toxins produced by filamentous fungi or bacteria, for example, mycotoxins contaminate about a quarter of worldwide grains (Hussein and Brasel 2001). Development of accurate and reliable biosensors for toxin detection has been a challenge, due to greater degree of diversity in the nature of toxin molecules and difficulties to extract low levels of toxins (in the order of $\leq$ ng) from food matrices (Ranjan et al. 2016). The conventional method for detection of bacterial toxins is based on ELISA tests. These tests typically take about 2 hours of incubation time for the samples to equilibrate before reading and are relatively sensitive, with an LOD and dynamic range of 1–100 ng/mL for Staphylococcal enterotoxin B (Han et al. 2013; Mabry et al. 2006). Nanobiosensors show great potential for use in diverse biosensing strategies, they are rapid, sensitive, and present specific detection of contaminants over the existing conventional methods. For toxin detection, the most common strategies include antibodies or aptamers with specificity to the toxin that will be detected. The toxin functionalizes the magnetic nanoparticles, and the sample separation from the matrix is performed using nanoparticle-based magnetic solid phase extraction or immunomagnetic separation (Duncan 2011). The immunological-based sensing offers high sensitivity and selectivity owing to the site-specific binding of antibodies to unique biomarkers (Sutarlie et al. 2017). Additionally from using antibodies/aptamers as a molecular recognition element, specific detection of bacterial toxins can be achieved by utilizing the enzymatic activities of some toxins, for example, botulinum toxin (Shi et al. 2015b), or specific receptors, such as the ganglioside GM1 receptor for cholera toxin (Viswanathan et al. 2006).

Detection of bacterial toxins includes, in many cases, the same methods for bacterial sensing. Recently, Sharma et al. (2015) evaluated the sensitivity of electrochemical and fluorescence immunoassay methods using zinc sulfide (ZnS) quantum dots to detect Staphylococcal enterotoxin B. The authors concluded that electrochemical assay is faster, more sensitive (LOD 0.02 ng/mL), requires low-cost instrument, and therefore, represents the best alternative method as compared to the existing ones such as ELISA test. SERS probe method has been applied for detection of enterotoxin B and uses a peptide ligand (aptamer) functionalized magnetic gold nanorods. In this method, the LOD for the homogeneous assay was determined as 224 aM (ca. 2697 enterotoxin B molecules/20 μL sample volume). According to the authors, the developed nanosensor can be applied for the quantitative analysis of enterotoxin B in complex matrices (Temur et al. 2012). Optimal results of LOD were obtained for detection of cholera toxin, using an immunosensor that combined the advantages of AuNPs with non-conducting films (polytyramine) to design a biocompatible interface for the immobilization of antitoxin antibody, obtained a sub-attomolar LOD of 0.09 aM. This immunosensor was successfully applied for the detection of cholera toxin in turbid water sample (Loyprasert et al. 2010).

Mycotoxins are typically small hydrophobic molecules that can be better detected through labels like enzymes, nanoparticles, redox molecules, and fluorophores. Conventionally, mycotoxins are detected using liquid chromatography assisted with molecular fluorescence detection and mass spectrometry or mycotoxin ELISA kits

(Chauhan et al. 2016). Although, these methods are well known for their accurate and precise detection of mycotoxins in food or feed samples, they require skilled operators, extensive sample preparation, equipment, and may lack accuracy at low analytic concentration (Cigić and Prosen 2009; Goryacheva et al. 2007).

The recent biosensor techniques for mycotoxins detection commonly use receptor biomolecules (e.g., antibodies, DNA, or enzymes) and synthetic chemicals (e.g., aptamers, mimotopes) for specific recognition. Magnetic bead micro/nanoparticles can be also used in the separation process because they offer great advantages such as easy handling, reusability, and homogeneous dispersity (Aguilar-Arteaga et al. 2010). Competitive binding assays are frequently used with SERS, fluorometric, electrochemical, or electrochemiluminescence for mycotoxin detection (Sutarlie et al. 2017). In the competitive assays, two types of protocols known as "indirect" and "direct" methods are followed. In the "indirect" method, the electrode surface is coated with a saturated concentration of labeled analyte-protein conjugate and competition takes place between the free analyte and the immobilized labeled analyte-protein conjugate, for the fixed amount of antibody. In the "direct" mode, free sample analyte competes with the absorbed labeled analyte-protein conjugate for the fixed amount of immobilized antibody, while a transducer monitors the target analyte concentration present in the solution (Chauhan et al. 2016).

Table 13.3 presents some recent works about mycotoxin nanosensor developments. Multiple research works demonstrate that nanomaterials such as quantum dots and AuNPs coated with antigens or a secondary antibody can perform the response signal for mycotoxin sensing (Bonel et al. 2010). Urusov et al. (2011) developed an immunoanalytical system composed by a surface plasmon resonance sensor and amplified by the anti-species antibody-conjugated with AuNPs. This system archived a signal amplification of more than 10 and results in a LOD of 60 pg/mL for ochratoxin A.

Gold nanoparticle-based immunochromatographic strip methods have been employed for the detection of aflatoxin M1 in milk. Milk samples contaminated with

**TABLE 13.3**
**Examples of Nanoparticles-Based Detection of Toxins**

| Nanoparticles (NPs) | Target Compound | Method/Technique | References |
|---|---|---|---|
| Magnetic NPs | Aflatoxin B1 | Colorimetric | Urusov et al. (2014) |
| Gold NPs | Ochratoxin A | Fluorescence | Chen et al. (2014) |
| CuTe quantum dots/gold NPs | Aflatoxin B1 | FRET | Sabet et al. (2017) |
| Gold NPs/quantum dots | Botulinum toxin | FRET | Lee et al. (2015) |
| Gold nanorods | Aflatoxin B1 | Colorimetric | Xu et al. (2013) |
| Silica NPs | Cholera toxin, SEB | Fluorescence | Lian et al. (2010) |
| Graphene oxide NPs | BoNT/A | FRET | Shi et al. (2015b) |
| Silver NPs | Citrinin | SERS | Singh et al. (2014) |
| Gold NPs | Ochratoxin A | Colorimetric | Xiao et al. (2015) |
| Gold NPs | Aflatoxin B1 | Colorimetric | Wang et al. (2014) |
| Fluospheres® | Ochratoxin A | Fluorescence | Hayat et al. (2015) |

*Note:* BoNT/A—botulinum neurotoxin A; SEB—staphylococcal enterotoxin B; CuTe—copper telluride.

the aflatoxin M1 exhibit a colorless zone on the strip, while in its absence, a red color band appears (Wang et al. 2011c). Recently, a FRET-based method has been developed using a nanobiosensor for detection of aflatoxin B1 in agricultural foods, based on interactions of aptamers conjugated (quantum dots) with AuNPs that lead to quenching effect on quantum dots fluorescence and to its recovery when the aptamers are attracted to the toxin (Sabet et al. 2017). Gan et al. (2013) employed magnetic $Fe_3O_4$-graphene oxides as the absorbent and antibody-labeled with cadmium telluride (CdTe) quantum dots as the signal tag for aflatoxin M1 detection and achieved the LOD of 0.3 pg/mL.

The detection of mycotoxins can be enhanced by concentrating the toxin using antibody-functionalized magnetic nanoparticles. Recently, Urusov et al. (2014) showed the adsorption of immunoglobulins on the surface of magnetic nanoparticles to determine aflatoxin B1 (Figure 13.4). This approach provided a significant reduction in the incubation period required during the competitive interaction stage of the ELISA and a very low LOD (i.e., 20 pg/mL).

### 13.4.3 Detection of Pesticides and Others Hazards in Food

The presence of chemicals in food is a public health concern and represents a recognized obstacle for trade (WHO 2017). Therefore, the main food contaminants or adulterants (e.g., pesticides, melamine, acrylamide, nitrite, and toxic metals) that can be found in food, as well as the main conventional and emergent techniques used for their detection are detailed below (Lin 2014).

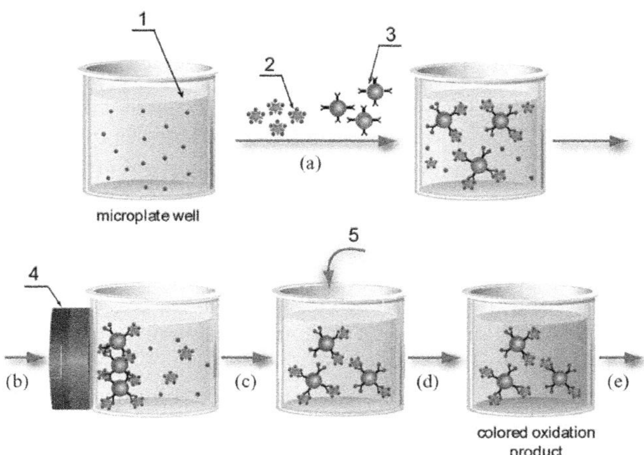


**FIGURE 13.4** Scheme of ELISA method using magnetic nanoparticles. 1–sample containing AFB1; 2–AFB1-peroxidase conjugate; 3–MNP conjugate with antibodies against aflatoxin B1 (AFB1); 4–magnet; and 5–peroxidase substrate. In the step (a), free AFB1 contained in the test sample competes with peroxidase-labeled AFB1 for binding sites on the antibodies adsorbed on the MNP surface; step (b) magnet separation of MNP; step (c) MNPs are washed; step (d) is added the peroxidase substrate to the MNP suspension; and step (e) the absorbance of the peroxidase reaction product is recorded; this result reflects by inverse proportion the AFB1 content in the sample. (Reproduced from Urusov, A. E. et al., *Sensors*, 14, 21843–21857, 2014.)

#### 13.4.3.1 Pesticides

The use of pesticides in agriculture raises public concern regarding the safety of food products and the contamination of the environment. Among pesticides, organophosphorus and carbamates are the most widely employed around the world and might present a potential risk to human health and environment (Kumar et al. 2010). Gas chromatography-mass spectrometry (GC-MS) and high-performance liquid chromatography (HPLC) are generally used to detect pesticides. However, these analytical assays require complex sample treatment procedures and expensive equipment, resulting in high-cost assays.

Nanoparticles have been used for the detection of pesticides, fertilizers, and other toxic chemicals. The strategies devised for detection of food adulterants or contaminants include colorimetric, fluorometric, and electrochemical methods. Compared to optical methods, electrochemical approach may prove to be more useful for food matrices because the problem of light scattering and absorption from various food ingredients can be avoided (Duncan 2011). Most of the works on biosensors for organophosphorus pesticides are based on the inhibition of acetylcholine esterase (AChE) enzyme. Apart from AChE, fluorescence assays, based on specific recognition of organophosphates by organophosphorus hydrolase enzyme, have also been developed (Wang et al. 2002).

A nanoparticle-based (AuNPs) optical biosensor (paper dipstick) for the direct detection of organophosphate chemical and pesticides was developed by Luckham and Brennan (2010). In that work, the authors obtained greatest sensitivity to paraoxon pesticide detection (minimum detection limit of 500 nM) using a silica support for AuNPs conjugated with enzymes. Another gold nanoparticle-based electrochemical biosensor for pesticide detection was developed by Liu et al. (2012), using rhodamine B-covered gold nanoparticle as colorimetric and fluorometric sensors for the detection of organophosphorus and carbamate pesticides. This assay is based on the AChE inhibition by pesticides, thus preventing the generation of thiocholine, which turns the nanoparticle solutions blue and affects the fluorescence of rhodamine B. Carbon nanotubes-based bionanocomposites or devices have been used for detection of pesticides due to their unique mechanical, physical, and chemical properties (Cui 2007). A multi-walled carbon nanotube-electrode was grafted by molecular imprinting to develop a high sensitive potentiometric biosensor for organochlorine pesticides, based on the modification of $\gamma$-hexachlorocyclohexane imprinted polymer film onto the surface of Cu electrode (Anirudhan and Alexander 2015). In another work, multi-walled carbon nanotube/polyaniline composite film was prepared by electrochemical polymerization and used as support for immobilized AChE for sensing organophosphate pesticides (Chen et al. 2010). Quantum dots can also be used to examine pesticides with high sensitivity and specificity. Detection of the organophosphorous was achieved using an optical transducer of CdTe semiconductor quantum dots integrated with AChE for fluorometric detection of organophosphorous in real samples of vegetables and fruits (Zheng et al. 2011). Other approaches include the FRET phenomenon and quantum dots to sensing pesticides. Arvand and Mirroshandel (2017) developed a FRET-based aptasensor to detect edifenphos fungicide that enables the energy transfer from the quantum dots to graphene oxide sheets, quenching the fluorescence of quantum dots. However, when the graphene oxide was replaced by the fungicide in solution, the fluorescence of quantum dots was restored, and its intensity was proportional to the edifenphos concentration. In another work, synthesized carbon quantum dots were used for the detection of organophosphorous. The fluorescence emission of carbon quantum dots could be effectively quenched by AuNPs via FRET, thiocholine was used to recover the quenched fluorescence emission of carbon quantum dots, but due to the inhibition of the thiocholine by the organophosphorous, it was possible to establish a relation of the concentration of the organophosphorous by the fluorescence change of carbon quantum dots (Wu et al. 2017).

#### 13.4.3.2 Melamine

Like pesticides, the excessive use of fertilizers also raises safety concerns. Melamine is a fertilizer that has reported as adulterant in protein-rich products such as egg, biscuits, candy, and coffee drinks (Vasimalai and Abraham 2013). Traditional analytical methods for testing melamine include the Kjeldahl method, GC–MS and HPLC, which are time consuming and expensive. Therefore, it is of great importance to develop rapid, simple, reliable, and sensitive methods to detect melamine contamination in foods. Gold nanoclusters, AuNPs, and quantum dots have attracting features due to their unique electronic and optical properties. Based on the variation of some properties of the particles that make up the sensor, color changes can be detected by instrumentation or by the naked eye. Colorimetric methods to detect melamine include unmodified AuNPs, which show a color change from red-to-blue in solution when melamine was added, due to melamine-induced nanoparticle aggregation (Li et al. 2010; Xing et al. 2013). Recently, SERS method was included to colorimetric unmodified gold nanoparticle method to overcome some limitations, such as false positive and inaccurate signal in the presence of interfering compounds (Lang et al. 2015). Peng et al. (2016) developed a sensitive and reliable electrochemical sensor for detection of melamine based on AuNPs deposited on a graphene doped carbon paste electrode. Melamine sensing was achieved, based on the interaction between melamine molecules and AuNPs, causing suppression in the peak current. This decrease in the value of the electric current showed a linear relationship with the melamine concentration (Peng et al. 2016). More recently, Kalaiyarasan et al. (2017) report a ratiometric nanosensor for selective detection of melamine based in fluorescence sensing by the use of glutathione-stabilized gold nanoclusters, due to melamine-induced aggregation and quenching of fluorescence intensity in nanoclusters. This nanosensor was successfully applied to determine melamine in cow milk.

#### 13.4.3.3 Acrylamide

Acrylamide is a neurotoxin and a potential carcinogen (Exon 2006). Large amounts of acrylamide were found in thermally processed food especially french fries, baked bread, and potato-based snacks (Mottram et al. 2002). Considering its toxicity, the rapid and sensitive detection of acrylamide in food has become a very important issue in food safety. To overcome the limitations of high cost and time demand of the traditional methods to determine acrylamide (i.e., gas chromatography coupled to mass spectrometry [GC-MS] and liquid chromatography coupled to tandem mass spectrometry [LC-MS/MS]), different kinds of detectors were developed. These include a: (i) nanostructured cell (hemoglobin-gold–nanoparticles-glass) based in the interaction between the amino groups of the N-terminal valine in the hemoglobin structure and the acrylamide molecule (Garabagiu and Mihailescu 2011); (ii) electrochemical biosensor constituted by a multi-walled carbon nanotube/copper nanoparticles/polyaniline composite with covalent immobilized hemoglobin onto its surface and electrodeposited onto pencil graphite electrode (Batra et al. 2013); and (iii) glassy carbon electrode modified with single-walled carbon nanotubes (Krajewska et al. 2008). Recently, Hu et al. (2014) developed a fluorescent labels sensing method based on acrylamide polymerization-induced distance increase between quantum dots for detection of acrylamide. The quantum dots modified with N-acryloxysuccinimide were successfully used for detection of acrylamide in potato chips and cookies with a LOD of 3.5 μg/mL.

#### 13.4.3.4 Nitrite

Nitrite and nitrate exist widely in the environment and food products, being recognized as hazardous because they act as a precursor for the production of highly carcinogenic N-nitrosamines upon interaction with proteins (Song et al. 2015). Numerous methods have been used for the detection and determination of nitrite and/or nitrate, including spectrophotometric, electrochemical, and chromatographic techniques. In the field of nanotechnology, most of the works are based in electrochemical devices due to their potential low-cost and portability, using metal oxide nanoparticles, nanoclusters, carbon nanotubes, organic and inorganic electro-polymerized films, and combinations of these for nitrite detection (Wang et al. 2017). Metallic nanoparticles, such as gold, platinum, and palladium can be used to increase electrochemical activities and performances of catalysis and mass transport (Welch and Compton 2006). Cobalt phthalocyanine-supported palladium nanoparticle was synthesized by using as modifier of glassy carbon electrode to fabricate a sensitive and selective electrochemical nitrite sensor. The electrode exhibits enhanced electro-catalytic behavior to the oxidation of nitrite (Song et al. 2017). An electrochemical sensor (paste carbon electrode) for analysis of nitrite in foodstuff was developed by Gupta et al. (2017) using CdO-decorated single-wall carbon nanotube incorporated with 1-methyl-3-butylimidazolium bromide. The results revealed that the nanostructure shows high electro-catalytic activity toward electro-oxidation of nitrite. Xue et al. (2013) developed an electrochemical sensor for the determination of nitrite based on a glassy carbon electrode modified with graphene-chitosan and AuNPs. This sensor showed optimal electrochemical catalytic activities toward sulfite and nitrite. Others approaches include fluorescence detection of nitrite by functionalized silver nanoclusters that interact with peroxynitrous acid for quenching of nanoclusters fluorescence (Chen et al. 2016b) and the use of functionalized quantum dots for electrochemiluminescent detection (Yao et al. 2013; Yin et al. 2013).

#### 13.4.3.5 Metals

Several metal ions such as arsenic, cadmium, copper, mercury, and lead are present into the environment and can be found as residues in food. Exposure excess to toxic metal ions can cause neurological, reproductive, cardiovascular, and developmental disorders (Liu et al. 2011; Shah et al. 2012). Conventional methods for determination of individual metals in food products include: titration, colorimetric analysis, UV-vis spectroscopy, and either flame or graphite furnace atomic absorption spectrometry. Nanosensors for detection of heavy metals are based on noble metal nanoparticles like Ag, Au, and Cu due to their unique property of surface plasmon resonance (Ajay et al. 2017), and metallic nanoparticles functionalized with ionic liquids have also been used in the magnetic-based dispersive microsolid-phase extraction of metals from food matrix (Hernández et al. 2017). This last method has been reported for selective extraction of food contaminants, such as cadmium (Mirabi et al. 2015) copper (Farahani et al. 2015) and lead (Pirouz et al. 2015; Ramandi and Shemirani 2015). Functionalized gold nanoparticle-based colorimetric detection was also demonstrated for arsenic (Weng et al. 2014; Zhan et al. 2014), mercury (Guo et al. 2011; You et al. 2013), chromium (Wang et al. 2015; Zhao et al. 2012), and lead (Li and Wang 2010; Ratnarathorn et al. 2014). AuNPs are under continuous research as high sensitive method for detection of heavy metals based in the fact that aggregation of nanoparticles induced by interaction with specific metal ions results in color change.

## 13.5 CONCLUSIONS AND FUTURE PERSPECTIVES

The advances in nanotechnology provide an outstanding assortment of nanostructures as potential carriers for preservatives in food. Several natural and food grade antimicrobials, antioxidants, and flavors have been effectively formulated as nanostructures, and comprehensive research is developed on active nanocomposite films and coatings. Important advances in the development of nanodevices for detection of pathogens, toxins, and other hazards in food have been described, thus providing powerful tools to improve food safety and preservation. This variety of nanostructured materials is available for development of a new generation of safe foods and innovative food packaging systems. Further studies in real food systems are necessary to certify the effectiveness and safety of nanomaterials. Information about the toxicity of nanoparticles is relatively scarce in relation to their specific characteristics in food, where interactions with food matrices and modifications of nanoparticles during the transit in the digestive tract may represent a key role in the assessment of consumer risks.

## REFERENCES

Abbaspour, A., F. Norouz-Sarvestani, A. Noon, and N. Soltani. 2015. "Aptamer-conjugated silver nanoparticles for electrochemical dual aptamer—Based sandwich detection of *Staphylococcus aureus*." *Biosensors and Bioelectronics* no. 68:149–155.

Abreu, S., M. A. S. Oliveira, M. Rodrigues, M. Cerqueira, A. Vicente, and A. Machado. 2015. "Antimicrobial nanostructured starch based films for packaging." *Carbohydrate Polymers* no. 129:127–134.

Acevedo-Fani, A., L. Salvia-Trujillo, M. A. Rojas-Graü, and O. Martín-Belloso. 2015. "Edible films from essential-oil-loaded nanoemulsions: Physicochemical characterization and antimicrobial properties." *Food Hydrocolloids* no. 47:168–177.

Afonso, S., B. Perez-Lopez, R. C. Faria, C. Mattoso, M. Hernandez-Herrero, A. X. Roig-Sagues, M. M. Costa, and A. Merkoci. 2013. "Electrochemical detection of *Salmonella* using gold nanoparticles." *Biosensors and Bioelectronics* no. 40:121–126.

Aguiar, J., B. N. Estevinho, and L. Santos. 2016. "Microencapsulation of natural antioxidants for food application—The specific case of coffee antioxidants—A review." *Trends in Food Science & Technology* no. 58:21–39.

Aguilar-Arteaga, K., J. A. Rodriguez, and E. Barrado. 2010. "Magnetic solids in analytical chemistry: A review." *Analytica Chimica Acta* no. 674:157–165.

Ajay, P., J. Printo, D. S. Kiruba, L. Susithra, K. Takatoshi, and M. Sivakumar. 2017. "Colorimetric sensors for rapid detection of various analytes." *Materials Science and Engineering C* no. 78:1231–1245.

Alexandre, E. M. C., R. V. Lourenço, A. M. Q. B. Bittante, I. C. F. Moraes, and P. J. A. Sobral. 2016. "Gelatin-based films reinforced with montmorillonite and activated with nanoemulsion of ginger essential oil for food packaging applications." *Food Packaging and Shelf Life* no. 10:87–96.

Alipoormazandarani, N., S. Ghazihoseini, and A. N. Nafchi. 2015. "Preparation and characterization of novel bionanocomposite based on soluble soybean polysaccharide and halloysite nanoclay." *Carbohydrate Polymers* no. 134:745–751.

Alves, A. C. S., R. M. Mainardes, and N. M. Khalil. 2016. "Nanoencapsulation of gallic acid and evaluation of its cytotoxicity and antioxidant activity." *Materials Science and Engineering C* no. 60:126–134.

Anbinder, P., P. Peruzzo, M. Martino, and J. Amalvy. 2015. "Effect of antioxidant active films on the oxidation of soybean oil monitored by Fourier transform infrared spectroscopy." *Journal of Food Engineering* no. 151:43–50.

Anirudhan, T. S., and S. Alexander. 2015. "Design and fabrication of molecularly imprinted polymer-based potentiometric sensor from the surface modified multiwalled carbon nanotube for the determination of lindane (γ-hexachlorocyclohexane), an organochlorine pesticide." *Biosensors and Bioelectronics* no. 64:586–593.

Appendini, P., and J. H. Hotchkiss. 2002. "Review of antimicrobial food packaging." *Innovative Food Science & Emerging Technologies* no. 3:113–126.

Arrieta, M. P., E. Fortunati, F. Dominici, E. Rayón, J. López, and J. M. Kenny. 2014. "Multifunctional PLA–PHB/cellulose nanocrystal films: Processing, structural and thermal properties." *Carbohydrate Polymers* no. 107:16–24.

Arrieta, M. P., E. Fortunati, F. Dominici, E. Rayón, J. López, and J. M. Kenny. 2015. "Bionanocomposite films based on plasticized PLA-PHB/cellulose nanocrystal blends." *Carbohydrate Polymers* no. 121:265–275.

Arvand, M., and A. A. Mirroshandel. 2017. "Highly-sensitive aptasensor based on fluorescence resonance energy transfer between cysteine capped ZnS quantum dots and graphene oxide sheets for the determination of edifenphos fungicide." *Biosensors and Bioelectronics* no. 96:324–331.

Azam, A., A. S. Ahmed, M. Oves, M. S. Khan, S. S. Habib, and A. Memic. 2012. "Antimicrobial activity of metal oxide nanoparticles against gram-positive and gram-negative bacteria: A comparative study." *International Journal of Nanomedicine* no. 7:6003–6009.

Azeredo, H. M. C. 2013. "Antimicrobial nanostructures in food packaging." *Trends in Food Science & Technology* no. 30:56–69.

Banerjee, K., S. Banerjee, S. Das, and M. Mandal. 2015. "Probing the potential of apigenin liposomes in enhancing bacterial membrane perturbation and integrity loss." *Journal of Colloids and Interface Science* no. 453:48–59.

Baser, K. H. C., and G. Buchbauer. 2009. "*Handbook of Essential Oils: Science, Technology, and Applications*." Boca Raton, FL: CRC Press.

Bassolé, I. H. N., and H. R. Juliani. 2012. "Essential oils in combination and their antimicrobial properties." *Molecules* no. 17:3989–4006.

Batra, B., S. Lata, M. Sharma, and C. Pundir. 2013. "An acrylamide biosensor based on immobilization of haemoglobin onto multiwalled carbon nanotube/copper nanoparticle/polyaniline hybrid film." *Analytical Biochemistry* no. 433:210–217.

Biddeci, G., G. Cavallarob, F. Di Blasia, G. Lazzarab, M. Massaroc, S. Miliotob, F. Parisib, S. Rielac, and G. Spinelli. 2016. "Halloysite nanotubes loaded with peppermint essential oil as filler for functional biopolymer film." *Carbohydrate Polymers* no. 152:548–557.

Bindhu, M. R., and M. Umadevi. 2014. "Antibacterial activities of green synthesized AuNPs." *Materials Letters* no. 120:122–125.

Bonel, L., C. Vidal, P. Duato, and J. R. Castillo. 2010. "Ochratoxin A nanostructured electrochemical immunosensors based on polyclonal antibodies and gold nanoparticles coupled to the antigen." *Analytical Methods* no. 2:335–341.

Bonilla, J., and P. J. A. Sobral. 2017. "Antioxidant and physicochemical properties of blended films based on gelatin-sodium caseinate activated with natural extracts." *Journal of Applied Polymer Science* no. 134:44467.

Bonilla, J., E. Talón, L. Atarés, M. Vargas, and A. Chiralt. 2013. "Effect of the incorporation of antioxidants on physicochemical and antioxidant properties of wheat starch-chitosan films." *Journal of Food Engineering* no. 118:271–278.

Bost, M., S. Houdart, M. Oberli, E. Kalonji, J. F. Huneau, and I. Margaritis. et al. 2016. "Dietary copper and human health: Current evidence and unresolved issues." *Journal of Trace Elements in Medicine and Biology* no. 35:107–115.

Brandelli, A. 2015. "Nanobiotechnology strategies for delivery of antimicrobials in food and agriculture." in *Nanotechnologies in Food and Agriculture*, edited by M. Rai, C. Ribeiro, L. Mattoso, and N. Duran, 119–139. New York: Springer.

Brandelli, A., and T. M. Taylor. 2015. "Nanostructured and nanoencapsulated natural antimicrobials for use in food products." in *Handbook of Natural Antimicrobials for Food Safety and Quality*, edited by T. M. Taylor, 229–257. Oxford, UK: Woodhead Publishing.

Brandelli, A., and S. M. M. Meira. 2016. "Applications of renewable polymers incorporating nanocomposites." in *Green Polymer Composites Technology: Properties and Applications*, edited by I. Inamuddin, 149–162. Boca Raton, FL: CRC Press.

Brandelli, A., L. F. W. Brum, and J. H. Z. Santos. 2017. "Nanostructured bioactive compounds for ecological food packaging." *Environmental Chemistry Letters* no. 15:193–204.

Bruno, J. 2014. "Application of DNA aptamers and quantum dots to lateral flow test strips for detection of foodborne pathogens with improved sensitivity versus colloidal gold." *Pathogens* no. 3:341–355.

Bruno, J., T. Phillips, A. Richarte, T. Montez, A. Garcia, and J. Sivils. 2016. "Fluorescent DNA aptamer-magnetic bead sandwich assays and portable fluorometer for sensitive and rapid foodborne pathogen detection and epidemiology." *Journal of Infectious Diseases and Epidemiology* no. 1:173–183.

Campos-Requena, V.H., B.L. Rivas, M.A. Pérez, and E.D. Pereira. 2016. "Short- and long-term loss of carvacrol from polymer/clay nanocomposite film - a chemometric approach." *Polymer International* no. 65:483–490.

Chatterjee, A. K., R. K. Sarkar, A. P. Chattopadhyay, P. Aich, R. Chakraborty, and T. Basu. 2012. "A simple robust method for synthesis of metallic copper nanoparticles of high antibacterial potency against *E. coli*." *Nanotechnology* no. 23:085–103.

Chauhan, R., J. Singh, T. Sachdev, T. Basu, and B. D. Malhotra. 2016. "Recent advances in mycotoxins detection." *Biosensors and Bioelectronics* no. 81:532–545.

Chen, D., C. Chen, and D. Du. 2010. "Detection of organophosphate pesticide using polyaniline and carbon nanotubes composite based on acetylcholinesterase inhibition." *Journal of Nanoscience and Nanotechnology* no. 1:5662–5666.

Chen, G. G., X. M. Qi, M. P. Li, Y. Guan, J. Bian, F. Peng, C. L. Yao, and R. C. Sun. 2015. "Hemicelluloses/montmorillonite hybrid films with improved mechanical and barrier properties." *Scientific Reports* no. 9:16405.

Chen, H., X. Hu, E. Chen, S. Wu, D. J. McClements, and S. Liu. 2016a. "Preparation, characterization, and properties of chitosan films with cinnamaldehyde nanoemulsions." *Food Hydrocolloids* no. 61:662–671.

Chen, J., S. Pang, L. He, and S. R. Nugen. 2016b. "Highly sensitive and selective detection of nitrite ions using $Fe_3O_4$@$SiO_2$/Au magnetic nanoparticles by surface-enhanced Raman spectroscopy." *Biosensors and Bioelectronics* no. 85:726–733.

Chen, J., X. Zhang, S. Cai, D. Wu, M. Chen, S. Wang, and J. Zhang. 2014. "A fluorescent aptasensor based on DNA-scaffolded silver-nanocluster for ochratoxin A detection." *Biosensors and Bioelectronics* no. 57:226–231.

Cho, I. H., and S. Ku. 2017. "Current technical approaches for the early detection of foodborne pathogens: challenges and opportunities." *International Journal of Molecular Sciences* no. 18:2078.

Chopra, M., P. Kaur, M. Bernela, and R. Thakur. 2014. "Surfactant assisted nisin loaded chitosan-carrageenan nanocapsule synthesis for controlling food pathogens." *Food Control* no. 37:158–164.

Chorianopoulos, N. G., D. S. Tsoukleris, E. Z. Panagou, P. Falaras, and G.-J. E. Nychas. 2011. "Use of titanium dioxide ($TiO_2$) photocatalysts as alternative means for *Listeria monocytogenes* biofilm disinfection in food processing." *Food Microbiology* no. 28:164–170.

Cigić, I. K., and H. Prosen. 2009. "An overview of conventional and emerging analytical methods for the determination of mycotoxins." *International Journal of Molecular Sciences* no. 10:62–115.

Córdoba, L. and P. Sobral. 2017. "Physical and antioxidant properties of films based on gelatin, gelatin-chitosan or gelatin-sodium caseinate blends loaded with nanoemulsified active compounds." *Journal of Food Engineering* no. 213:47–53.

Cui, D. 2007. "Advances and prospects on biomolecules functionalized carbon nanotubes." *Journal of Nanoscience and Nanotechnology* no. 7:1298–1314.

Dhall, R. K. 2013. "Advances in edible coatings for fresh fruits and vegetables: A review." *Critical Reviews in Food Science and Nutrition* no. 53(5):435–450.

Dammak, I., R. A. de Carvalho, C. S. Trindade, R. Lourenço, and P. J. A. Sobral. 2017. "Properties of active gelatin films incorporated with rutin-loaded nanoemulsions." *International Journal of Biological Macromolecules* no. 98:39–49.

Duan, N., B. Xu, S. Wu, and Z. Wang. 2016. "Magnetic nanoparticles-based aptasensor using gold nanoparticles as colorimetric probes for the detection of *Salmonella typhimurium*." *Analytical Science* no. 32:431–436.

Duan, Y. F., Y. Ning, Y. Song, and L. Deng. 2014. "Fluorescent aptasensor for the determination of *Salmonella typhimurium* based on a graphene oxide platform." *Microchimica Acta* no. 181:647–653.

Duncan, T. V. 2011. "Applications of nanotechnology in food packaging and food safety: Barrier materials, antimicrobials and sensors." *Journal of Colloid and Interface Science* no. 363:1–4.

Eksi, H., R. Guzel, B. Guven, I. H. Boyaci, and A. O. Solak. 2015. "Fabrication of an electrochemical *E. coli* biosensor in biowells using bimetallic nanoparticle-labelled antibodies." *Electroanalysis* no. 27:343–352.

Elsabee, M. Z., and E. S. Abdou. 2013. "Chitosan based edible films and coatings: A review." *Materials Science and Engineering C* no. 33:1819–1841.

Esfandyari-Manesha, M., Z. Ghaedib, M. Asemic, M. Khanavic, A. Manayic, H. Jamalifard, F. Atyabia, and R. Dinarvand. 2013. "Study of antimicrobial activity of anethole and carvone loaded PLGA nanoparticles." *Journal of Pharmacy Research* no. 7:290–295.

Exon, J. H. 2006. "A review on the toxicology of acrylamide." *Journal of Toxicology and Environmental Health B: Critical Reviews* no. 9:397–412.

Farahani, M. D., F. Shemirani, N. F. Ramandi, and M. Gharehbaghi. 2015. "Ionic liquid as a ferrofluid carrier for dispersive solid phase extraction of copper from food samples." *Food Analytical Methods* no. 8:1979–1989.

Fortunati, E., S. Rinaldi, M. Peltzer, N. Bloise, L. Visai, I. Armentano, A. Jiménez, L. Latterini, and J. M. Kenny. 2014. "Nano-biocomposite films with modified cellulose nanocrystals and synthesized silver nanoparticles." *Carbohydrate Polymers* no. 101:1122–1133.

Gahruie, H., E. Ziaee, M. H. Eskandari, and S. M. Hosseini. 2017. "Characterization of basil seed gum-based edible films incorporated with *Zataria multiflora* essential oil nanoemulsion." *Carbohydrate Polymers* no. 166:93–103.

Gan, N., J. Zhou, P. Xiong, F. Hu, Y. Cao, T. Li, and Q. Jiang. 2013. "An ultrasensitive electrochemiluminescent immunoassay for aflatoxin M1 in milk, based on extraction by magnetic graphene and detection by antibody-labelled CdTe quantum dots-carbon nanotubes nanocomposite." *Toxins* no. 5:865–883.

Gao, X., and S. Nie 2003. "Molecular profiling of single cells and tissue specimens with quantum dots." *Trends in Biotechnology* no. 21(9):371–373.

Garabagiu, S., and G. Mihailescu. 2011. "Simple hemoglobin–gold nanoparticles modified electrode for the amperometric detection of acrylamide." *Journal of Electroanalytical Chemistry* no. 659:196–200.

Ghanbarzadeh, B., S. A. Oleyaei, and H. Almasi. 2015. "Nanostructured materials utilized in biopolymer-based plastics for food packaging applications." *Critical Reviews in Food Science and Nutrition* no. 55:1699–1723.

Ghayempour, S., M. Montazer, and M. M. Rad. 2015. "Tragacanth gum as a natural polymeric wall for producing antimicrobial nanocapsules loaded with plant extract." *International Journal of Biological Macromolecules* no. 81:514–520.

Ghorbanzade, T., S. M. Jafari, S. Akhavan, and R. Hadavi. 2017. "Nano-encapsulation of fish oil in nano-liposomes and its application in fortification of yogurt." *Food Chemistry* no. 216:146–152.

Gokhale, A. A., and I. Lee. 2014. "Recent advances in the fabrication of nanostructured barrier films." *Journal of Nanoscience and Nanotechnology* no. 14:2157–2177.

Gomes, C., R. G. Moreira, and E. Castell-Perez. 2011. "Poly(DL-lactide-co-glycolide) (PLGA) nanoparticles with entrapped trans-cinnamaldehyde and eugenol for antimicrobial delivery applications." *Journal of Food Science* no. 76:16–24.

Gong-Jun, Y., H. Jin-Lin, M. Wen-Jing, S. Ming, and J. Xin-An. 2009. "A reusable capacitive immunosensor for detection of *Salmonella* spp. based on grafted ethylene diamine and self-assembled gold nanoparticle monolayers." *Analytica Chimica Acta* no. 647:159–166.

Goryacheva, I. Y., S. De Saeger, I. S. Nesterenko, S. A. Eremin, and C. Van Peteghem. 2007. "Rapid all-in-one three-step immunoassay for non-instrumental detection of ochratoxin A in high-coloured herbs and spices." *Talanta* no. 72:1230–1234.

Guo, Y., Z. Wangb, W. Qub, H. Shao, and X. Jiang. 2011. "Colorimetric detection of mercury, lead and copper ions simultaneously using protein-functionalized gold nanoparticles." *Biosensors and Bioelectronics* no. 26:4064–4069.

Gupta, V. K., M. A. Khalilzadeh, A. Rudbaraki, S. Agarwal, M. L. Yola, and N. Atar. 2017. "Fabrication of highly sensitive nitrite electrochemical sensor in foodstuff using nanostructure sensor." *International Journal of Electrochemical Science* no. 12:3931–3940.

Han, H. J., J. Lee, S. Park, J. Ahn, and H. G. Lee. 2015. "Extraction optimization and nanoencapsulation of jujube pulp and seed for enhancing antioxidant activity." *Colloids and Surfaces B: Biointerfaces* no. 130:93–100.

Han, J.-H., H.-J. Kim, L. Sudheendra, and S. J. Gee. 2013. "Photonic crystal lab-on-a chip for detecting staphylococcal enterotoxin B at low attomolar concentration." *Analytical Chemistry* no. 85:3104–3109.

Hannon, J. C., J. Kerry, M. Cruz-Romero, M. Morris, and E. Cummins. 2015. "Advances and challenges for the use of engineered nanoparticles in food contact materials." *Trends in Food Science & Technology* no. 43:43–62.

Hayat, A., R. Mishra, G. Catanante, and J. Mart. 2015. "Development of an aptasensor based on a fluorescent particles-modified aptamer for ochratoxin A detection." *Analytical and Bioanalytical Chemistry* no. 407:7815–7822.

He, X., and H. Hwang. 2016. "Nanotechnology in food science: Functionality, applicability, and safety assessment." *Journal of Food and Drug Analysis* no. 24:671–681.

Hernández, A., R. Álvarez, E. Contreras, K. Aguilar, and A. Castañeda. 2017. "Food analysis by microextraction methods based on the use of magnetic nanoparticles as supports: Recent advances." *Food Analytical Methods* no. 10: 2974–2993.

Hill, L. E., T. M. Taylor, and C. Gomes. 2013. "Antimicrobial efficacy of poly (DL-lactide-co-glycolide) (PLGA) nanoparticles with entrapped cinnamon bark extract against *Listeria monocytogenes* and *Salmonella typhimurium*." *Food Science* no. 78:626–632.

Hu, Q., X. Xu, Z. Li, Y. Zhang, J. Wang, and Y. Fu. 2014. "Detection of acrylamide in potato chips using a fluorescent sensing method based on acrylamide polymerization-induced distance increase between quantum dots." *Biosensors and Bioelectronics* no. 54:64–71.

Huang, A., Z. Qiu, M. Jin, Z. Shen, X. Chen, X. Wang, and J. W. Li. 2014. "High-throughput detection of food-borne pathogenic bacteria using oligonucleotide microarray with quantum dots as fluorescent labels." *International Journal of Food Microbiology* no. 185:27–32.

Hussein, S., and M. Brasel. 2001. "Toxicity, metabolism, and impact of mycotoxins on human and animals." *Toxicology* no. 167:101–134.

Ibarguren, C., P. M. Naranjo, C. Stötzel, M. C. Audisio, E. L. Sham, E. M. F. Torres, and F. A. Müller. 2014. "Adsorption of nisin on raw montmorillonite." *Applied Clay Science* no. 90:88–95.

Imran, M., A. M. Revol-Junelles, C. Paris, E. Guedon, M. Linder, and S. Desobry. 2015. "Liposomal nanodelivery systems using soy and marine lecithin to encapsulate food biopreservative nisin." *LWT Food Science and Technology* no. 62:341–349.

Jafarzadeh, S., F. Ariffin, S. Mahmud, A. F. Alias, S. F. Hosseini, and M. Ahmad. 2017. "Improving the physical and protective functions of semolina films by embedding a blend nanofillers (ZnO-nr and nano-kaolin)." *Food Packaging and Shelf Life* no. 12:66–75.

Jemaa, M. B., H. Falleh, M. A. Neves, H. Isoda, M. Nakajima, and R. Ksouri. 2017. "Quality preservation of deliberately contaminated milk using thyme free and nanoemulsified essential oils." *Food Chemistry* no. 217:726–734.

Kalaiyarasan, G., K. Anusuya, and J. James. 2017. "Melamine dependent fluorescence of glutathione protected gold nanoclusters and ratiometric quantification of melamine in commercial cow milk and infant formula." *Applied Surface Science* no. 420:963–969.

Khalaf, H. H., A. M. Sharoba, H. H. El-Tanahi, and M. K. Morsy. 2013. "Stability of antimicrobial activity of pullulan edible films incorporated with nanoparticles and essential oils and their impact on turkey deli meat quality." *Journal of Food and Dairy Science* no. 4:557–573.

Khoshakhlagh, K., A. Koocheki, M. Mohebbi, and A. Allafchian. 2017. "Development and characterization of electrosprayed *Alyssum homolocarpum* seed gum nanoparticles for encapsulation of D-limonene." *Journal of Colloid and Interface Science* no. 490:562–575.

Krajewska, A., J. Radecki, and H. Radecka. 2008. "A voltammetric biosensor based on glassy carbon electrodes modified with single-walled carbon nanotubes/hemoglobin for detection of acrylamide in water extracts from potato crisps." *Sensors* no. 8:5832–5844.

Kumar, S. V., M. Fareedullah, Y. Sudhakar, B. Venkateswarlu, and E. A. Kumar. 2010. "Current review on organophosphorus poisoning." *Archives of Applied Scientific Research* no. 2:199–215. http://scholarsresearchlibrary.com/archive.html.

Lang, T., S. Pang, and L. He. 2015. "Integration of colorimetric and SERS detection for rapid screening and validation of melamine in milk." *Analytical Methods* no. 7:6426–6431.

Lauri, A., and P. Mariani. 2009. "Potentials and limitations of molecular diagnostic methods in food safety." *Genes & Nutrition* no. 4:1–12.

Lee, J., M. Brennan, R. Wilton, C. Rowland, and E. Rozhkova. 2015. "Fast ratiometric FRET from quantum dot conjugated stabilized single chain variable fragments for quantitative botulinum neurotoxin sensing." *Nano Letters* no. 15:7161–7167.

Li, L., B. Li, D. Cheng, and L. Mao. 2010. "Visual detection of melamine in raw milk using gold nanoparticles as colorimetric probe." *Food Chemistry* no. 122:895–900.

Li, W., L. Li, Y. Cao, T. Lan, H. Chen, and Y. Qin. 2017. "Effects of PLA film incorporated with ZnO nanoparticle on the quality attributes of fresh-cut apple." *Nanomaterials* no. 7:207.

Li, X., and Z. Wang. 2010. "Gold nanoparticle-based colorimetric assay for determination of lead(II) in aqueous media." *Chemical Research in Chinese Universities* no. 26:194–197.

Lian, W., D. Wu, D. V. Lim, and S. Jin. 2010. "Sensitive detection of multiplex toxins using antibody microarray." *Analytical Biochemistry* no. 401:271–279.

Lin, M. 2014. "Nanotechnology and its applications to improve the detection of chemical hazards in foods," in *Food Chemical Hazard Detection:Development and Application of New Technologies*, edited by S. Wang, 249–261. Chichester, England: John Wiley & Sons, Ltd.

Lima, E., R. Guerra, V. Lara, and A. Guzmán. 2013. "AuNPs as efficient antimicrobial agents for *Escherichia coli* and *Salmonella typhi*." *Chemistry Central Journal* no. 7:1–7.

Liu, D., W. Chen, J. Wei, X. Li, Z. Wang, and X. Jiang. 2012. "A highly sensitive, dual-readout assay based on AuNPs for organophosphorus and carbamate pesticides." *Analytical Chemistry* no. 84:4185–4189.

Liu, D., Y. Dong, D. Bhattacharyya, and G. Sui. 2017b. "Novel sandwiched structures in starch/cellulose nanowhiskers (CNWs) composite films." *Composites Communications* no. 4:5–9.

Liu, J., Y. Hu, G. Zhu, and X. Zhou. 2014. "Highly sensitive detection of zearalenone in feed samples using competitive surface-enhanced Raman scattering immunoassay." *Journal of Agricultural Food Chemistry* no. 62:8325–8332.

Liu, Y., L. Li, N. Pan, Y. Wang, X. Ren, Z. Xie, G. Buschle-Diller, and T. S. Huang. 2017a. "Antibacterial cellulose acetate films incorporated with N-halamine-modified nano-crystalline cellulose particles." *Polymers for Advanced Technologies* no. 28:463–469.

Liu, Y., Z. Liu, Y. Wang, J. Dai, J. Gao, and J. Xie. 2011. "A surface ion-imprinted mesoporous sorbent for separation and determination of Pb(II) ion by flame atomic absorption spectrometry." *Microchimica Acta* no. 172:309–317.

Liu, Y., Y. Sun. Y. X. Xu, H. Feng, S. D. Fu, J. W. Tang, W. Liu, D. C. Sun, H. Jiang, and S. S. Xu. 2013. "Preparation and evaluation of lysozyme-loaded nanoparticles coated with poly-γ-glutamic acid and chitosan." *International Journal of Biological Macromolecules* no. 59:201–207.

Lopes, N. A., and A. Brandelli. 2017. "Nanostructures for delivery of natural antimicrobials in food." *Critical Reviews in Food Science and Nutrition* no. 10:1–11.

Loyprasert, S., M. Hedström, P. Thavarungkul, P. Kanatharana, and B. Mattiasson. 2010. "Sub-attomolar detection of cholera toxin using a label-free capacitive immunosensor." *Biosensors and Bioelectronics* no. 25:1977–1983.

Luckham, R. E., and J. D. Brennan. 2010. "Bioactive paper dipstick sensors for acetylcholinesterase inhibitors based on sol-gel/enzyme/gold nanoparticle composites." *Analyst* no. 135:2028–2035.

Ma, X., L. Song, L. Xia, C. Jiang, and Z. Wang. 2017. "A novel colorimetric detection of *S. typhimurium* based on $Fe_3O_4$ magnetic nanoparticles and gold nanoparticles." *Food Analytical Methods* no. 10:2735–2742.

Mabry, R., K. Brasky, R. Geiger, and R. Carrion. 2006. "Detection of anthrax toxin in the serum of animals infected with *Bacillus anthracis* by using engineered immunoassays." *Clinical and Vaccine Immunology* no. 13:671–677.

Martínez-Hernández, G. B., M. L. Amodio, and G. Colelli. 2017. "Carvacrol-loaded chitosan nanoparticles maintain quality of fresh-cut carrots." *Innovative Food Science and Emerging Technologies* no. 41:56–63.

Maurer, J. 2011. "Rapid detection and limitations of molecular techniques." *Annual Review in Food Science and Technology* no. 2:259–279.

McClements, D. J. 2011. "Edible nanoemulsions: Fabrication, properties, and functional performance." *Soft Matter* no. 7:2297–2316.

McVey, C., F. Huang, C. Elliott, and C. Cao. 2017. "Endonuclease controlled aggregation of gold nanoparticles for the ultrasensitive detection of pathogenic bacterial DNA." *Biosensors and Bioelectronics* no. 92:502–508.

Mello, M. B., P. S. Malheiros, A. Brandelli, N. P. Silveira, M. M. Jantzen, and A. S. Motta. 2013. "Characterization and antilisterial effect of phosphatidylcholine nanovesicles containing the antimicrobial peptide pediocin." *Probiotics and Antimicrobial Proteins* no. 5:43–50.

Mirabi, A., Z. Dalirandeh, and A. S. Rad. 2015. "Preparation of modified magnetic nanoparticles as a sorbent for the preconcentration and determination of cadmium ions in food and environmental water samples prior to flame atomic absorption spectrometry." *Journal of Magnetism and Magnetic Materials* no. 381:138–144.

Mohanty, A. K., M. Misra, and H. Nalwa. 2009. *Packaging Nanotechnology*. Los Angeles, CA: American Scientific Publishers.

Mosquera, M., B. Giménez, I. M. Silva, J. F. Boelter, P. Montero, C. Gómez-Guillén, and A. Brandelli, 2014. "Nanoencapsulation of an active peptidic fraction from sea bran scales collagen." *Food Chemistry* no. 156:144–150.

Mothershed, E., and A. Whitney. 2006. "Nucleic acid-based methods for the detection of bacterial pathogens: Present and future considerations for the clinical laboratory." *Clinical Chimica Acta* no. 363:206–220.

Mottram, D. S., B. L. Wedzicha, and A. T. Dodson. 2002. "Acrylamide is formed in the Maillard reaction." *Nature* no. 419:448.

Mozafari, M. R., J. Flanagan, L. Matia-Merino, A. Awati, A. Omri, Z. E. Suntres, and H. Singh. 2006. "Recent trends in the lipid-based nanoencapsulation of antioxidants and their role in foods." *Journal of the Science of Food and Agriculture* no. 86:2038–2045.

Nakagawa, K. 2014. "Nano- and microencapsulation of flavor in food systems." in *Nano- and Microencapsulation for Foods*, edited by H. S. Kwak, 249–271. Chichester, UK: John Wiley & Sons.

Norman, S., W. Stone, A. Gole, J. Murphy, and L. Sabo-Attwood. 2008. "Targeted photothermal lysis of the pathogenic bacteria, *Pseudomonas aeruginosa*, with gold nanorods." *Nano Letters* no. 8:302–306.

Oroian, M., and I. Escriche. 2015. "Antioxidants: Characterization, natural sources, extraction and analysis." *Food Research International* no. 74:10–36.

Osorio-Tobón, J. F., E. K. Silva, and M. A. A. Meireles. 2016. "Nanoencapsulation of flavors and aromas by emerging technologies." in *Encapsulations*, edited by A. Grumezescu, 89–126. Oxford, UK: Elsevier.

Pathakoti, K., M. Manubolu, and H. Hwang. 2017. "Nanostructures: Current uses and future applications in food science." *Journal of Food and Drug Analysis* no. 25:245–253.

Peng, J., Y. Feng, X. Han, and Z. Gao. 2016. "Sensitive electrochemical detection of melamine based on gold nanoparticles deposited on a graphene doped carbon paste electrode." *Analytical Methods* no. 8:2526–2532.

Peng, S., L. Zou, W. Liu, L. Gan, W. Liu, R. Liang, C. Liu, J. Niu, Y. Cao, Z. Liu, and X. Chen. 2015. "Storage stability and antibacterial activity of eugenol nanoliposomes prepared by an ethanol injection-dynamic high-pressure microfluidization method." *Journal of Food Protection* no. 78:22–30.

Pereira, M. C., D. A. Oliveira, L. E. Hill, R. C. Zambiazi, C. D. Borges, M. Vizzotto, S. Mertens-Talcott, S. Talcott, and C. L. Gomes. 2018. "Effect of nanoencapsulation using PLGA on antioxidant and antimicrobial activities of guabiroba fruit phenolic extract." *Food Chemistry* no. 240:396–404.

Pérez-Lopez, B., and A. Mercoçi. 2011. "Nanomaterials based biosensors for food analysis applications." *Trends in Food Science & Technology* no. 22:625–639.

Pirouz, M. J., M. H. Beyki, and F. Shemirani. 2015. "Anhydride functionalised calcium ferrite nanoparticles: A new selective magnetic material for enrichment of lead ions from water and food samples." *Food Chemistry* no. 170:131–137.

Pradhan, N., S. Singh, N. Ojha, A. Shrivastava, A. Barla, V. Rai, and S. Bose. 2015. "Facets of nanotechnology as seen in food processing, packaging, and preservation industry." *BioMed Research International* no. 2015:365672.

Prombutara, P., Y. Kulwatthanasal, N. Supaka, I. Sramala, and S. Chareonpornwattana. 2012. "Production of nisin-loaded solid lipid nanoparticles for sustained antimicrobial activity." *Food Control* no. 24:184–190.

Rai, M., A. P. Ingle, I. Gupta, and A. Brandelli. 2015. "Bioactivity of noble metal nanoparticles decorated with biopolymers and their application in drug delivery." *International Journal of Pharmaceutics* no. 496:159–172.

Ramandi, N. F., and F. Shemirani. 2015. "Selective ionic liquid ferrofluid based dispersive-solid phase extraction for simultaneous preconcentration/separation of lead and cadmium in milk and biological samples." *Talanta* no. 131:404–411.

Ramezanzade, L., S. F. Hosseini, and M. Nikkhah. 2017. "Biopolymer-coated nanoliposomes as carriers of rainbow trout skin-derived antioxidant peptides." *Food Chemistry* no. 234:220–229.

Ranjan, S., N. Dasgupta, A. R. Chakraborty, S. M. Samuel, C. Ramalingam, R. Shanker, and A. Kumar. 2014. "Nanoscience and nanotechnologies in food industries: Opportunities and research trends." *Journal of Nanoparticle Research* no. 16:2464.

Ranjan, S., N. Dasgupta, and E. Lichtfouse. 2016. "*Nanoscience in food and agriculture 2*." Cham, Switzerland: Springer.

Ratnarathorn, N., O. Chailapakul, and W. Dungchai. 2014. "Highly sensitive colorimetric detection of lead using maleic acid functionalized gold nanoparticle." *Talanta* no. 132:613–618.

Reddy, J. P., and J. W. Rhim. 2014. "Characterization of bionanocomposite films prepared with agar and paper-mulberry pulp nanocellulose." *Carbohydrate Polymers* no. 110:480–488.

Rhim, J. W., H. M. Park, and C. S. Ha. 2013. "Bio-nanocomposites for food packaging applications." *Progress in Polymer Science* no. 38:1629–1652.

Rohde, A., J. Hammerl, B. Appel, R. Dieckmann, and S. Al Dahouk. 2015. "FISHing for bacteria in food—A promising tool for the reliable detection of pathogenic bacteria?" *Food Microbiology* no. 4:395–407.

Ruengvisesh, S., A. Loquercio, E. Castell-Perez, and T. M. Taylor. 2015. "Inhibition of bacterial pathogens in medium and on spinach leaf surfaces using plant-derived antimicrobials loaded in surfactant micelles." *Journal of Food Science* no. 80:2522–2529.

Sabet, F., M. Hosseini, H. Khabbaz, M. Dadmehr, and M. Ganjali. 2017. "FRET-based aptamer biosensor for selective and sensitive detection of aflatoxin B1 in peanut and rice." *Food Chemistry* no. 220:527–532.

Sadegh-Hassani, F., and A. Mohammadi Nafchi. 2014. "Preparation and characterization of bionanocomposite films based on potato starch/halloysite nanoclay." *International Journal of Biological Macromolecules* no. 67:458–462.

Salgado, P. R., C. M. Ortiz, Y. M. Musso, Y. Di Giorgio, and A. M. Mauri. 2015. "Edible films and coatings containing bioactives." *Current Opinion in Food Science* no. 5:86–92.

Salmieri, S., F. Islam, R. A. Khan, F. M. Hossain, H. M. M. Ibrahim, C. Miao, W. Y. Hama, and M. Lacroix. 2014. "Antimicrobial nanocomposite films made of poly(lactic acid)-cellulose nanocrystals (PLA-CNC) in food applications: Part A—Effect of nisin release on the inactivation of *Listeria monocytogenes* in ham." *Cellulose* no. 21:1837–1850.

Shah, B. R., C. Zhang, Y. Li, and B. Li. 2016. "Bioaccessibility and antioxidant activity of curcumin after encapsulated by nano and Pickering emulsion based on chitosan-tripolyphosphate nanoparticles." *Food Research International* no. 89:399–407.

Shah, F., M. Soylak, T. G. Kazi, and I. Afridi. 2012. "Single step in-syringe system for ionic liquid based liquid microextraction combined with flame atomic absorption spectrometry for lead determination." *Journal of Analytical Atomic Spectrometry* no. 27:1960–1965.

Shahidi, F., and Y. Zhong. 2015. "Measurement of antioxidant activity." *Journal of Functional Foods* no. 18:757–781.

Sharma, A., V. K. Rao, D. V. Kamboj, R. Gaur, S. Upadhyay, and M. Shaik. 2015. "Relative efficiency of zinc sulfide (ZnS) quantum dots (QDs) based electrochemical and fluorescence immunoassay for the detection of staphylococcal enterotoxin B (SEB)." *Biotechnology Reports* no. 6:129–136.

Shi, J., C. P. Chan, Y. Pang, W. Ye, F. Tian, J. Lyu, Y. Zhang, and M. Yang. 2015a. "A fluorescence resonance energy transfer (FRET) biosensor based on graphene quantum dots (GQDs) and gold nanoparticles (AuNPs) for the detection of *mecA* gene sequence of *Staphylococcus aureus*." *Biosensors and Bioelectronics* no. 67:595–600.

Shi, J., J. Guo, G. Bai, and C. Chan. 2015b. "A graphene oxide based fluorescence resonance energy transfer (FRET) biosensor for ultra-sensitive detection of botulinum neurotoxin A (BoNT/A) enzymatic activity." *Biosensors and Bioelectronics* no. 65:238–244.

Silva, I. M., J. F. Boelter, N. P. Silveira, and A. Brandelli. 2014. "Phosphatidylcholine nanovesicles coated with chitosan or chondroitin sulfate as novel devices for bacteriocin delivery." *Journal of Nanoparticle Research* no. 16:2479.

Singh, K., E. O. Ganbold, E. M. Cho, and K. H. Cho. 2014. "Detection of the mycotoxin citrinin using silver substrates and Raman spectroscopy." *Journal of Hazardous Materials* no. 265:89–95.

So, H. M., D. W. Park, E. K. Jeon, Y. H. Kim, B. S. Kim, C. K. Lee, S. Y. Choi, S. C. Kim, H. Chang, and J. O. Lee. 2008. "Detection and titer estimation of *Escherichia coli* using aptamer-functionalized single-walled carbon-nanotube field-effect transistors." *Small* no. 4:197–201.

Song, H., L. Gao, Y. Li, L. Mao, and J. Yang. 2017. "A sensitive and selective electrochemical nitrite sensor based on a glassy carbon electrode modified with cobalt phthalocyanine-supported Pd nanoparticles." *Analytical Methods* no. 9:3166–3171.

Song, P., L. Wu, and W. Guan. 2015. "Dietary nitrates, nitrites, and nitrosamines intake and the risk of gastric cancer: A meta-analysis." *Nutrients* no. 7:9872–9895.

Sorrentino, A., G. Gorrasi, and V. Vittoria. 2007. "Potential perspectives of bio-nanocomposites for food packaging applications." *Trends in Food Science & Technology* no. 18:84–95.

Sozer, N., and J. L. Kokini. 2008. "Nanotechnology and its applications in the food sector." *Trends in Biotechnology* no. 2:82–89.

Sun, D. W. 2014. "*Emerging Technologies for Food Processing*." 2nd Ed. London, UK: Elsevier.

Sutarlie, L., S. Y. Ow, and X. Su. 2017. "Nanomaterials-based biosensors for detection of microorganisms and microbial toxins." *Biotechnology Journal* no. 12:1500459.

Tastan, Ö., G. Ferrarib, T. Baysal, and F. Donsì. 2016. "Understanding the effect of formulation on functionality of modified chitosan films containing carvacrol nanoemulsions." *Food Hydrocolloids* no. 61:756–771.

Tavassoli-Kafrani, E., H. Shekarchizadeh, and M. Masoudpour-Behabadi. 2016. "Development of edible films and coatings from alginates and carrageenans." *Carbohydrate Polymers* no. 137:360–374.

Temur, E., A. Zengin, I. H. Boyac, F. C. Dudak, H. Torul, and U. Tamer. 2012. "Attomole sensitivity of staphylococcal enterotoxin B detection using an aptamer-modified surface-enhanced Raman scattering probe." *Analytical Chemistry* no. 84:10600–10606.

Unalan, U. I., G. Cerri, E. Marcuzzo, C. A. Cozzolino, and S. Farris. 2014. "Nanocomposite films and coatings using inorganic nanobuilding blocks (NBB): Current applications and future opportunities in the food packaging sector." *RSC Advances* no. 4:29393–29428.

Urusov, E., S. Kostenkoa, G. Sveshnikovb, V. Zherdeva, and B. Dzantiev. 2011. "Ochratoxin A immunoassay with surface plasmon resonance registration: Lowering limit of detection by the use of colloidal gold immunoconjugate." *Sensors and Actuators B* no. 156:343–349.

Urusov, A. E., A. V. Petrakova, M. V. Vozniak, A. V. Zherdev, and B. B. Dzantiev. 2014. "Rapid immunoenzyme assay of aflatoxin B1 using magnetic nanoparticles." *Sensors* no. 14:21843–21857.

Vasimalai, N., and J. S. Abraham. 2013. "Picomolar melamine enhanced the fluorescence of gold nanoparticles: Spectrofluorometric determination of melamine in milk and infant formulas using functionalized triazole capped gold nanoparticles." *Biosensors and Bioelectronics* no. 42:267–272.

Velusamy, V., K. Arshak, O. Korostynska, K. Oliwa, and C. Adley. 2010. "An overview of foodborne pathogen detection: in the perspective of biosensors." *Biotechnology Advances* no. 28:232–254.

Viswanathan, S., L.-C. Wu, M.-R. Huang, and J.-A. Ho. 2006. "Electrochemical immunosensor for cholera toxin using liposomes and poly(3,4-ethylenedioxythiophene)-coated carbon nanotubes." *Analytical Chemistry* no. 78:1115–1121.

Viter, R., A. Tereshchenko, V. Smyntyna, J. Ogorodniichuk, N. Starodub, R. Yakimova, V. Khranovskyy, and A. Ramanavicius. 2017. "Toward development of optical biosensors based on photoluminescence of $TiO_2$ nanoparticles for the detection of *Salmonella*." *Sensors and Actuators B: Chemical* no. 252:95–102.

Wang, A., A. Mulchandani, and W. Chen. 2002. "Specific adhesion to cellulose and hydrolysis of organophosphate nerve agents by a genetically engineered *Escherichia coli* strain with a surface-expressed cellulose-binding domain and organophosphorus hydrolase." *Applied and Environmental Microbiology* no. 68:1684–1689.

Wang, H., Y. Li, A. Wang, and M. Slavik. 2011b. "Rapid, sensitive, and simultaneous detection of three foodborne pathogens using magnetic nanobead-based immunoseparation and quantum dot-based multiplex immunoassay." *Journal of Food Protection* no. 74:2039–2047.

Wang, J., B. H. Liu, Y. T. Hsu, and F. Y. Yu. 2011c. "Sensitive competitive direct enzyme-linked immunosorbent assay and gold nanoparticle immunochromatographic strip for detecting aflatoxin M1 in milk." *Food Control* no. 22:964–969.

Wang, J., R. Krause, K. Block, M. Musameh, A. Mulchandani, and M. J. Schöning. 2002. "Flow injection amperometric detection of OP nerve agents based on an organophosphorus-hydrolase biosensor detector." *Biosensors and Bioelectronics* no. 18:255–260.

Wang, Q. H., L. J. Yu, Y. Liu, L. Lin, and R. G. Lu. 2017. "Methods for the detection and determination of nitrite and nitrate: A review." *Talanta* no. 165:709–720.

Wang, X., R. Niessner, and D. Knopp. 2014. "Magnetic bead-based colorimetric immunoassay for aflatoxin B1 using gold nanoparticles." *Sensors* no. 14:21535–21548.

Wang, X., Y. Wei, S. Wang, and L. Chen. 2015. "Red-to-blue colorimetric detection of chromium via Cr(III)-citrate chelating based on Tween 20-stabilized gold nanoparticles." *Colloids and Surfaces A:Physicochemical and Engineering Aspects* no. 472:57–62.

Wang, X., Y. Du, Y. Li, D. Li, and R. Sun. 2011a. "Fluorescent identification and detection of staphylococcus aureus with carboxymethyl chitosan/CdS quantum dots bioconjugates." *Journal of Biomaterials Science Polymer* no. 22:1881–1893.

Warriner, K., S. M. Reddy, A. Namvar, and S. Neethirajan. 2014. "Developments in nanoparticles for use in biosensors to assess food safety and quality." *Trends in Food Science and Technology* no. 40:183–199.

Wei, D., W. Sun, W. Qian, Y. Ye, and X. Ma. 2009. "The synthesis of chitosan-based silver nanoparticles and their antibacterial activity." *Carbohydrate Research* no. 344:2375–2382.

Welch, C. M., and R. G. Compton. 2006. "The use of nanoparticles in electroanalysis: A review." *Analytical and Bioanalytical Chemistry* no. 384:601–619.

Wen, J., S. Zhou, and Y. Yuan. 2014. "Graphene oxide as nanogold carrier for ultrasensitive electrochemical immunoassay of *Shewanella oneidensis* with silver enhancement strategy." *Biosensors and Bioelectronics* no. 52:44–49.

Weng, C., J. Cang, J. Chang, T. Hsiung, B. Unnikrishnan, and Y. Hung. 2014. "Detection of arsenic(III) through pulsed laser-induced desorption/ionization of gold nanoparticles on cellulose membranes." *Analytical Chemistry* no. 86:3167–3173.

WHO. 2017. "*Food Safety: Chemical Risks in Food.*" http://www.who.int/foodsafety/areas_work/chemical-risks/en/. (accessed 22 October 2017).

Wu, S., N. Duan, Z. Shi, C. Fang, and Z. Wang. 2014. "Simultaneous aptasensor for multiplex pathogenic bacteria detection based on multicolor upconversion nanoparticles labels." *Analytical Chemistry* no. 86:3100–3107.

Wu, S., Y. Wang, N. Duan, H. Ma, and Z. Wang. 2015. "Colorimetric aptasensor based on enzyme for the detection of *Vibrio parahemolyticus*." *Journal of Agricultural Food Chemistry* no. 63:7849–7854.

Wu, X., Y. Song, X. Yan, C. Zhu, Y. Ma, D. Du, and Y. Lin. 2017. "Carbon quantum dots as fluorescence resonance energy transfer sensors for organophosphate pesticides determination." *Biosensors and Bioelectronics* no. 94:292–297.

Wu, Y., Y. Luo, and Q. Wang. 2012. "Antioxidant and antimicrobial properties of essential oils encapsulated in zein nanoparticles prepared by liquid–liquid dispersion method." *Food Science and Technology* no. 48:283–290.

Xiao, R., D. Wang, Z. Lin, B. Qiu, M. Liu, L. Guo, and G. Chen. 2015. "Disassembly of gold nanoparticle dimers for colorimetric detection of ochratoxin A." *Analytical Methods* no. 7:842–825.

Xing, H., Y. Wu, S. Zhan, and P. Zhou. 2013. "A rapid colorimetric detection of melamine in raw milk by unmodified gold nanoparticles." *Food Analytical Methods* no. 6:1441–1447.

Xu, W., W. Xie, X. Huang, X. Chen, N. Huang, X. Wang, and J. Liu. 2017. "The graphene oxide and chitosan biopolymer loads $TiO_2$ for antibacterial and preservative research." *Food Chemistry* no. 221:267–277.

Xu, X., X. Liu, Y. Li, and Y. Ying. 2013. "A simple and rapid optical biosensor for detection of aflatoxin B1 based on competitive dispersion of gold nanorods." *Biosensors and Bioelectronics* no. 47:361–367.

Xue, W., L. Hui, W. Min, G. Shu-Li, and Z. Yan. 2013. "Simultaneous electrochemical determination of sulphite and nitrite by a gold nanoparticle/graphene-chitosan modified electrode." *Chinese Journal of Analytical Chemistry* no. 41:1232–1237.

Yang, M., Y. Xia, Y. Wang, X. Zhao, Z. Xue, and F. Quan. 2016. "Preparation and property investigation of crosslinked alginate/silicon dioxide nanocomposite films." *Journal of Applied Polymer Science* no. 133:43489–43497.

Yao, X., P. Yan, K. Zhang, and J. Li. 2013. "Preparation of water-soluble CdSe quantum dots and its application for nitrite detection in the anodic electrochemiluminescence." *Luminescence* no. 28:551–556.

Yashin, A., Y. Yashin, J. Wang, and B. Nemzer. 2013. "Antioxidant and antiradical activity of coffee." *Antioxidants* no. 2:230–245.

Yin, X., Q. Chen, H. Song, M. Yang, and H. Wang. 2013. "Sensitive and selective electrochemiluminescent detection of nitrite using dual-stabilizer-capped CdTe quantum dots." *Electrochemical Communications* no. 34:81–85.

You, J., H. Hu, P. Zhou, L. Zhang, Y. Zhang, and T. Kondo. 2013. "Novel cellulose polyampholyte-gold nanoparticle-based colorimetric competition assay for the detection of cysteine and mercury(II)." *Langmuir* no. 29:5085–5092.

Zambrano-Zaragoza, L., E. Mercado-Silva, A. Del Real, E. Gutiérrez-Cortez, M. A. Cornejo-Villegas, and D. Quintanar-Guerrero. 2014. "The effect of nano-coatings with α-tocopherol and xanthan gum on shelf-life and browning index of fresh-cut 'Red Delicious' apples." *Innovative Food Science & Emerging Technologies* no. 22:188–196.

Zawistowski, J., C. G. Biliaderis, and N. A. M. Eskin. 1991. "Polyphenol oxidases." in *Oxidative Enzymes in Foods*, edited by D. S. Robinson, and N. A. M. Eskin, 217–273. London, UK: Elsevier.

Zhan, S., M. Yu, L. Lv, L. Wang, and P. Zhou. 2014. "Colorimetric detection of trace arsenic(III) in aqueous solution using arsenic aptamer and gold nanoparticles." *Australian Journal of Chemistry* no. 67:813–818.

Zhang, W., J. Chen, Y. Chen, W. Xia, Y. L. Xiong, and H. Wang. 2016a. "Enhanced physicochemical properties of chitosan/whey protein isolate composite film by sodium laurate-modified $TiO_2$ nanoparticles." *Carbohydrate Polymers* no. 138:59–65.

Zhang, H., X. Ma, Y. Liu, and N. Duan. 2016b. "Simultaneous detection of *Staphylococcus aureus* and *Salmonella typhimurium* using multicolor time-resolved fluorescence nanoparticles as labels." *International Journal of Food Microbiology* no. 237:172–179.

Zhang, X., G. Xiao, Y. Wang, Y. Zhao, H. Su, and T. Tan. 2017. "Preparation of chitosan-$TiO_2$ composite film with efficient antimicrobial activities under visible light for food packaging applications." *Carbohydrate Polymers* no. 169:101–107.

Zhang, Y., Y. Niu, Y. Luo, M. Ge, T. Yang, L. L. Yu, and Q. Wang. 2014. "Fabrication, characterization and antimicrobial activities of thymol-loaded zein nanoparticles stabilized by sodium caseinate-chitosan hydrochloride double layers." *Food Chemistry* no. 142:269–275.

Zhao, L., Y. Jin, Z. Yan, Y. Liu, and H. Zhu. 2012. "Novel, highly selective detection of Cr(III) in aqueous solution based on a gold nanoparticle colorimetric assay and its application for determining Cr(VI)." *Analytica Chimica Acta* no. 731:75–81.

Zhao, Y., M. Ye, Q. Chao, N. Jia, Y. Ge, and H. Shen. 2009. "Simultaneous detection of multifood-borne pathogenic bacteria based on functionalized quantum dots coupled with immunomagnetic separation in food samples." *Journal of Agricultural Food Chemistry* no. 57:517–524.

Zheng, Z., Y. Zhou, X. Li, S. Liu, and Z. Tang. 2011. "Highly-sensitive organophosphorous pesticide biosensors based on nanostructured films of acetylcholinesterase and CdTe quantum dots." *Biosensors and Bioelectronics* no. 26:3081–3085.

Zhou, J. J., S. Y. Wang, and S. Gunasekaran. 2009. "Preparation and characterization of whey protein film incorporated with $TiO_2$ nanoparticles." *Journal of Food Science* no. 74:50–56.

# Section V

## Future Perspectives

# 14 Advanced Methods for the Detection of Micro- and Nanosystems in Food

*Rosa Busquets*

## CONTENTS



## 14.1 INTRODUCTION

The analysis of nanosystems in food products and packaging is becoming more and more necessary due to the increasing use of nanosystems in food products and their commercialization. Nanotechnology in food is being accepted once it has not been involved in controversial applications to date, in contrast to the other disruptive technologies, such as genetically modified crops, which are generating rejection by the consumers. With all, the food industry is being cautious, and not completely open to discuss its activities in this field to avoid rejection (Editorial from Nature Nanotechnology 2010), which is holding back progress. The potential risks of the intake of nanomaterials and the limited knowledge about their effects in living organisms [there are risks of cytotoxicity and systemic toxicity (Whitby and Busquets 2013; Lacey 2017)] are slowing the progress in the nanofood sector. Risk assessment should be done on case by case basis (European Commission 2013) because the behavior of engineered nanomaterials is difficult to predict.

A limited number of commercial food products incorporating nanomaterials are in the market, and these are being successful. An example is chocolate with nano and micro $TiO_2$, which represent an estimated intake of 2–3 mg $TiO_2$/Kg (body mass) child (<10 years) in the United Kingdom (Weir et al. 2012). The Nanodatabase is an excellent on-line resource that compiles commercial products, including food, incorporating nanomaterials (DTU 2017). Analytical needs will increase in parallel with a more generalized presence of nanosystems in food and the need to enforce regulations about their use.

Defining which aspects of nanosystems in food need to be characterized requires understanding of the differential features, with respect to common ingredients, that could be related with their toxicity and enhanced activity. Among the added properties associated with organic micro- and nanosystems are the encapsulation and transport of functional ingredients. Indeed, nanostructures can make possible the integration of high loadings of an active principle in the food, which boost the ingredient's functionality (Rasti et al. 2017); improve the dispersion of ingredients in food media where they have some incompatibilities; or control the release of food ingredients (Comunian et al. 2017; Lei et al. 2017). Nanosystems are also useful to protect sensitive components from the surrounding environment during food processing, storage, and digestion (Lei et al. 2017) or have the potential to make the products cost effective by providing greater sensorial properties with less amount of substance. The encapsulation method is chosen based on the bioactive component and matrix, and these aspects have recently been reviewed (Ângelo Cerqueira et al. 2017; Dias et al. 2017). Natural polymers (polysaccharides, proteins, lipids), which are "generally recognized as safe," and combinations of them, are making up organic micro- and nanosystems in food applications. In contrast, the use of synthetic polymers for very similar purposes than in food technology, such as improved loading, bioavailability, pharmacokinetics, and transport to target sites, is restricted to pharmaceutical formulations. The natural polymers in nanoingredients have the form of supramolecular structures named nanocapsules, nanohydrogels, nanoemulsions, lipid nanoparticles, and micelles (de Souza Simões et al. 2017) and have been discussed elsewhere in this volume. Carbohydrates and proteins are the most commonly used encapsulating polymers. Their selection influences the size, shape, and stability under different environment in the food product (Dias et al. 2017). Among polysaccharides, starch is the most widely used, alone, or in combination with others, leading to nanosystems with different structures and polarities. Starch-based nanocapsules can be used to entrap macromolecules like lipids to smaller molecules such as polyphenols (Zhu 2017). Alginate is another carbohydrate frequently used (Comunian et al. 2017; Mokhtari et al. 2017; Lei et al. 2017).

Besides organic nanosystems, inorganic nanostructures can be part of innovative packaging materials (Luna and Vilchez 2017) and inks (Bautista et al. 2017), both sectors are having lot of strength because of their contribution to the enhancement of shelf life thanks to their capacity to reduce contact with oxygen, control bacterial growth, and also can improve mechanical properties from the packaging. Inorganic nanomaterials are also present as additives in food, such as $TiO_2$ for its whitening and brightening properties (Dudefoi et al. 2017).

## 14.2 ANALYTICAL NEEDS

The analytical approach is designed to get key information with reliability. Information from the content/function of the micro- and nanosystems is needed when developing the formulation of a new ingredient. The stability and ageing of the nanosystem within the matrix needs to be studied, and the possible toxicity of the nanofood and its compliance with the current legislation needs to be assessed. Hence, the most important properties that could be related to some sort of toxicity and thus need to be determined are particle size distribution, structure, and loading capacity, which are factors related with the enhanced properties attributed to nanomaterial. Besides these, physical characteristics of the micro- and nanosystems, evidence of their internal chemical composition, details of the interaction between the micro-, nanosystem, and the active ingredient encapsulated, as well as the interaction of the nanosystem with cells/tissues, will provide important information about their toxicity and the bioavailability of the entrapped active ingredients. Finally, data regarding the chemical composition of the surface of the micro- and nanosystems can indicate their degree of hydrophilicity and interaction with the surrounding matrix. Changes in the physical and chemical characteristics of the nanosystems can alter their toxicity, and for that reason, it is important to capture all these features in the analysis.

The existence of legislation is the driving force that encourages the development of suitable analytical methods. There is no regulation devoted specifically to the inclusion of nanosystems in food, however, nanosystems are included in other existing legislation or recommendations, hence nanofoods are controlled by the general food safety principles established by international regulatory organizations (Bownman and Ludlow 2017). The European Union and Switzerland have additionally incorporated nano-specific provisions regarding the inclusion of nanomaterials in agri/feed/food in existing legislation (Amenta et al. 2015). There are distinct risk assessment procedures and regulations depending on whether the nanosystems are the main ingredient (classified as novel foods), when used as an additive, or as part of food contact materials (Gallocchio et al. 2015). Food that newly incorporate nanoingredients require a pre-market assessment and authorization by the European Food Safety Authority (EFSA) [Article 12 from the Regulation (European Union) No1333/2008/EC, 257/2010/EC], organization that will need to measure the characteristics defining the nanoingredients including particle size and physicochemical characteristics as per their definition (European Commission, 2011). These ingredients present in the form of engineered nanomaterials will need to be clearly indicated in the list of ingredients, and their name will be followed by the word “nano” in brackets (European Parliament 2011). There is legislation to ensure that the substances migrating from food contact materials to food do not endanger the consumer’s health or change the food properties. This is comprised in the European Regulation 1935/2004, where four food contact materials (plastics, ceramics, regenerated cellulose, and active intelligent materials) have specific measures. In addition to these measures concerning the chemical composition of the packaging, the labeling of food contact materials should not be misleading, therefore, its inclusion in the label is mandatory (Regulation 1169/2011 by the European Parliament) and analytical methodology should exist for the determination of nanosystems in that type of food product. In food contact materials, the use of nanomaterials is regulated in plastics only, but these must have been previously specified on an authorization list (European Parliament 2016). Regarding the implementation of the European Regulation 1935/2004 law, businesses have indicated that material-specific analytical methods to test composition, migration, and risk assessment should be standardized (harmonized), and this would facilitate applying the same standards across Europe and compliance (European Parliament 2016).

There are difficulties when trying to evaluate the safety of food product regarding the presence of nanosystems. Harmonized analytical methods are not yet available today, and this situation limits the reliability of the measurements and delays having appropriate contaminant limits in food. An additional difficulty found when studying the contamination of food by nanomaterials migrated from the packaging is the limited of information available regarding the nature of food contact materials (European Parliament 2016). For monitoring nanomaterials migrated to food from inks and contact materials, routine and rapid quantitative analysis of nanomaterials in the different food matrices is needed. Nanomaterials from packaging are mainly inorganic such as nano- $TiO_2$, $SiO_2$, ZnO, $Fe_3O_4$, Ag, and nanoclay, but also can include organic nanomaterials such as nanocellulose in different forms (crystalline or in fibers) or nanochitosan (Bautista et al. 2017; Luna and Vilchez 2017). Nanomaterials in inks are also mainly inorganic, such as the conductive nano- Ag or Cu, and these typical nanomaterials could be expanded to organic nanomaterials (carbon nanotubes, graphene) which are being studied (Bautista et al. 2017; Luna and Vilchez 2017). The analysis of the nanomaterials that could migrate to food has high cost in terms of access to analytical equipment, expertise, and preparation, as identified by businesses (European Parliament 2016), however, the expense will be at similar level than the already required routine analysis of pesticides in food carried out by solid phase extraction and chromatography coupled to mass spectrometry. Therefore, it is "affordable" and possible to have such methodology ready. Standardized methodology will be available soon given the favorable conditions, worldwide, the food industry and relevant authorities have aligned needs (EFSA. Scientific Committee and Emerging Risks Unit 2017), and there is technical ability to make it possible. However, the development of analytical procedures aiming at guaranteeing the safety of consumers should be done following procedures that would allow measuring the key properties of nanomaterials related with their toxicology in complex matrices, these procedures would need to be validated before their use in routine food control analysis. There is scarcity of both suitable reference materials to be used in quality assurance and validated methods. This situation is bringing laboratories to make their own internal reference materials to assess the quality parameters of their analytical methods (Linsinger et al. 2011; Linsinger et al. 2014; Dudkiewicz et al. 2015). Feasibility studies toward preparing reference materials are carried out and difficulties inherent to the changing nature of nanosystems in food are being identified. For instance, nanosystems can agglomerate once they are in the food matrix, hence the particle sizes in the food can be different to the size distribution of nanosystems in the solution used to spike the food when preparing a laboratory reference material (Grombe et al. 2015). Following, analytical approaches used for the characterization of micro- and nanosystems in food will be discussed.

## 14.3 SAMPLE PREPARATION AND ITS IMPLICATIONS IN MEASUREMENTS

Following the sampling stage, the analysis includes a series of steps to purifying and isolate the analytes (nanosystems in this case) from the rest of the sample. The analysis of nanosystems in food has different requirements than the analysis of traditional molecular contaminants such as pesticides. This is because particles and molecules interact very differently with the solvents and sorbents used for the purification. However, the analysis of either nanomaterials or molecules can be affected by substances present in the sample matrix and could lead to low accuracy in the analysis. Therefore, extraction and purification steps will improve the trueness of the measured values from nanosystems as isolated entities. In addition, precautions to preserve environmental factors which can alter the properties of the nanosystems, and maintain the interaction between the nanomaterial and the matrix, will add value to the characterization.

Treatments carried out to reduce the presence of matrix in the purified sample will define the information that can be obtained. Purification and pre-concentration of the micro- and nanosystems will be required when assessing their migration to food, or characterizing nano-food, as the food samples may have high matrix content. In this scenario, complex matrices could reduce accuracy in quantitative analysis when using main quantitative techniques [i.e., inductively coupled plasma-mass spectrometry (ICP-MS), liquid chromatography-mass Spectrometry (LC-MS), gas chromatography-mass spectrometry (GC-MS), porosimetry] or introduce artifacts in qualitative analysis [i.e., Raman spectroscopy, IR spectroscopy, dynamic light scattering (DLS), UV spectroscopy, scanning electron microscopy (SEM)]. Particles will need to be separated and washed from the matrix, despite that the purification will alter the disposition of the nanosystems in the food environment. Keeping the nanosystems within the matrix during the analysis can be achieved by sacrificing quantitative results or using highly selective techniques [environmental SEM (ESEM), confocal laser scanning microscopy (CLSM), X-ray diffraction (XRD), X-ray photoelectron spectroscopy]. However, there are cases where sample treatment has not been necessary despite using a technique that would commonly require working with purified samples. For instance, the effect of antioxidants in nanoform dispersed in an active coating was assessed through the oxidation degree of the surface of an active coating with IR. The assessment was carried out by comparing the ratio of the intensities of the bands corresponding to O-H stretching (3300 $cm^{-1}$), with the band from the C-O stretch (1140 $cm^{-1}$), which was assumed to remain unaltered by the presence of antioxidants (López-Córdoba et al. 2017). Lower intensity of the O-H band was found with presence of the antioxidant. In this case, purification steps were not needed, given that the active coating did not contain food matrix, and the signal studied was highly related to the effect of antioxidants.

Sample treatment has high relevance when the procedure applied can affect the accuracy of the determination of the particle size of micro- and nanosystems. This is because particle size is one of the most important characteristics measured to define the population of nanoparticles, being the one mainly responsible for their special properties and also a main factor determining their toxicity. The most established technique for measuring the particle size distribution of nanomaterials is DLS. DLS requires the dispersion of particles in liquid, where they present random (Brownian) movement. The movement of particles is monitored by irradiating them with a laser, and the temporal fluctuation of scattered radiation is transformed into an estimation of their hydrodynamic diameter (which includes the particle and solvation sphere and constitutes an estimation of the particle size). This technique assumes that the particles are spherical as described by Stokes-Einstein equation, and in cases where these are not, there will be major discrepancy between the estimated size by DLS and microscopy (Mbundi et al. 2014). The theory of different modalities of light scattering has been the objective of a review (Brar and Verma 2011).

The determination of the particle size distribution will probably require purification of the nanosystems because the analysis can be greatly affected by surrounding particles or macromolecules. The bigger components of the sample need to be separated because they would lead to multiple scattering, rather than the required single scattering, and reduce inter-particle interactions, which would also lead to inaccurate measurement: this can be done by filtering or centrifuging the samples. The purification required should not alter those factors that affect the dynamic circumference of the nanosystems: their diameter, shape, charge, and electrical mobility of the particles. Temperature, pH, ionic strength, and viscosity of the media may affect the dynamic sphere. Therefore, preserving factors in the matrix affecting its dynamic circumference is a priority in this analysis.

Dilution of the particles will also reduce multiple scattering. The dilution can induce change in the morphology of organic nanosystems. For instance, some polymers, when diluted in aqueous media, can change toward orientating the most hydrophilic groups toward the exterior of the particle; and hydrophobic groups would orientate toward the inner part of the nanosystem or evolve toward forming agglomerates. If the dilution is carried out with the same solvent as in the samples, the organic nanosystems will not rupture or change shape. An example of critical dilution step carried out was the determination of the size distribution of nanoemulsions containing ß-carotene when they were subject to conditions in *in vitro* simulated gastro-intestinal tract. The sample containing nanosystems was diluted ten times with saliva fluid, gastric fluid, and buffer at pH 7, to mimic the intestinal phase, prior to the analysis with DLS (Gasa-Falcon et al. 2017). In some cases, surfactant, such as the non-ionic Tween 20, assisted in dispersing nanodroplets and preventing their coalescence. However, substances such as bile salts, phospholipid, and lipase, which are present in the intestinal phase, can displace Tween 20 and lead to increased droplet sizes, as found in investigations studying changes in nanoemulsions during the digestion (Gasa-Falcon et al. 2017). Besides the addition of a surfactant, the application of ultrasounds before measurements with DLS can reduce agglomeration, but the dispersion achieved will decrease with time, and it could also de-agglomerate nanosystems as they were in food, which would be undesirable.

The measurement of the Z-potential of the system (potential difference between the media and the stationary layer of fluid associated to the particle) with laser Doppler microelectrophoresis, can be carried out with the same instrument than DLS and will show if the nanosystems are stable under the conditions of the measurement or if, on the contrary, there are inter-particle interactions leading to agglomeration. Z-potential is typically measured when formulating and measuring the stability of emulsions (Zhu et al. 2018). Z-potential can change with the adsorption of biomolecules, and through this parameter, the effect of the different gastrointestinal phases on the physicochemical properties of nanoemulsions can be monitored. For instance, a study found changes in the Z-potential along the gastrointestinal tract, especially in the stomach phase, which led to a reduction of the negative charge possibly because salts present could shield electrostatic interactions. On the contrary, the intestinal phase led to more negative Z-potential, reaching values as high as the initial state or in the mouth phase, possibly because the adsorption of bile salts or phospholipids from intestinal fluids (Gasa-Falcon et al. 2017). This example illustrates how the composition of the solvent can affect the properties measured in nanoemulsions.

The pH of the media used for the DLS and Z-potential measurements can also have an impact in the shape of the nanoparticle in solution, as what was studied in the particular case of the nanomaterial graphene oxide (Whitby et al. 2011). The effect of the pH will be more prominent in nanosystems with ionizable functional groups. Therefore, the dilution of the sample prior measurements with DLS can be necessary for the estimation of the particle size distribution, however, it can also induce changes in the shape and size of the hydrodynamic sphere of the nanosystem. Currently, the smallest hydrodynamic spheres that can be detected are in the range of 0.3 nm (Malvern Instruments Limited 2014), which is actually an overestimation of the particle size given that the hydrodynamic sphere includes solvent.

Microscopy imaging is considered a standard technique in the characterization of nanomaterials (EFSA Scientific Committee 2011). It allows studying the direct interaction of the nanosystems with the matrix and provides information of their size and shape. transmission electron microscopy (TEM) and SEM are the techniques most widely used in recent investigations. SEM micrographs originate from low energy secondary electrons scattered off from the sample after being scanned with a low energy beam of electrons (1–30 keV). SEM provides great depth of field (images in 3D). In TEM, a high energy electron beam (80–300 keV) is transmitted through a very thin sample providing images with high resolution (Dudkiewicz et al. 2011; Busquets 2017). The resolution achieved with state-of-the art TEM is below 0.1 nm, and it is favored by thinner samples and electron beam with high accelerating voltage. For soft samples such as food, which can become damaged during imaging, accelerating voltages of up to 100 KeV are recommended (Dudkiewicz et al. 2011).

The sample can be bulky and prepared without difficulties for SEM analysis. In contrast, thin sample are required in TEM, and these are more challenging to prepare. Both techniques work under high vacuum and require dry samples. Other modalities of microscopy are more suitable than SEM and TEM for imaging in moist environment [environmental (E-), liquid-, wet-SEM/ TEM], or image under cryogenic conditions, which requires high vacuum and frozen specimens. Cryo-sectioning is useful for imaging semi-liquid samples or samples that cannot be fixed due to their composition; for scanning the internal structure of nanosystems with SEM; or when preserving the sample matrix is a priority (Dudkiewicz et al. 2011). Environmental SEM does not need coated samples, and can be used to imaging food in their natural state, and although it can achieve resolution below 1 nm, it offers less resolution than standard SEM. The wet-modality requires the samples to be encapsulated, and it is especially useful for imaging nanoparticles of metals in liquid food samples in their native state (Mbundi et al. 2014). These capsules can be centrifuged and coated which would allow to enrich a membrane with nanosystems (Dudkiewicz et al. 2011). However, these microscopy techniques that make possible imaging hydrated samples such as food do not have widespread use yet maybe because of the highly specialized equipment needed.

The preparation of the specimens with nanosystems for imaging can consist of relatively mild treatments such as: fixating the protein structure with glutaraldehyde; treating the lipid structure with osmium tetroxide; dehydrating with ethanol; and cryo-fracturing (Dudkiewicz et al. 2011); embedding in resin; leaving the specimen to dry on air; freeze-drying; absorbing liquid with filter paper in contact with the sample drop to avoid agglomeration (Novak et al. 2001); or dispersing the nanosystems with surfactant (i.e., 0.1% sodium dodecyl sulphate) before drying (Mokhtari et al. 2017). Liquid food samples can be encapsulated in agar prior to the standard pre-treatments (Dudkiewicz et al. 2011). Specimens containing metallic nanoparticles, or specimens that can be treated with heavy-metal stain, can be imaged through high energy back scattered electrons in SEM to improve the contrast between elements with different atomic number within a complex matrix. This strategy offers clearer interpretation of the data, however, it is then recommendable to compare the image with a stained control sample.

To minimize charging effects and improve contrast in SEM, specimens can be coated with a conductive layer, typically from metal or carbon [i.e., non-conductive starch films were coated with a thin layer (<50 nm) of gold] (Dudkiewicz et al. 2015; López-Córdoba et al. 2017). A main electron source in SEM is field emission. Field emission SEM (FESEM) is commonly used to obtain high-quality micrographs from soft substrates, such as rosemary nanoparticles or echium oil by scanning with low voltage (Comunian et al. 2017; López-Córdoba et al. 2017). FESEM results in low electrical charging and does not make necessary sputtering the samples with conductive coating. The sample preparation steps listed in this section involve mild treatments that preserve with certain extent the environment of the micro- and nanosystems within the food matrix and are appropriate for imaging samples that contain relatively high concentration of nanomaterials. However, the usual case when studying nanoparticles that have migrated to food is having samples with low abundance of nanomaterials, and this will translate into greater difficulty when having to locate them with the microscope, carrying a greater statistical uncertainty to the measurement.

Indeed, microscopic techniques have the limitation that they require a very small sample (i.e., a droplet of ~10 μl) which can lead to inadequate statistical representativity of the bulk sample (Dudkiewicz et al. 2011). Furthermore, imaging can also be carried out in a very localized area of the specimen, and if the concentration of particles in the sample is low, detecting enough particles may become too challenging. If the number of particles was not enough for their robust measurement, pre-concentrating should be considered. Hence, the development of protocols to recover enough particles for imaging from liquid and solid food samples are very important

(Lari and Dudkiewicz 2014). Following are examples of such strategies that are illustrated through procedures to recover and pre-concentrate synthetic amorphous silica from tomato soup and spherical silver nanoparticles from meat while trying to preserve their clustering state in the samples. These procedures were selected by the authors after having tested others such as drying or ultracentrifuging. Soup samples were diluted with borate buffer at pH 8, conditions that led to a negative charged sample that is beneficial for electron microscopy analysis. A drop of the pre-treated soup sample was placed onto a TEM grid coated in 0.1% solution of skin porcine gelatine. For SEM analysis, the samples were attached with carbon glue to the stub and coated with Platinum/Palladium. Frozen meat was diluted with the same borate buffer and homogenized. The homogenized samples spiked with particles were centrifuged in tubes which contained hydrophobic TEM grids supported onto agar supports. These protocols were found advantageous with respect to resin embedding and cryo-sectioning in terms of preparation time, less need of specialized equipment, and increasing sample volume which increases the representativity of the sample (Dudkiewicz et al. 2015).

An excellent work assessing the preparation of samples for electron microscopy identified that the number of particles analyzed was not a main contributor in the uncertainty associated with the measurement of their size. The number of particles that needs to be analyzed to achieve uncertainty below 5% ranged from 38 to 359 for particle sizes ranging from 34 to 11 nm, respectively (Dudkiewicz et al. 2015). In contrast, recent works tend to assess particle size distribution with lower number nanosystems (Comunian et al. 2017; Rasti et al. 2017); guidelines informing about harmonized procedures to characterize particles with different techniques would assist the diverse community of scientists working in the field of food nanotechnology. In contrast, the homogeneity of the initial sample was found to be a main contribution in the uncertainty associated with the determination of the particle size distribution (Dudkiewicz et al. 2015). Hence, digesting the sample matrix or extracting the particles for greater homogeneity would be advantageous, although it would reduce the meaning of the information. Imaging from greater number of independent sample replicates would effectively reduce uncertainty. Importantly, the food matrix could affect the reproducibility of the measurement of the particle size in SEM and TEM, the measurement was affected significantly just in one of the studied matrices (Dudkiewicz et al. 2015), which is in agreement with a previous study measuring Ag nanoparticles in meat (Grombe et al. 2015). Interestingly, the reproducibility obtained for the analysis of Ag nanoparticles when embedded in meat (relative standard deviation, RSD 3%) was 3 time better than in stock solution. This could be because the meat matrix would have minimized particle clustering (Dudkiewicz et al. 2015). An evaluation of food sample preparation methods suitable for electron microscopy, as well as the establishment of a selection tree to aid in the selection of imaging methods have been published by Dudkiewicz et al. (2011). Careful considerations must be taken with the sample treatment strategy because it can alter the structure of the food matrix and agglomeration of the particles. It is recommendable to image the matrix following a range of sample preparation steps to realize the implications of these pre-treatments in the information obtained.

## 14.4 SEPARATION AND DETECTION OF NANOSYSTEMS

Separation techniques have been used when quantifying the loading capacity of nanosystems. In this context, the amount of active principle encapsulated is analyzed with methods developed for the determination of the molecules after breaking the nanocapsules. For instance, the concentration of polyphenols (synaptic acid and quercetin) and echium oil (rich in Ʊ-3 fatty acids) in microcapsules was quantified by rupturing the capsules and extracting the active principles with liquid-liquid extraction using methanol. Polyphenols were quantified in the alcohol extract with UV-Vis using two different wavelengths, whereas the fatty acids were isolated using an extraction with hexane and evaporation to dryness (Comunian et al. 2017). In cases where the analytical test was highly selective regarding a property of the nanosystems, a simple separation has been carried out. For instance, the release of rosemary nanoparticles from cassava starch film was assessed by shaking the film in food simulant and analyzing the release nanoparticles in solution with Folin Ciocalteu UV-Vis assay selective to polyphenols, without needing to separate other molecules from solution (López-Córdoba et al. 2017).

The separation of a mixture of compounds integrating micro- and nanosystems or the separation of markedly different micro- and nanosystems from the same food matrix is scarce in the literature, but it holds the key to solve complex problems that simple liquid-liquid extraction and UV-Vis analysis cannot solve. The quantification of molecular components of organic nanosystems can be carried out by rupturing the nanosystems and separating them with traditional liquid chromatography, gas chromatography (if the components are volatile or can be derivatized to volatile substances), and by capillary electrophoresis. A modality of capillary electrophoresis (micellar capillary electrophoresis) would allow the analysis of micelles directly. The development and validation of the analytical methods by these traditional separation techniques is neither challenging nor time consuming. The most suitable detection systems for these separation techniques are UV/fluorescence/mass spectrometry (for liquid chromatography and electrophoresis) and mass spectrometry (for gas chromatography).

There is the need to separate nanosystems based on their size, shape, and differentiate between their agglomerate estates. These techniques should be high-throughput, ideally. The separation of the nanosystems can be done with size exclusion chromatography (SEC), which working range is 0.5–10 nm and hydrodynamic chromatography (10 nm–2 μm) (Peters et al. 2011). In SEC, the separation of particles is based on the nanosystems' hydrodynamic volumes, and not on the interaction of these with the stationary phase like in other chromatographic modalities. The separation in SEC is carried out using a packed beads column with porous beads. The separation of nanosystems based on their shape is possible with SEC, for instance, rod and spherical gold nanoparticles could be separated thanks to the addition of mixtures of surfactants in the mobile phase (Wei et al. 1999). To minimize sorption of the nanosystems onto the stationary phase, surfactants such as sodium dodecyl sulphate may be added to the mobile phase, and the separation can notably be improved (Wei and Liu 1999). SEC has been used for the separation of inorganic nanomaterials (Kowalczyk et al. 2011), but it is not commonly used for the analysis of organic nanosystems purified from food yet (Busquets 2017). In hydrodynamic chromatography, the stationary phase is constituted by non-porous packed beads, and therefore the matrix will not affect the separation, which makes it advantageous for the analysis of purified extract for food. Typical detection systems in hydrodynamic chromatography are UV, DLS, and MS (Philippe and Schaumann 2014). Therefore, it can be used for both organic and inorganic nanosystems although, like SEC, its use is still rare in the analysis of organic nanosystems, but it may progress thanks to the advantages it offers for the analysis of complex food matrices. Hydrodynamic chromatography (HDC) has proven to be useful when separating mixtures of nanoparticles (i.e., ZnO, $TiO_2$) with high presence of organic matter and salts. It can separate by size and quantify nanoparticles with sensitivity in the part per billion level when coupled to mass spectrometry. The separation of polystyrene nanoparticles with HDC showed that it is possible to keep agglomerates during the separation, even when the interaction between particles is weak, possibility that makes it very promising for the study of nanofood (Philippe and Schaumann 2014). Field flow fractionation (FFF) can separate macromolecules, microorganism, or particles (1 nm–1 μm) based on their different mobilities. In this case, the particles advance through a channel where there is aqueous mobile phase pumped through two tightly packed polymeric layers and the action of a field perpendicular to the hydrodynamic flow. The perpendicular field can be gravity (flow FFF), a centrifugation force (sedimentation FFF), which can have a greater resolution capacity than FFF, among other modalities (Fedotov et al. 2011). The detection of particles following FFF can be carried out with UV, fluorescence, DLS, or MS, consequently, it can be used for both inorganic and organic particles. FFF is a very mature and robust technique that has great potential for the separation of nanosystems, the channel is relatively simple to operate, and even to make, however, it requires method development, and it is not widely available in the laboratories dealing with food technology. This may be holding back establishing this technique as a reference one for the separation of nanosystems in food.

## 14.5 COMPLEMENTARY ANALYTICAL TECHNIQUES

Every analytical technique can be applied within a defined working range of conditions or concentrations. Microscopy techniques are very important in the nanofood context because they can be used to measure direct properties in nanomaterials, unlike many other approaches that offer indirect information. Microscopy has drawbacks, such as the localized analysis and small specimens which can lead to problems of representativity of the whole sample, or the very high number of micrographs that need to be treated for establishing the particle size and its uncertainty. The dependence of the RSD of mean particle size (pm), where particle size had been estimated from the equivalent circular diameter of the particle as projected in a 2D image, with the number of particles (N) and interquartile range of particle size distributions (IQR %) is given in the equation 1 (Dudkiewicz et al. 2015).

$$RSDpm = 10071 \times \mathrm{N}^{-0.553} \times \mathrm{IQR}\ \% \tag{14.1}$$

Equation (14.1) was obtained from the measurement of a population of 1388 particles randomly selected from 200 images from the analysis of reference food materials (chicken paste and soup) spiked with silver and silica nanoparticles. The smallest number of particles required for an IQR (%) of particle size 111 nm, with an RSDpm of 5% was found to be 359 particles (Dudkiewicz et al. 2015).

The sample preparation method may be selected after trying several approaches for a nanosystem/food matrix to understand how preparation can affect the details in the image. It is highly recommendable to characterize nanosystems with a range of techniques for both sample treatment and determination.

An example of the advantages of the analysis with complementary microscopy techniques is the optimization of a nanoemulsion-filled hydrogel, developed to improve the bioavailability of nobiletin, which is a flavone with pharmaceutical properties (Lei et al. 2017). This example is shown in Figure 14.1. A hydrogel filled with nanoemulsion containing nobiletin was freeze-dried, and its morphology examined with SEM. The loading of the active principle of the hydrogel was found to affect the morphology (undulation) of the hydrogel with SEM. A detailed morphological examination of the crystals of the active principle dispersed in the hydrogel was carried out with optical and fluorescent microscopy. With optical microscopy, the crystals presented filament structures and were especially visible at the higher loading concentrations of the drug (indicated with arrows in Figure 14.1). A convenient pre-treatment was carried out to observe the nanoemulsion within the hydrogel: a fluorescent hydrophobic dye (nile red) was dispersed in the nanoemulsion before drying the hydrogel. This pre-treatment led to a very clear picture of the distribution of the dye, which could interact with the hydrophobic active principle within the hydrogel. The crystals of the hydrophobic drug seemed to favor coalescence of hydrophobic droplets around them. In addition, the analysis of the hydrogel with XRD indicated that the active principle was mainly in amorphous form within the hydrogel and in less extent as crystals (Lei et al. 2017). This had implications in control release of the drug. An alternative technique that could analyze crystalline samples, through interference contrast, is high resolution TEM (Dudkiewicz et al. 2011).

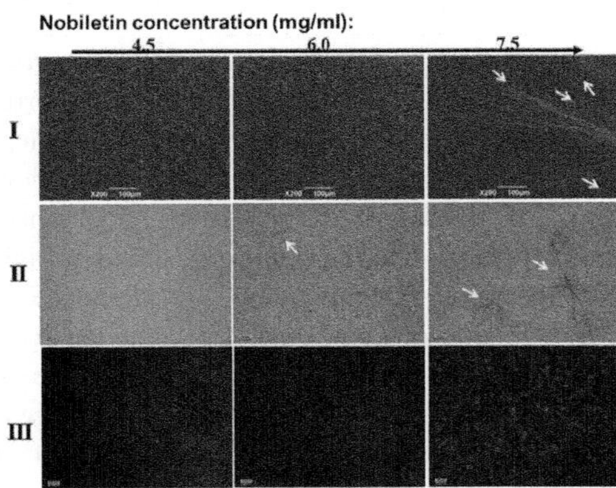


**FIGURE 14.1** Microstructure of nobiletin-loaded nanoemulsion-filled alginate hydrogels, I: SEM images of the hydrogel surface, II: images by optical microscopy, and III: images by fluorescent microscopy. Arrows indicate the nobiletin crystals. The scale bar in I and II is unclear. (Reprinted with permission from Lei, L. et al., *LWT Food Sci. Technol.*, 82, 260–267, 2017.)

The analysis of alginate nano/microspheres loaded with peppermint phenolic extract carried out with SEM, TEM, and DLS (Mokhtari et al. 2017) showed the advantages of a multianalytical approach to characterize nanocapsules (shown in Figure 14.2). In SEM, the alginate hydrogel is shown as a microparticle (>1 μm) that may be constituted from agglomerated sub-particles. The agglomerate may be an

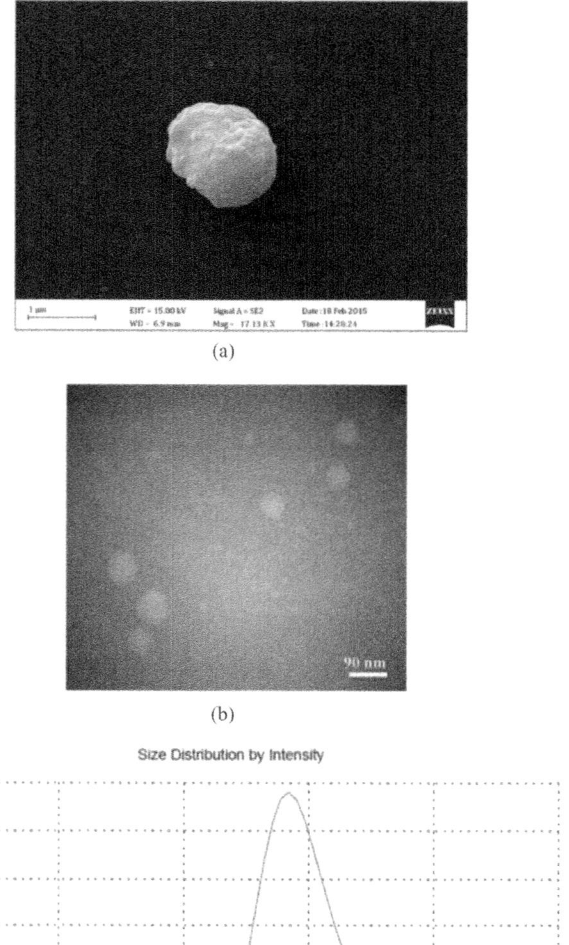


**FIGURE 14.2** Alginate nanospheres added with peppermint phenolic extract: (a) SEM photomicrograph, (b) TEM photomicrograph, and (c) Size distribution graph. The scale bar in (a) corresponds to 1 μm and in (b) corresponds to 90 nm. (Reprinted with permission from Mokhtari, S. et al., *Food Chem.* 229: 286–295, 2017.)

artifact which may have formed when drying the sample on air. We assume that that micrograph is representative of the sample, but certainly, additional images from the nanocapsules would be informative. The micrograph was obtained with rather high accelerating voltage (15 kV) given that alginate is a soft material, and the specimen could suffer modifications by the electron beam during imaging: the selected voltage has to be high enough to achieve optimal resolution, but low enough to not alter the sample and prevent charging. In contrast to the result obtained with SEM, the TEM micrograph shows a 2D image of a population of nanocarriers with a range of particle sizes, after having treated the sample with surfactant. The surfactant stabilized the emulsion droplets and minimized coalescence, but may have de-agglomerated existing clusters in the original sample. The particle size distribution shown by dark-field TEM (detection of the fraction of the beam diffracted by the sample) agrees with the size distribution of the hydrodynamic sphere obtained with DLS. The measurement with DLS was probably carried out after a filtration step to eliminate bigger particles.

CLSM is an advantageous scanning probe microscopy technique. It can achieve poorer spatial resolutions (50–100 nm) and lower magnifications than SEM or TEM, but it can be used to image nanosystems in food samples that have been de-hydrated and fixed onto a slide or even hydrated samples. It is possible to obtain images in 3D and in color when different parts of the sample have been dyed with auto fluorescent dyes (Prasad et al. 2007; Mbundi et al. 2014). CLSM can be very useful to image nanosystems within food matrix (Salvia-Trujillo et al. 2016), and also to study the fate of nanosystems in cells and tissues when investigating their safety.

A complementary technique to DLS and microscopy that allows establishing the particle size distribution is nanoparticle tracking analysis (NTA), which started to be commercialized in 2006. This technique combines laser light scattering microscopy with a charge-coupled device camera that records the trajectory of nanoparticles which have Brownian movement when suspended in solution. The movement of the particle can be related with their size with a formula derived from the Stokes-Einstein equation. The particle size range of NTA (30 nm–1 μm) is slightly shorter than electron microscopy and DLS (1 nm–1 μm), and it cannot detect sub-nanometer particles like TEM (Filipe et al. 2010). The concentration range where NTA operates ($10^7$–$10^9$ particles/ml) is narrower than the range for DLS ($10^8$–$10^{12}$ particles/ml) (Filipe et al. 2010). NTA is particularly useful for characterizing monodisperse and polydisperse samples and can have superior peak resolution than DLS. Different populations of particles can become very well defined with NTA, and the presence of bigger particles does not affect the detection of the smaller ones, unlike in DLS, this is an important advantage. NTA also allows studying aggregation at different temperatures with the instrument and provides information about the aggregation kinetics. A limitation is that the analysis time with NTA (5–60 min) can be longer than with DLS (2–5 min) (Filipe et al. 2010). But overall, it is a very powerful characterization technique, which is not widely used in the characterization of nanosystems in food and their aggregation behavior, possibly because it is relatively new in the market and DLS is, in contrast, a very well-established technique. The current definition of nanomaterial indicates that 50% of the particles, in either free, aggregates, or agglomerates form, possess structures in the critical size range (below 100 nm) (Potocnik 2011). Consequently, the capacity to measure size and size-range of the particles needs to be prioritized when deciding on the method and technique to characterize nanotechnology-based materials, and both NTA and DLS offer this possibility, whereas it would be an enormous task by microscopy as vast number of micrographs would need to be treated.

A study compared the uncertainty of the measurement of particle size of pristine silica particles with SEM, DLS, and gas electrophoretic mobility molecular analyzer (GEMMA). In GEMMA, single charged analytes are produced by the action of an electrospray and charge reduction with polonium-210. Following, charged nanoparticles are separated by their electrophoretic mobility (Allmaier et al. 2008). These three techniques showed an uncertainty of 3%–6% in the measurement. In contrast, when comparing DLS, GEMMA, and TEM for the analysis of Ag nanoparticles in aqueous dispersion, the uncertainty obtained with TEM (8%–21%) was like with DLS and about two times greater than with GEMMA. The cause of the relatively high dispersion of results could be sample inhomogeneity, sample preparation, or data treatment. TEM was selected instead of SEM in this case because it gave greater contrast between the nanomaterials, which were imaged as dark spots, and the matrix, in bright-field TEM.

Quantitative analysis of silica nanoparticles in soup and Ag nanoparticles in meat was carried out with FFF-ICP-MS and single particle-ICP-MS, respectively, following matrix digestion. The analysis of Ag nanoparticles with single particle-ICP-MS leads to up to 5% uncertainty (compared to up to 19% with TEM). The lower uncertainty achieved with the hyphenated techniques compared to microscopy was attributed to the higher homogeneity of the sample due to the digestion being carried out. The analysis of silica nanoparticles with FFF-ICP-MS led to up to 21% uncertainty, which was similar to SEM. This high dispersion of the results could be due to intrinsic inhomogeneity of the sample (Dudkiewicz et al. 2015). Overall, hyphenated techniques can be advantageous with respect to microscopy: they reduce the effect of the matrix, and increase representativity of the sample, although method development with hyphenated techniques is time consuming. A scheme displaying the capabilities of a range of techniques discussed in this chapter is shown in Figure 14.3. SEM-EDS

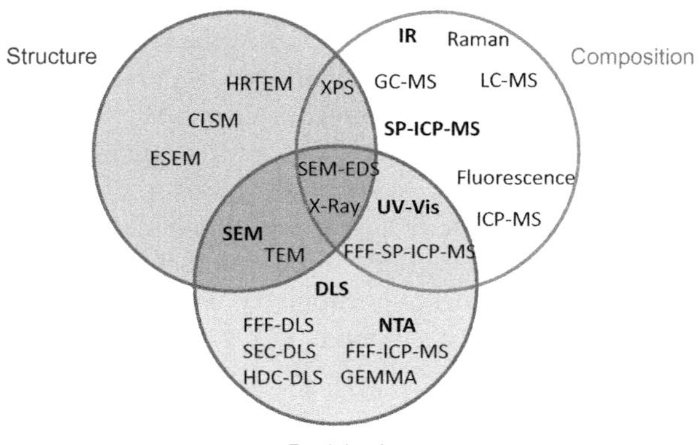


**FIGURE 14.3** Classification of the scope of techniques used in the characterization of organic or inorganic micro—and nanosystems in food. The most commonly used techniques within the scope of this chapter appear in bold.

and XRD have the capacity to offer structural and compositional information (metals). These, and UV-Vis, could also be employed for the quantification of particle sizes, although this is normally carried out by DLS, which is not restricted by the composition of the particles and does not need high number of acquisitions (as in microscopy) or crystallinity (like XRD). Likewise, CLSM, ESEM, and high resolution TEM are mainly, but infrequently, used for providing qualitative information of the structure of nanosystems, and are seldomly employed for the measurement of particle size distribution. It is predicted that with the development and validation of analytical methods involving separation of particles using FFF, SEC, and HDC, the analysis with hyphenated techniques will become more generalized.

## 14.6 CONCLUSIONS AND FUTURE PERSPECTIVES

Particle size, shape, and the stability, distribution, and evolution of nanosystems as well as the active principles that they may contain, within food products need to be established. Every analytical technique offers partial information of the situation in the nanofood or food packaging, and the limits of the information that every technique can offer with reliability are being defined. It is highly recommendable to characterize nanosystems with a range of techniques for both sample treatment and determination. SEM and TEM are widely used because they can show the shape and detail of the nanosystems, although advances that both techniques can incorporate for imaging hydrated samples are not fully exploited. Confocal microscopy can also be employed to characterize nanosystems in moist samples despite that it has limitations regarding the magnification that it provides. Major disadvantages of microscopy in quantitative analysis are the high number of samples that need to be imaged and treated to determine particle size and minimize problems of sample representativity that result from the small sample volumes required. The sample preparation method needs to be optimized for every study nanosystem/matrix, as it is crucial to obtain accurate information in microscopy, but also in every analytical technique analyzing food. DLS and NTA are excellent approaches to measure size distribution of nanoparticles. NTA is more robust than DLS in the sense that NTA's measurements are less affected by the presence of small amounts of large particles. Methods including hyphenated techniques can minimize matrix effects and separate particles by their shape and size and quantify nanosystems with high sensitivity (comparable to the analysis of organic molecules and metals). However, more efforts are needed to develop methods that would facilitate the use of hyphenated techniques for the characterization of nanosystems in food. Separation techniques such as HDC and sedimentation FFF coupled to mass spectrometry or DLS have a brilliant future ahead in the analysis of nanosystems in food.

## REFERENCES

Allmaier, G., C. Laschober, and W. W. Szymanski. 2008. "Nano ES GEMMA and PDMA, New Tools for the Analysis of Nanobioparticles-Protein Complexes, Lipoparticles, and Viruses." *Journal of the American Society for Mass Spectrometry* 19 (8): 1062–1068. doi:10.1016/j.jasms.2008.05.017.

Amenta, V., K. Aschberger, M. Arena, H. Bouwmeester, F. B. Moniz, P. Brandhoff, S. Gottardo et al. 2015. "Regulatory Aspects of Nanotechnology in the Agri/feed/food Sector in EU and Non-EU Countries." *Regulatory Toxicology and Pharmacology* 73 (1): 463–476. doi:10.1016/j.yrtph.2015.06.016.

Bautista, L., L. Molina, S. Niembro, J. M. García, J. López, and A. Vílchez. 2017. "Coatings and Inks for Food Packaging Including Nanomaterials." In *Emerging Nanotechnologies in Food Science*, edited by Rosa Busquets, 1st ed., pp. 149–173. Amsterdam,the Netherlands: Elsevier.

Bownman, D., and K. Ludlow. 2017. "Ensuring Food Safety: General Principles for Safeguarding What You Eat Including the Role of Food Labels." In *Emerging Nanotechnologies in Food Science*, edited by Rosa Busquets, 1st ed., pp. 175–193. Amsterdam, the Netherlands: Elsevier.

Brar, S. K., and M. Verma. 2011. "Measurement of Nanoparticles by Light-Scattering Techniques." *TrAC—Trends in Analytical Chemistry* 30 (1): 4–17. doi:10.1016/j.trac.2010.08.008.

Busquets, R. 2017. "Analysis of Nanomaterials in Food." In *Emerging Nanotechnologies in Food Science*, edited by Rosa Busquets, pp. 53–80. Amsterdam, the Netherlands: Elsevier.

Cerqueira, M. A., A. C. Pinheiro, O. L. Ramos, H. Silva, A. I. Bourbon, and A. A. Vicente. 2017. "Advances in Food Nanotechnology." In *Emerging Nanotechnologies in Food Science*, edited by Rosa Busquets, pp. 11–38. Amsterdam, the Netherlands: Elsevier.

Comunian, T. A., R. Ravanfar, I. A. de Castro, R. Dando, C. S. Favaro-Trindade, and A. Abbaspourrad. 2017. "Improving Oxidative Stability of Echium Oil Emulsions Fabricated by Microfluidics: Effect of Ionic Gelation and Phenolic Compounds." *Food Chemistry* 233: 125–134. doi:10.1016/j.foodchem.2017.04.085.

Dias, D. R., D. A. Botrel, R. V. De Barros Fernandes, and S. V. Borges. 2017. "Encapsulation as a Tool for Bioprocessing of Functional Foods." *Current Opinion in Food Science* 13: 31–37. doi:10.1016/j.cofs.2017.02.001.

DTU Environment, and Danish Consumer Council. 2017. The Nanodatabase. http://nanodb.dk/en/search-database/ (accessed August 2017).

Dudefoi, W., K. Moniz, E. Allen-Vercoe, M.-H. Ropers, and V. K. Walker. 2017. "Impact of Food Grade and Nano-$TiO_2$ Particles on a Human Intestinal Community." *Food and Chemical Toxicology* 106: 242–249. doi:10.1016/j.fct.2017.05.050.

Dudkiewicz, A., A. B. A. Boxall, Q. Chaudhry, K. Mølhave, K. Tiede, P. Hofmann, and T. P. J. Linsinger. 2015. "Uncertainties of Size Measurements in Electron Microscopy Characterization of Nanomaterials in Foods." *Food Chemistry* 176: 472–479. doi:10.1016/j.foodchem.2014.12.071.

Dudkiewicz, A., K. Tiede, K. Loeschner, L. H. S. Jensen, E. Jensen, R. Wierzbicki, A. B. A. Boxall, and K. Molhave. 2011. "Characterization of Nanomaterials in Food by Electron Microscopy." *TrAC—Trends in Analytical Chemistry* 30 (1): 28–43. doi:10.1016/j.trac.2010.10.007.

Editorial from Nature Nanotechnology. 2010. "Nanofood for Thought." *Nature Nanotechnology* 5 (2): 89. doi:10.1038/nnano.2010.22.

European Commision, UE. 2013. Research in Nanoscience & Technologies-Policy Issues. Research & Innovation, Key Enabling Technologies.http://ec.europa.eu/research/industrial_technologies/index_en.html.

European Commission. 2011. Comission recommendation of 18 October 2011 on the definition of nanomaterial. Off. J.Eur. Union 2011/696/ EU, L275/38-L274/40. https://ec.europa.eu/research/industrial_technologies/pdf/policy/commission-recommendation-on-the-definition-of-nanomater-18102011_en.pdf (accessed 14 May 2019).

European Food Safety Authrority (EFSA) Scientific Committee. 2011. "Guidance on the Risk Assessment of the Application of Nanoscience and Nanotechnologies in The Food and Feed Chain." *EFSA Journal* 9 (5): 1–35.

European Food Safety Authrority (EFSA) Scientific Committee and Emerging Risks Unit. 2017. "Network & Working Group on Nanotechnologies in Food and Feed." In *Network & Working Group on Nanotechnologies in Food and Feed*. Parma. http://www.efsa.europa.eu/sites/default/files/event/171128-1-a.pdf (accessed 14 May 2019).

European Parliament. 2013. Regulation (EU) No 1169/2011 of the European Parliament and of the Council of 25 October 2011 on the provision of food information to consumers, amending Regulations (EC) No 1924/2006 and (EC) No 1925/2006 of the European Parliament and of the Council, and repealing Commission Directive 87/250/EEC, Council Directive 90/496/EEC, Commission Directive 1999/10/EC, Directive 2000/13/EC of the European Parliament and of the Council, Commission Directives 2002/67/EC and 2008/5/EC and Commission Regulation (EC) No 608/2004.

European Parliament. 2016. Food Contact Materials—Regulation (EC) 1935/2004. http://www.europarl.europa.eu/RegData/etudes/STUD/2016/581411/EPRS_STU%282016%29581411_EN.pdf (accessed 14 May 2019).

Fedotov, P. S., N. G. Vanifatova, V. M. Shkinev, and B. Y. Spivakov. 2011. "Fractionation and Characterization of Nano- and Microparticles in Liquid Media." *Analytical and Bioanalytical Chemistry* 400 (6): 1787–1804. doi:10.1007/s00216-011-4704-1.

Filipe, V., A. Hawe, and W. Jiskoot. 2010. "Critical Evaluation of Nanoparticle Tracking Analysis (NTA) by NanoSight for the Measurement of Nanoparticles and Protein Aggregates." *Pharmaceutical Research* 27 (5): 796–810. doi:10.1007/s11095-010-0073-2.

Gallocchio, F., S. Belluco, and A. Ricci. 2015. "Nanotechnology and Food: Brief Overview of the Current Scenario." *Procedia Food Science* 5: 85–88. doi:10.1016/j.profoo.2015.09.022.

Gasa-Falcon, A., I. Odriozola-Serrano, G. Oms-Oliu, and O. Martín-Belloso. 2017. "Influence of Mandarin Fiber Addition on Physico-Chemical Properties of Nanoemulsions Containing β-Carotene under Simulated Gastrointestinal Digestion Conditions." *LWT—Food Science and Technology* 84: 331–337. doi:10.1016/j.lwt.2017.05.070.

Grombe, R., G. Allmaier, J. Charoud-Got, A. Dudkiewicz, H. Emteborg, T. Hofmann, E. H. Larsen et al. 2015. "Feasibility of the Development of Reference Materials for the Detection of Ag Nanoparticles in Food: Neat Dispersions and Spiked Chicken Meat." *Accreditation and Quality Assurance* 20 (1): 3–16. doi:10.1007/s00769-014-1100-5.

https://eur-lex.europa.eu/legal-content/EN/TXT/PDF/?uri=CELEX:32011R1169&from=EN (accessed 14 May 2019).

Kowalczyk, B., I. Lagzi, and B. A. Grzybowski. 2011. "Nanoseparations: Strategies for Size and/or Shape-Selective Purification of Nanoparticles." *Current Opinion in Colloid and Interface Science* 16 (2): 135–148. doi:10.1016/j.cocis.2011.01.004.

Lacey, J. 2017. "Bioavailability of Nanomaterials and Interaction with Cells." In *Emerging Nanotechnologies in Food Science*, edited by Rosa Busquets, 1st ed., pp. 81–96. Amsterdam, the Netherlands: Elsevier.

Lari, L., and A. Dudkiewicz. 2014. "Sample Preparation and EFTEM of Meat Samples for Nanoparticle Analysis in Food." In *Electron Microscopy and Analysis Group Conference. Journal of Physiscs: Conference Series*, pp. 1–4. IOP Publishing. doi:10.1088/1742-6596/522/1/012057.

Lei, L., Y. Zhang, L. He, S. Wu, B. Li, and Y. Li. 2017. "LWT—Food Science and Technology Fabrication of Nanoemulsion- Filled Alginate Hydrogel to Control the Digestion Behavior of Hydrophobic Nobiletin." *LWT—Food Science and Technology* 82: 260–267. doi:10.1016/j.lwt.2017.04.051.

Linsinger, T. P. J., G. Roebben, C. Solans, and R. Ramsch. 2011. "Reference Materials for Measuring the Size of Nanoparticles." *TrAC—Trends in Analytical Chemistry* 30 (1): 18–27. doi:10.1016/j.trac.2010.09.005.

Linsinger, T. P. J., R. Peters, and S. Weigel. 2014. "International Interlaboratory Study for Sizing and Quantification of Ag Nanoparticles in Food Simulants by Single-Particle ICPMS Characterisation of Nanomaterials in Biological Samples." *Analytical and Bioanalytical Chemistry* 406 (16): 3835–3843. doi:10.1007/s00216-013-7559-9.

López-Córdoba, A., C. Medina-Jaramillo, D. Piñeros-Hernandez, and S. Goyanes. 2017. "Cassava Starch Films Containing Rosemary Nanoparticles Produced by Solvent Displacement Method." *Food Hydrocolloids* 71: 26–34. doi:10.1016/j.foodhyd.2017.04.028.

Luna, J., and A. Vilchez. 2017. "Polymer Nanocomposites for Food Packaging." In *Emerging Nanotechnologies in Food Science*, edited by Rosa Busquets, 1st ed., pp. 119–147. Oxford, UK: Elsevier.

Marlvern Instruments Limited. 2015. Accuracy and Reproducibility in Automated Dynamic Light Scattering Measurements. https://particular.ie/wp-content/uploads/2014/05/Accuracy-and-reproducibility-in-automated-DLS-measurements.pdf (accessed 14 May 2019).

Mbundi, L., H. Gallar-Ayala, M. R. Khan, J. L. Barber, S. Losada, and R. Busquets. 2014. "Advances in the Analysis of Challenging Food Contaminants: Nanoparticles, Bisphenols, Mycotoxins, and Brominated Flame Retardants." In *Advances in Molecular Toxicology* 8, edited by J. C. Fishbein and J. M. Heilman, pp. 35–105. Elsevier. doi:10.1016/B978-0-444-63406-1.00002-7.

Mokhtari, S., S. M. Jafari, and E. Assadpour. 2017. "Development of a Nutraceutical Nano-Delivery System through Emulsification/Internal Gelation of Alginate." *Food Chemistry* 229: 286–295. doi:10.1016/j.foodchem.2017.02.071.

Novak, J. P., C. Nickerson, S. Franzen, and D. L. Feldheim. 2001. "Purification of Molecularly Bridged Metal Nanoparticle Arrays by Centrifugation and Size Exclusion Chromatography." *Analytical Chemistry* 73 (23): 5758–5761. doi:10.1021/ac010812t.

Peters, R., G. ten Dam, H. Bouwmeester, H. Helsper, G. Allmaier, F. vd Kammer, R. Ramsch et al. 2011. "Identification and Characterization of Organic Nanoparticles in Food." *Trends in Analytical Chemistry* 30 (1): 100–112. doi:10.1016/j.trac.2010.10.004.

Philippe, A., and G. E. Schaumann. 2014. "Evaluation of Hydrodynamic Chromatography Coupled with Uv-Visible, Fluorescence and Inductively Coupled Plasma Mass Spectrometry Detectors for Sizing and Quantifying Colloids in Environmental Media." *PLoS ONE* 9 (2): 1–9. doi:10.1371/journal.pone.0090559.

Potocnik, J. 2011. Commission Recommendation, no. June 2010: L275/38-L275/40. doi:10.2777/13162.

Prasad, V., D. Semwogerere, and E. W. Weeks. 2007. "Confocal Microscopy of Colloids." *Journal of Physics: Condensed Matter* 19 (11): 113102.

Rasti, B., A. Erfanian, and J. Selamat. 2017. "Novel Nanoliposomal Encapsulated Omega-3 Fatty Acids and Their Applications in Food." *Food Chemistry* 230: 690–696. doi:10.1016/j.foodchem.2017.03.089.

Salvia-Trujillo, L., E. A. Decker, and D. J. McClements. 2016. "Influence of an Anionic Polysaccharide on the Physical and Oxidative Stability of Omega-3 Nanoemulsions: Antioxidant Effects of Alginate." *Food Hydrocolloids* 52: 690–698. doi:10.1016/j.foodhyd.2015.07.035.

Souza Simões, L. de, D. A. Madalena, A. C. Pinheiro, J. A. Teixeira, A. A. Vicente, and Ó. L. Ramos. 2017. "Micro- and Nano Bio-based Delivery Systems for Food Applications: *In Vitro* Behavior." *Advances in Colloid and Interface Science* 243 (May): 23–45. doi:10.1016/j.cis.2017.02.010.

Wei, G.-T., and F.-K. Liu. 1999. "Separation of Nanometer Gold Particles by Size Exclusion Chromatography." *Journal of Chromatography A* 836 (2): 253–260. doi:10.1016/S0021-9673(99)00069-2.

Wei, G.-T., F.-K. Liu, and C. R. C. Wang. 1999. "Shape Separation of Nanometer Gold Particles by Size-Exclusion Chromatography." *Analytical Chemistry* 71 (11): 2085–2091.

Weir, A., P. Westerhoff, L. Fabricius, K. Hristovski, and N. von Goetz. 2012. "Titanium Dioxide Nanoparticles in Food and Personal Care Products." *Environmental Science And Technology* 46 (4): 2242–2250.

Whitby, R. L. D., A. Korobeinyk, V. M. Gun'ko, R. Busquets, A. B. Cundy, K. László, J. Skubiszewska-Zięba et al. 2011. "pH-Driven Physicochemical Conformational Changes of Single-Layer Graphene Oxide." *Chemical Communications (Cambridge, England)* 47 (34): 9645–9647. doi:10.1039/c1cc13725e.

Whitby, R. L. D., and R. Busquets. 2013. "Nanomaterials and the Environment: Global Impact of Tiny Materials." *Nanomaterials and the Environment* 1: 1–2. doi:10.2478/nanome-2012-0001.

Zhu, F. 2017. "Encapsulation and Delivery of Food Ingredients Using Starch Based Systems." *Food Chemistry* 229: 542–552. doi:10.1016/j.foodchem.2017.02.101.

Zhu, X.-F., J. Zheng, F. Liu, C.-Y. Qiu, W.-F. Lin, and C.-H. Tang. 2018. "Freeze-Thaw Stability of Pickering Emulsions Stabilized by Soy Protein Nanoparticles. Influence of Ionic Strength before or after Emulsification." *Food Hydrocolloids* 74: 37–45. doi:10.1016/j.foodhyd.2017.07.017.

# 15 New Research Trends and Future Perspective in Bio-based Nanosystems Produced by Electrohydrodynamic Processing for Applications in the Food Industry

*María A. Busolo and Cristina Prieto López*

**CONTENTS**

## 15.1 NOVEL RESEARCH TRENDS AND RECENT ADVANCES RELATED TO FOOD INDUSTRY

Nanostructures and nanomaterials exhibit physical, chemical, and biological properties that are significantly different from their bulk counterparts. The current and potential applications of nanotechnology in food sector include the improvement of food safety, food packaging, and food processing, being nanoparticles, liposomes, and nanoemulsions the most significant nanostructured systems for the food industry (Pathakoti et al. 2017).

Nanoencapsulation of active substances is one of the most versatile applications of nanostructures in the food industry. This technique results in the protection of compounds against degradation, longer shelf life, controlled release, and solubility improvement (Jafari and McClements 2017). Electrospinning has been proposed as a feasible route to encapsulate.

Nanotechnology can be implemented in practically every segment related to food industry such as feed additives, food ingredients and additives, food contact materials, and nutrient supplements—nutraceuticals. The use of nanostructures in the food industry is mainly focused in increasing the stability of substances and their bioavailability, enhancing food security by extending the shelf life, improving flavor and nutrient delivery, and serving functional foods (see Figure 15.1). However, the lack of a common worldwide regulatory framework for appropriate guidance regarding manufacture, safety use, risk assessment, and disposal of nanomaterials is a limiting factor for their application in the food industry.

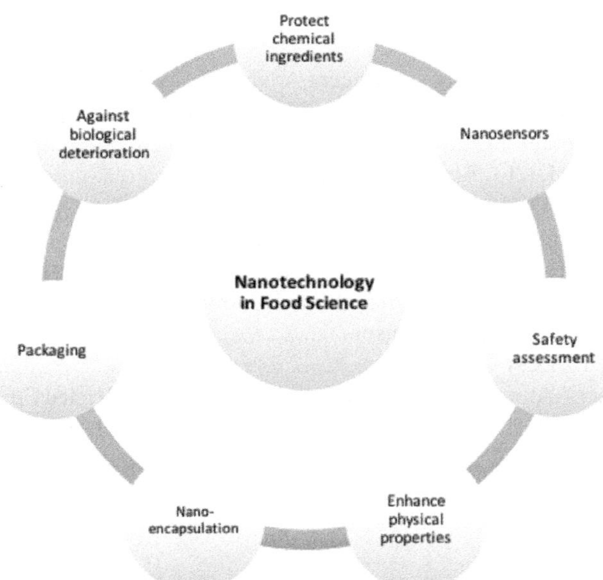


**FIGURE 15.1** Scheme of functionality, applications, and safety issues of nanotechnology in Food science. (From He, X. and Hwang, H.-M., *J. Food Drug Anal.*, 24, 671–681, 2016.)

This text reviews recent advances and trends in development of bio-based capsules and fibers obtained by electrohydrodynamic techniques for food-related applications.

### 15.1.1 Nanomaterials Production Processes by Electrohydrodynamic Processing

Typically, encapsulation processes comprise spray drying, spray cooling, extrusion, emulsion techniques, fluidized bed coating, coacervation, liposome entrapment, inclusion complexation, etc. (Katouzian and Jafari 2016, Nedovic et al. 2011, Paximada et al. 2017, Perez-Masia et al. 2015). However, these techniques mostly require heating and pressure and the use of strong and toxic organic solvents or expensive equipment. Electrohydrodynamic (EHD) processing, has emerged as an advantageous alternative technology for encapsulation that needs neither temperature nor expensive equipment, and use of toxic organic solvents can be avoided by adjusting some processing conditions (i.e., use of molten polymers). EHD constitutes the basis for electrospinning and electrospray.

#### 15.1.1.1 Electrospinning

This technique is a straightforward, versatile, and simple approach to the manufacturing of nanofibers with high specific surface areas, high porosities, and controllable compositions from both organic and inorganic materials for a wide range of applications in the industry (Chakraborty et al. 2009, Ding et al. 2010, Srivastava 2017, Wang et al. 2013). The electrospinning process consists of applying a high-voltage electric field to charge the droplet of a polymer solution at the end of a capillary tube. The hemispherical droplet at the tip of the needle elongates forming a conical shape (Taylor cone). If the concentration of the solution or the molecular chain entanglement in the liquid is high, and the electric force overcomes the surface tension of the viscous solution, a jet projection of fibers emerges and moves toward the conductive collector (Katouzian and Jafari 2016). These fibers stretch and elongate causing most of polymer solution evaporation, thereby solidification of the fibers occurs before they are collected on the screen in the form of non-woven mats (Aruna et al. 2017, Ghorani and Tucker 2015), as shown in Figure 15.2.

Nearly all soluble and fusible polymers are susceptible to be electrospun. The final morphology and dimensions of nanofibers will depend on the proper setting of solution and polymer parameters as well as processing and operating conditions (Aruna et al. 2017, Ghorani and Tucker 2015, Greiner and Wendorff 2007). Besides pure fiber structures, many other morphologies (i.e., pearl-necklace-like beaded fiber, highly porous fiber, grafted fiber, hollow interior micro tubes, and twisted fibers) can be achieved by tuning operating and processing conditions.

The scale up of nanofibers through single jet is not economically and technically feasible, and most of the electrospun fiber applications require large quantities of material (Persano et al. 2013). Depending on the solution properties, the throughput of a single-jet set up varies from 0.01 to 10 mL/min, which is a limiting factor to industrial scale up where mass production is needed (Bhardwaj and Kundu 2010,

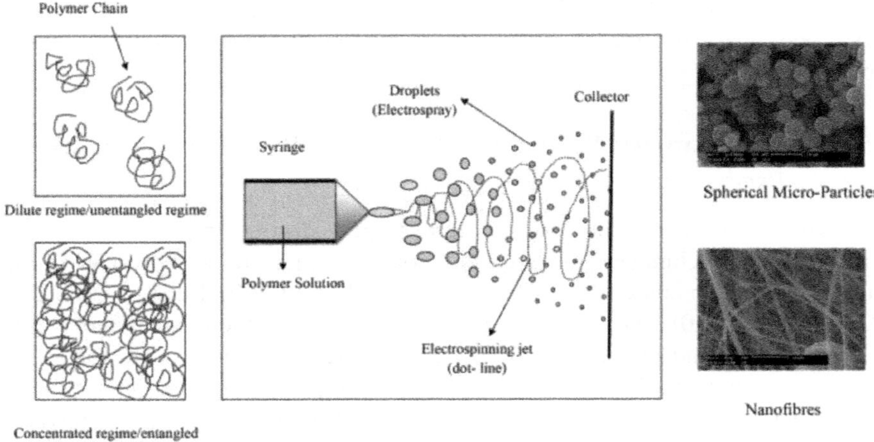


**FIGURE 15.2** Left: Schematic of physical representation at the molecular level of entanglement regimes for dilute and concentrated polymer concentration. Middle: Schematic diagram of a basic electrospinning (jet formation) and electrospraying (liquid-droplet atomization) process. Right: Examples of SEM image of microspheres (electrospraying) and nanofibers (electrospinning). (Reprinted with permission from Ghorani, B. and Tucker, N., *Food Hydrocolloid.*, 51, 227–240, 2015.)

Molnar and Nagy 2016, Theron et al. 2005). Scaling up by a multi-nozzle technology is then feasible, but requires some adjustments since jets in a multiple arrangement can interact, undergo bending instabilities, and lead to repulsion because of Coulombic forces (Theron et al. 2005). Since more recently, companies like Bioinicia S.L., MECC Co. Ltd, Elmarco, Inovenso Co., ANSTCO, Electrospunra, and Fmn Co., among others, commercialize EHD processing machines to cover from research to industrial production. Fluidnatek® is the brand name of electrospinning and electrospraying equipment designed by Bioinicia (Bioinicia 2017) which has recently received the GMP approval for their manufacturing facilities.

### 15.1.1.2 Electrospray

Electrospinning and electrospraying are "sister" technologies, and the difference between them is based on the degree of molecular cohesion in the raw material, which is basically controlled by the concentration of the polymeric solution (Ghorani and Tucker 2015). For low-concentrated polymer solutions, when the electrostatic force in the droplets overcomes the cohesion force, the polymer jet breaks up in fine particles due to the low viscoelasticity of the solution, thus nanoparticles are gathered in the grounded or oppositely charged collector (García-Moreno et al. 2016, Subbiah et al. 2005) as shown in Figure 15.2. In this case, the process is called *electrospray*, because of the non-continuous nature of the structures obtained (López-Rubio and Lagaron 2012). The charge of droplets produced by electrospray makes impossible the droplet agglomeration and coagulation and high deposition efficiency is achieved (Faridi Esfanjani and Jafari 2016). Electrospray shows high encapsulation efficiency (more than 80%), sustained release of encapsulated material, enhanced thermal, light, and storage stability, and improved protection of bioactives from chemical degradation over conventional encapsulation technologies (Echegoyen et al. 2017).

Commercially available one-needle electrospray machines have been used for pilot scale production, such as Fluidnatek LE-10 and LE-500 (Bioinicia 2017, Gómez-Mascaraque et al. 2016, Paximada et al. 2017, Pérez-Masiá et al. 2015) and MECC NF-102 from the Japanese company MECC Co. Ltd. (Fukui et al. 2010). Mass production of electrosprayed capsules cannot be simply achieved by increasing the flow rate of spraying solution, but increasing the number of needles in parallel (higher amount of Taylor cones).

## 15.1.2 Nanomaterials Applications

### 15.1.2.1 Food Packaging

Active food packaging addresses the changing demands of the food industry and consumers as well as the increasing regulatory and legal requirements about food safety (Realini and Marcos 2014), providing several functions such as oxygen scavenging, antimicrobial activity, or free radical trapping (Ahmed et al. 2017, Hurme et al. 2002, Restuccia et al. 2010). Active agents, such as antioxidants, can be directly incorporated into the packaging material, remain stable there, and finally be released from the packaging material in a controlled way to inhibit the oxidation of sensitive components (Busolo and Lagaron 2015). However, many active agents are thermally sensitive and cannot be directly incorporated using the conventional processing methods (Fabra et al. 2016). The immobilization by encapsulation using electrospinning aims at protecting sensitive substances from oxidation, heat, or extreme conditions during the processing because no severe conditions are needed in EHD techniques. Some of recent studies involving electrospun nanofibers for active substances encapsulation for promising active packaging applications are listed in the Table 15.1.

Some studies involve the use of essential oils, volatile compounds, and phenolic compounds for producing active electrospun fibers. These active nanostructures, once incorporated into a polymer layer, can be integrated in a multilayer system with controlled antimicrobial properties and used as antimicrobial or antioxidant food packaging. For instance, (R)-(+)-limonene was encapsulated in a poly(vinyl alcohol) (PVA) fibrous matrix for potential applications in various fields, such as cosmetics or food packaging (Camerlo et al. 2013). Cerqueira et al. (2016) electrospun zein ultra-thin fibers containing cinnamaldehyde as antimicrobial agent onto polyhydroxybutyrate-co-valerate (PHBV) and developed active multilayer structures by intercalation of zein-cinnamaldehyde nanofibers with PHBV or alginate layers. A controlled release of the aldehyde was achieved, avoiding the rapid volatilization and burst release. An inclusion complex made of cinnamon essential oil and β-cyclodextrin was prepared and then incorporated into poly(lactic acid) (PLA) nanofibers via electrospinning (Wen et al. 2016). The resulting nanofilm showed strong antimicrobial activity against *Staphylococcus aureus* and *Escherichia coli*, as well as ability for extending the shelf life of meat products. In another study, electrospun active nanofibers mats were successfully fabricated from chitosan/PVA/β-cyclodextrin (CH/PVA/β-CD) solution with

**TABLE 15.1**
**Active Substances-Loaded Nanofibers of Interest for Potential Active Food Packaging**

| Wall Material/Matrix | Active Substance | Packaging Material | References |
|---|---|---|---|
| PVA | R(+) limonene | – | Camerlo et al. (2013) |
| Zein | Cinnamaldehyde | PHBV | Cerqueira et al. (2016) |
| PLA | Cinnamon essential oil-β-cyclodextrin | – | Wen et al. (2016) |
| Chitosan-PVA | Cinnamon essential oil-β-cyclodextrin<br>Oregano essential oil-β-cyclodextrin | – | Munhuweyi et al. (2018) |
| PLA | Cyclodextrin-linalool inclusión complex | – | Aytac et al. (2017) |
| PCL, corn starch-sodium caseinate | Carvacrol | – | Tampau et al. (2017) |
| PEO | Liposome-eugenol-$SiO_2$ | – | Cui et al. (2017) |
| WPI, zein, SPI | α-Tocopherol | Wheat gluten | Fabra et al. (2016) |
| PCL | α-Tocopherol | – | Dumitriu et al. (2017) |
| PUL-CMC | Tea polyphenols | – | Shao et al. (2018) |
| PHBV | ZnO | PHBV | Castro-Mayorga et al. (2017) |

*Note:* PVA, poly(vinyl alcohol); PHBV, polyhydroxybutyrate-co-valerate; PLA, poly(lactic acid); PCL, polycaprolactone; PEO, polyethylene oxide; WPI, whey protein isolate; SPI, soy protein isolate; PUL-CMC, pullulan-carboxymethylcellulose sodium.

cinnamon and oregano essential oils (Munhuweyi et al. 2018). Three types of modified cyclodextrins were also used to electrospin nanofibrous webs of cyclodextrin/linalool-inclusion complex (CD/linalool-IC-NFs) obtaining high loading capacity and preserving the antimicrobial properties of linalool (Aytac et al. 2017). A different approach was evaluated for preservation of properties of volatile substances and getting better physicochemical properties and physical stability during processing and storage. Eugenol, a volatile and thermally instable substance, was encapsulated in liposomes and subsequently absorbed onto silica nanoparticles ($SiO_2$) before immobilization in polyethylene oxide (PEO) nanofibers (Cui et al. 2017). The physical stability of liposomes containing $SiO_2$-eugenol was significantly improved by the presence of the silica nanoparticles. Liposomes containing $SiO_2$-eugenol-loaded electrospun nanofibrous membranes exhibited excellent antioxidant activity on beef.

The encapsulation of antioxidant compounds in hydrocolloid-based fibers have been reported as potential systems for the development of bioactive packaging materials. A strong natural antioxidant molecule, α-tocopherol, was encapsulated in whey protein isolate (WPI), zein, and soy protein isolate (SPI) nanofibers which were directly electrospun as a coating onto on wheat gluten films (Fabra et al. 2016). The hydrocolloid matrices were able to protect the antioxidant compound from degradation during a typical sterilization process and affect the release of the antioxidant to aqueous media. More recently, tea polyphenols have been incorporated into pullulan-carboxymethylcellulose sodium solutions for obtaining active electrospun nanofiber films (Shao et al. 2018). As expected, the morphology of fibers was tuned by adjusting relevant process parameters (concentration of polymer solution, applied voltage, and feeding rate). In packaging tests performed using strawberries as model, after 10 days of storage at 4°C the quality of fruit was improved when protected with the pullulan-carboxymethylcellulose sodium packaging. The findings demonstrate a facile packaging route to improve food sustainability and reduce waste.

Nanosized inorganic particles have been also assessed for potential antimicrobial food packaging applications due to their processing convenience (high thermal resistance), strong antimicrobial performance, and high surface to volume ratio that allows to enhance the antimicrobial effect at low concentration. Zinc oxide (ZnO) nanoparticles were incorporated into PHBV nanofibers and subsequently used as coating of PHBV films (Castro-Mayorga et al. 2017). The authors confirmed a suitable distribution of ZnO within the PHBV fibers and some loss of transparency regarding neat PHBV film. However, the active film exhibited suitable release of zinc (below 25 mg/Kg food simulant imposed by the European Union [EU] regulation) (European Commission 2011) and bactericidal effect against *L. monocytogenes*.

#### 15.1.2.2 Encapsulated Food Components

Consumers' interest in the relationship between diet, well-being, and health has increased the demand for information and offer of functional foods since the early 1990s (Ayelén Vélez et al. 2017) and represents a sustainable trend in a multi-niche market. Functional foods provide consumers with an alternative way to achieve a healthy lifestyle that differs from conventional healthy diets. Electrospinning of biopolymers for the encapsulation of food ingredients, enzymes, probiotics, and other active compounds related to food industry, has been intensely studied over the last years, but drastically increased recently because of the market trends, being the preservation of active compounds the most widely investigated topic (Faridi Esfanjani and Jafari 2016, Ghorani and Tucker 2015, López-Rubio et al. 2012, Nedovic et al. 2011). The advantages of electrospinning technique are not only the production of very thin fibers with large surface areas, but also the possibility of large-scale productions combined with the simplicity of the process. Natural biopolymers, proteins, and carbohydrates are commonly used as wall materials not only because their sustained release behavior of the incorporated compound and biocompatibility, but also because they are often in themselves valuable dietary supplements and functional food enhancers (Ghorani and Tucker 2015). Common protein-based wall materials used for electrospinning and electrospraying are WPI, whey protein concentrate (WPC), soy isolate, gelatin, zein, and casein. Common polysaccharides used in electrohydrodynamic processing (EHDP) are chitosan, alginates, cellulose, and its derivatives. Synthetic polymers such as PEO or PVA, when combined with biopolymers, improve the fiber forming ability of the blended solution (Anu Bhushani and Anandharamakrishnan 2014). Table 15.2 displays some of the most recent studies involving the immobilization of substances for potential applications as food additives.

**TABLE 15.2**
**Encapsulation of Food Components, Additives, and Nutraceutics in Electrospun Nanofibers**

| Matrix | Food Substance/Additive/ Nutraceutic | References |
|---|---|---|
| PEO/gelatin | Catechin | Nagir and Spriani (2017) |
| PVA/PEO | β-Carotene-nanoliposomes | De Freitas Zômpero et al. (2015) |
| Zein | Omega-3 | Moomand and Lim (2014) |
| Zein-PVP | Omega-3 | Yang et al. (2017b) |
| Zein | Omega-3–ferulic acid | Yang et al. (2017a) |
| Zein | β-carotene | Fernandez et al. (2009) |
| Zein | Tannin from *S. adstringens* bark | de Oliveira Mori et al. (2014) |
| Zein | Gallic acid | Neo et al. (2013) |
| PVA | Fish oil | García-Moreno et al. (2016) |
| PUL-amaranth protein isolate | Quercetin, ferulic acid | Aceituno-Medina et al. (2015) |
| – | HPβCD-Vitamin E inclusion complex | Celebioglu and Uyar (2017) |
| – | Cineole-cyclodextrine inclusion complex<br>p-Cymene-cyclodextrine inclusión complex | Celebioglu et al. (2017) |
| PVA | *B. animalis* Bb12 | López-Rubio et al. (2009) |
| PEC-PUL | *Lactobacillus rhamnosus GG* | Liu et al. (2016) |

PUL, pullulan; HPβCD, hydroxypropyl-β-cyclodextrin; PEC, pectin.

Catechin-gelatin nanofibers were obtained by electrospinning process with PEO as spinnability improver polymer (Nasir and Apriani 2017). The obtained nanofibers showed to have very smooth morphology (no beads), and any chemical changes in the chemical structure of fiber components were also discarded by FTIR analysis. In order to overcome the limitations of using β-carotene in water-based formulations regarding to the hydrophobic nature and low photostability of the substance, β-carotene-loaded nanoliposomes were incorporated into polyvinyl alcohol (PVA) and PEO nanofibers (de Freitas Zômpero et al. 2015). FTIR analysis and liposomal release studies confirmed the presence of phospholipid molecules inside the electrospun fibers. In further research activities, this kind of hybrid structure can be obtained by substitution of a part of polymer (PEO and PVA) by suitable protein food-grade wall materials.

Encapsulation in zein electrospun nanofibers has shown to be an efficient strategy for protecting fish oil and omega-3 fatty acids against oxidative degradation, to avoid undesirable fishy odor when used as nutraceutical, and to preserve their nutritional properties until incorporation in food preparations. Zein is a maize storage prolamine of great interest in many industrial applications such as food, food coating, and food packaging, but also in encapsulation of bioactive substances for generation of

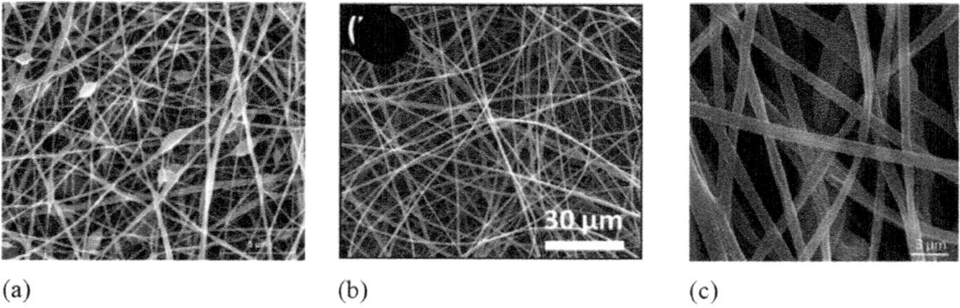


(a) (b) (c)

**FIGURE 15.3** Encapsulated food components in microfibers: (a) SEM micrograph of PVA electrospun fibers containing *Bifidobacterium animalis* Bb12 obtained through coaxial electrospinning. (Reprinted with permission from López-Rubio, A. et al., *Biomacromolecules*, 10, 2823–2829, 2009. Copyright 2009 American Chemical Society). (b) Representative SEM image of Vitamin E/HPβCD-IC nanofiber. (Reprinted with permission from Celebioglu, A. and Uyar, T. 2017. *J. Agric. Food Chem.* 65, 5404–5412, 2017. Copyright 2017 American Chemical Society. (c) Morphological characterization via SEM of zein fibers with 30% fish oil loading. (Adapted from Moomand and Lim 2014. With permission.)

electrospun nanofibers with unique features and properties (Fernandez et al. 2009, Moomand and Lim 2014, Parris et al. 2005, Torres-Giner et al. 2008). Moomand and Lim (2014) reported high encapsulation efficiency of fish oil in zein fibers and greater oxidative stability in comparison to non-encapsulated fish oil (Figure 15.3). Yang et al. (2017b) improved the oxidative and thermal stability of fish oil by encapsulation in zein-polyvinylpyrrolidone (PVP) nanofibers obtained by coaxial electrospinning. Even though the oxidative stability of encapsulated fish oil in the coaxial nanofibers was enhanced, the release behavior of encapsulated fish oil was significantly less than that of single nanofibers. Ferulic acid was incorporated to zein and fish oil solution to fabricate composite single nanofibrous mat (Yang et al. 2017a). The addition of ferulic acid into the nanofibrous mat not only improved the oxidative stability of encapsulated fish oil, but also increased the nutritional value of the nanofibrous mat due to the synergic effect of fish oil and ferulic acid. Zein has been also used for encapsulation of other functional agents of interest in food applications. β-Carotene was incorporated in zein nanofibers for protection against the oxidation and provide an alternative for nutraceutical formulations (Fernandez et al. 2009). Tannin from *Stryphnodendron adstringens* bark was also encapsulated in zein nanofibers in order to protect the compound antimicrobial activity during potential food applications (de Oliveira Mori et al. 2014). Gallic acid was successfully incorporated into zein ultra-fine fibers (Neo et al. 2013). The produced fibers exhibit nanosized diameters, and antioxidant assays showed that gallic acid retained its antioxidant activity after incorporation in zein electrospun fibers. Fish oil was encapsulated via emulsion electrospinning in PVA nanofibers, using WPI or fish protein hydrolysate (FPH) as emulsifiers (García-Moreno et al. 2016). Independently of the emulsifier used, PVA concentration had a high influence on fiber morphology: fibers without bead defects were only produced for solutions with 10.5% PVA. High omega-3 encapsulation efficiency was obtained for fibers produced from PVA emulsion blend stabilized with WPI, but with low oil load capacity. Moreover, the encapsulated oil was randomly distributed as small droplets inside the fibers. However, the electrospun fibers presented a higher content of hydroperoxides and secondary oxidation products compared to emulsified and unprotected fish oil.

Besides common wall materials, other materials are being studied because of their local availability and nutritional properties. For instance, quercetin and ferulic acid were incorporated into a blend of pullulan-amaranth protein isolate ultra-thin fibers, being amaranth a traditional Mexican crop with high nutritional value (Aceituno-Medina et al. 2015). The authors obtained a sustained release of both antioxidants from fibers and observed that substances kept to a greater extent their antioxidant capacity in comparison with the non-encapsulated compounds.

The electrospinnability of cyclodextrins has been taken into consideration because their ability to form inclusion complexes with functional food substances, as well as the stability and sustained release from these complexes. Similarly to common polymeric systems, factors such as type of solvent used, solution concentration, and intermolecular interaction between cyclodextrin molecules play an important role in the electrospinning process of fibers (Anu Bhushani and Anandharamakrishnan 2014). These functional fibers may find practical application in the food industry. The electrospinning of polymer-free nanofibrous mats from inclusion complex (IC) between hydroxypropyl-β-cyclodextrin (HPβCD) and vitamin E was demonstrated (Celebioglu and Uyar 2017) (Figure 15.3). The authors observed that, while pure vitamin E is insoluble in water, vitamin E/HPβCD-IC nanofibers displayed fast-dissolving behavior, which greatly enhanced the antioxidant activity of vitamin E. Additionally; vitamin E/HPβCD-IC nanofibers provided enhanced photo-stability for the highly sensitive vitamin E even after exposure to UV-light. Electrospun nanofibers containing cineole and p-cymene-cyclodextrin IC exhibited fast-dissolving behavior in water and enhanced thermal stability (Celebioglu et al. 2017).

Despite not being a nanometric example, probiotics have been used in supplements and food preparations for a long time. Viability and stability of probiotic bacteria during food processing and storage, as well as their survival while passing upper gastrointestinal tract, is a challenge for the food industry (Ghorani and Tucker 2015). In that regard, coaxial electrospinning of PVA was also applied for the encapsulation and stabilization of the bifidobacterial strain *B. animalis* Bb12 (López-Rubio et al. 2009) (see Figure 15.3). The obtained electrospun fibers showed lower melting point and crystallinity, but higher glass transition temperature compared to net PVA fibers. Results also shown that encapsulated strain within the electrospun PVA fibers remained viable up to 130 days, depending on the storage conditions. Liu et al. (2016) used an aqueous solution containing pectin (PEC) and pullulan (PUL) for encapsulation of probiotic bacteria *Lactobacillus rhamnosus* GG as a model of bioactive compound. The electrospun PEC/PUL fibers containing the bacteria were cross-linked by soaking in a saline solution. Bacteria showed 90% viability after electrospinning and cross-linking, which demonstrates the potential use of edible polysaccharides as bacteria carriers, even though further research needs to be carried out to determine the bacteria viability in storage.

Electrospray capsules are generally preferred over electrospun fibers for food and nutraceutical applications, since apart from facilitating handling and subsequent incorporation into different products, they also present greater surface to volume ratio and, thus, are expected to have better release profiles than fibers

(Hong et al. 2008). Bulk additives such as vitamins, antioxidants, preservatives, and more recently functional components, are added to food preparations to improve the food product itself and to provide benefits beyond basic nutrition. Most nanotechnology applications in food production are addressed to improve the stability of food during processing and storage, to enhance product characteristics, or to increase the potency and bioavailability of nutrients in the food (Peters et al. 2016). Functional ingredients such as carotenoids, probiotics, fish oils, proteins, and peptides have been incorporated in nanodelivery systems to improve their bioavailability, functionality, and stability (Pathakoti et al. 2017). By reducing the particle size of ingredients via encapsulation, solubility can be improved through an increase of the surface area-to-volume ratio, leading to an increase in bio-accessibility (He and Hwang 2016). Table 15.3 shows the latest publications related to encapsulation of food components, additives, and nutraceutics in electrosprayed capsules.

Electrospraying has been deeply used to obtain nanocapsules of bioactive agents for enhancing their stability and functionality. It seems there is no limitation in terms of the substance to encapsulate or wall materials that can be used. However, the encapsulation matrices intended for food incorporation or food-contact articles should contain food-grade ingredients, generally recognized as safe (GRAS) substances or authorized substances (Anu Bhushani and Anandharamakrishnan 2014).

**TABLE 15.3**
**Latest Publications Related to Encapsulation of Food Components, Additives, and Nutraceutics in Electrosprayed Capsules**

| Matrix | Food Substance/Additive/ Nutraceutic | References |
|---|---|---|
| Gelatin | EGCG | Gómez-Mascaraque et al. (2015) |
| Zein | *Sarcopoterium spinosum* extract | Faridi Esfanjani and Jafari (2016) |
| Zein | Curcumin | Gómez-Estaca et al. (2012) |
| Gelatin, zein | Green tea extract | Gómez-Mascaraque et al. (2017) |
| Bacterial cellulose, proteins | EGCG | Paximada et al. (2017) |
| Chocolate | – | Luo et al. (2012) |
| Cocoa butter | – | Bocanegra et al. (2005) |
| Stearic acid | Ethylvanillin | Eltayeb et al. (2016) |
| Gelatin, WPC, SPI | α-Linolenic acid | Gómez-Mascaraque and López-Rubio (2016) |
| WPC, PUL | *Bifidobacterium* strains | López-Rubio et al. (2012) |
| WPC | *Lactobacillus plantarum* | Gómez-Mascaraque et al. (2016b) |
| Alginate, zein | *Lactobacillus acidophilus* | Laelorspoen et al. (2014) |
| Sodium alginate-citric pectin | *Lactobacillus plantarum* | Coghetto et al. (2016) |
| PVP, PVA, barley starch, maltodextrin, WPC | *Aloe vera* juice | Torres-Giner et al. (2017) |

Common food grade substances for encapsulation of bioactives are proteins, polysaccharides, but also combinations of materials to improve the processability of materials, encapsulation efficiency, and stability of the contained bioactive.

In this sense, electrospraying has been used for nanoencapsulation of a wide range of bioactive products of interest in controlled delivery. For instance, antioxidants such as epigallocatechin gallate (EGCG) was encapsulated in gelatin nanocapsules with almost 100% encapsulating efficiency (Gómez-Mascaraque et al. 2015). Paximada et al. (2017) applied emulsion electrospray as one-step technique to produce EGCG-loaded sub-micron particles bacterial cellulose and protein blends. They studied the stability of EGCG at different storage conditions and found that the capsules tend to collapse at high relative humidity, but encapsulation provides EGCG great stability at neutral and basic conditions, and at 37°C/60°C, comparatively with non-encapsulated EGCG. *Sarcopoterium spinosum* extract is a phenolic-rich extract, and its bioavailability and stability were enhanced by encapsulation in zein nanoparticles produced by electrospray (Faridi Esfanjani and Jafari 2016). Green tea extract was encapsulated within electrosprayed gelatin and zein microparticles (Gómez-Mascaraque et al. 2017). The extract encapsulation efficiency resulted around 90% and showed to be effective in stabilization of the catechins during thermal treatment (180°C, 12 min). The green tea microcapsules were added to a food preparation, but no significant protection of the extract was allowed during the food preparation. Emulsion electrospraying of gelatin, WPC, and a SPI was applied for the microencapsulation and enhanced protection of α-linolenic acid as model of thermosensitive hydrophobic bioactive, achieving microencapsulation efficiencies of up to 67% (Gómez-Mascaraque and López-Rubio 2016). More recently, Torres-Giner et al. (2017) also used a pilot line equipment to nanoencapsulate *aloe vera* juice in both synthetic polymer nanofibers, i.e., PVP and PVA, and naturally occurring polymers, i.e., barley starch (BS), maltodextrin, and WPC.

Electrospray has turned out to be an effective method to encapsulate aqueous-based food ingredients such as flavors and aromas, but also suitable for processing of chocolate, colorants, or other food ingredients (Bocanegra et al. 2005). This is an interesting approach taking into account that new techniques prevail in the *haute cuisine* and can be a strategy to help professional chefs to innovate in a highly demanding market. Even though some systems obtained using electrospray are not in the nano-range, they deserve to be mentioned because of the potentiality of the technique for being applied in non-scientific or technological fields. Chocolate microspheres were obtained through electrospray process, and the effects of process parameters such as sugar concentration, addition of electrolytes, flow rate, applied voltage, and collection distance on the production and morphology of as-sprayed chocolate particles were studied (Luo et al. 2012). Cocoa butter microcapsules containing an aqueous solution or an oil-in-water emulsion containing sugar, colorants, and emulsifiers, were produced via coaxial electrospray (Bocanegra et al. 2005).

Parameters such as thickness of the shell or number of inner cores in the microcapsules were easily controlled by properly adjusting the flow rates. In those particular cases, nanosized particles were not required since the detectable size in the tongue is around 20 μm (Weidner 2009). Electrospray was also used to encapsulate curcumin into zein nanoparticles for tuning chromaticities of milk-based products through the addition of various amounts of these nanoparticles (Gómez-Estaca et al. 2012). Ethylvanillin (EV) was encapsulated in core-shell nanoparticles by using stearic acid, both substances are representatives of typical hydrophobic coating and hydrophilic flavor component of the food industry (Eltayeb et al. 2016). The resulting nanoparticles exhibited a core-shell structure, and the thickness of the outer layer depended on the concentration of lipid in the processed solution. The release of EV was consistent with the diffusion through a lipid membrane model.

When probiotics are added to food products, they may lose their viability, thus several techniques for the microencapsulation of cells have been attempted as a form of cell protection. Some studies reported the microencapsulation as an alternative for the encapsulation/protection of probiotics, protecting cells against environmental stress such as extreme pH, temperature, excessive salinity, and enzyme degradation, thus increasing the cell viability (Coghetto et al. 2016, Nualkaekul and Charalampopoulos 2011). New technologies for microencapsulation of bacteria are being developed, however, electrospray has emerged as very convenient because enables the production of small capsules varying from the micro to the sub-micro sizes. Due to the micrometric size of bacteria, nanoencapsulation of bacteria is not possible. Despite of the advantages of electrospraying as a method for the protection of probiotics, research efforts are still needed to minimize the viability loss observed during the processing of sensitive strains and to maximize productivity (Gómez-Mascaraque et al. 2016). *Bifidobacterium* strains encapsulation has been carried out through electrospraying using WPC and PUL (López-Rubio et al. 2012). WPC showed to have greater protective ability as encapsulation material than PUL, as it effectively prolonged the viability of cells even at high relative humidity. It was found that electrospraying processing can reduce in some extension the viability of non-commercial probiotic cultures. Beside this, the process parameters and the properties of the probiotic feed suspension have an impact on the productivity of the electrospraying technique, as expected in EHD processes (Gómez-Mascaraque et al. 2016, López-Rubio et al. 2012). *Lactobacillus plantarum* was used as model probiotic microorganism for the optimization of the microencapsulation electrospraying conditions in WPC matrix (Gómez-Mascaraque et al. 2016). The results showed that the increase of applied voltage, surfactant concentration, and prebiotic addition, increased the product yield. Bacterial viability, on the other hand, remained below 1 log10 CFU/g in all tests.

The survival of encapsulated probiotic at simulated digestive process conditions has been also studied. For instance, *Lactobacillus acidophilus* was encapsulated by using a combination of techniques, electrospraying and alcoholic zein solution acidification, in alginate-zein core-shell microcapsules (Laelorspoen et al. 2014). The proposed technique helped to improve the survival of encapsulated probiotics in simulated gastric fluids up to 5-folds, thus demonstrating the potential for effective probiotics delivery vehicle in gastro intestinal-tract. Electrospraying was used to microencapsulate *Lactobacillus plantarum* in sodium alginate or in sodium alginate-citric pectin matrixes (Coghetto et al. 2016). The survival of immobilized cells was tested at simulated gastric acid and intestinal juices. Results showed lower viability reduction in the immobilized cells respecting the control when exposed to gastric acid and intestinal juices as well as a survival of 21 days under refrigeration storage. Librán et al. (2017) presented a new encapsulation concept to enhance the viability of freeze-dried probiotic strains based on electrospraying. This method, termed *electrospray coating atomization* (*ECA*), consisted in electrospraying a homogeneous coating of ultra-fine particles of different food hydrocolloids on freeze-dried powder of a probiotic strain. PVP was used as pharma-approved reference material. Both protected and uncoated microorganisms were stored at different conditions, and significant enhanced survivability of the coated freeze-dried strain was found during storage at stressing conditions in comparison with the uncoated counterpart (see Figure 15.4).

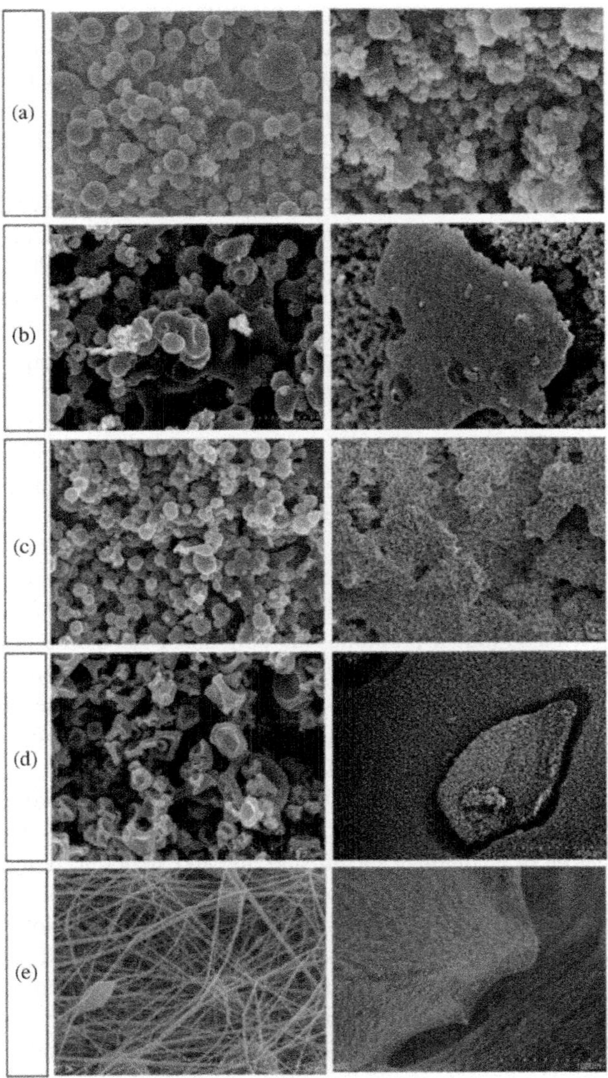


**FIGURE 15.4** Scanning electron microscopy images of the electrosprayed biomaterials (left column) and freeze-dried microorganisms ECA with the corresponding biopolymer. (a–e): WPC, Fibersol®, maltodextrin, zein ,and PVP, respectively. (Reprinted with permission from Librán, C.M. et al., *Innov. Food Sci. Emerg. Technol.*, 39, 216–222, 2017.)

#### 15.1.2.3 Nanosensors

Food products are susceptible to contamination by microorganisms, which are responsible of many foodborne diseases in humans, as well as to lose their nutritional properties due to temperature variations during storage and distribution stages. Traditional passive packaging systems protect food products from moisture, contamination, and spoilage, acting as a passive barrier against external agents. However, the passive packaging systems fail to address increasing concerns of food safety (Kumar et al. 2017). Intelligent packaging provides information about the product quality and involves internal and external indicators that monitor interaction between the food, the packaging, and the environment (Fuertes et al. 2016). The package will provide information not only about the product itself, but will also be able to inform about the history of the product (storage conditions, headspace composition, microbial growth, etc.) (Realini and Marcos 2014). The intelligent function can be obtained by indicators, sensors, and/or devices able to communicate information about the packaging system (Realini and Marcos 2014).

Nanotechnology enables the application of nanosensors in smart food packaging to control their quality, during the various stages of the logistic process, and to ensure product quality to the final consumer (Pathakoti et al. 2017). The design and preparation of an optimum interface between the biocomponent and the detector material is the major challenge as well as the key part of sensor development (Kossek et al. 1996). In this context, nanostructured substrates for nanosensors with large surface can be prepared by electrospinning (Li et al. 2006). Li et al. developed a preliminary biosensor to detect *E. coli* DNA using an electrospun PLA nanofiber membrane as substrate (Li et al. 2006). Mihindukulasuriya and Lim developed an ultraviolet oxygen indicator based on $TiO_2$ nanoparticles by electrospinning (Mihindukulasuriya and Lim 2013). The electrospun indicators were more sensitive to ultraviolet irradiation than the continuous film indicators prepared by casting.

Another characteristic of the smart food packaging is the capacity for energy storage. For instance, biodegradable matrices such as polycaprolactone (PCL), PLA, and zein have been used to encapsulate a phase changing material (PCM), specifically dodecane, by means of electrospinning technique for the development of coating materials with energy storage capacity for thermal insulation applications (Perez-Masia et al. 2013a, 2013b). Chalco-Sandoval et al. also studied the temperature buffering capacity of nanostructured materials containing PCM (Chalco-Sandoval et al. 2015). They developed polystyrene (PS)-based multilayer structures using PCL for the encapsulation of a commercial blend of paraffins as PCM, by applying high throughput electrohydrodynamic processing. In a further study, it was developed a PS foam tray prototype containing an ultra-thin fiber-structured PS/PCM coating for providing heat management capacity to the packaging system (Chalco-Sandoval et al. 2017) (see Figure 15.5). The results showed high encapsulation efficiency of the PCM inside the PS matrix and superior heat storage capacity of the developed material. These results encourage to perform additional investigation to improve the efficiency of the developed materials.

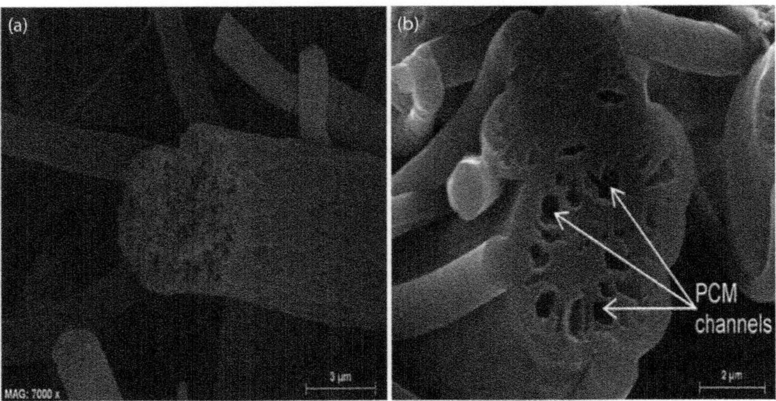


**FIGURE 15.5** Surface (a) and cross-section (b) SEM images of the PS tray with the ultra-thin fiber-structured PS/PCM coating. Scale markers correspond to 20 and 200 mm for the surface and cross-section, respectively. (Reprinted with permission from Chalco-Sandoval, W. et al., *J. Food Eng.*, 192, 122–128, 2017.)

#### 15.1.2.4 Nano-food

The demand for meat and milk protein is growing as world population is increasing, and it is getting more and more difficult to meet the demand of nutritionally complete protein (containing all essential amino acids). Appetizing alternatives for meat, which are nutritionally, texturally, and taste-wise appealing, are necessary to feed the world population in the longer term (Nieuwland et al. 2013). Even though there are alternative sources of protein from plants and insects containing high quality proteins as well, developing palatable products is, however, still a challenge. Electrospinning of fibrillar structures from food grade biopolymers is an interesting technological alternative because production of foods with novel textures, foods from renewable resources, special foods with concentrated food component(s), or enhanced bioavailability of the components may be possible (Liu et al. 2016). As protein replacer, the food-grade mat should be made from biopolymers, be edible, not require the use of toxic solvents, and able to be electrospun to give fibers without the need to introduce man-made polymers in the mixture. The mechanisms behind the electrospinning of proteins, as well as the properties of the obtained fibers have been deeply studied (Dror et al. 2008, Ramji and Shah 2014, Tonda-Turo et al. 2013, Wang et al. 2014, Wu et al. 2016). In general, proteins must be more or less unfolded depending on their specific nature and several parameters must be taken into account to process them, i.e., solvent, addition of denaturing agents, and heat (Mendes et al. 2017). The limitations related to fiber stability in aqueous media and sufficient mechanical strength can be improved by cross-linking or by addition of polymers to the fiber matrix. However, as far as it is known, very few studies have been carried out in order to obtain edible electrospun mats for protein-based food products replacement purposes. This is mainly due to the limitations of using food-grade solvents, cross-linkers, and carriers to achieve processability and suitable fiber properties.

The feasibility of obtaining aligned fibers in a food-grade way by means of electrospinning from globular proteins was demonstrated using gelatin as a carrier polymer (Nieuwland et al. 2013). The spun fibrils, of interest for meat replacers, were soluble in water. In order to use these protein fibers in a food product, the solubility has to be decreased, e.g., by cross-linking using food-grade reagents, such as ferulic acid, or enzymes and glucose (Han and Zhao 2016). Zein and gelatin were mixed with protein (sodium caseinate, WP, ovalbumin) to test their ability as carriers to these proteins for electrospinning under food-grade conditions (Heuvel et al. 2013) The results showed that zein is a poor carrier of proteins for electrospinning while gelatin was able to form fibers with up to 17.5% whey protein content. This demonstrates an opportunity to fabricate meat substitutes that mimic the texture and bite of meat, but further research must be done in this area.

## 15.2 CONSUMERS' ATTITUDE TOWARD NANOTECHNOLOGY IN FOOD-RELATED PRODUCTS

Nanomaterials are being currently used in food industry to impart foods improved organoleptic properties (Amenta et al. 2015, Camerlo et al. 2013, Luo et al. 2012), shelf life extension through active and passive agents in packaging materials (Busolo and Lagaron 2015, Cui et al. 2017, Fernandez et al. 2009, Garber 2006, Realini and Marcos 2014, Torres-Giner et al. 2017), and other nutritional qualities such as antioxidant or specific bioactive compounds to be delivered in a controlled way (García-Moreno et al. 2017, Gómez-Estaca et al. 2012, Moomand and Lim 2014). The global nanocapsules market size was valued at USD 1.9 billion in 2015 and is expected to increase by 7.9% over the next 10 years (Grand View Research 2017). Healthcare, food, cosmetics, and agriculture industries constitute the major application areas of nanocapsules. The public perception of nanotechnology in general is positive, but at the same time consumers are concerned about its use in food products. They do not have enough information to make decisions and clarify doubts related to the behavior of nanoparticles in the body and the toxic effects they could have (Benetti et al. 2016). Limitations, advantages, and present and potential applications in the food industry are not fully understood, not only by consumers, but also by the scientific community. Research is being mainly focused on the functionality of food nanotechnology, and only a few studies have assessed the potential toxicity by exposure to nanoparticles, either intended or unintended, contained in food products and food packaging (He and Hwang 2016). Taking into account the unique physicochemical and functionality of engineered nanomaterials, they may be responsible for potentially adverse effects because of their undefined biological hazards to environment and humans (Ciappellano et al. 2016, Kulkarni et al. 2016, Manickam et al. 2017). Nanomaterials can be completely metabolized, excreted, or accumulated within the body (Amenta et al. 2015). The potential for genotoxicity is very high among the food and beverage industry as these products are consumed directly. Until now, there are ambiguities, gaps in knowledge or very little information on safe consuming and use of nano-scaled food materials and fortified foods, and their possible side effects in humans (Katouzian and Jafari 2016, Kulkarni et al. 2016). Some aspects in which there is a need to understand the associated risks are: (1) migration patterns of nanoparticles from food contact materials, which may vary depending on the nanoparticle nature and food properties; (2) nanoparticle properties and their behavior in the specific matrix containing them, including stability during the food processing and storage; and (3) fate of ingested nanomaterial: digestion, absorption, bioavailability, metabolism, excretion, and bioaccumulation should be fully understood (Kulkarni et al. 2016). There is an urgent need to study the as-described aspects for complete assessment of the biodistribution properties, toxicological effects, and improper alterations of the nanoengineered materials used in food applications (Katouzian and Jafari 2016).

Toxicity testing of nanomaterials is carried out by using *in vitro* and *in vivo* assays and establishing a dose-response relationship, corresponding to the likelihood of adverse health effects at varying degrees of exposure (Ciappellano et al. 2016). Oxidative stress has been shown to be an underlying mechanism of possible toxicity of nanomaterials, causing both immunotoxicity and genotoxicity (Dusinska et al. 2017). Immunotoxicity can be given by the aggregation of nanosized-particles, which have previously evaded the biological defensive mechanisms, causing the effective sequestering by immune cell. Genotoxicity may have implications for risks of cancer and possibly other chronic diseases, influencing the health not only of individuals, but also of the next generation (Dusinska et al. 2017). The OECD's Working Party on Manufactured Nanomaterials (WPMN) launched on 2007 the Sponsorship Programme for the Testing of Manufactured Nanomaterials to ensure that the tests used to address the safety of manufactured nanomaterials are consistent and defensible. The tests have been analyzed using OECD Guidelines for the Testing of Chemicals and comprise nanomaterial physical-chemical properties, environmental fate, toxicological and eco-toxicological effects, mammalian toxicology, and material safety (OECD 2017). The European Food Safety Authority (EFSA) has developed a practical approach for assessing potential risks arising from applications of nanomaterials in the food and feed chain (Committee 2011). This approach involves a complete guidance for the physicochemical characterization of engineered nanomaterials and testing procedures of *in vitro* genotoxicity, absorption, distribution, metabolism, and excretion and repeated-dose studies in rodents.

Societal and consumer acceptance or rejection of food products involving nanotechnology are barriers both to the implementation of these technological innovations and to their subsequent exploitation and commercialization in the form of tangible food products which can be sold to consumers. It was found that nanotechnology in packaging is perceived as being more beneficial and acceptable than in food preparations (Siegrist et al. 2007). In a study where socio-psychological factors were taken into account, some factors influencing societal acceptability of development and applications of nanotechnology were identified (Gupta et al. 2012). The results showed that general public differentiates nanotechnology applications based on the extent to which they are beneficial, useful, necessary, or real, and also on the extent to which the end user is physically close to them. In addition, it was detected a societal demand for concrete and necessary benefits provided by nanomaterials, so the experts who participated in this study suggested the development of "consumer led" products strategy on the part of the stakeholders for commercialization of nanotechnology. How to create public awareness, handle public perception, and gain consumer trust and acceptance of the use of nanotechnology in the food industry are important challenges. It is important to generate information and make it available for consumers, in order to provide enough information related to risks, but also benefits of products, and to create confidence in actors related to food nanotechnology system (i.e., researchers, food producers, manufacturing companies).

## 15.3 EU REGULATORY FRAMEWORK FOR NANOTECHNOLOGY IN FOOD-RELATED PRODUCTS

Commercially available nutraceuticals containing nanomaterials need to be assessed in terms of their safety, and producers must present relative dossiers to national authorities on demand. Besides the hard law tools represented by European Directives and Regulations, the EFSA provides a soft approach to nanomaterials safety regulation through scientific opinions, the risk assessment guidelines, and the technical support to companies and notifiers. These activities are carried out as an independent authority and under the law, they are influencing the EU approach toward nanosafety in food. For this, it is necessary to establish a set of protocols and regulations on the food security.

There are a few studies related to the potential toxicity of the presence of nanomaterials in foods and food packaging even though the human exposure to nanomaterials is expected to increase. Little is known about the bioavailability, biodistribution, routes of nanomaterials, and the ultimate toxicity upon exposure to them (He and Hwang 2016). Nanocapsules that are used as food additives come in direct contact with human organs, which may result in higher levels of exposure depending on their concentration in food and the amount of food consumed. The Danish Environmental Protection Agency (Danish Ministry of the Environment 2015) found a relatively high potential for consumer exposure in the Danish market to nanomaterials in food and beverages, coming from nano-ingredients, food supplements, and nanomaterials in packaging. The primary exposure route is oral, as the products are intended to be ingested. Metallic elements (silver, platinum, palladium, and gold) claimed to be in nano-form as food supplements were identified in the range of 10 to <500 ppm. Some coloring or anticaking additives were determined to possibly contain nanoparticles of silicon dioxide, titanium dioxide, calcium carbonate, and vegetable carbon. In the Danish study, a nanomaterial exposure up to 3 mg/kg of body weight has been estimated due to the content of nanosized particles in these additives.

European Commission published in December 18, 2013, a proposal for a regulation on novel foods, which also addresses engineered nanomaterials. These nanomaterials, in accordance with Regulation EU 1169/2011, must be assessed and authorized under the proposed regulation before marketing. The new regulation does not contemplate the use of nanomaterials in food contact materials, which continue to require individual authorization by the European Commission under regulation EC 10/2011. However, the present regulation forms part of an integrated effort of adapting EU laws to the new challenges posed by the use of engineered nanomaterials.

The EFSA established in 2010 the Network for Risk Assessment of Nanotechnologies in Food and Feed ("Nano Network") in order to enhance cooperation with EU Member States on nanomaterials. Nano Network facilitates the exchange of information between EFSA and Member States, as well as the prioritization of risk assessment activities (European Food Safety and Schoonjans 2016).

In the last Nano Network meeting, held in 2016 in Madrid, the creation of a new working group to update its 2011 guidance on risk assessment of nanotechnologies in food and feed as well as the potential to launch a COST action on nanomaterials in food were discussed. A public consultation on the draft guidance regarding nanotechnologies risk assessment is planned in 2018. Following the discussions at the 2016 Nano Network Meeting, a list of research proposals under H2020 relating specifically to nanomaterials in food (i.e., measuring the physicochemical properties in food matrices, *in vitro* digestion, and bioavailability/toxicity of engineered nanomaterials in the food matrix) was analyzed. As such, the use of nanomaterials in food is at present underrepresented in the spectrum of ongoing and scheduled EU research activities (European Food Safety and Schoonjans 2016).

Rauscher et al. have reviewed the regulatory aspects of nanomaterials in the European Union (Rauscher et al. 2017). There is not a regulatory framework for the use of engineered nanomaterials for food contact materials in the EU, and the EFSA scientific committees sustain that a case-by-case approach. This is, nanomaterials used in food contact materials must be explicitly authorized and a specific risk assessment is required (Rauscher et al. 2017).

The unusual physicochemical properties of engineered nanomaterials are attributable to their small size, chemical composition, surface structure, solubility, shape, and aggregation (Arora et al. 2012). As a result, their properties differ substantially from the bulk material with the same composition as conductivity, reactivity, and optical sensitivity. Possible adverse results of these features are harmful interactions with biological systems and the environment, with the potential to generate toxicity. As the size of a particle decreases, its surface area increases and also allows a greater proportion of its atoms or molecules to be displayed on the surface rather than the interior of the material (Nel et al. 2006). As with any other man-made materials, both *in vitro* and *in vivo* studies on biological effects of nanoparticles need to be performed (Arora et al. 2012). Their use in food and pharmaceutics is more diversified and difficult to assess. Nanomaterials made from biological molecules such as lipids, sugars, or proteins, are intended to encapsulate fragile molecules such as flavors or vitamins to protect them during gastrointestinal transit. It is likely interesting, but the risk may be a modification in the intestinal absorption of the active ingredient transported. Metallic nanoparticles are more problematic, their physicochemical properties and, in particular, their surface reactivity are the causes for their biological reactivity and their potential capacity to overcome barriers and penetrate into the organism. These nanometals are able to generate oxidative stress and induce multiple cellular responses including inflammation and genotoxicity (Marano and Guadagnini 2013).

Size is a key factor in evaluating the potential toxicity of a particle. However, it is not the only important factor. Other properties of nanomaterials that influence toxicity include: the shape of the particles, the chemical composition, such as the polymers and surfactants used, as well as the organic solvents used during the synthesis process, solubility, and presence or absence of functional groups of other chemicals (Balogh et al. 2007, Chen et al. 2014, Kotsilkova et al. 2001). The large number of variables influencing toxicity means that it is difficult to generalize about health risks associated with exposure to nanomaterials, since each factor must be assessed individually and all material properties must be taken into account (Chen et al. 2014).

## 15.4 CONCLUSIONS AND FUTURE PERSPECTIVES

The social demand for new products based on nanomaterials has led to the expansion of the nanotechnology market not only in the development of new energetic materials or electronic devices, but also in the healthcare, food, cosmetic, or agrochemical industries, due to the well-known benefits that this new technology could provide with respect to their bulk counterparts. Numerous are the possibilities of applying these new materials in the food sector, from the development of new packaging, to the creation of nanosensors, encapsulated bioactive components, or the incorporation of new ingredients. All of them could contribute to improve the organoleptic properties and/or the nutritional quality of a food product, its shelf life, as well as its food safety. For these reasons, industry is asking for new nano-manufacturing processes, easily scalable and environmentally friendly. In this regard, electrohydrodynamic processes, electrospinning and electrospray, have proven to be an excellent alternative to existing technologies, as they are simple and versatile processes that do not require the use of high temperature or pressure, toxic organic solvents, or expensive equipment. In addition, the availability of equipment for processing from laboratory scale to industrial scale, such as those developed by Bioinicia, ensure a rapid industrial implementation. However, the lack of a global regulatory framework to guide manufacturing, safety use, risk management, and the disposal of these materials is a limiting factor for its industrial application. Nevertheless, the enforcement of the new European regulation of novel foods (EC 2015/2283), and the creation of the European Nano Network, are small advances toward the nanotechnology revolution in the food industry.

## REFERENCES


Aceituno-Medina, Marysol, Sandra Mendoza, José María Lagaron, and Amparo López-Rubio. 2015. "Photoprotection of folic acid upon encapsulation in food-grade amaranth (Amaranthus hypochondriacus L.) protein isolate—Pullulan electrospun fibers." *LWT—Food Science and Technology* 62 (2):970–975. doi:10.1016/j.lwt.2015.02.025.

Ahmed, Ishfaq, Hong Lin, Long Zou, Aaron L. Brody, Zhenxing Li, Ihsan M. Qazi, Tushar R. Pavase, and Liangtao Lv. 2017. "A comprehensive review on the application of active packaging technologies to muscle foods." *Food Control* 82 (Supplement C):163–178. doi:10.1016/j.foodcont.2017.06.009.

Amenta, Valeria, Karin Aschberger, Maria Arena, Hans Bouwmeester, Filipa Botelho Moniz, Puck Brandhoff, Stefania Gottardo et al. 2015. "Regulatory aspects of nanotechnology in the agri/feed/food sector in EU and non-EU countries." *Regulatory Toxicology and Pharmacology* 73 (1):463–476. doi:10.1016/j.yrtph.2015.06.016.

Anu Bhushani, J. and Chinnaswamy Anandharamakrishnan. 2014. "Electrospinning and electrospraying techniques: Potential food based applications." *Trends in Food Science & Technology* 38 (1):21–33. doi:10.1016/j.tifs.2014.03.004.

Arora, Sumit, Jyutika M. Rajwade, Kishore M. Paknikar. 2012. "Nanotoxicology and in vitro studies: The need of the hour." *Toxicology and Applied Pharmacology* 258 (2):151–165. doi:10.1016/j.taap.2011.11.010.

Aruna, Singanahally Thippareddy, L. S. Balaji, Shanmugam Senthil Kumar, and B. Shri Prakash. 2017. "Electrospinning in solid oxide fuel cells—A review." *Renewable and Sustainable Energy Reviews* 67:673–682. doi:10.1016/j.rser.2016.09.003.

Ayelén Vélez, María, María Cristina Perotti, Liliana Santiago, Ana María Gennaro, and Erica Hynes. 2017. "6—Bioactive compounds delivery using nanotechnology: Design and applications in dairy food A2—Grumezescu, Alexandru Mihai." In *Nutrient Delivery*, 221–250. Academic Press Elsevier, New York.

Aytac, Zeynep, Zehra Irem Yildiz, Fatma Kayaci-Senirmak, Turgay Tekinay, and Tamer Uyar. 2017. "Electrospinning of cyclodextrin/linalool-inclusion complex nanofibers: Fast-dissolving nanofibrous web with prolonged release and antibacterial activity." *Food Chemistry* 231 (Supplement C):192–201. doi:10.1016/j.foodchem.2017.03.113.

Balogh, Lajos, Shraddha S.Nigavekar, Bindu M.Nair, Wojciech Lesniak, Chunxin Zhang, Lok Yun Sung, Muhammed S.T.Kariapper et al. 2007. "Significant effect of size on the in vivo biodistribution of gold composite nanodevices in mouse tumor models." *Nanomedicine: Nanotechnology, Biology and Medicine* 3 (4):281–296. doi:10.1016/j.nano.2007.09.001.

Benetti, Federico, Christian Micheletti, and Laura Manodori. 2016. "*Regulatory Perspectives on Nanotechnology in Nutraceuticals* --Grumezescu, Alexandru Mihai". In *Nutraceuticals*, pp. 183–230. Academic Press, Elsevier, New York.

Bhardwaj, Nandana, and Subhas Kundu. 2010. "Electrospinning: A fascinating fiber fabrication technique." *Biotechnology Advances* 28, 325–347.

Bioinicia 2017. https://bioinicia.com/.

Bocanegra, Rodrigo, Anikumar G. Gaonkar, Antonio Barrero, Ignacio G. Loscertales, David Pechack, and Manuel Marquez. 2005. "Production of cocoa butter microcapsules Using an electrospray process." *Journal of Food Science* 70 (8):e492–e497. doi:10.1111/j.1365-2621.2005.tb11520.x.

Busolo, María Antonieta, and José María Lagaron. 2015. "Antioxidant polyethylene films based on a resveratrol containing clay of interest in food packaging applications." *Food Packaging and Shelf Life* 6 (Supplement C):30–41. doi:10.1016/j.fpsl.2015.08.004.

Camerlo, Agathe, Corinne Vebert-Nardin, René M. Rossi, and Ana M. Popa. 2013. "Fragrance encapsulation in polymeric matrices by emulsion electrospinning." *European Polymer Journal* 49 (12):3806–3813. doi:10.1016/j.eurpolymj.2013.08.028.

Castro-Mayorga, Jineth Lorena, María José Fabra, Amir Masoud Pourrahimi, Richard. T. Olsson, and José María Lagaron. 2017. "The impact of zinc oxide particle morphology as an antimicrobial and when incorporated in poly(3-hydroxybutyrate-co-3-hydroxyvalerate) films for food packaging and food contact surfaces applications." *Food and Bioproducts Processing* 101:32–44. doi:10.1016/j.fbp.2016.10.007.

Celebioglu, Asli, and Tamer Uyar. 2017. "Antioxidant vitamin E/cyclodextrin inclusion complex electrospun nanofibers: Enhanced water solubility, prolonged shelf life, and photostability of vitamin E." *Journal of Agricultural and Food Chemistry* 65 (26):5404–5412. doi:10.1021/acs.jafc.7b01562.

Celebioglu, Asli, Zehra Irem Yildiz, and Tamer Uyar. 2017. "Electrospun nanofibers from cyclodextrin inclusion complexes with cineole and p-cymene: Enhanced water solubility and thermal stability." *International Journal of Food Science & Technology*. doi:10.1111/ijfs.13564.

Cerqueira, Miguel A., María José Fabra, Jinneth Lorena Castro-Mayorga, Ana I. Bourbon, Lorenzo M. Pastrana, António A. Vicente, and Jose M. Lagaron. 2016. "Use of electrospinning to develop antimicrobial biodegradable multilayer systems: Encapsulation of cinnamaldehyde and their physicochemical characterization." *Food and Bioprocess Technology* 9 (11):1874–1884. doi:10.1007/s11947-016-1772-4.

Chakraborty, Syandan, I. Chien Liao, Andrew Adler, and Kam W. Leong. 2009. "Electrohydrodynamics: A facile technique to fabricate drug delivery systems." *Advanced Drug Delivery Reviews* 61 (12):1043–1054. doi:10.1016/j.addr.2009.07.013.

Chalco-Sandoval, Wilson, María José Fabra, Amparo López-Rubio, and Jose M. Lagaron. 2015. "Development of polystyrene-based films with temperature buffering capacity for smart food packaging." *Journal of Food Engineering* 164 (Supplement C):55–62. doi:10.1016/j.jfoodeng.2015.04.032.

Chalco-Sandoval, Wilson, María José Fabra, Amparo López-Rubio, and Jose M. Lagaron. 2017. "Use of phase change materials to develop electrospun coatings of interest in food packaging applications." *Journal of Food Engineering* 192:122–128. doi:10.1016/j.jfoodeng.2015.01.019.

Chen, Hongda, James N. Seiber, and Matt Hotze. 2014. "ACS select on nanotechnology in food and agriculture: A perspective on implications and applications." *Journal of Agriculture and Food Chemistry* 62 (6):1209–1212. doi:10.1021/jf5002588.

Ciappellano, Silvia Gabriella, Erik Tedesco, Marco Venturini, and Federico Benetti. 2016. "In vitro toxicity assessment of oral nanocarriers." *Advanced Drug Delivery Reviews* 106 (Part B):381–401. doi:10.1016/j.addr.2016.08.007.

Coghetto, Chaline Caren, Graziela Brusch Brinques, Nataly Machado Siqueira, Jéssica Pletsch, Rosane Michele Duarte Soares, and Marco Antônio Záchia Ayub. 2016. "Electrospraying microencapsulation of Lactobacillus plantarum enhances cell viability under refrigeration storage and simulated gastric and intestinal fluids." *Journal of Functional Foods* 24 (Supplement C):316–326. doi:10.1016/j.jff.2016.03.036.

Commission, European. 2011. "Commission Regulation (EU) No 10/2011 of 14 January 2011 on plastic materials and articles intended to come into contact with food." *Official Journal of the European Union*.

Committee, EFSA Scientific. 2011. "Guidance on the risk assessment of the application of nanoscience and nanotechnologies in the food and feed chain." *EFSA Journal* 9 (5). doi:10.2903/j.efsa.2011.2140.

Cui, Haiying, Lu Yuan, Wei Li, and Lin Lin. 2017. "Antioxidant property of $SiO_2$-eugenol liposome loaded nanofibrous membranes on beef." *Food Packaging and Shelf Life* 11 (Supplement C):49–57. doi:10.1016/j.fpsl.2017.01.001.

de Freitas Zômpero, Rafael Henrique, Amparo López-Rubio, Samantha Cristina de Pinho, José María Lagaron, and Lucimara Gaziola de la Torre. 2015. "Hybrid encapsulation structures based on β-carotene-loaded nanoliposomes within electrospun fibers." *Colloids and Surfaces B: Biointerfaces* 134 (Supplement C):475–482. doi:10.1016/j.colsurfb.2015.03.015.

de Oliveira Mori, Cláudia L. S., Nathália Almeida dos Passos, Juliano Elvis Oliveira, Luiz Henrique Capparelli Mattoso, Fábio Akira Mori, Amélia Guimarães Carvalho, Alessandra de Souza Fonseca, and Gustavo Henrique Denzin Tonoli. 2014. "Electrospinning of zein/tannin bio-nanofibers." *Industrial Crops and Products* 52 (Supplement C):298–304. doi:10.1016/j.indcrop.2013.10.047.

Ding, Bin, Moran Wang, Xianfeng Wang, Jianyong Yu, and Gang Sun. 2010. "Electrospun nanomaterials for ultrasensitive sensors." *Materials Today* 13 (11):16–27. doi:10.1016/S1369-7021(10)70200-5.

Dror, Yael, Tamar Ziv, Vadim Makarov, Hila Wolf, Arie Admon, and Eyal Zussman. 2008. "Nanofibers made of globular proteins." *Biomacromolecules* 9 (10):2749–2754. doi:10.1021/bm8005243.

Dumitriu, Raluca P., Geoffrey R. Mitchell, Fred J. Davis, and Cornelia Vasile. 2017. "Functionalized coatings by electrospinning for anti-oxidant food packaging." *Procedia Manufacturing* 12 (Supplement C):59–65. doi:10.1016/j.promfg.2017.08.008.

Dusinska, Maria, Jana Tulinska, Naouale El Yamani, Miroslava Kuricova, Aurelia Liskova, Eva Rollerova, Elise Rundén-Pran, and Bozena Smolkova. 2017. "Immunotoxicity, genotoxicity and epigenetic toxicity of nanomaterials: New strategies for toxicity testing?" *Food and Chemical Toxicology* 109 (Part 1):797–811. doi:10.1016/j.fct.2017.08.030.

Echegoyen, Yolanda, María José Fabra, Jineth Lorena Castro-Mayorga, Adriane Cherpinski, and José María Lagaron. 2017. "High throughput electro-hydrodynamic processing in food encapsulation and food packaging applications: Viewpoint." *Trends in Food Science & Technology* 60:71–79. doi:10.1016/j.tifs.2016.10.019.

Eltayeb, Megdi, Eleanor Stride, Mohan Edirisinghe, and Anthony Harker. 2016. "Electrosprayed nanoparticle delivery system for controlled release." *Materials Science and Engineering: C* 66 (Supplement C):138–146. doi:10.1016/j.msec.2016.04.001.

EUROPEAN COMMISSION. 2011. "COMMISSION REGULATION (EU) No 10/2011 of 14 January 2011 on plastic materials and articles intended to come into contact with food. Official Journal of the European Union 02011R0010-20160914."

European Food Safety, Authority, and Reinhilde Schoonjans. 2016. "Annual report of the EFSA scientific network of risk assessment of nanotechnologies in food and feed for 2016." *EFSA Supporting Publications* 13 (12):1145E. doi:10.2903/sp.efsa.2016.EN-1145.

Fabra, María José, Amparo López-Rubio, and Jose M. Lagaron. 2016. "Use of the electrohydrodynamic process to develop active/bioactive bilayer films for food packaging applications." *Food Hydrocolloids* 55:11–18. doi:10.1016/j.foodhyd.2015.10.026.

Faridi Esfanjani, Afshin, and Seid Mahdi Jafari. 2016. "Biopolymer nano-particles and natural nano-carriers for nano-encapsulation of phenolic compounds." *Colloids Surf B Biointerfaces* 146:532–543. doi:10.1016/j.colsurfb.2016.06.053.

Fernandez, Avelina, Sergio Torres-Giner, and Jose Maria Lagaron. 2009. "Novel route to stabilization of bioactive antioxidants by encapsulation in electrospun fibers of zein prolamine." *Food Hydrocolloids* 23 (5):1427–1432. doi:10.1016/j.foodhyd.2008.10.011.

Fuertes, Guillermo, Ismael Soto, Raul Carrasco, Manuel Vargas, Jorge Sabattin, and Carolina Lagos. 2016. "Intelligent packaging systems: Sensors and nanosensors to monitor food quality and safety." *Journal of Sensors* 2016:8. doi:10.1155/2016/4046061.

Fukui, Yu, Tatsuo Maruyama, Yuko Iwamatsu, Akihiro Fujii, Tsutomu Tanaka, Yoshikage Ohmukai, and Hideto Matsuyama. 2010. "Preparation of monodispersed polyelectrolyte microcapsules with high encapsulation efficiency by an electrospray technique." *Colloids and Surfaces A: Physicochemical and Engineering Aspects* 370 (1):28–34. doi:10.1016/j.colsurfa.2010.08.039.

Garber, C. 2006. "Nanotechnology food coming to a fridge near you." https://www.nanowerk.com/spotlight/spotid=1360.php.

García-Moreno, Pedro J., Necla Özdemir, Karen Stephansen, Ramona V. Mateiu, Yolanda Echegoyen, Jose M. Lagaron, Ioannis S. Chronakis, and Charlotte Jacobsen. 2017. "Development of carbohydrate-based nano-microstructures loaded with fish oil by using electrohydrodynamic processing." *Food Hydrocolloids* 69:273–285. doi:10.1016/j.foodhyd.2017.02.013.

García-Moreno, Pedro J., Karen Stephansen, Jules van der Kruijs, Antonio Guadix, Emilia M. Guadix, Ioannis S. Chronakis, and Charlotte Jacobsen. 2016. "Encapsulation of fish oil in nanofibers by emulsion electrospinning: Physical characterization and oxidative stability." *Journal of Food Engineering* 183 (Supplement C):39–49. doi:10.1016/j.jfoodeng.2016.03.015.

Ghorani, Behrouz, and Nick Tucker. 2015. "Fundamentals of electrospinning as a novel delivery vehicle for bioactive compounds in food nanotechnology." *Food Hydrocolloids* 51:227–240. doi:10.1016/j.foodhyd.2015.05.024.

Gómez-Estaca, Joaquín, Mari Pau Balaguer, Rafael Gavara, and Pilar Hernandez-Munoz. 2012. "Formation of zein nanoparticles by electrohydrodynamic atomization: Effect of the main processing variables and suitability for encapsulating the food coloring and active ingredient curcumin." *Food Hydrocolloids* 28 (1):82–91. doi:10.1016/j.foodhyd.2011.11.013.

Gómez-Mascaraque, Laura G., and Amparo López-Rubio. 2016. "Protein-based emulsion electrosprayed micro- and submicroparticles for the encapsulation and stabilization of thermosensitive hydrophobic bioactives." *Journal of Colloid and Interface Science* 465 (Supplement C):259–270. doi:10.1016/j.jcis.2015.11.061.

Gómez-Mascaraque, Laura G., Russell Cruz Morfin, Rocío Pérez-Masiá, Gloria Sanchez, and Amparo Lopez-Rubio. 2016. "Optimization of electrospraying conditions for the microencapsulation of probiotics and evaluation of their resistance during storage and in-vitro digestion." *LWT—Food Science and Technology* 69 (Supplement C):438–446. doi:10.1016/j.lwt.2016.01.071.

Gómez-Mascaraque, Laura G., Marai Hernández-Rojas, Paula Tarancón, Mathieu Tenon, Nicolas Feuillère, Jorge F. Vélez Ruiz, Susana Fiszman, and Amparo López-Rubio. 2017. "Impact of microencapsulation within electrosprayed proteins on the formulation of green tea extract-enriched biscuits." *LWT—Food Science and Technology* 81 (Supplement C):77–86. doi:10.1016/j.lwt.2017.03.041.

Gómez-Mascaraque, Laura G., José María Lagarón, and Amparo López-Rubio. 2015. "Electrosprayed gelatin submicroparticles as edible carriers for the encapsulation of polyphenols of interest in functional foods." *Food Hydrocolloids* 49 (Supplement C):42–52. doi:10.1016/j.foodhyd.2015.03.006.

Gottschalk, Fadri, Bernd Nowack, Carsten Lassen, Jesper Kjolholt, Frans Christensen, 2015. "Nanomaterials in the Danish Environment. Modelling exposure of the Danish environment to selected nanomaterials." *Environmental project* No. 1639. https://www2.mst.dk/udgiv/publications/2015/01/978-87-93283-60-2.Pdf.

Grand View Research. 2017. http://www.grandviewresearch.com/industry-analysis/global-nanocapsules-market.

Greiner, Andreas, and Joachim H. Wendorff. 2007. "Electrospinning: A fascinating method for the preparation of ultrathin fibers." *Angewandte Chemie International Edition* 46 (30):5670–5703.

Gupta, Nidhi, Arnout R. H. Fischer, Ivo A. van der Lans, and Lynn J. Frewer. 2012. "Factors influencing societal response of nanotechnology: An expert stakeholder analysis." *Journal of Nanoparticle Research* 14 (5):857. doi:10.1007/s11051-012-0857-x.

Han, Yan-Ping, and Xin-Huai Zhao. 2016. "Properties of bovine gelatin cross-linked by a mixture of two oxidases (horseradish peroxidase and glucose oxidase) and glucose." *CyTA—Journal of Food* 14 (3):457–464. doi:10.1080/19476337.2015.1134671.

He, Xiaojia, and Huey-Min Hwang. 2016. "Nanotechnology in food science: Functionality, applicability, and safety assessment." *Journal of Food and Drug Analysis* 24 (4):671–681. doi:10.1016/j.jfda.2016.06.001.

Heuvel, M., P. Geerdink, P. Brier, P. Eijnden, J. Henket, M. Langelaan, N. Stroeks, H. Deventer, and A. Martin. 2013. "Food-grade electrospinning of proteins." *InsideFood Symposium 2013*, Leuven, Belgium., 9–12 April, 2013.

Hong, Youliang, Yanyan Li , Yizi Yin, Dongmei Li, Guangtian Zou. 2008. "Electrohydrodynamic atomization of quasi-monodisperse drug-loaded spherical/wrinkled microparticles." *Journal of Aerosol Science* 39 (6):525–536. doi:10.1016/j.jaerosci.2008.02.004.

Hurme, E., Sipiläinen-Malm Thea, R. Ahvenainen, and T. Nielsen. 2002. "5—Active and intelligent packaging." In *Minimal Processing Technologies in the Food Industries*, pp. 87–123. Woodhead Publishing Cambridge, UK.

Jafari, Seid Mahdi, and David Julian McClements. 2017. "Chapter one—Nanotechnology approaches for increasing nutrient bioavailability." In *Advances in Food and Nutrition Research*, edited by Fidel Toldrá, 1–30. Academic Press, Elservier, New York.

Katouzian, Iman, and Seid Mahdi Jafari. 2016. "Nano-encapsulation as a promising approach for targeted delivery and controlled release of vitamins." *Trends in Food Science & Technology* 53 (Supplement C):34–48. doi:10.1016/j.tifs.2016.05.002.

Kossek, S., C. Padeste, L. Tiefenauer, and W.H. Scouten. 1996. "Immobilization of streptavidin for immunosensors on nanostructured surfaces." *Journal of Molecular Recognition* 9 (5–6):485–487. doi:10.1002/(SICI)1099-1352(199634/12)9:5/6<485:AID-JMR288>3.0.CO;2-R.

Kotsilkova R., V. Petkova, Y. Pelovski. 2001. "Thermal analysis of polymer-silicate nanocomposites." *Journal of Thermal Analysis and Calorimetry* 64:591–598. doi:10.1023/A:1011563521316.

Kulkarni, Aditya S., Padmini S. Ghugre, and Shobha A. Udipi. 2016. "15—Applications of nanotechnology in nutrition: Potential and safety issues A2—Grumezescu, Alexandru Mihai." In *Novel Approaches of Nanotechnology in Food*, 509–554. Academic Press Elservier, New York.

Kumar, Vineet, Praveen Guleria, and Surinder Kumar Mehta. 2017. "Nanosensors for food quality and safety assessment." *Environmental Chemistry Letters* 15 (2):165–177. doi:10.1007/s10311-017-0616-4.

Laelorspoen, Nalin, Saowakon Wongsasulak, Tipaporn Yoovidhya, and Sakamon Devahastin. 2014. "Microencapsulation of Lactobacillus acidophilus in zein–alginate core–shell microcapsules via electrospraying." *Journal of Functional Foods* 7 (Supplement C):342–349. doi:10.1016/j.jff.2014.01.026.

Li, Dapeng, Margaret W. Frey, and Antje J. Baeumner. 2006. "Electrospun polylactic acid nanofiber membranes as substrates for biosensor assemblies." *Journal of Membrane Science* 279 (1):354–363. doi:10.1016/j.memsci.2005.12.036.

Librán, Celia María, Sergio Castro, and José María Lagaron. 2017. "Encapsulation by electrospray coating atomization of probiotic strains." *Innovative Food Science and Emerging Technologies* 39:216–222. doi:10.1016/j.ifset.2016.12.013.

Liu, Shih-Chuan, Ran Li, Peggy M. Tomasula, Ana M. M. Sousa, and Linshu Liu. 2016. "Electrospun food-grade ultrafine fibers from pectin and pullulan blends." *Food and Nutrition Sciences* 7 (7):11. doi:10.4236/fns.2016.77065.

López-Rubio, Amparo, and Jose M. Lagaron. 2012. "Whey protein capsules obtained through electrospraying for the encapsulation of bioactives." *Innovative Food Science & Emerging Technologies* 13 (Supplement C):200–206. doi:10.1016/j.ifset.2011.10.012.

López-Rubio, Amparo, Ester Sanchez, Yolanda Sanz, and Jose M. Lagaron. 2009. "Encapsulation of living bifidobacteria in ultrathin PVOH electrospun fibers." *Biomacromolecules* 10 (10):2823–2829. doi:10.1021/bm900660b.

López-Rubio, Amparo, Ester Sanchez, Sabina Wilkanowicz, Yolanda Sanz, and Jose Maria Lagaron. 2012. "Electrospinning as a useful technique for the encapsulation of living bifidobacteria in food hydrocolloids." *Food Hydrocolloids* 28 (1):159–167. doi:10.1016/j.foodhyd.2011.12.008.

Luo, C. J., Shirin Loh, Eleanor Stride, and Mohan Edirisinghe. 2012. "Electrospraying and electrospinning of chocolate suspensions." *Food and Bioprocess Technology* 5 (6):2285–2300. doi:10.1007/s11947-011-0534-6.

Manickam, Venkatraman, Ranjith Kumar Velusamy, Rajeeva Lochana, Amiti, Bhavapriya Rajendran, and Ramasamy Tamizhselvi. 2017. "Applications and genotoxicity of nanomaterials in the food industry." *Environmental Chemistry Letters* 15 (3):399–412. doi:10.1007/s10311-017-0633-3.

Marano, Francelyne, Rina Guadagnini. 2013. "Les nanoparticules dans l'alimentation: quels risques pour le consommateur?." *Cahiers de Nutrition et de Diétetique* 48 (3):142–150. doi:10.1016/j.cnd.2013.01.005.

Mendes, Ana Carina, Karen Stephansen, and Ioannis. S. Chronakis. 2017. "Electrospinning of food proteins and polysaccharides." *Food Hydrocolloids* 68:53–68. doi:10.1016/j.foodhyd.2016.10.022.

Mihindukulasuriya, Suramya D. F., and Loong-Tak Lim. 2013. "Oxygen detection using UV-activated electrospun poly(ethylene oxide) fibers encapsulated with $TiO_2$ nanoparticles." *Journal of Materials Science* 48 (16):5489–5498. doi:10.1007/s10853-013-7343-4.

Molnar, Kolos, and Zsombor K. Nagy. 2016. "Corona-electrospinning: Needleless method for high-throughput continuous nanofiber production." *European Polymer Journal* 74:279–286. doi:10.1016/j.eurpolymj.2015.11.028.

Moomand, Khalid, and Loong-Tak Lim. 2014. "Oxidative stability of encapsulated fish oil in electrospun zein fibres." *Food Research International* 62 (Supplement C):523–532. doi:10.1016/j.foodres.2014.03.054.

Munhuweyi, Karen, Oluwafemi J. Caleb, Albert J. van Reenen, and Umezuruike Linus Opara. 2018. "Physical and antifungal properties of β-cyclodextrin microcapsules and nanofibre films containing cinnamon and oregano essential oils." *LWT—Food Science and Technology* 87 (Supplement C):413–422. doi:10.1016/j.lwt.2017.09.012.

Muhamad Nasir, and Dita Apriani. 2017. "Synthesis of catechin-gelatin nanofiber by electrospinning." *Materials Science Forum* 887:96–99.

Nedovic, Viktor, Ana Kalusevic, Verica Manojlovic, Steva Levic, and Branko Bugarski. 2011. "An overview of encapsulation technologies for food applications." *Procedia Food Science* 1 (Supplement C):1806–1815. doi:10.1016/j.profoo.2011.09.265.

Nel, Andre, Tian Xia, Lutz Madler, Ning Li. 2006. "Toxic potential of materials at the nanolevel." *Science* 311 (5761):622–627. doi:10.1126/science.1114397.

Neo, Yung Pin, Sudip Ray, Jianyong Jin, Marija Gizdavic-Nikolaidis, Michel K. Nieuwoudt, Dongyan Liu, and Siew Yong Quek. 2013. "Encapsulation of food grade antioxidant in natural biopolymer by electrospinning technique: A physicochemical study based on zein-gallic acid system." *Food Chemistry* 136 (2):1013–1021. doi:10.1016/j.foodchem.2012.09.010.

Nieuwland, Maaike, Peter Geerdink, P. Brier, P. van den Eijnden, Jolanda T. M. M. Henket, Marloes L. P. Langelaan, Niki Stroeks, Henk C. van Deventer, and Anneke H. Martin. 2013. "Food-grade electrospinning of proteins." *Innovative Food Science & Emerging Technologies* 20 (Supplement C):269–275. doi:10.1016/j.ifset.2013.09.004.

Nualkaekul, Sawaminee, and Dimitris Charalampopoulos. 2011. "Survival of Lactobacillus plantarum in model solutions and fruit juices." *International Journal of Food Microbiology* 146 (2):111–117. doi:10.1016/j.ijfoodmicro.2011.01.040.

OECD. 2017. "Testing Programme of Manufactured Nanomaterials." accessed 2nd November 2017. http://www.oecd.org/chemicalsafety/nanosafety/overview-testing-programme-manufactured-nanomaterials.htm.

Parris, Nicholas, Peter H. Cooke, and Kevin B. Hicks. 2005. "Encapsulation of essential oils in zein nanospherical particles." *Journal of Agricultural and Food Chemistry* 53 (12):4788–4792. doi:10.1021/jf040492p.

Pathakoti, Kavitha, Manjunath Manubolu, and Huey-Min Hwang. 2017. "Nanostructures: Current uses and future applications in food science." *Journal of Food and Drug Analysis* 25 (2):245–253. doi:10.1016/j.jfda.2017.02.004.

Paximada, Paraskevi, Yolanda Echegoyen, Apostolos A. Koutinas, Ioanna G. Mandala, and Jose M. Lagaron. 2017. "Encapsulation of hydrophilic and lipophilized catechin into nanoparticles through emulsion electrospraying." *Food Hydrocolloids* 64 (Supplement C):123–132. doi:10.1016/j.foodhyd.2016.11.003.

Perez-Masia, Rocío, Rubén Lopez-Nicolas, María Jesús Periago, Gaspar Ros, José María Lagaron, and Amparo Lopez-Rubio. 2015. "Encapsulation of folic acid in food hydrocolloids through nanospray drying and electrospraying for nutraceutical applications." *Food Chemistry* 168:124–133. doi:10.1016/j.foodchem.2014.07.051.

Perez-Masia, Rocío, Amparo Lopez-Rubio, María José Fabra, and José María Lagaron. 2013a. "Biodegradable polyester-based heat management materials of interest in refrigeration and smart packaging coatings." *Journal of Applied Polymer Science* 130 (5):3251–3262. doi:10.1002/app.39555.

Pérez-Masiá, Rocío, Amparo López-Rubio, and José María Lagarón. 2013b. "Development of zein-based heat-management structures for smart food packaging." *Food Hydrocolloids* 30 (1):182–191. doi:10.1016/j.foodhyd.2012.05.010.

Pérez-Masiá, Rocío, Rubén López-Nicolás, Maria Jesús Periago, Gaspar Ros, Jose M. Lagaron, and Amparo López-Rubio. 2015. "Encapsulation of folic acid in food hydrocolloids through nanospray drying and electrospraying for nutraceutical applications." *Food Chemistry* 168 (Supplement C):124–133. doi:10.1016/j.foodchem.2014.07.051.

Persano, Luana, Andrea Camposeo, Cagri Tekmen, and Dario Pisignano. 2013. "Industrial upscaling of electrospinning and applications of polymer nanofibers: A review." *Macromolecular Materials and Engineering* 298 (5):504–520. doi:10.1002/mame.201200290.

Peters, Ruud J. B., Hans Bouwmeester, Stefania Gottardo, Valeria Amenta, Maria Arena, Puck Brandhoff, Hans J. P. Marvin et al. 2016. "Nanomaterials for products and application in agriculture, feed and food." *Trends in Food Science & Technology* 54 (Supplement C):155–164. doi:10.1016/j.tifs.2016.06.008.

Ramji, Karpagavalli, and Ramille N. Shah. 2014. "Electrospun soy protein nanofiber scaffolds for tissue regeneration." *Journal of Biomaterials Applications* 29 (3):411–422. doi:10.1177/0885328214530765.

Rauscher, Hubert, Kirsten Rasmussen, and Birgit Sokull-Klüttgen. 2017. "Regulatory aspects of nanomaterials in the EU." *Chemie Ingenieur Technik* 89 (3):224–231. doi:10.1002/cite.201600076.

Realini, Carolina E., and Begonya Marcos. 2014. "Active and intelligent packaging systems for a modern society." *Meat Science* 98 (3):404–419. doi:10.1016/j.meatsci.2014.06.031.

Restuccia, Donatella, U. Gianfranco Spizzirri, Ortensia I. Parisi, Giuseppe Cirillo, Manuela Curcio, Francesca Iemma, Francesco Puoci, Giuliana Vinci, and Nevio Picci. 2010. "New EU regulation aspects and global market of active and intelligent packaging for food industry applications." *Food Control* 21 (11):1425–1435. doi:10.1016/j.foodcont.2010.04.028.

Shao, Ping, Ben Niu, Hangjun Chen, and Peilong Sun. 2018. "Fabrication and characterization of tea polyphenols loaded Pullulan-CMC electrospun nanofiber for fruit preservation." *International Journal of Biological Macromolecules*. doi:10.1016/j.ijbiomac.2017.10.054.

Siegrist, Michael, Marie-Eve Cousin, Hans Kastenholz, and Arnim Wiek. 2007. "Public acceptance of nanotechnology foods and food packaging: The influence of affect and trust." *Appetite* 49 (2):459–466. doi:10.1016/j.appet.2007.03.002.

Srivastava, R.K. 2017. "16—Electrospinning of patterned and 3D nanofibers A2—Afshari, Mehdi." In *Electrospun Nanofibers*, 399–447. Woodhead Publishing Cambridge, UK.

Subbiah, Thandavamoorthy, G. S. Bhat, R. W. Tock, S. Parameswaran, and S. S. Ramkumar. 2005. "Electrospinning of nanofibers." *Journal of Applied Polymer Science* 96 (2):557–569. doi:10.1002/app.21481.

Tampau, Alina, Chelo González-Martinez, and Amparo Chiralt. 2017. "Carvacrol encapsulation in starch or PCL based matrices by electrospinning." *Journal of Food Engineering* 214 (Supplement C):245–256. doi:10.1016/j.jfoodeng.2017.07.005.

Theron, S. A., Alexander. L. Yarin, Eyal Zussman, and Ehud Kroll. 2005. "Multiple jets in electrospinning: Experiment and modeling." *Polymer* 46 (9):2889–2899. doi:10.1016/j.polymer.2005.01.054.

Tonda-Turo, Chiara, Elisa Cipriani, Sara Gnavi, Valeria Chiono, Clara Mattu, Piergiorgio Gentile, Isabelle Perroteau, Marco Zanetti, and Gianluca Ciardelli. 2013. "Crosslinked gelatin nanofibres: Preparation, characterisation and in vitro studies using glial-like cells." *Materials Science and Engineering: C* 33 (5):2723–2735. doi:10.1016/j.msec.2013.02.039.

Torres-Giner, Sergio, Enrique Gimenez, and José María Lagaron. 2008. "Characterization of the morphology and thermal properties of Zein Prolamine nanostructures obtained by electrospinning." *Food Hydrocolloids* 22 (4):601–614. doi:10.1016/j.foodhyd.2007.02.005.

Torres-Giner, Sergio, Sabina Wilkanowicz, Beatriz Melendez-Rodriguez, and José María Lagaronn. 2017. "Nanoencapsulation of aloe vera in synthetic and naturally occurring polymers by electrohydrodynamic processing of interest in food technology and bioactive packaging." *Journal of Agriculture and Food Chemistry* 65 (22):4439–4448. doi:10.1021/acs.jafc.7b01393.

Wang, Xianfeng, Bin Ding, Gang Sun, Moran Wang, and Jianyong Yu. 2013. "Electro-spinning/netting: A strategy for the fabrication of three-dimensional polymer nano-fiber/nets." *Progress in Materials Science* 58 (8):1173–1243. doi:10.1016/j.pmatsci.2013.05.001.

Wang, Xiaoyuan, Yahong Yuan, Xiaochen Huang, and Tianli Yue. 2015. Controlled release of protein from core–shell nanofibers prepared by emulsion electrospinning based on green chemical. *Journal of Applied Polymer Science* 132 (16):41811–41814. doi:10.1002/app.41811.

Weidner, Eckhard. 2009. "High pressure micronization for food applications." *The Journal of Supercritical Fluids* 47 (3):556–565. doi:10.1016/j.supflu.2008.11.009.

Wen, Peng, Ding-He Zhu, Kun Feng, Fang-Jun Liu, Wen-Yong Lou, Ning Li, Min-Hua Zong, and Hong Wu. 2016. "Fabrication of electrospun polylactic acid nanofilm incorporating cinnamon essential oil/β-cyclodextrin inclusion complex for antimicrobial packaging." *Food Chemistry* 196 (Supplement C):996–1004. doi:10.1016/j.foodchem.2015.10.043.

Wu, Hong, Kun Feng, Ding He Zhu, Huan Yang, Peng Wen, and Min Hua Zong. 2016. "Progress of electrospun protein and polysaccharide nanofiber application in food industry." *Modern Food Science and Technology* 32 (7):295–303. doi:10.13982/j.mfst.1673-9078.2016.7.044.

Yang, Huan, Kun Feng, Peng Wen, Min-Hua Zong, Wen-Yong Lou, and Hong Wu. 2017a. "Enhancing oxidative stability of encapsulated fish oil by incorporation of ferulic acid into electrospun zein mat." *LWT—Food Science and Technology* 84 (Supplement C):82–90. doi:10.1016/j.lwt.2017.05.045.

Yang, Huan, Peng Wen, Kun Feng, Min H. Zong, Wen Y. Lou, and Hong Wu. 2017b. "Encapsulation of fish oil in a coaxial electrospun nanofibrous mat and its properties." *RSC Advances* 7 (24):14939–14946. doi:10.1039/C7RA00051K.

# Index

**Note:** Page numbers in italic and bold refer to figures and tables, respectively.

## I



## L



## M



## N

## O

## P



## R



## S